KERATOCONUS
DIAGNOSIS AND MANAGEMENT

KERATOCONUS
DIAGNOSIS AND MANAGEMENT

LUIS IZQUIERDO Jr., MD, MSc, PhD
Professor of Ophthalmology
Universidad Nacional Mayor de San Marcos;
Chair, Department of Ophthalmology
Oftalmosalud Instituto de Ojos
Lima, Peru

MARIA A. HENRIQUEZ, MD, MSc, PhD
Chief of Research and Visual Science Department
Oftalmosalud Instituto de Ojos;
Professor of Ophthalmology
Oftalmosalud Instituto de Ojos
Lima, Peru

MARK J. MANNIS, MD
Professor and Chair
Department of Ophthalmology & Vision Science
University of California, Davis
Sacramento, California
United States

ELSEVIER

Elsevier
1600 John F. Kennedy Blvd.
Ste 1800
Philadelphia, PA 19103-2899

KERATOCONUS

ISBN: 978-0-323759786

Content Strategist: Kayla Wolfe
Content Development Specialist: Shweta Pant
Publishing Services Manager: Shereen Jameel
Project Manager: Gayathri S
Design Direction: Amy Buxton

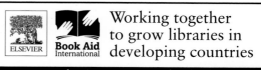

Printed in India
Last digit is the print number: 9 8 7 6 5 4 3 2 1

Roberto Albertazzi, MD
Medical Director
Quilmes Eye Center
Quilmes;
Keratoconus consultant
Zaldivar Institute,
Buenos Aires City, Buenos Aires
Argentina

Timothy J. Archer, MA(Oxon)
London Vision Clinic
London, United Kingdom

Mouhamed Al-Aqaba, FRCOphth, PhD
Academic Ophthalmology
Division of Clinical Neuroscience
School of Medicine
University of Nottingham;
Department of Ophthalmology
Queen's Medical Centre
Nottingham, United Kingdom

Jorge L. Alió, MD, PhD, FEBO
Professor and Chairman of Ophthalmology
Department of Pathology and Surgery
Universidad Miguel Hernandez,
Elche, Alicante;
Cornea, Cataract and Refractive Surgery Unit
Vissum Corporation,
Alicante, Spain

Renato Ambrósio Jr., MD, PhD
Adjunct Professor
Ophthalmology
Federal University of the State of Rio de
    Janeiro;
Affiliated Professor
Ophthalmology
Federal University of São Paulo;
Founder and Research Director
Rio de Janeiro Corneal Tomography and
    Biomechanics Study Group;
Clinical Director
Cornea and Refractive Surgery
Instituto de Olhos Renato Ambrosio
Rio de Janeiro, Brazil

Carlos G. Arce, MD, MS(Ophthalmology)
Director
Eye Clinic of Sousas, Campinas;
Ophthalmologist
Cornea, Refractive Surgery, Contact Lens and
    Development Sectors
Ophthalmic Hospital and Eye Bank of
    Sorocaba
Sorocaba, Brazil
Consultant
Ziemer Ophthalmic Systems AG
Port, Switzerland

Shady Awwad, MD
Professor of Clinical Ophthalmology;
Head, Cornea and Refractive Surgery Division;
Director, Laser Eye Center;
Department of Ophthalmology
American University of Beirut Medical Center
Beirut, Lebanon

Nelson Batista Sena Jr., MD
Rio de Janeiro Corneal Tomography and
    Biomechanics Study Group;
Department of Ophthalmology, Federal
    University the State of Rio de Janeiro
    (UNIRIO)
Rio de Janeiro, Brazil

Jorge L. Alió del Barrio, MD, PhD, FEBOS-CR
Cornea, Cataract and Refractive Surgery Unit
Vissum Corporación
Alicante, Spain

Or Ben-Shaul, MD
Cornea and External Disease Unit
Ophthalmology Department
Carmel Medical Center
Haifa, Israel

Melissa Barnett, OD, FAAO, FSLS, FBCLA
Principal Optometrist
Department of Ophthalmology & Vision
    Science
University of California, Davis
Sacramento, California,
United States

Michael W. Belin, MD
Professor of Ophthalmology & Vision Science
Ophthalmology
University of Arizona,
Tucson, Arizona
United States

Andrea L. Blitzer, MD
Fellow, Cornea and External Disease
Department of Ophthalmology and Visual
    Sciences
University of Chicago Medical Center,
Chicago, Illinois
United States

Yelena Bykhovskaya, PhD
Assistant Professor
Department of Surgery and BOG
    Regenerative Medicine Institute
Cedars-Sinai Medical Center,
Los Angeles, California
United States

Mauro Campos, MD
Ophthalmologist
Associated Professor and Postgraduate
    Supervisor Professor
Federal University of São Paulo
São Paulo, Brazil

Efekan Coşkunseven, MD
Associate Professor
Department of Refractive Surgery
Dunyagoz Etiler Hospital;
Faculty of Health Sciences
Istanbul Rumeli University
Istanbul, Turkey

Arthur Mauricio Delgadillo, Ing
National University of San Marcos
San Marcos, Lima
Peru

**Victoria Grace C. Dimacali, BSc (Hons.), MD,
MRCSOphth (Ed)**
Cornea and External Diseases Department
National Eye Centre
Singapore

Harminder S. Dua, MD, FRCOphth, PhD
Chair and Professor of Ophthalmology
Ophthalmology
University of Nottingham;
Consultant Ophthalmologist

Queens Medical Centre
Nottingham, Nottinghamshire
United Kingdom

Daniel Elies, MD
Cornea and Refractive Surgery Unit,
Institute of Ocular Microsurgery (IMO)
    Grupo Miranza,
Barcelona, Spain,
European School for Advanced Studies in
    Ophthalmology (ESASO),
Lugano, Switzerland;
Universidad Autónoma de Barcelona (UAB),
Barcelona, Spain

Louise Pellegrino Gomes Esporcatte, MD, MSc
Rio de Janeiro Corneal Tomography
    and Biomechanics Study Group,
    Rio de Janeiro;
Renato Ambrosio Eye Institute,
    Rio de Janeiro;
PhD Student
Department of Ophthalmology
Federal University of São Paulo
São Paulo, Brazil

**Fernando Faria-Correia, MD, PhD, FEBOS-CR,
PCEO**
Cataract and Refractive Surgery Consultant
Ophthalmology
CUF Porto
Porto, Portugal

Asim V. Farooq, MD
Assistant Professor
Department of Ophthalmology and Visual
    Science
University of Chicago
Chicago, Illinois
United States

Joaquin Fernandez, MD, PhD
Qvision
Deparment of Ophthalmology
Hospital Vithas Virgen del Mar
Almeria, Spain

Rajesh Fogla, FRCSEd, FRCOphth, FACS, MMed
Director Cornea Clinic
Eye Department
Apollo Hospitals
Hyderabad, Telangana
India

Javier García-Montesinos, MD, PhD
Department of Ophthalmology
Regional University Hospital of Málaga,
Málaga, Spain

Arkasubhra Ghosh, MSc, PhD
Director
GROW Research Laboratory
Narayana Nethralaya Foundation
Bangalore, Karnataka
India

Isabel Gomez, MD
Cornea and Refractive Surgery fellow
Instituto de Ojos Oftalmosalud
Lima, Peru;
Universidad Pontificia Bolivariana
Medellin, Colombia

José Alvaro Pereira Gomes, MD, PhD
Associate Professor
Cornea and External Disease Service
Department of Ophthalmology and Visual
   Sciences
Paulista Medical School
Federal University of São Paulo (EPM/
   UNIFESP)
São Paulo, Brazil

Enrique O. Graue-Hernández, MD, MSc
Director
Department of Cornea and Refractive Surgery
Institute of Ophthalmology
"Conde de Valenciana"
Mexico City, Mexico

Jose Güel, MD, PhD
Director
Cornea and Refractive Surgery Unit
Instituto de Microcirugia Ocular
Associate Professor of Ophthalmology
Autonoma University of Barcelona
Barcelona, Spain;
Lead Professor and Coordinator
Anterior Segment Diseases
European School for Advanced Studies in
   Ophthalmology (ESASO)
Lugano, Switzerland

Ilyse D. Haberman, MD
Department of Ophthalmology
New York University Langone Health
New York, United States

Jorge Haddad, MD
Rio de Janeiro Corneal Tomography and
   Biomechanics Study Group
Cornea and Cataract Department
Paulista Ophthalmological Institute
São Paulo, Brazil

Farhad Hafezi, MD, PhD, FARVO
Laboratory for Ocular Cell Biology;
ELZA Institute
Dietikon, Zurich
Switzerland;
Roski Eye Institute
University of Southern California
Los Angeles, California
United States;
Department of Ophthalmology
Wenzhou Medical University
Wenzhou, China;
Faculty of Medicine
University of Geneva
Geneva, Switzerland

Maria A. Henriquez, PhD
Chief of Research and Visual Science
   Department
Oftalmosalud Instituto de Ojos;
Professor of Ophthalmology
Oftalmosalud Instituto de Ojos
Lima, Peru

Mark Hillen, PhD
ELZA Institute
Dietikon, Zurich
Switzerland

Luis Izquierdo Jr., MD, PhD
Professor of Ophthalmology
Universidad Nacional Mayor de San Marcos;
Chair
Department of Ophthalmology
Oftalmosalud Instituto de Ojos
Lima, Peru

Nicolás Kahuam-López, MD , PhD
Department of Cornea and Refractive Surgery
Institute of Ophthalmology "Conde de
   Valenciana"
Mexico City, Mexico

Belma Kayhan, MD
Ophthalmology Department
Sultan 2. Abdulhamid Khan Training and
   Research Hospital
University of Health Sciences
Istanbul, Turkey

Pooja Khamar, PhD
Department of Cornea and Refractive Surgery
Narayana Nethralaya
Bangalore, India

Mark Krauthammer, M
Anterior Segment and Refractive Surgery Unit
Ophthalmology Department
Hadassah Medical Center, Jerusalem;
Ophthalmology Department
Tel Aviv Sourasky Medical Center
Tel Aviv, Israel

Gairik Kundu, MS
Department of Cornea and Refractive Surgery
Narayana Nethralaya
Bangalore, India

Karen Lee, OD, FAAO, FSLS
Clinical Assistant Professor
University of Houston College of Optometry
Houston, Texas
United States

W. Barry Lee, MD, FACS
Partner
Cornea, External Disease & Refractive Surgery
Eye Consultants of Atlanta—Piedmont
   Hospital;
Medical Director
Georgia Eye Bank
Atlanta, Georgia
United States

Marian S. Macsai, MD
Professor of Ophthalmology
Ophthalmology
University of Chicago Pritzker School of
   Medicine
Chicago, Illinois;

Chief
Division of Ophthalmology
Northshore University HealthSystems
Evanston, Illinois
United States

Felicidad Manero, MD
Cornea and Refractive Surgery Unit
Institute of Ocular Microsurgery (IMO)
   Grupo Miranza;
Autonomous University of Barcelona (UAB)
Barcelona, Spain

Mark J. Mannis, MD
Professor and Chair
Department of Ophthalmology & Vision
   Science
Davis Sacramento, California
United States

David Mauricio, DSc
Arthur Mauricio Delgadillo, Ing
National University of San Marcos
San Marcos, Lima
Peru

**Jodhbir S. Mehta, BSc (Hons.), MBBS, PhD,
FRCOphth, FRCSOphth (Ed), FAMS**
Cornea and External Diseases Department
Singapore National Eye Centre;
Tissue Engineering and Cell Therapy Group
   Singapore Eye Research Institute;
Duke-National University of Singapore
   Graduate Medical School;
School of Material Science and Engineering
Nanyang Technological University
Singapore

Milad Modabber, MD, MSc, FRCSC
Associate surgeon
Herzig Eye Institute
Toronto, Ontario
Canada

Merce Morral, MD, PhD
Cornea, Cataract and Refractive Surgery
   Specialist
Cornea and Refractive Surgery
Instituto de Microcirugia Ocular
Barcelona, Spain
European School for Advanced Studies in
   Ophthalmology (ESASO)
Lugano, Switzerland

Nuno Moura-Coelho, MD, MMed, FEBO
Cornea and Refractive Surgery Unit
Instituto de Microcirugía Ocular (IMO)
    Grupo Miranza
Barcelona, Spain;
European School for Advanced Studies in
    Ophthalmology (ESASO)
Lugano, Switzerland;
NOVA Medical School
Faculty of Medical Sciences
New University of Lisbon (NMS | FCM - UNL)
Lisbon, Portugal

Alejandro Navas, MD, PhD
Associate Professor
Department of Cornea and Refractive Surgery
Institute of Ophthalmology Conde de
    Valenciana
Mexico City, Mexico

Shyam Patel, MD
Cornea Service
Eye Consultants of Atlanta
Piedmont Healthcare
Atlanta, Georgia
United States

Nicolas Cesário Pereira, MD, PhD
Head
Cornea and External Disease
Sorocaba Eye Bank, Sorocaba;
Department of Ophthalmology
Federal University of São Paulo
São Paulo, Brazil

Diana Quintanilla Perez, Ing
National University of San Marcos
San Marcos, Lima
Peru

Claudia Perez-Straziota, MD
Cole Eye Institute
Cleveland Clinic
Cleveland, Ohio
United States

Claudia E. Perez Straziota, MD
Cole Eye Institute
Cleveland Clinic
Cleveland, Ohio
United States

Roberto Pineda, MD
Associate Professor
Ophthalmology
Massachusetts Eye & Ear;
Harvard Medical School
Boston, Massachusetts
United States

Yaron S. Rabinowitz, MD
Director of Ophthalmology Research
Department of Surgery and BOG
    Regenerative Medicine Institute
Cedars-Sinai Medical Center;
Cornea Genetic Eye Institute
Beverly Hills, California
United States

Manuel Ramirez, MD, FACS
Professor
APEC
Professor, Corneal Imaging
Universidad Nacional Autonoma de Mexico
Mexico City, Mexico

J. Bradley Randleman, MD
Professor
Ophthalmology
Cleveland Clinic Lerner College of Medicine;
Refractive Surgeon
Cole Eye Institute
Cleveland Clinic
Cleveland, Ohio
United States

Dan Z. Reinstein, MD, MA(Cantab), FRCSC, FRCOphth
Medical Director
Refractive Surgery
London Vision Clinic
London, United Kingdom;
Columbia University Medical Center
New York, USA;
Sorbonne Université
Paris, France;
School of Biomedical Sciences
University of Ulster
Coleraine, United Kingdom

Jose Luis Reyes Luis, MD
Cornea
Massachusetts Eye and Ear
Boston, Massachusetts
United States;
Ophthalmological Clinic Durango
AMCCI Specialty Hospital
Durango, Mexico City
Mexico

Cynthia J. Roberts, PhD
Professor
Ophthalmology & Visual Sciences, and
    Biomedical Engineering
The Ohio State University
Columbus, Ohio
United States

Pablo Felipe Rodrigues, MD, PhD
student
Cornea and External Disease Service
Department of Ophthalmology and Visual
    Sciences
Paulista Medical School
Federal University of São Paulo (EPM/
    UNIFESP)
São Paulo, Brazil

Dalia G. Said, FRCOphth, MD
Academic Ophthalmology
Division of Clinical Neuroscience
School of Medicine
University of Nottingham;
Department of Ophthalmology
Queen's Medical Centre
Nottingham, United Kingdom

Gustavo Hernandez Sahagún, MD
Research Department
Oftalmosalud Institute of Eyes
Lima, Peru

Marcella Salomão, MD
Rio de Janeiro Corneal Tomography and
    Biomechanics Study Group;
Instituto Benjamin Constant
Rio de Janeiro, Brazil

Marcony R. Santhiago, MD, PhD
Faculty member
Department of Ophthalmology
University of São Paulo
São Paulo, Brazil

Enrica Sarnicola, MD
Ophthalmologist
Struttura Complessa Oculistica 2
Ospedale Oftalmico di Torino
Turin, Italy;
Ophthalmologist
Clinica degli Occhi Sarnicola
Grosseto, Italy

Ivan R. Schwab, MD, FACS
Professor of Ophthalmology
Department of Ophthalmology & Vision
    Science
University of California, Davis
Sacramento California
United States

Theo Seiler, MD, PhD
Institute for Refractive and Ophthalmic
    Surgery (IROC)
Zurich, Switzerland

Theo G. Seiler, MD
Institute for Refractive and Ophthalmic
    Surgery (IROC)
Zurich, Switzerland;
Ophthalmology Clinic
University Hospital Dusseldorf
Duesseldorf, Germany;
University Clinic for Ophthalmology
Inselspital Bern
Bern, Switzerland

Swaminathan Sethu, BDS, MSc, PhD
Scientist
GROW Research Lab
Narayana Nethralaya Foundation
Bangalore, Karnataka
India

Rohit Shetty, FRCS, PhD
Vice Chairman
Ophthalmology
Narayana Nethralaya
Bangalore, Karnataka
India

David Smadja, MD
Ophthalmology Department
Hadassah Medical Center
Jerusalem, Israel

Darren S. J. Ting, FRCOphth, PhD
Academic Ophthalmology
Division of Clinical Neuroscience
School of Medicine
University of Nottingham;
Department of Ophthalmology
Queen's Medical Centre
Nottingham, United Kingdom

Taíse Tognon, MD, PhD
Ophthalmologist
Instituto Penido Burnier and Acuitè
    Oftalmoclínica
Campinas, Brazil

Emilio A. Torres-Netto, MD, PhD
Center for Applied Biotechnology and
    Molecular Medicine
University of Zurich
Zurich, Switzerland;
Department of Ophthalmology
Federal University of São Paulo
São Paulo, Brazil;
Faculty of Medicine
University of Geneva
Geneva, Switzerland

Mauricio Vélez, MD
Cornea Specialist and Cornea Director
Bolivarian Pontifical University
Medellín, Colombia

Ryan S. Vida, OD, FAAO
London Vision Clinic
London, United Kingdom

Madeline Yung, MD
Assistant Professor of Ophthalmology
Department of Ophthalmology
University of California
San Francisco, California
United States

Mona Zarif, MSc, OD, PhD
Division of Ophthalmology
Universidad Miguel Hernández
Alicante, Spain

Since its first description in the literature of ophthalmology, keratoconus has remained a source of fascination for the cornea specialist. Over the past several decades, our understanding of this disorder has been clarified with new genetic insights, a better understanding of corneal biology and the physical properties of the cornea, and a much more detailed understanding of corneal optics. Nonetheless, the ramifications of this disease for patients remain profound, appearing as it does in youth and following a progressive course.

New modalities have emerged that have provided greatly enhanced sensitivity and diagnostic accuracy. Our enhanced understanding of keratoconus has also been accompanied by an array of new therapies, both optical and surgical, that afford the patient significant improvement in vision and lifestyle. Yet the fascination with keratoconus remains, and its mysteries are still being unraveled.

In this volume, we have gathered authorities from around the world to provide a detailed contemporary assessment of the diagnostic and therapeutic options available to today's practitioners. It is our hope that this text will serve as a guide to the practitioner, as well as the student of vision science. We have sought to marry our understanding of the basic science of keratoconus with its clinical manifestations and to provide the reader with the most thorough possible discussion of the disorder, its diagnosis, and management.

Luis Izquierdo Jr.
Maria A. Henriquez
Mark J. Mannis

ACKNOWLEDGMENTS

First and foremost, we wish to thank the many authors who labored over the chapters that make this text so unique. Writing chapters for a textbook has to be a labor of love. It is time consuming—demanding detail, precise annotation, and clarity. We cannot thank the contributing authors enough for their hard work and for bringing their expertise to this project.

We would also like to thank the team at Elsevier for their guidance and support, with special thanks to Kayla Wolfe, who supported this project from the beginning and who provided sage guidance throughout the process.

As always, we want to thank our families for giving us the time to work on this volume. In many ways, this is their accomplishment.

And finally, we thank the readers for whom we hope this will be a useful source of information about a subject important to all of us.

Luis Izquierdo Jr.
Maria A. Henriquez
Mark J. Mannis

CONTENTS

Keratoconus Principles

CHAPTER 1

Keratoconus: A Brief History

Mark J. Mannis

The disorder now known as keratoconus has fascinated and perplexed clinicians for more than three centuries.[1-3] Recognized as early as the 1700s, its pathophysiology remains both curious and frustrating, and, during the last century, its clinical management has considerably changed, improving the lives of afflicted patients. Keratoconus is a disease that can be managed in many ways, ranging from optical correction to a variety of surgical interventions, and it is, at the same time, a disorder whose core etiology continues to elude us. Even today, with the tools of molecular genetics that have pinpointed single nucleotides as the source of many disorders—several of which are associated with keratoconus—the disorder cannot be traced to a consistent, single genetic abnormality and is considered to be both genetic and environmental in origin.[4]

In the Beginning: 17th and 18th Centuries

The first mention of what is identifiable as keratoconus is from the records of Benedict Duddell (c. 1696–1760). Duddell, practicing in Nottingham, England, went to Paris to study with the famous English oculist, John Thomas Woolhouse (1660–1734) and subsequently returned to England where he practiced in Hammersmith, near London. Among the treatises that he wrote between 1729 and 1736, he described corneal anatomy in detail. In his 1736 treatise, Duddell described the case of a young boy with prominent cone-shaped corneas (Fig. 1.1). The findings were also in the context of albinism and nystagmus, and, although not identified specifically as keratoconus, this is likely the first description of the disorder.[3,5]

The flamboyant and opportunistic itinerant oculist, Chevalier John Taylor (1708–1772), who despite his education and prominence is largely regarded as a quack, has been the subject of many descriptions that point both to his erudition and to his blatant dishonesty and charlatanism.[6] Taylor served as oculist to King George II of England as well as to other European royal families. Whatever is said about his honesty, it is likely that Taylor was an astute observer. In 1766 he wrote a description of a condition he called "ochlodes" and described it as a conical deformation of the cornea with a blunted apex with the base of the cone equal to the diameter of the cornea. His description is consistent with advanced keratoconus.

Burkhard David Mauchart (1696–1751) was appointed court physician in Tübingen (1723) and was professor at the university after completing his education in Tübingen, Paris, and Strasbourg. He described what he termed "cornea diaphanum," which may have been an early description of keratoconus, differentiating this from other forms of staphylomatous corneal protrusion, although current evidence suggests that he could not be credited with the early description of keratoconus.[3,7]

The 19th Century: The Age of Description

NEW OBSERVATIONS

The first half of the 19th century witnessed newer descriptions of conical cornea. Case histories of patients with what appeared to be a conical cornea were documented by Antonio Scarpa (1801),

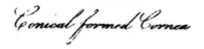

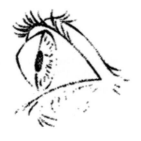

Fig. 1.1   Drawing from James Wardrop, 1808.

James Wardrop (1808), Pierre Demours (1818), and R. Lyall (1789-1831), who presented four cases of "staphyloma pellucidum conicum" to the Edinburgh Medical and Surgical Society.[3]

Interestingly, Sir William Adams (1817) reported surgical procedures rendering aphakic two patients with conical cornea. The resulting improvement in vision suggested that the hyperopic shift from cataract extraction in these patients represented a surgical treatment for the myopia induced by the conical cornea.[8]

William McKenzie (1761–1868) described conical cornea in his *Practical Treatise on the Diseases of the Eye* (1830). McKenzie served as the Surgeon Oculist to Queen Victoria and was founder of the Glasgow Eye Infirmary. His descriptions of the cornea in this condition included a corneal apex that could be eccentric, apical opacification in some cases, and the progressive myopic shift that occurs with progression of the disease. He accurately pointed out that the disease typically had its onset in puberty and was often asymmetrical. He did not associate the disease with inflammation, pain, or elevation in intraocular pressure. Essentially his description of keratoconus was much as we describe it today.[9]

The frustration with keratoconus as an entity difficult to manage is described best by JH Pickford (1844) when he wrote: "There is no disease to which the eye is subject, hitherto so rebellious to medicine, so intractable in its nature, and, at the same time, so fatal to vision, as conical cornea; and not one, the pathology and treatment of which are so little understood." This discouraging statement can be understood in an era decades before contact lenses and a century before keratoplasty would be available to these patients.[10] This pessimism is also reflected in the work of von Ammon, who provided detailed descriptions of keratoconus and concluded that the prognosis for treatment was very poor. The first use of the term "keratoconus" was by von Ammon in 1828.[11]

THE WORK OF JOHN NOTTINGHAM

Although there were several descriptions of what was surely keratoconus over the preceding 50 years, it was the extensive treatise by John Nottingham (1854) that collected the accounts of keratoconus and its consequences and merged them into a comprehensive description of the disease.[12] Nottingham (1810–1895) studied medicine in London and Paris and practiced in Liverpool, UK where he was a surgeon at Southern Hospital.

He based his work on the collective descriptions of predecessors including, among others, Scarpa, von Ammon, von Carion, McKenzie, along with his own clinical observations of the disease. In his monumental 270-page treatise entitled *Practical Observations on Conical Cornea and on the Short Sight and Other Defects of Vision Connected With It*, Nottingham described the epidemiology and clinical presentation of the disease, and contemporary treatments (Fig. 1.2).

In his treatise, Nottingham described keratoconus as a relatively rare disorder with a predilection for Asian races. His clinical description included apical thinning and protrusion of the cornea, and he described corneal hydrops with loss of transparency and edema. As is the case in contemporary ophthalmology, Nottingham could not identify a singular cause for the disease but rather suggested the possibility of an inherited component in addition to the influence of environmental exogenous factors, including inflammation, alternations in nutrition, and anomalies of the nervous system, among others.

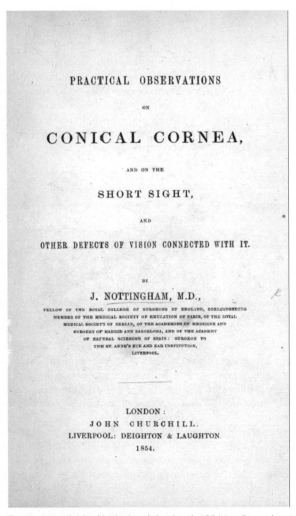

Fig. 1.2 Frontispiece of John Nottingham's landmark 1854 treatise on keratoconus.

With regard to treatment, Nottingham suggested three general approaches: (1) *Optical* management (including biconcave lenses, Galilean telescopes, pinhole goggles, and contact lenses "in concept"); (2) *Medical* management (systemic administration of zinc sulfate, arsenic, myrrh, and others, as well as topical nitric oxide of mercury); and (3) *Surgical* management (including anterior chamber paracentesis, pupilloplasty to form an eccentric pupil, and excision of the corneal apex), although he recommended surgery only after all other treatments were undertaken.

Remarkably, Nottingham's extensive treatise described keratoconus much as we do today, with the difference being our repertoire of effective optical and surgical treatments of the disease.

Late 19th and Early 20th Centuries: The Period of Emerging Therapies

As the disease became better characterized, clinicians began turning their attention to more effective therapies: medical, optical, and surgical.

MEDICAL THERAPY

Of the approaches to medical therapy employed in the 19th century, few had any significant rationale or effectiveness and bear the least emphasis in our discussion. These included, among others, the use of emetics, purgatives, systemic calomel for fluid absorption, iodine collyrium, zinc sulfate, silver or iodine ointment applied to the lids, prolonged patching with miotics, and leeches applied to the lower lid or temple. Several devices were also employed to exert extended pressure on the corneas in an attempt to effect flattening of the anterior curvature. Needless to say, none of these remedies had a significant positive impact on the course of the disease.

OPTICAL THERAPY

Optical treatments employed included concave lenses, spherocylindrical spectacles, stenopaic slits, blocking lenses, pinhole glasses, Raehlman hyperbolic lenses (1878), and the hydrodiascope (1892).

Concave lenses were recommended early on by McKenzie[9] and were likely useful for the progressive myopia experienced by keratoconic patients but became less effective with the progression of the disease.[9] Raehlman (1879) developed hyperbolic lenses, which were designed to optically neutralize the progressively astigmatic corneas of the patient. These lenses were custom made for each patient and had the significant limitation that when the patient looked through any but the central portion of the lens, the effect was negated.[13]

Another optical device peculiar to keratoconus and what may seem today as a bizarre solution to the problem was the hydrodiascope, introduced in 1896.[14–16] Designed as a goggle that was filled with fluid and worn over one eye, the device was originally described and was able to improve visual acuity to a normal level by neutralization of irregular astigmatism and spectacle magnification. Its principal disadvantage was its poor cosmetic appearance and the high demand that it placed on accommodation. With the advent of contact lenses, the hydrodiascope fell into disuse (Fig. 1.3).

The appearance of contact lens technology would transform the management of keratoconus. In 1888 Adolph Eugen Fick in Zurich published his work on the development of a contact lens. In his series, one patient had keratoconus, a disease in which he was very interested.[17,18] A year later in 1889, Eugene Kalt in Paris investigated contact lenses as an "orthopedic appliance" for the treatment of keratoconus; this was, in fact, the first form of orthokeratology.[19] The early scleral lenses made of fenestrated glass (Fig. 1.4) would ultimately be reborn as the contemporary gas-permeable scleral lenses that have revolutionized the care of this disorder. In the interim,

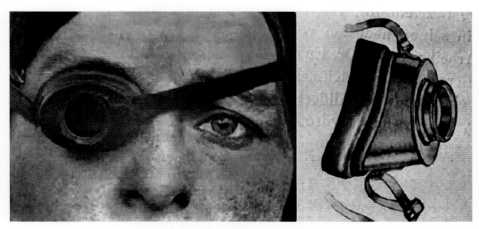

Fig. 1.3 Hydrodiascope for the optical treatment of the keratoconic cornea.

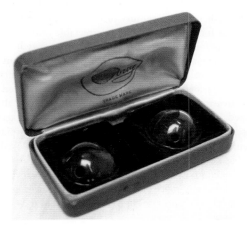

Fig. 1.4 Early fenestrated scleral lenses.

prior to the "reinvention" of the scleral lens, multiple contact lens approaches have been specifically designed for keratoconus, including specially designed soft contact lenses, rigid lenses with curvatures designed for the keratoconic cornea (e.g., Soper Cone lens, the Rose K lens), hybrid lenses, and piggyback lenses, among others. These will be reviewed later in this volume as we discuss contemporary contact lens care.

THE EVOLUTION OF SURGERY FOR KERATOCONUS

Surgery for keratoconus has undergone a steady evolution over the past 150 years. Surgical approaches to the disorder can be divided into three general periods: (1) 1800 to 1906; (2) 1906 to 1990; and (3) 1990 to 2020.

The first of these periods (1800–1906) included methods of flattening the conical cornea either via cautery or cone resection or by producing an optical bypass eccentrically.[20,21] During this period, the primary surgical approach to the management of keratoconus was thermal keratoplasty. Heated cautery was applied to the surface to scarify and flatten the central cornea, and some surgeons favored perforation of the cornea with the cautery at the time of surgery[22] (Fig. 1.5). This

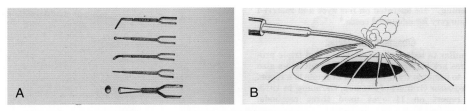

Fig. 1.5 (A) Knapp cautery points for flattening the conical cornea. (B) Diagrammatic central flattening with corneal cautery.

procedure resulted in a firm leukoma centrally, often requiring an optical iridectomy at a later date. Over this period, surgeons developed multiple variations of the procedure, including the transition to galvanocautery, localized thermal applications to modulate astigmatism, and combination surgery with optical iridectomy. Interestingly, thermal flattening of the cornea would survive as a treatment for keratoconus, although uncommonly used in the late 20th century.[23]

The second of these three periods (1906–1990) was heralded by the landmark case report in 1906 by Eduard Zirm,[24,25] ushering in a century of penetrating keratoplasty, which became the surgical treatment of choice for disease no longer correctable optically. Other techniques were introduced, including various forms of lamellar and epikeratoplasty.[26] Nonetheless, penetrating keratoplasty would become the mainstay of surgical therapy of keratoconus for close to a century.[27]

In the third phase of surgical development (1990–2020) with the resurgence of selective layered keratoplasty, deep anterior lamellar keratoplasty (DALK) moved into primary position as the preferred surgical treatment of the disease. During this period, alternative surgical techniques were also developed, including the notably unsuccessful internal keratotomy,[28] intracorneal rings,[29] femtosecond laser–assisted keratoplasty,[30] Bowman's layer transplantation,[31] and collagen cross-linking.[32] Collagen cross-linking is currently most widely employed in patients with early keratoconus to prevent disease progression.

The contemporary keratoconus patient has a wide variety of therapeutic choices ranging from specialized contact lens correction to corneal curvature restructuring (collagen cross-linking, intracorneal rings, Bowman's layer transplant) or to replacement of the defective cornea with deep anterior lamellar or penetrating keratoplasty.

The history of keratoconus is a fascinating tale of progression from the initial observation of findings to the development of optical and surgical management techniques and to a broadening but incomplete understanding of genetic and environmental factors.[33] In subsequent chapters, we will explore the current understanding of the disease and will look to present management and techniques to be developed in the future.

References

1. McGhee CN. 2008 Sir Norman McAlister Gregg Lecture: 150 years of practical observations on the conical cornea–what have we learned? *Clin Exp Ophthalmol.* 2009;37:160–176.
2. Ali NQ, Patel DV, Lockington D, McGhee CN. Citation analysis of keratoconus 1900-2013: the most influential publications, authors, institutions, and journals. *Asia Pac J Ophthalmol (Phila).* 2014;3(2):67–73.
3. Grzybowski A, McGhee CN. The early history of keratoconus prior to Nottingham's landmark 1854 treatise on conical cornea: a review. *Clin Exp Optom.* 2013;96(2):140–145.
4. Ferrari G, Rama P. The keratoconus enigma: a review with emphasis on pathogenesis. *Ocul Surf.* 2020;18(3):363–373.
5. McGhee CNJ. Keratoconus: the arc of past, present and future. *Clin Exp Optom.* 2013;96:137–139.
6. Albert DM, Atzen SL, *Chevalier John Taylor: England's Early Oculist: Pretender or Pioneer?* Madison, WI: Parallel Press; 2011.

7. Grzybowski A. Mauchart did not give the first description of keratoconus. *Acta Ophthalmol.* 2014;92:e84–e85.
8. Adams W. On the restoration of vision, when injured or destroyed in consequence of the cornea having assumed a conical form. *J Sci Arts.* 1817;2:402–417.
9. McKenzie W. Partial and general enklargements of the eyeball, effusions, and tunours with in the coats. In: *A Practical Treatise on the Diseases of the Eye.* London: Longman, Rees, Orme, Brown, and Green; 1830:526–566.
10. Pickford JH. On conical cornea. *Dublin J Med Sci.* 1824;24:355–387.
11. von Ammon FA. Hornhautauswuchs–Hyperkeratosis. In: Busch DWH, von Graefe CF, Horn E, Link HF, Mueller J, Osann E, eds. *Encyclopaedisches Woerterbuch Der Medicinischen Wissenschaften.* Berlin: Verlag von Weit et Comp; 1838:17–24.
12. Gokul A, Patel DV, McGhee CNJ. Dr John Nottingham's 1854 landmark treatise on conical cornea considered in the context of the current knowledge of keratoconus. *Cornea.* 2016;35:673–678.
13. Raehlmann E. Ueber die Anwendung der hyperbolischen Linsen be Keratoconus und unregelmassig. *Astigmatismus Klin Monbl Augenheilkd.* 1898;36:33–47.
14. Pearson RM. An appraisal of the optics of the hydrodiascope. *Cont Lens Anterior Eye.* 2008;31:65–72.
15. Pearson RM. Addenda to paper entitled: an appraisal of the optics of the hydrodiascope. *Cont Lens Anterior Eye.* 2018;41:315–316.
16. Faber S. Hydradiaskop und keratoconus. *Klin Monbl Augenheilkd.* 1906;44:93–109.
17. Fick AE. A Contact lens. *Arch Ophthalmol.* 1888;19:215–226.
18. Efron N. Centenary Celebration of Fick's *Eine Contactbrille Arch Ophthalmol.* 1988;106:1370–1372.
19. Pearson RM. Kalt, keratoconus, and the contact lens. *Optom Vis Sci.* 1989;66:643–646.
20. Sekundo W, Stevens JD. Surgical treatment of keratoconus at the turn of the 20th century. *J Refract Surg.* 2001;17:69–73.
21. Wray C. The operative treatment of keratoconus. *Proc R Soc Med.* 1913;7:152–157.
22. Critchett A. *Conical Cornea: Its Surgical Evolution.* London: Morton & Burt; 1903.
23. Gasset AR, Kaufman HE. Thermokeratoplasty for keratoconus. *Am J Ophthalmol.* 1975;79:226–228.
24. Zirm E. Eine erfolgreiche totale Keratoplastik. *Albrecht Von Graefes Arch Ophthalmol.* 1906;64:580–593.
25. Zirm EK. Eine Erfolgreiche totale Keratoplastik. *J Refract Corneal Surg.* 1989;5:258–261.
26. McDonald MB, Kaufman HE, Durrie DS, Keates RH, Sanders DR. Epikeratophakia for keratoconus. *Arch. Ophthalmol.* 1986;104:1294–1297.
27. Kirkness CM, FIcker LA, Stable AD, Rice NS. The success of penetrating keratoplasty for keratoconus. *Eye (Lond.).* 1990;4:673–675.
28. Sato T. Posterior incision of hte cornea: surgical treatment for cornea and astigmatism. *Am J Ophthalmol.* 1950;33:943–948.
29. Colin J, Cochener B, Savary G, Malet F. Correcting keratoconus with intracorneal rings. *J Cataract Refract Surg.* 2000;26:1117–1122.
30. Farid M, Steinert RF. Deep anterior lamellar keratoplasty performed with the femtosecond laser zigzag incision for the treatment of stromal corneal pathology and ectatic disease. *J Cataract Refract Surg.* 2009;35:809–813.
31. Dragnea DC, Birbal RS, Ham L, et al. Bowman layer transplantation in the treatment of keratoconus. *Eye Vis (Lond).* 2018;5:24.
32. Wollensak G, Spoerl E, Seiler T. Riboflavin/ultraviolet-A—induced collagen crosslinking for the treatment of keratoconus. *Am J Ophthalmol.* 2003;135:620–627.
33. Mas Tur V, MacGregor C, Jayaswal R, et al. A review of keratoconus: diagnosis, pathophysiology, and genetics. *Surv Ophthalmol.* 2017;62:770–783.

CHAPTER 2

Keratoconus: Definitions

Maria A. Henriquez ■ J. Bradley Randleman

KEY CONCEPTS

- Keratoconus (KC) is described as a condition in which the cornea assumes a conical shape with coinciding corneal stromal thinning inducing irregular astigmatism, myopia, and protrusion.
- Forme fruste is an atypical or attenuated manifestation of a disease or syndrome, with the implications of incompleteness, partial presence, or aborted state.
- Suspicious topography is defined as a corneal topography that presents signs of abnormality that are not enough to claim keratoconus.

Keratoconus: Definitions

Keratoconus (KC) is a condition in which the cornea assumes a conical shape with coinciding corneal stromal thinning. This process induces irregular astigmatism, myopia, and protrusion, leading to mild to markedly impaired visual quality.[1,2] KC is a progressive disorder that typically affects both eyes, although disease presentation can be highly asymmetric, and only one eye may be affected clinically.[3-5] Symptoms are highly variable and, in part, depend on the stage of the disease progression. Early in the disease there may be no specific symptoms, and KC may be noted by the ophthalmologist simply because the patient cannot be refracted to a clear 20/20 corrected vision. In advanced disease there is significant distortion of vision accompanied by profound visual loss.

The diagnosis of KC, in its earliest stages, remains challenging and controversial. In 2015 a consensus of ophthalmologists from around the world used a Delphi panel approach to put forward opinions regarding KC and ectatic diseases, focusing on definition, clinical management, and surgical treatments. The experts determined that KC is an ectatic disorder in which abnormal posterior ectasia, abnormal corneal thickness distribution, and clinical noninflammatory corneal thinning are essential findings for diagnosis.[6]

Other authors, however, have questioned these diagnostic criteria. Neither Bae et al.[7] nor Ruisenor et al.[8] found that posterior corneal or regional thickness metrics successfully identified the clinically unaffected eye in patients with highly asymmetric KC, whereas Hwang et al.[9] and Golan et al.[10] both found combined metric strategies to distinguish between the clinically unaffected eye and a normal cohort. However, neither analysis found posterior corneal metrics or regional thickness metrics to be effective in their modeling.

Although the classical KC definition refers to it as a non inflammatory disorder, enough information exists for inflammation to be considered as a significant component of the pathophysiology of KC. The inflammation observed in KC resembles the chronic inflammation associated with systemic diseases rather than acute inflammation.[11] This is evidenced by the fact that cytokines that make up the acute phase reaction, such as tumor necrosis factor alpha (TNF-α), are not overly expressed in KC, but chronic inflammation-associated target genes such as matrix metalloproteinase-9 (MMP-9) are significantly high.[12] Also, KC corneas have a reduction in collagen fibril-maturating enzyme lysyl oxidase (LOX), a cross-linking enzyme involved in the formation of a fibrillar extracellular matrix through the oxidative linkage of collagen. Specifically, a significant reduction of transcript levels in KC corneal epithelia and LOX activity in KC tears correlated with disease severity have been reported.[13,14]

Initially, the diagnosis of KC was based on slit-lamp examination and clinical signs, and then topographic signs were included as diagnostic criteria. The diagnosis of clinical KC is based on classic corneal biomicroscopic and topographic characteristics[15–17] including the presence of one or more clinical signs (corneal stromal thinning, Vogt striae, Fleischer ring, scissoring of the red reflex, or oil droplet sign identified by retinoscopy) and the presence of topographic characteristics (an increased area of corneal power surrounded by concentric areas of decreasing power, inferior-superior [I-S] power asymmetry, and skewing of the steepest radial axes above and below the horizontal meridian). Fig. 2.1 shows an advanced case of KC, in which all these topographic characteristics are present.

More recently, with the advent of Scheimpflug imaging analysis and anterior segment optical coherence tomography (OCT), early diagnosis of the disease was achieved with information such as pachymetry, epithelial, elevation, and aberrometry data (Figs. 2.1 and 2.2).[18–24] As a result of the early diagnosis provided by these new devices, many terms have come to life such as subclinical keratoconus (SCK), and forme fruste keratoconus (FFKC). A variety of indicators have been suggested to diagnose these entities; however, there is a lack of unified criteria to define them.[25]

SUBCLINICAL KERATOCONUS

The term "subclinical" by dictionary definition[26] is "not detectable or producing effects that are not detectable by the usual clinical tests." Currently, the usual tests for KC diagnosis include corneal topography and tomography. Therefore although many papers today may use the term "subclinical" to mean disease evident on imaging but not on "clinical" examination, this definition appears to be incorrect and outdated.

Henriquez et al,[25] in a review concerning the definitions used in published articles for the terms SCK and FFKC, noted that the most frequently cited criteria combinations used to define SCK are normal-appearing cornea on slit-lamp biomicroscopy, keratometry, retinoscopy, and ophthalmoscopy plus I-S asymmetry and/or bow-tie pattern with skewed radial axis plus diagnosis of KC in the fellow eye. Table 2.1 shows the frequency of parameters used in the definition of SCK in published studies. Table 2.2 shows the most commonly used combinations to define SCK in the studies.[25]

Currently, SCK definition refers to those eyes with normal slit-lamp examination, topographic/tomographic signs of KC or suspicious topography (but not enough to define as KC), and KC in the fellow eye. Figs. 2.3 and 2.4 show an example of SCK in which the right eye is a subclinical KC case and the left eye has a clear KC (Box 2.1).

FORME FRUSTE KERATOCONUS

Forme fruste (from French, "crude, or unfinished, form"; pl., formes frustes) is an atypical or attenuated manifestation of a disease or syndrome, with the implications of incompleteness, partial presence, or aborted state. Marc Amsler in 1938 used photographic Placido disk to describe early corneal topographic changes and coined the term "FFKC."[27,28] Fig. 2.5 and Fig. 2.6 shows an example of FFKC in the right eye and clear KC in the left eye.

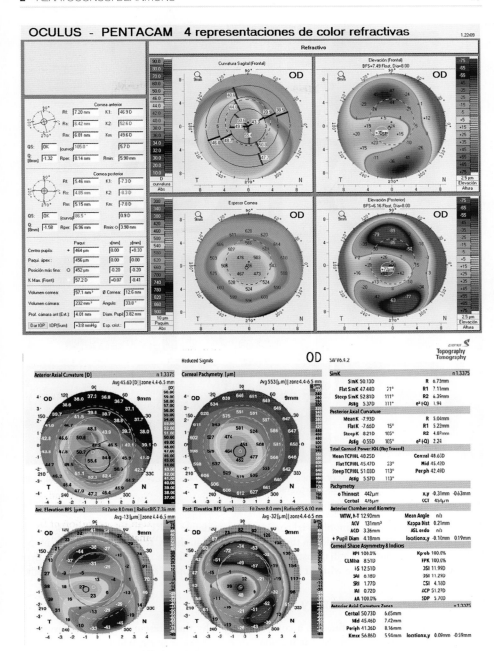

Fig. 2.1 Refractive maps including the curvature axial map, anterior and posterior elevation, and pachymetric map from a keratoconus cornea using the Pentacam AXL *(up)* and the Galilei 700 *(down)*.

According to our review,[25] the most frequently cited criteria combinations used to define FFKC have been normal topography, normal slit-lamp examination, and KC in the fellow eye. Table 2.3 shows the frequency of parameters used in defining FFKC in published studies, and

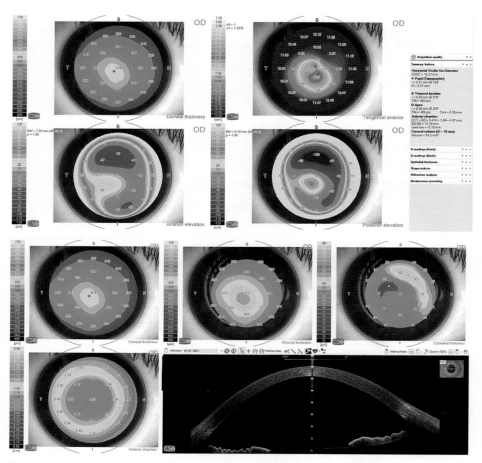

Fig. 2.2 Anterior segment optical coherence tomography using the MS-39 device, in which the epithelial map of the same patient with keratoconus is presented.

Table 2.2 lists the most commonly used combinations to define FFKC in the studies[25] (Box 2.2). The majority of the papers included in the review—72.72% in the SCK papers and 77.27% in the FFKC papers—included as a diagnostic criterion having KC in the fellow eye. This means that early diagnosis of the disease without bilateral clinical/topographic expression remains difficult.

Suspicious Topography Criteria

Suspicious topography is defined as a corneal topography that presents signs of abnormality that are not enough to claim KC; it includes an *asymmetric bow tie*, which is an asymmetric steepening in any direction greater than 0.5 diopters (D) but less than 1.0 D compared with the region 180 degrees opposite the steepest region with no skewed radial axis. It may also refer to *inferior steepening/skewed radial axis*, which includes significant skewed radial axis (20 degrees or greater) with or without inferior steepening or 1.0 D or more of inferior

TABLE 2.1 ■ **Frequency of Parameters Used in the Definition of Subclinical Keratoconus in the Analyzed Studies**

Parameter	Frequency
Diagnosis of KC in the fellow eye	72.72% (24/33)
Normal-appearing cornea on slit-lamp biomicroscopy, keratometry, retinoscopy, and ophthalmoscopy	45.45% (15/33)
Inferior-superior (I-S) asymmetry and/or bow-tie pattern with skewed radial axes	36.36% (12/33)
Lack of any KC-related findings/signs in the slit-lamp biomicroscopy	33.33% (11/33)
No history of contact lens use, ocular surgery, or trauma	21.21% (7/33)
Corneal topography showing an abnormal localized steepening or central/inferior steepening or asymmetric bow-tie pattern or claw-shaped pattern on topography	21.71 (7/33)
One of the following signs: steep keratometric curvature greater than 47 D, oblique cylinder greater than 1.5 D, central corneal thickness less than 500 μm	12.12% (4/33)
I-S lower than 1.4 D and/or maximum keratometry lower than or equal to 47 D	12.12% (4/33)
Keratoconus percentage index (KISA) between 60% and 100% in the SCK eye	9.09% (3/33)
Keratoconus percentage index (KISA) lower than 60%	9.09% (3/33)
Normal topography (with no asymmetric bow tie and no focal or inferior steepening pattern)	9.09% (3/33)
No topography finding significant enough to be diagnosed as clinical	6.06% (2/33)
Keratoconus severity score (no specified number was used for SCK definition)	6.06% (2/33)
Abnormal biomicroscopic findings including Vogt's striae and Fleischer ring >2 mm or skewed radial axis (SRAX) >21 degrees or >20 degrees, or keratoconus predicting index (KPI) >30% or >0.3 or keratoconus severity index (KSI) >30%, and abnormal keratoconus index (KCI)	6.06% (2/33)
Corrected distance visual acuity (CDVA) of 20/20 or better (Snellen)	6.06% (2/33)
Keratoconus severity score (KSS) 0, 1, or 2	6.06% (2/33)
Paracentral I-S dioptric asymmetry difference in 1.4 to 1.9 D gradient	6.06% (2/33)
Belin/Ambrósio Enhanced Ectasia total deviation index (BAD-D) from the Pentacam <1.60 standard deviations	3.03% (1/33)
Corvis biomechanical index (CBI) score of greater than 0.5 in both eyes	3.03% (1/33)
Simulated central corneal power greater than 47.2 D but less than 48.7 D	3.03% (1/33)
Maximum keratometry ≥47 D/47.2 D	3.03% (1/33)
Elevation of the posterior corneal surface (unspecified quantitative value)	3.03% (1/33)

KC, keratoconus; *SCK,* subclinical keratoconus; *μm,* microns.
Henriquez MA, Hadid M, Izquierdo L Jr. A systematic review of subclinical keratoconus and forme fruste keratoconus. *J Refract Surg.* 2020;36(4):270–279.

steepening compared with the region 180 degrees opposite the steepest region and an I-S value less than 1.4 D.[25] Therefore some of the topographic parameters used for both definitions (SCK and FFKC) are not clearly diagnostic criteria for "KC" and can overlap the "suspicious topographic definition."[29]

TABLE 2.2 ■ Most Frequently Cited Criteria Combinations Used to Define Subclinical Keratoconus and FFKC

Frequently Cited Criteria Combinations Including Three Parameters	Studies That Used This Combination
To Define Subclinical Keratoconus (SCK)	
Normal-appearing cornea on slit-lamp biomicroscopy, keratometry, retinoscopy, and ophthalmoscopy	21.71% (7/33)
Inferior-superior asymmetry and/or bow-tie pattern with skewed radial axes	
Diagnosis of KC in the fellow eye	
Inferior-superior asymmetry and/or bow-tie pattern with skewed radial axes	12.12% (4/33)
No history of contact lens use, ocular surgery, or trauma.	
Diagnosis of keratoconus (KC) in the fellow eye	
Normal-appearing cornea on slit-lamp biomicroscopy, keratometry, retinoscopy, and ophthalmoscopy	12.12% (4/33)
Corneal topography showing an abnormal localized steepening or central/inferior steepening or asymmetric bow-tie pattern or claw-shape pattern on topography	
Diagnosis of KC in the fellow eye	
To Define Forme Fruste Keratoconus (FFKC)	
Normal topography	31.81% (7/22)
Normal slit-lamp examination	
Keratoconus KC in the fellow eye	
Lack of any KC-related findings/signs in the slit-lamp biomicroscopy	9.09% (2/22)
Keratoconus percentage index (KISA) values between 60% and 100%	
KC in the fellow eye	

Note: All other combinations that included at least three criteria were used in fewer than three studies for SCK definitions and in only one study in the FFKC definitions.
Henriquez MA, Hadid M, Izquierdo L Jr. A systematic review of subclinical keratoconus and forme fruste keratoconus. *J Refract Surg*. 2020;36(4):270–279.

Unilateral KC

Over time, information regarding the altered biomechanics in the "normal topographic eye" of FFKC[19] and the importance of "between eye asymmetry" analysis in the diagnosis of KC make it clear that KC is a bilateral disease,[20,30] and consensus was achieved regarding the statement "true unilateral KC does not exist."

Consensus Needed in the Future

The literature review reflects some gaps in information. Certain criteria related to epithelial imaging,[17] wavefront aberrations,[18,19] corneal biomechanics,[15] and posterior elevation[20] that have been associated with early diagnosis of KC have not been included as inclusion criteria in the majority of the studies to define SCK and FFKC.

However, consensus has not been reached about how many and which signs of a suspicious topography are necessary to distinguish SCK or FFKC from "KC suspect or abnormal topography" in a patient in whom neither of the eyes has over KC. Thus the differentiation between an early form of KC and an abnormal topography remains a challenge and will require consensus on what features are relevant.

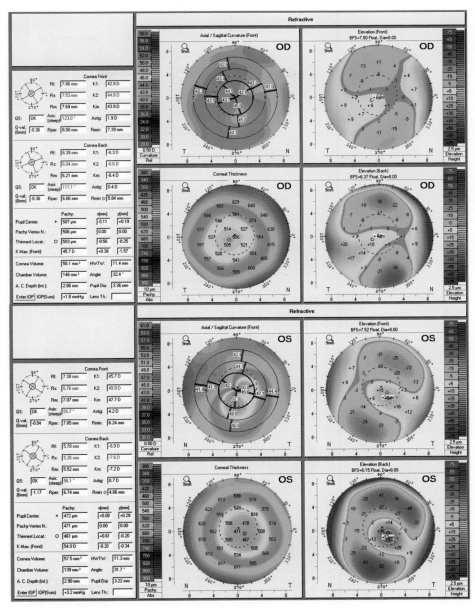

Fig. 2.3 Refractive maps of subclinical keratoconus in the right eye and keratoconus in the left eye. Note the abnormal topography in the right eye owing to abnormal localized inferior steepening, and inferior-superior asymmetry (lower than 1.4 D).

Finally, it remains doubtful if the term "SCK" is adequate, considering that KC is a bilateral disease. Clinical signs of KC in the fellow eye would mean that the disease is no longer subclinical in its presentation.

Acknowledgment

We would like to thank Marta Hadid, MD, for bibliographic research.

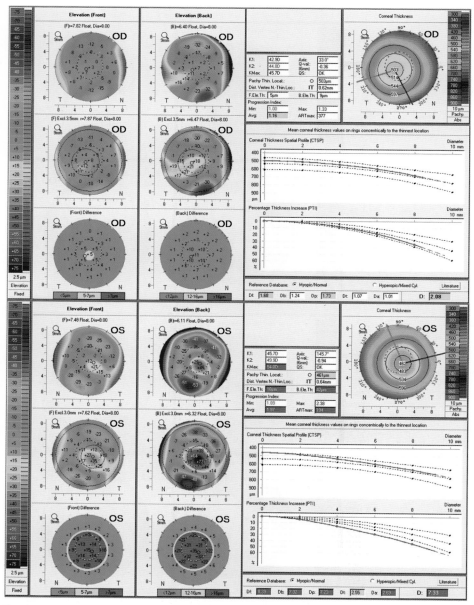

Fig. 2.4 Belin/Ambrósio Enhancement Display of the patient presented in Fig. 2.3. Final D from the right eye is suspicious whereas the Final D from the left eye is abnormal.

BOX 2.1 ■ Subclinical Keratoconus

- Normal slit-lamp examination
- Topographic/tomographic signs of keratoconus (KC) or suspicious topography (but not enough to define as KC)
- KC in the fellow eye

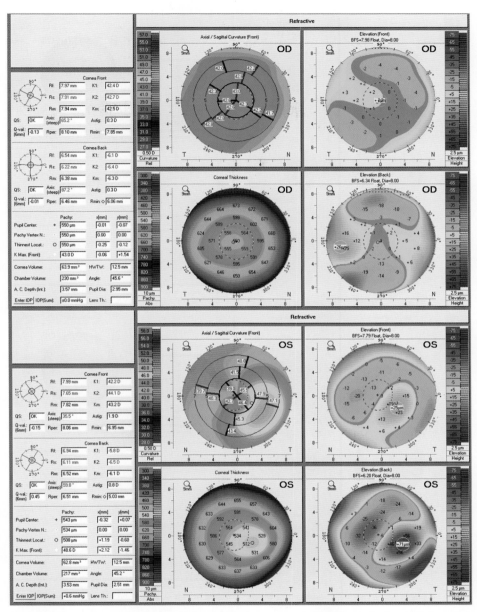

Fig. 2.5 Refractive maps of a patient with forme fruste keratoconus in the right eye *(top)* and keratoconus in the left eye *(bottom)*.

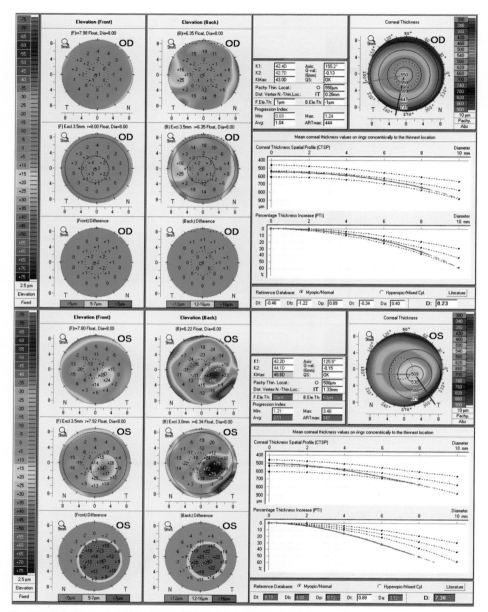

Fig. 2.6 Belin/Ambrosio Enhancement Display for patient presented if Fig. 2.5, where Final D value is lower than 1.6, considering as normal in the right eye and the Final D from the left eye is abnormal.

TABLE 2.3 ■ Frequency of Parameters Used in the Definition of Forme Fruste Keratoconus in the Analyzed Studies

Parameter	Frequency
Keratoconus (KC) in the fellow eye	77.27% (17/22)
Normal topography	59.09% (13/22)
Normal slit-lamp examination	40.90% (9/22)
Lack of any KC-related findings/signs in the slit-lamp biomicroscopy	13.63% (3/22)
Superior-inferior (I-S) power difference in 4-mm central zone more than 1.5 D	9.09% (2/22)
Keratoconus percentage index (KISA) values between 60% and 100%	9.09% (2/22)
Nidek corneal navigator (NCN) score: nonnull score similarity to KC for the contralateral eyes	9.09% (2/22)
Mean keratometry <47 D	4.54% (1/22)
Paracentral I-S dioptric asymmetry ≤1.4	4.54% (1/22)
Apex of the cone not centered at the 6 o'clock semimeridian	4.54% (1/22)
Corneal thickness at the apex of the cone is approximately 30 mm thinner than the corresponding distance above the pupil center	4.54% (1/22)
Area of inferior or superior steepening (unspecific value) or minor topographic asymmetry	4.54% (1/22)
Corneal steepness higher than 47.00 D	4.54% (1/22)
Keratoconus percentage index (KISA) less than 60%	4.54% (1/22)
Keratoconus severity score (KSS) of 1 or 2, regardless of the status of the fellow eye	9.09% (2/22)
Oblique cylinder greater than 1.5 D	4.54% (1/22)
NCN score: null score similarity to suspect KC and KC	4.54% (1/22)
KSS could be 0, 1, or 2 as long as the other eye with KC has a KSS greater than or equal to 3	4.54% (1/22)
Asymptomatic Pentacam tomography and elevation	4.54% (1/22)

Henriquez MA, Hadid M, Izquierdo L Jr. A systematic review of subclinical keratoconus and forme fruste keratoconus. J Refract Surg. 2020;36(4):270–279.

BOX 2.2 ■ Forme Fruste Keratoconus

- Normal topography
- Normal slit-lamp examination
- Keratoconus in the fellow eye

References

1. Krachmer JH, Feder RS, Belin MW. Keratoconus and related noninflammatory corneal thinning disorders. *Surv Ophthalmol*. 1984;28:293–322.
2. Rabinowitz YS. Keratoconus. *Surv Ophthalmol*. 1998;42(4):297–319.
3. Mas Tur V, MacGregor C, Jayaswal R, O'Brart D, Maycock N. A review of keratoconus: diagnosis, pathophysiology, and genetics. *Surv Ophthalmol*. 2017;62(6):770–783.
4. Lee LR, Hirst LW, Readshaw G. Clinical detection of unilateral keratoconus. *Aust N Z J Ophthalmol*. 1995;23:129–133.

5. Rabinowitz YS, Nesburn AB, McDonnell PJ. Videokeratography of the fellow eye in unilateral keratoconus. *Ophthalmology*. 1993;100:181–186.
6. Gomes JA, Tan D, Rapuano CJ, et al. Group of Panelists for the Global Delphi Panel of Keratoconus and Ectatic Diseases. Global consensus on keratoconus and ectatic diseases. *Cornea*. 2015;34(4):359–369.
7. Bae GH, Kim JR, Kim CH, Lim DH, Chung ES, Chung TY. Corneal topographic and tomographic analysis of fellow eyes in unilateral keratoconus patients using Pentacam. *Am J Ophthalmol*. 2014;157:103–109.e1.
8. Ruiseñor Vázquez PR, Galletti JD, Minguez N, et al. Pentacam Scheimpflug tomography findings in topographically normal patients and subclinical keratoconus cases. *Am J Ophthalmol*. 2014;158:32–40.e2.
9. Hwang ES, Perez-Straziota CE, Kim SW, Santhiago MR, Randleman JB. Distinguishing highly asymmetric keratoconus eyes using combined Scheimpflug and spectral domain OCT analysis. *Ophthalmology*. 2018;125(12):1862–1871.
10. Golan O, Piccinini AL, Hwang ES, et al. Distinguishing highly asymmetric keratoconus eyes using dual Scheimpflug/Placido analysis. *Am J Ophthalmol*. 2019;201:46–53.
11. Feghali CA, Wright TM. Cytokines in acute and chronic inflammation. *Front Biosci*. 1997;2:d12–d26.
12. Shetty R, Ghosh A, Lim RR, et al. Elevated expression of matrix metalloproteinase-9 and inflammatory cytokines in keratoconus patients is inhibited by cyclosporine A. *Invest Ophthalmol Vis Sci*. 2015;56:738–750.
13. Shetty R, Sathyanarayanamoorthy A, Ramachandra RA, et al. Attenuation of lysyl oxidase and collagen gene expression in keratoconus patient corneal epithelium corresponds to disease severity. *Mol Vis*. 2015;21:12–25.
14. Pahuja N, Kumar NR, Shroff R, et al. Differential molecular expression of extracellular matrix and inflammatory genes at the corneal cone apex drives focal weakening in keratoconus. *Invest Ophthalmol Vis Sci*. 2016;57(13):5372–5382.
15. Maeda N, Klyce S, Smolek M. Comparison of methods for detecting keratoconus using videokeratography. *Arch Ophthalmol*. 1995;113(7):870–874.
16. Maeda N, Klyce S, Smolek M, Thompson H. Automated keratoconus screening with corneal topography analysis. *Invest Ophthalmol Vis Sci*. 1994;35(6):2749–2757.
17. Rabinowitz YS, Garbus J, McDonnell PJ. Computer-assisted corneal topography in family members of patients with keratoconus. *Arch Ophthalmol*. 1990;108(3):365–371.
18. Ambrósio R Jr, Alonso RS, Luz A. Coca Velarde LG. Corneal-thickness spatial profile and corneal-volume distribution: tomographic indices to detect keratoconus. *J Cataract Refract Surg*. 2006;32(11):1851–1859.
19. Luz A, Lopes B, Hallahan KM, et al. Enhanced combined tomography and biomechanics data for distinguishing forme fruste keratoconus. *J Refract Surg*. 2016;32(7):479–494.
20. Henriquez MA, Izquierdo L Jr, Mannis MJ. Intereye asymmetry detected by Scheimpflug imaging in subjects with normal corneas and keratoconus. *Cornea*. 2013;32(6):779–782.
21. Silverman RH, Urs R, RoyChoudhury A, Archer TJ, Gobbe M, Reinstein DZ. Combined tomography and epithelial thickness mapping for diagnosis of keratoconus. *Eur J Ophthalmol*. 2017;27(2):129–134.
22. Saad A, Gatinel D. Evaluation of total and corneal wavefront high order aberrations for the detection of forme fruste keratoconus. *Invest Ophthalmol Vis Sci*. 2012;53(6):2978–2992.
23. Alió JL, Shabayek MH. Corneal higher order aberrations: a method to grade keratoconus. *J Refract Surg*. 2006;22(6):539–545.
24. Villavicencio OF, Gilani F, Henriquez MA, Izquierdo L Jr, Ambrósio RR Jr, Belin MW. Independent population validation of the Belin/Ambrósio Enhanced Ectasia Display: implications for keratoconus studies and screening. *Int J Keratoconus Ectatic Corneal Diseases*. 2014;3(1):1–8.
25. Henriquez MA, Hadid M, Izquierdo L Jr. A systematic review of subclinical keratoconus and forme fruste keratoconus. *J Refract Surg*. 2020;36(4):270–279.
26. Randleman JB, Trattler WB, Stulting RD. *Merriam-Webster's Collegiate Dictionary*. 3rd ed. Springfield, MA: Merriam-Webster Incorporated; 2008.
27. Amsler M. Le kératocône fruste au Javal. *Ophthalmologica*. 1938;96(2):77–83.
28. Amsler M. Kératocône classique et kératocône fruste; arguments unitaires. *Ophthalmologica*. 1946;111(2-3):96–101.
29. Randleman JB, Trattler WB. Stulting RD. Validation of the ectasia risk score system for preoperative laser in situ keratomileusis screening. *Am J Ophthalmol*. 2008;145(5):813–818.
30. Henriquez MA, Izquierdo L Jr, Belin MW. Intereye asymmetry in eyes with keratoconus and high ammetropia: Scheimpflug imaging analysis. *Cornea*. 2015;34(suppl 10):S57–S60.

CHAPTER 3

Epidemiology of Keratoconus

José Alvaro Pereira Gomes ■ Pablo Felipe Rodrigues

KEY CONCEPTS

- Epidemiological studies describe the distribution of disease, identify factors that influence that distribution, and measure the impact and morbidity of disease in a defined population.
- Population-based screening studies are the best methodology to assess the true prevalence of the disease.
- Modern imaging technology has made an earlier diagnosis of keratoconus easier, even before the loss of visual acuity.
- An inverse relationship between age and the keratoconus severity has been reported. Corneal collagen interfibrillar space decreases with age, and the collagen bundles become thicker, modifying the biomechanical properties of the cornea.
- The presence of estrogen, progesterone, and androgen receptors in epithelial corneal cells and keratocytes raises the possibility of a relationship between hormones and biomechanical properties of the cornea at different stages of life.
- Genetic and hereditary links to keratoconus have also been studied. Most familial keratoconus is autosomal dominant.
- Eye rubbing, allergy, and environmental factors also contribute to keratoconus pathogenesis.

Introduction

Epidemiological studies describe the distribution of disease, identify factors that influence that distribution, and measure the impact and morbidity of disease in a defined population.[1] They can recognize vulnerable groups, helping to define more transparent and consistent designs to health programs and services. The introduction of cutting-edge technology, both in disease diagnosis and data analysis, has further refined the epidemiological process, allowing a more efficient formulation of health policies.[2] In this sense, the technological revolution provided by new diagnostic imaging devices in assessing the cornea and anterior segment and by innovative artificial intelligence algorithms has significantly changed the way we identify and treat vision-threatening conditions such as keratoconus.[3]

Incidence and Prevalence

Attempts to establish prevalence and incidence estimates of keratoconus in the population have shown great variability over the last century. Among the possible factors for this variability are the heterogeneity of types of epidemiologic studies and the lack of well-defined criteria for keratoconus definition.[4]

Most of the prevalence studies have been carried out in hospitals or clinics, because of the ability to collect data.[5] However, they usually underestimate the prevalence of the disease, as patients are commonly symptomatic, and the early and more subtle forms can be missed.[5] One of the most commonly cited publications on the epidemiology of keratoconus is the study by Kennedy et al.[6] in Minnesota, United States, who found a prevalence of 0.054% based on the clinical diagnosis made by the findings of scissoring movement in retinoscopy and keratometry. This number was similar to those reported in Finland[7] and Denmark[8] but much higher than those reported in Russia, at 0.0004%.[9] and 0.0068% in Macedonia.[5] More recently, a large-scale evaluation from the Netherlands mandatory health insurance database showed prevalence approximately fivefold higher than previous reports, at around 0.27%, or 1:375 patients[10] (Table 3.1).

Population-based screening studies are the best methodology to assess the true prevalence of the disease. Cross-sectional surveys enroll people who volunteer to participate in the investigation.[5] Selection bias may also occur, as diseased individuals might not be interested in participating. However, others who are not aware of the condition may volunteer, counterbalancing the possibility of a significant error.[5,17] The first cross-sectional study was published by Hofstetter in 1959.[18] Twenty-five optometrists used Placido disk images to analyze 13,395 eyes and confirmed the diagnosis of the disease by the presence of oval or keratoconic-type pattern images.[18]

TABLE 3.1 ■ **Hospital/Clinic-Based Epidemiological Studies of Keratoconus**

Author	Location	Age in Years	Sample Size	Incidence/ 100,000	Prevalence/ 100,000	Method
Tanabe et al. (1985)[11]	Muroran, Japan	10–60	2601		9	Keratometry
Kennedy et al. (1986)[6]	Minnesota, USA	12–77	64	2	54.5	Keratometry + retinoscopy
Ihalainen (1986)[7]	Finland	15–70	294	1.5	30	Keratometry + retinoscopy
Gorskova and Sevost'ianov (1998)[9]	Urals, Russia				0.2–0.4	Keratometry
Pearson et al. (2000)[12]	Midlands, UK	10–44	382	4.5 – W 19.6 – A	57 229	Keratometry + retinoscopy
Ota et al. (2002)[13]	Tokyo, Japan		325	9		Keratometry
Georgiou et al. (2004)[14]	Yorkshire, UK		74	3.3 – W 25 – A		Clinical examination
Assiri et al. (2005)[15]	Asir, Saudi Arabia	8–28	125	20		Keratometry
Nielsen et al. (2007)[8]	Denmark		NA	1.3	86	Clinical indices + topography
Ljubic (2009)[5]	Skope, Macedonia		2254		6.8	Keratometry
Ziaei et al. (2012)[16]	Yazd, Iran	25.7 ± 9	536	22.3		Topography

A, Asian (Indian, Pakistani, and Bangladeshi); *KC,* keratoconus; *NA,* not available; *P,* patient; *W,* White.
This table was modified from Gordon-Shaag A, Millodot M, Kaiserman I, et al. Risk factors for keratoconus in Israel: a case-control study. *Ophthalmic Physiol Opt.* 2015;35(6):673–681.

The estimated prevalence of keratoconus was 0.6% in the American population. The elliptical or "irregular" pattern was observed in 0.1% of patients between 0 and 19 years and 7.4% between 70 and 79 years old, with a preponderance in females.[18]

An important population-based study including 4667 subjects was conducted in central India.[19] Using keratometric values of more than 48 diopters (D) as a cutoff, the authors found a prevalence of keratoconus of 2.3%. Considering that keratometry measures only the central corneal power, it is possible that cases of inferior ectasia were missed. Another similar study carried out in Beijing, China with 3468 people reported a prevalence of 1% of corneas with more than 48 D,[20] using optical low coherence reflectometry biometry of the right eyes. An investigation of French army recruits using corneal topography found a prevalence of keratoconus of 1.2%.[5]

Other prevalence studies, including population-based surveys from Asia and the Middle East using corneal topographic and tomographic values, found a higher prevalence of keratoconus in these parts of the world, ranging from 0.9% to 3.3% (Table 3.2). In 2018 Torres-Netto et al. performed a cross-sectional, observational, multicenter study collecting data from 522 pediatric patients from 6 years to 21 years of age who were seen at multiple nonophthalmic emergency departments in Saudi Arabia.[21] Bilateral corneal measurements were performed using a Scheimpflug corneal tomography system. Two masked examiners established the diagnosis of keratoconus using both objective and subjective screening criteria. Final keratoconus prevalence was 4.79% (95% confidence interval [CI]: 2.96 - 6.62) or 1:21 patients, the highest reported so far.[21]

Epidemiological Characteristics and Risk Factors for Keratoconus

AGE

Keratoconus is believed to affect adolescents and young adults with a higher incidence occurring between 20 and 30 years of age.[4] Some studies suggest an average age of 20 years old (±6.4)[26] and 24.05 years old (±8.97).[27]

Better access to modern imaging technology has provided an earlier diagnosis of keratoconus even before the loss of visual quality.[5] Such characteristics have allowed both diagnosis at an earlier age and earlier therapeutic intervention. The rate of progression of keratoconus in children is higher when compared with adults in the same time interval.[28,29] One possible explanation for this observation is the association of young patients with allergic conditions and eye rubbing.

The diagnosis of keratoconus in patients older than 50 years has not been significant, ranging between 7.4% and 15%.[30,31] An inversed relationship between age and the keratoconus severity has been reported. Corneal collagen interfibrillar space decreases with age and the collagen bundles become thicker, modifying the biomechanical properties of the cornea. This increment in corneal rigidity with age can explain the decrease in keratoconus with increasing age.

SEX GENDER AND HORMONES

Several groups have sought to understand the relationship between gender and keratoconus. Some authors reported a preponderance of females, with rates of 53% to 66%,[16,32,33] whereas others found a higher prevalence of keratoconus in males, with values of 53% to 62%.[33,34] The Collaborative Longitudinal Evaluation of Keratoconus (CLEK) study reported functional discomfort more frequently in women. This difference, however, was not reproduced in clinical examination.[35]

The discovery that estrogen, progesterone, and androgen receptors are present in epithelial corneal cells and keratocytes raises the possibility of a relationship between hormones and biomechanical properties of the cornea at the different stages of life.[36] The classic example is the positive correlation between the role of hormones during pregnancy in inducing corneal biomechanical

TABLE 3.2 ■ Population-Based Epidemiological Studies of Keratoconus

Author	Location	Age in Years (Mean)	Sample Size	Prevalence/ 100,000	Method	Sampling Method
Hofstetter (1959)[18]	Indianapolis, USA	1–79	13345	120	Placido disk[a]	Rural volunteers
Santiago et al. (1995)[5]	France	18–22	670	1190	Topography	Army recruits
Jonas et al. (2009)[19]	Maharashtra, India	>30 (49.4 ± 13.4)	4667	2300	Keratometry[a]	Rural volunteers (eight villages)
Millodot et al. (2011)[17]	Jerusalem, Israel	18–54 (24.4 ± 5.7)	981	2340	Topography	Urban volunteers (one college)
Waked et al. (2012)[22]	Beirut, Lebanon	22–26	92	3300	Topography	Urban volunteers (one college)
Xu et al. (2012)[20]	Beijing, China	50–93 (64.2 ± 9.8)	3166	900	Optical low coherence reflectometry[a]	Rural + urban volunteers
Hashemi et al. (2013)[23]	Shahrud, Iran	50.83 ± 0.12	4592	760	Topography	Urban volunteers from random cluster
Hashemi et al. (2013)[24]	Tehran, Iran	14–81 (40.8 ± 17.1)	426	3300	Topography	Urban volunteers (stratified cluster)
Gordon-Shaag et al. (2015)[5]	Haifa, Israel	18–60 (25.05 ± 8.83)	314	3180	Topography	Urban volunteers (one college)
Hashemi et al. (2014)[25]	Mashhad, Iran	20–34 (26.1 ± 2.3)	1073	2500	Topography	Urban volunteers (stratified cluster in one university)
Torres Netto et al. (2018)[21]	Riyadh, Saudi Arabia	6–21 (16.8 ± 4.2)	1044	4790	Rotational Scheimpflug corneal tomography system	Patients who were seen at emergency rooms for nonophthalmic appointments at four locations in the Kingdom of Saudi Arabia

[a]The methods for detecting keratoconus used in these studies have limitations and results should be interpreted with caution.
This table was modified from Gordon-Shaag A, Millodot M, Kaiserman I, et al. Risk factors for keratoconus in Israel: a case-control study. Ophthalmic Physiol Opt. 2015;35(6):673–681.

changes, post-LASIK changes, and progression in patients with keratoconus.[37] Estrogen receptors are present in the keratocytes of the human cornea and high estrogen levels during pregnancy (100 times higher) impair corneal biomechanics and thickness.[38,39] Various studies have demonstrated that serum levels of matrix metalloproteinases (MMPs) are increased and serum levels of tissue inhibitors of matrix metalloproteinases (TIMPs) are decreased during pregnancy.[40,41] This implies that increased levels of proteolytic enzymes and decreased levels of their inhibitors during pregnancy can play an important role in the progression of keratoconus. Another recent clinical example of this influence was a report of the rapid progression of keratoconus in a 49-year-old woman on selective tissue estrogenic activity regulator (STEAR) therapy for endometriosis.[30,42]

GENETICS AND HEREDITY

Genetics and heredity seem to contribute to the pathogenesis of keratoconus.

Most familial keratoconus is autosomal dominant. Moreover, monozygotic twins present greater concordance with the topographic pattern of keratoconus than dizygotic twins.[43] Family-based linkage studies have identified more than 19 candidate genetic loci that present mutations for keratoconus indicating genetic heterogeneity. Additionally, keratoconus can present with different grades of severity, even bilaterally for the same individual.[44,45] Such characteristics reveal the influence of cofactors in the phenotypic presentation of this corneal ectasia.

The association of keratoconus with a predisposing family history has also been investigated. The presence of a positive association, however, has shown wide variability,[16,29,46,47] ranging from 5% to 27.9%. Large population-based studies such as the CLEK study have shown a positive family history of keratoconus in 13.5% of patients.[35] In the Dundee University Scottish Keratoconus Study (DUSKS),[48] the rate was 5% for Caucasians but 25% for the Asian subgroup. This result reflects a higher level of positive family history in populations with a higher prevalence of keratoconus. Similar results can be observed in studies involving keratoconus patients in families with multiple children, as found in northern Finland, where prevalence was 19% versus 9% in southern Finland, where families had few children.[7] The genetic influence is also strongly present when observing a higher prevalence of keratoconus in communities with inbreeding relationships.[49]

ENVIRONMENTAL FACTORS

As we previously mentioned, keratoconus prevalence is not the same in different parts of the world. Northern Europe, the Urals, northern United States, and Japan have a low prevalence.[6,7,9,12–14,50] In contrast to these low numbers, keratoconus prevalence is relatively high in countries of the Middle East,[15–17,19,23–25] India,[19] and China.[20] A common characteristic of the Middle Eastern countries and some areas in India is the hot and dry climate for most parts of the year. The oxidative damage secondary to excessive sun exposure, to ultraviolet (UV) light, may in part explain these numbers. The ethnic background or different lifestyles including nutrition habits can also play a role in keratoconus pathogenesis[51] (Table 3.3).

TABLE 3.3 ■ The Main Environmental Factors Associated With Keratoconus[47]

	Normal Controls (n = 183)	Keratoconus (n = 218)
Allergy	66 (35%)	96 (44%) $P < 0.105$ (NS)
Joint hypermobility	10 (12%)	34 (15%) $P < 0.305$ (NS)
Eye rubbing	106 (58%)	174 (80%) $P = 0.001$
Positive family history	1 (0.05%)	22 (10%) $P = 0.001$

NS, Not significant.

EYE RUBBING AND ATOPY

Eye rubbing is considered one of the most important risk factors for inducing keratoconus and is often associated with ocular allergy or intellectual disability.[52] Furthermore, it has been reported that people with Down syndrome frequently rub their eyes,[31] which is a habit linked to keratoconus and associated with an inflammation process and biomechanical alterations.

Approximately 70% (ranging from 12% to 80%) of keratoconus patients report rubbing their eyes. There are some variations in this association, including whether the eye rubbing is gentle or vigorous[53] and the length of rubbing. The CLEK study reported that 48% of keratoconus patients rubbed both eyes vigorously, whereas 2.2% rubbed only one eye.[35] It is important to mention that there are reports of cases of asymmetric keratoconus in which the most affected eye was the one that was rubbed most vigorously. The mechanism that explains this association starts with the microtrauma to the ocular surface produced by eye rubbing.[54] This trauma induces epithelial and stromal cells to secrete MMP-1 and MMP-13, which, together with the release of inflammatory mediators such as interleukins 1 and 6 and tumor necrosis factor (TNF-α), lead to apoptosis of keratocytes resulting in progressive loss of the stromal collagen and corneal thinning.[54]

Atopy is an exaggerated immunoglobulin E (IgE)-mediated immune response that commonly affects the nose, eyes, skin, and lungs causing allergic rhinitis, conjunctivitis, asthma, and eczema.[49] There is some controversy in the literature regarding the association between keratoconus and atopy.[54] A positive association has been reported,[55–58] but many reports did not find a significant association when compared with controls.[59–61] A multivariate logistic regression analysis confirmed the assumption that atopy was not truly associated with keratoconus but with eye rubbing.[61]

Allergy is an exaggerated immune response to a foreign antigen regardless of mechanism.[5] Allergy is frequently associated with keratoconus compared with controls or the general population.[7,31,48,52,55,56,62] About one-third of keratoconus patients are estimated to have allergy, but the percentage varies according to the study (see Table 3.3).

Moreover, one cannot forget the association between atopy/allergy and eye rubbing in response to environmental conditions that potentially augment the genetic predisposition to the development of keratoconus.

OTHER RISK FACTORS

Some studies show a positive correlation between keratoconus and Down syndrome,[31] mitral valve prolapse,[63] floppy eyelid syndrome,[64] obstructive sleep apnea,[30,65] and connective tissue disorders such as Ehlers-Danlos and Marfan syndromes, as well as osteogenesis imperfecta.[66]

Conclusion

The prevalence of keratoconus is variable, reaching almost 5% of the population in some regions of the world such as the Middle East. It affects men and women from all ethnic groups. Eye rubbing, allergy, environment, and genetic factors contribute to its pathogenesis. The refinement of prevalence studies with the incorporation of better imaging technology and artificial intelligence will help to improve early diagnostics, targeted therapeutics, and the visual prognosis of this corneal ectatic disease.

References

1. Stapleton F, Alves M, Bunya VY, et al. TFOS DEWS II Epidemiology Report. *Ocul Surf.* 2017;15(3):334–365.
2. Whiting PF, Davenport C, Jameson C, et al. How well do health professionals interpret diagnostic information? A systematic review. *BMJ Open.* 2015;5(7):e008155.

3. Salomão MQ, Esposito A, Dupps WJ Jr. Advances in anterior segment imaging and analysis. *Curr Opin Ophthalmol.* 2009;20(4):324–332.

4. Galvis V, Sherwin T, Tello A, Merayo J, Barrera R, Acera A. Keratoconus: an inflammatory disorder? *Eye (Lond).* 2015;29(7):843–859.

5. Gordon-Shaag A, Millodot M, Kaiserman I, et al. Risk factors for keratoconus in Israel: a case-control study. *Ophthalmic Physiol Opt.* 2015;35(6):673–681.

6. Kennedy RH, Bourne WM, Dyer JA. A 48-year clinical and epidemiologic study of keratoconus. *Am J Ophthalmol.* 1986;101(3):267–273.

7. Ihalainen A. Clinical and epidemiological features of keratoconus genetic and external factors in the pathogenesis of the disease. *Acta Ophthalmol Suppl.* 1986;178:1–64.

8. Nielsen K, Hjortdal J, Aagaard Nohr E, Ehlers N. Incidence and prevalence of keratoconus in Denmark. *Acta Ophthalmol Scand.* 2007;85(8):890–892.

9. Gorskova EN, Sevost'ianov EN. Epidemiology of keratoconus in the Urals. *Vestn Oftalmol.* 1998;114(4):38–40.

10. Godefrooij DA, de Wit GA, Uiterwaal CS, Imhof SM, Wisse RP. Age-specific incidence and prevalence of keratoconus: a nationwide registration study. *Am J Ophthalmol.* 2017;175:169–172.

11. Tanabe U, Fujiki K, Ogawa A, Ueda S, Kanai A. Prevalence of keratoconus patients in Japan. *Nippon Ganka Gakkai Zasshi.* 1985;89(3):407–411.

12. Pearson AR, Soneji B, Sarvananthan N, Sandford-Smith JH. Does ethnic origin influence the incidence or severity of keratoconus? *Eye (Lond).* 2000;14(Pt 4):625–628.

13. Ota R, Fujiki K, Nakayasu K. Estimation of patient visit rate and incidence of keratoconus in the 23 wards of Tokyo. *Nippon Ganka Gakkai Zasshi.* 2002;106(6):365–372.

14. Georgiou T, Funnell CL, Cassels-Brown A, O'Conor R. Influence of ethnic origin on the incidence of keratoconus and associated atopic disease in Asians and White patients. *Eye (Lond).* 2004;18(4):379–383.

15. Assiri AA, Yousuf BI, Quantock AJ, Murphy PJ. Incidence and severity of keratoconus in Asir province, Saudi Arabia. *Br J Ophthalmol.* 2005;89(11):1403–1406.

16. Ziaei H, Jafarinasab MR, Javadi MA, et al. Epidemiology of keratoconus in an Iranian population. *Cornea.* 2012;31(9):1044–1047.

17. Millodot M, Shneor E, Albou S, Atlani E, Gordon-Shaag A. Prevalence and associated factors of keratoconus in Jerusalem: a cross-sectional study. *Ophthalmic Epidemiol.* 2011;18(2):91–97.

18. Hofstetter HW. A keratoscopic survey of 13,395 eyes. *Am J Optom Arch Am Acad Optom.* 1959;36(1):3–11.

19. Jonas JB, Nangia V, Matin A, Kulkarni M, Bhojwani K. Prevalence and associations of keratoconus in rural Maharashtra in central India: the central India eye and medical study. *Am J Ophthalmol.* 2009;148(5):760–765.

20. Xu L, Wang YX, Guo Y, You QS, Jonas JB. Beijing Eye Study G. Prevalence and associations of steep cornea/keratoconus in Greater Beijing. The Beijing Eye Study. *PLoS One.* 2012;7(7):e39313.

21. Torres Netto EA, Al-Otaibi WM, Hafezi NL, et al. Prevalence of keratoconus in paediatric patients in Riyadh, Saudi Arabia. *Br J Ophthalmol.* 2018;102(10):1436–1441.

22. Waked N, Fayad AM, Fadlallah A, El Rami H. Keratoconus screening in a Lebanese students' population. *J Fr Ophtalmol.* 2012;35(1):23–29.

23. Hashemi H, Beiranvand A, Khabazkhoob M, et al. Prevalence of keratoconus in a population-based study in Shahroud. *Cornea.* 2013;32(11):1441–1445.

24. Hashemi H, Khabazkhoob M, Fotouhi A. Topographic keratoconus is not rare in an Iranian population: the Tehran Eye Study. *Ophthalmic Epidemiol.* 2013;20(6):385–391.

25. Hashemi H, Khabazkhoob M, Yazdani N, et al. The prevalence of keratoconus in a young population in Mashhad, Iran. *Ophthalmic Physiol Opt.* 2014;34(5):519–527.

26. Krachmer JH, Feder RS, Belin MW. Keratoconus and related noninflammatory corneal thinning disorders. *Surv Ophthalmol.* 1984;28(4):293–322.

27. Bilgin LK, Yilmaz S, Araz B, Yuksel SB. Sezen T. 30 years of contact lens prescribing for keratoconic patients in Turkey. *Cont Lens Anterior Eye.* 2009;32(1):16–21.

28. Chatzis N, Hafezi F. Progression of keratoconus and efficacy of pediatric [corrected] corneal collagen cross-linking in children and adolescents. *J Refract Surg.* 2012;28(11):753–758.

29. Leoni-Mesplie S, Mortemousque B, Touboul D, et al. Scalability and severity of keratoconus in children. *Am J Ophthalmol.* 2012;154(1):56–62, e51.

30. Pobelle-Frasson C, Velou S, Huslin V, Massicault B, Colin J. Keratoconus: what happens with older patients? *J Fr Ophtalmol*. 2004;27(7):779–782.
31. Zadnik K, Barr JT, Edrington TB, et al. Baseline findings in the Collaborative Longitudinal Evaluation of Keratoconus (CLEK) Study. *Invest Ophthalmol Vis Sci*. 1998;39(13):2537–2546.
32. Laqua H. Hereditary diseases in keratoconus. *Klin Monbl Augenheilkd*. 1971;159(5):609–618.
33. Amsler M. The "forme fruste" of keratoconus. *Wien Klin Wochenschr*. 1961;73:842–843.
34. Ertan A, Muftuoglu O. Keratoconus clinical findings according to different age and gender groups. *Cornea*. 2008;27(10):1109–1113.
35. Wagner H, Barr JT, Zadnik K. Collaborative Longitudinal Evaluation of Keratoconus (CLEK) Study: methods and findings to date. *Cont Lens Anterior Eye*. 2007;30(4):223–232.
36. Khaled ML, Helwa I, Drewry M, Seremwe M, Estes A, Liu Y. Molecular and histopathological changes associated with keratoconus. *Biomed Res Int*. 2017;2017:7803029.
37. Bilgihan K, Hondur A, Sul S, Ozturk S. Pregnancy-induced progression of keratoconus. *Cornea*. 2011;30(9):991–994.
38. Spoerl E, Zubaty V, Raiskup-Wolf F, Pillunat LE. Oestrogen-induced changes in biomechanics in the cornea as a possible reason for keratectasia. *Br J Ophthalmol*. 2007;91(11):1547–1550.
39. Gupta PD, Johar K Sr, Nagpal K, Vasavada AR. Sex hormone receptors in the human eye. *Surv Ophthalmol*. 2005;50(3):274–284.
40. Wang C, Li AL, Pang Y, Lei YQ, Yu L. Changes in intraocular pressure and central corneal thickness during pregnancy: a systematic review and meta-analysis. *Int J Ophthalmol*. 2017;10(10):1573–1579.
41. Pizzarello LD. Refractive changes in pregnancy. *Graefes Arch Clin Exp Ophthalmol*. 2003;241(6):484–488.
42. Torres-Netto EA, Randleman JB, Hafezi NL, Hafezi F. Late-onset progression of keratoconus after therapy with selective tissue estrogenic activity regulator. *J Cataract Refract Surg*. 2019;45(1):101–104.
43. Tuft SJ, Hassan H, George S, Frazer DG, Willoughby CE, Liskova P. Keratoconus in 18 pairs of twins. *Acta Ophthalmol*. 2012;90(6):e482–e486.
44. Ambrosio R Jr. Heritability of corneal shape in twin study. *Invest Ophthalmol Vis Sci*. 2014;55(12):8365.
45. McMahon TT, Shin JA, Newlin A, Edrington TB, Sugar J, Zadnik K. Discordance for keratoconus in two pairs of monozygotic twins. *Cornea*. 1999;18(4):444–451.
46. Fullerton J, Paprocki P, Foote S, Mackey DA, Williamson R, Forrest S. Identity-by-descent approach to gene localisation in eight individuals affected by keratoconus from north-west Tasmania, Australia. *Hum Genet*. 2002;110(5):462–470.
47. Rabinowitz YS. The genetics of keratoconus. *Ophthalmol Clin North Am*. 2003;16(4):607–620, vii.
48. Weed KH, MacEwen CJ, Giles T, Low J, McGhee CN. The Dundee University Scottish Keratoconus study: demographics, corneal signs, associated diseases, and eye rubbing. *Eye (Lond)*. 2008;22(4):534–541.
49. Gordon-Shaag A, Millodot M, Essa M, Garth J, Ghara M, Shneor E. Is consanguinity a risk factor for keratoconus? *Optom Vis Sci*. 2013;90(5):448–454.
50. Nielsen K, Hjortdal J, Pihlmann M, Corydon TJ. Update on the keratoconus genetics. *Acta Ophthalmol*. 2013;91(2):106–113.
51. Davidson AE, Hayes S, Hardcastle AJ, Tuft SJ. The pathogenesis of keratoconus. *Eye (Lond)*. 2014; 28(2):189–195.
52. McMonnies CW. Mechanisms of rubbing-related corneal trauma in keratoconus. *Cornea*. 2009; 28(6):607–615.
53. Weed KH, MacEwen CJ, McGhee CN. The variable expression of keratoconus within monozygotic twins: Dundee University Scottish Keratoconus Study (DUSKS). *Cont Lens Anterior Eye*. 2006;29(3):123–126.
54. Gordon-Shaag A, Millodot M, Shneor E, Liu Y. The genetic and environmental factors for keratoconus. *Biomed Res Int*. 2015;2015:795738.
55. Nemet AY, Vinker S, Bahar I, Kaiserman I. The association of keratoconus with immune disorders. *Cornea*. 2010;29(11):1261–1264.
56. Shneor E, Millodot M, Blumberg S, Ortenberg I, Behrman S, Gordon-Shaag A. Characteristics of 244 patients with keratoconus seen in an optometric contact lens practice. *Clin Exp Optom*. 2013;96(2):219–224.
57. Crews MJ, Driebe WT Jr, Stern GA. The clinical management of keratoconus: a 6 year retrospective study. *CLAO J*. 1994;20(3):194–197.

58. Kaya V, Karakaya M, Utine CA, Albayrak S, Oge OF, Yilmaz OF. Evaluation of the corneal topographic characteristics of keratoconus with Orbscan II in patients with and without atopy. *Cornea.* 2007;26(8):945–948.
59. Lowell FC, Carroll JM. A study of the occurrence of atopic traits in patients with keratoconus. *J Allergy.* 1970;46(1):32–39.
60. Gasset AR, Hinson WA, Frias JL. Keratoconus and atopic diseases. *Ann Ophthalmol.* 1978;10(8):991–994.
61. Bawazeer AM, Hodge WG, Lorimer B. Atopy and keratoconus: a multivariate analysis. *Br J Ophthalmol.* 2000;84(8):834–836.
62. Jordan CA, Zamri A, Wheeldon C, Patel DV, Johnson R, McGhee CN. Computerized corneal tomography and associated features in a large New Zealand keratoconic population. *J Cataract Refract Surg.* 2011;37(8):1493–1501.
63. Gomes JA, Rapuano CJ, Belin MW, Ambrosio R Jr. Group of panelists for the Global Delphi Panel of K. Ectatic D: Global Consensus on keratoconus diagnosis. *Cornea.* 2015;34(12):e38–e39.
64. Donnenfeld ED, Perry HD, Gibralter RP, Ingraham HJ, Udell IJ. Keratoconus associated with floppy eyelid syndrome. *Ophthalmology.* 1991;98(11):1674–1678.
65. Gokhale NS. Epidemiology of keratoconus. *Indian J Ophthalmol.* 2013;61(8):382–383.
66. Skoumal M, Haberhauer G, Mayr H. Concomitant diseases in primary joint hypermobility syndrome. *Med Klin (Munich).* 2004;99(10):585–590.

CHAPTER 4

Genetics of Keratoconus

Yelena Bykhovskaya ■ Yaron S. Rabinowitz

KEY CONCEPTS

- Keratoconus is a progressive corneal disease with genetic susceptibility.
- Genome-wide linkage studies have identified genes responsible for familial keratoconus.
- A number of keratoconus genes are also involved in other multisystem genetic disorders and ocular syndromes.
- Genome-wide association studies of keratoconus cases and population-wide studies of variation in central corneal thickness have identified new susceptibility genes and biological pathways.
- Transcriptomic and expression studies identify tissue-specific effects of keratoconus genes and noncoding RNAs.
- Genomic insights can be implemented into keratoconus clinical practice.

Evidence for Genetic Predisposition and Familial Inheritance of KC

Keratoconus (KC) is characterized by the progressive thinning and protrusion of the cornea, which assumes a conical shape in the most advanced cases (Box 4.1). It is most commonly detected at puberty and is progressive until the third to fourth decades of life, when it usually arrests.[1] Population prevalence of KC in different parts of the world ranges from 1:375 to 1:2000.[2-7] Some countries report higher prevalence owing to specific genetic and possibly environmental conditions.[8]

KC is a genetically heterogeneous disorder with family history being a major risk factor.[9] Having a first-degree relative with KC remains the most significant risk factor for developing KC.[1,10] The estimated KC prevalence in first-degree relatives was found to be 15 to 67 times higher than that in the general population.[11] Genetic contribution is further supported by higher concordance of KC severity in monozygotic twins versus dizygotic twins,[12] and consanguineous marriage (first-cousin marriage) is a risk factor for KC in the offspring.[13] Familial KC most commonly presents with an autosomal-dominant inheritance pattern and occasionally with a recessive pattern, especially in families with consanguineous marriages. Multiple segregation analyses in families have conclusively proved genetic determination and suggested complex genetic inheritance.[11,14]

Clinically, even in the absence of fully developed KC, abnormal corneal topography (KC suspect) is frequently diagnosed in family members of KC patients[15,16] (Fig. 4.1). In a longitudinal study, unaffected relatives with certain imaging parameters showed significantly greater risk of progression to KC.[17]

> ## BOX 4.1 ■ Features of Keratoconus
>
> - Complex/multifactorial
> - Genetically heterogeneous (familial transmission and "sporadic" presentation)
> - Gene-environmental interactions (i.e., eye rubbing)
> - Progressive
> - Population frequency between 1/375 and 1/2000 in different countries and ethnic groups
> - Clinically heterogeneous with variable age of onset and degree of visual acuity loss
> - Irreversible without treatment
> - If undiagnosed leads to post-LASIK ectasia

Example of the videokeratographs showing progression of keratoconus 'suspect' in a clinically normal fellow eye to KC over time (all maps are in the same 'absolute scale').

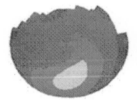 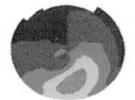 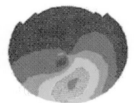

A: clinically normal fellow eye: 'keratoconus suspect' (Jul 1996): I-S value =2.14, KISA value=77.14%.

B: 'early' KC (keratoconus diagnosed by retinoscopy only otherwise clinically normal, 1 year later) (Nov, 1997): I-S value =3.24, KISA=122.93%.

C: KC (detectable by slit-lamp evaluation, 3 years later)(Mar 1999): I-S value=4.5, KISA value=204.00%

Fig. 4.1 Longitudinal study showing progression of clinically normal fellow eye of familial keratoconus patient to clinical keratoconus detectable by slit-lamp evaluation. (Adapted from Li X, Rabinowitz YS, Rasheed K, Yang H. Longitudinal study of the normal eyes in unilateral keratoconus patients. *Ophthalmology.* 2004;111(3):440–446.)

GENOME-WIDE LINKAGE STUDIES

Multiple genome-wide linkage studies (GWLS) in individual families and family sets have been undertaken. GWLS involve genotyping families affected by a certain disease using a collection of genetic markers across the genome and examining how those genetic markers segregate with the disease across multiple families. GWLS, also called linkage studies (Box 4.2), have been applied successfully to identify genetic variants that contribute to rare disorders such as familial breast cancer, Huntington disease, cystic fibrosis, and others (reviewed in Altshuler et al.).[18] For decades, these studies were generally conducted using 300 to 400 microsatellite markers spaced at 10 to 20 centimorgans (cM) apart. These multiallelic markers were robust and highly informative; however, their genotyping was a time-consuming process. Shortly after single nucleotide polymorphisms (SNPs) were discovered to be abundant polymorphic markers uniformly distributed throughout the human genome,[19] dense SNP arrays quickly became the genotyping platform of choice, owing to highly unparalleled interrogation and accurate scoring. Testing of genotyping data also evolved from being model based (recessive, dominant, etc.) to the use of robust nonparametric alternatives.[20]

GWLS analyses have identified a number of genomic loci linked with KC located on multiple chromosomes: 1p36.23-36.21, 2p24, 2q13, 3p14-q13, 5q14.3-q21.1, 5q21.2, 5q32-q33, 8q13.1-q21.11, 9q34, 13q32, 14q11.2, 14q24.3, 15q15.1, 15q22.33–24.2, 16q22.3-q23.1, and 20p13-p12.2,

20q12.[21] However, for the vast majority, identification of genomic positions of the KC genes did not lead to conclusive evidence for specific genes. Genes and variants started to be identified by implementing a tool testing for genetic association. Recent advances in next-generation sequencing (NGS) methods (allowing simultaneous interrogation of billions of nucleotides) and multiplex genotyping (allowing simultaneous interrogation of millions of nucleotides at the specific positions in the genome) led to the identification of mutations and variants (Table 4.1). Some of the identified genes and mutations were found to be located in the previously identified linkage regions.

NGS enables interrogation of genomic sequence in the absence of linkage. Whole exome sequencing (WES) is used to identify variants in the protein-coding regions (about 1% of the human genome), whereas whole genome sequencing (WGS) explores variants in the whole genome, as well as structural changes such as copy number variants.

BOX 4.2 ■ Genetic Studies

A **genetic linkage** study is a study aimed at identification of genetic markers inherited together with a locus for a specific trait or a disease, because of their proximity to one another on the same chromosome.

A **genetic association** study is a study aimed at testing whether genetic markers (i.e., single nucleotide polymorphisms [SNPs]) differ between two groups of individuals (cases vs. controls).

A **genomic sequencing** study is aimed at allowing researchers to identify complete nucleotide sequence of genes and intergenic regions of the genome.

A **genetic expression** study is aimed at detecting and quantifying messenger RNA (mRNA) levels of a specific gene.

A **genetic transcriptomic** study is aimed at detecting and quantifying the complete set of RNA transcripts that are produced by the genome.

A **genetic functional** study is aimed at studying the biochemical, cellular, and physiological properties of gene products, sometimes including intergenic regions of the genome.

TABLE 4.1 ■ Keratoconus Genes

Gene Name	Position	Variant(s)	Gene Function	Method	References
CAST	5q15	rs4434401	Calpain/calpastatin proteolytic degradation	GWLS, FM	101
COL4A3	2q36.3	Multiple	Collagen type IV, alpha-3 chain	S	102
COL4A4	2q36.3	Multiple	Collagen type IV, alpha-4 chain	S MA	102, 103, 58
COL5A1	9q34.2-34.3	Multiple	Collagen type V, alpha-1 chain	GWLS, FM, GWAS, MA, S	40, 43, 44, 58, 64, 104
DOCK9	13q32.3	c.2262A>C p.Gln754His	Guanine nucleotide exchange factor	GWLS, GWAS, S	27
FNDC3B	3q26.31	rs4894535	Fibronectin extracellular matrix protein	GWAS, MA	40, 58, 64, 70

Continued on following page

TABLE 4.1 ■ **Keratoconus Genes** (Continued)

Gene Name	Position	Variant(s)	Gene Function	Method	References
FOXO1	13q14.1	rs2721051	Transcription factor	GWAS, MA, TG	40, 58, 61, 64, 70, 105
HGF	7q21.1	rs3735520	Involved in corneal wound healing	GWAS, TG	56, 106, 107
IL1A	2q13	rs2071376	Interleukin 1 alpha, cytokine	TG, S	108–110
IL1B	2q13	Multiple	Interleukin 1 beta, cytokine	TG, S	110–112
IMMP2L	7q31.1	rs757219	Inner mitochondrial membrane peptidase subunit 2	GWAS, MA	57, 58
LOX	5q23.2	Multiple	Lysyl oxidase, participates in collagen cross-linking	GWLS, LD, FM, S, MA, TG	23, 30, 104, 107, 113–115
MAML2	11q21	rs10831500	Transcription factor	GWAS, TG	59, 60
MIR184	15q25.1	c.57 C>T	MicroRNA	GWLS, TG	33, 34
MPDZ/NF1B	9p23	rs1324183	Intergenic region	GWAS, TG	40, 61, 62, 70, 116, 117
PNPLA2	11p15.5	rs61876744	Participates in triglyceride hydrolysis	GWAS, TG	59, 60
PPIP5K2	5q21.2	Multiple	Kinase/phosphatase	GWLS, LD, FM, S	31
RAB3GAP1	2q21.3	rs4954218	Regulates exocytosis	GWAS, TG	57, 61, 118
SOD1	21q22.1	Multiple	Superoxide dismutase 1, cytoplasmic antioxidant enzyme	S	114, 119
TGFBI	5q31.1		Transforming growth factor beta induced	S	52, 120
TIMP3	22q12.3	c.476 C>T p.Pro458Ser	Tissue inhibitor of metalloproteinases	S	104
TSC1	9q34	Multiple	Hamartin, regulates cell growth	S	121
VSX1	20p11.2	Multiple	Visual system homeobox 1, transcription factor	S	122–126
WNT10A	2q35	rs12190810	WNT signaling	GWAS	127
ZEB1	10p11.2	c.1920G>T p.Gln640His	Zinc finger transcription factor	S	128, 129
ZNF469	16q24.2	Multiple	Transcription factor	GWAS, TG, S, TA	46, 58, 70, 116, 130

FM, Fine mapping; *GWAS,* genome-wide association studies; *GWLS,* genome-wide linkage studies; *LD,* linkage disequilibrium; *MA,* meta-analysis; *S,* sequencing; *TG,* targeted genotyping.

GENES FOR FAMILIAL KC

LOX

One of the first discovered and most promising KC genes is the one coding for the *LOX* (lysyl oxidase) gene. It is located in the 5q32-q33 genomic region identified by a two-stage GWLS.[22] Multiple SNPs rs10519694 and rs2956540 located in the intron (noncoding portion) of the *LOX* gene and SNPs rs1800449 and rs2288393 located in the exons (coding portion) of the gene were found to be genetically associated in KC families.[23] They were also found to be associated in case-control panels of KC patients without known family history. LOX initiates the cross-linking of collagens and elastin by catalyzing oxidative deamination of the epsilon-amino group in certain lysine and hydroxylysine residues.[24] LOX defects can potentially lead to the reduction of cross-linking of collagen fibers of the corneal stroma, thus leading to biomechanical weakening of the cornea. Multiple samples of independently collected KC patients around the world confirmed the *LOX* association (see Table 4.1). *LOX* involvement is also supported by functional data that showed its attenuation in the corneal epithelium of KC patients at levels corresponding to disease severity[25] and revealed changes in *LOX* distribution and its decreased activity in KC corneas.[26]

DOCK9

Single mutation rs191047852 (c.2262A > C, p.Gln754His) in the *DOCK9* (dedicator of cyto-kinesis 9) gene was identified by targeted Sanger sequencing of the 13q32 chromosomal region linked to KC in several Ecuadorian families. Dozens of affected individuals were found to carry this mutation whereas almost no controls were carriers.[27] Functional investigation in vitro found aberrant splicing of the *DOCK9* gene that leads to exon skipping, resulting in the introduction of a premature stop codon, disrupting the functional domains of DOCK9 protein, which may alter its biological function as an important regulator of corneal wound repair.[28]

PPIP5K2

Recently, two familial variants of a novel KC gene *PPIP5K2* (diphosphoinositol pentakisphos-phate kinase 2) were identified in a four-generation family identified in 1992,[29] linked by GWLS to 5q14.3-q21.1 (Tang et al.),[125] and by genetic association to the 95 to 100 Mb region on chro-mosome 5[30] and in another unrelated family (Fig. 4.2A and B). These two variants, rs35671301 (c.1255T > G, p.Ser419Ala, S419A) and rs781831998 (c.2528A > G, p.Asn843Ser, N843S), are located in the exonic portion of the *PPIP5K2* gene. Biochemical effects of these variants were investigated in vitro that identified significant reduction in the phosphatase activity and elevated levels of the kinase activity.[31] Further investigation in the mouse model carrying trun-cated *PPIP5K2* gene (in vivo) found irregularities on the anterior corneal surface, reduced anterior chamber depth, and corneal opacity in mice heterozygous and homozygous for the affected allele[31] (see Fig. 4.2C).

MIR184

MicroRNAs (miRNAs) are small noncoding RNAs that suppress posttranscriptional gene expres-sion by pairing with their target messenger RNAs (mRNAs), inducing either translational repres-sion or mRNA degradation of their targets.[32] The biologically active part of these molecules (seed) is only 18 to 25 nucleotides long. Mutation c.57 C > T in the seed region of miR-184 has been identified in familial hereditary ocular diseases, including familial KC with lens abnormalities and stromal thinning[33,34] and EDICT (endothelial dystrophy, iris hypoplasia, congenital cataract, and stromal thinning) syndrome.[35] This mutation represents a single known germline inherited miRNA defect associated with a variety of ocular abnormalities. Analysis of the biological effects of this mutation in human lens epithelial cells (in vitro) identified significantly altered expression of genes mostly coding for proteins of the cell membrane and those involved in calcium ion transfer.[36]

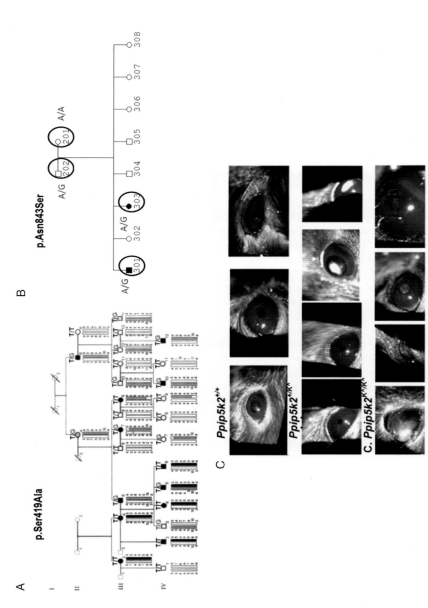

Fig. 4.2 Identification of variants in *PPIP5K2* gene. (A) The pedigree structure of the four-generation family with keratoconus with *PPIP5K2* variant (T/G, rs3567130, c.1255T > G, p.Ser419Ala, S419A). Generations are indicated by the roman numbers I, II, III, and IV. Linkage haplotypes are labeled under each individual. The gray haplotype is linked with keratoconus. (B) The pedigree structure of a second unrelated multiplex family and the genotypes of the *PPIP5K2* variant (A/G, rs781831998, c.2528A > G, p.Asn843Ser, N843S). (C) Slit-lamp biomicroscopic examination of mouse cornea. Images of mouse cornea at 3 months of age with normal gene (Ppip5k2+/+), heterozygous normal/truncated (Ppip5k2+/Kˆ), and homozygous truncated (Ppip5k2Kˆ/Kˆ) mice. (Adapted from Khaled ML, Bykhovskaya Y, Gu C, et al. *PPIP5K2* and *PCSK1* are candidate genetic contributors to familial keratoconus. *Sci Rep.* 2019;9(1):19406.)

BOX 4.3 ▪ Keratoconus-Related Disorders

##**Multisystem Disorders**
- Down syndrome
- Bardet-Biedl syndrome
- Nail-patella syndrome
- Ehlers-Danlos syndrome
- Alport syndrome
- Tuberous sclerosis complex
- Osteogenesis imperfecta

Ocular Disorders
- Congenital cataracts (*MIR184* mutation)
- Leber congenital amaurosis
- Retinitis pigmentosa
- Floppy eyelid syndrome
- Blue sclerae
- Aniridia
- Brittle cornea syndrome
- Corneal dystrophies including Avellino, lattice, deep filiform, posterior polymorphous, Fuchs

---

GENES INVOLVED IN KERATOCONUS AND OTHER SYNDROMES

In about 97% of cases, KC is seen in its non-syndromic form, that is, without involvement of other tissues; however, in about 3% of cases, it has been identified in patients with multisystem diseases such as Down syndrome,[37] Ehlers-Danlos syndrome (EDS), Bardet-Biedl syndrome, nail-patella syndrome, and others[1] (Box 4.3). A study has found that as many as 85% of the known KC-related genes may also be involved in connective tissue disorders or other ocular diseases[38] (Fig. 4.3).

COL5A1

Mutations in *COL5A1* and *COL5A2* genes, encoding the alpha-1 and the alpha-2 chain of type V collagen respectively, are identified in approximately 50% of patients with a clinical diagnosis of classic EDS.[39] EDS is a complex disease of the connective tissue, with joint hypermobility, high skin extensibility, and frequent bone defects. Notably, both generalized corneal thinning and KC have been frequently described in patients with EDS. Variants in and around *COL5A1* gene (rs1536482 and rs7044529) have been consistently identified to be involved in the regulation of central corneal thickness (CCT) by multiple genome-wide scans in multiple populations.[40–42] Targeted analysis of SNPs rs1536482 and rs7044529 found both of them to be consistently associated with KC in case-control panels as well as in a familial panel.[43] In addition, it has been shown that some family members of KC patients who carry minor alleles of *COL5A1* SNPs exhibit only diffuse corneal thinning with no evidence of focal ectasia (Fig. 4.4). Recently, a functional splice variant in *COL5A1* gene resulting in abnormal translation was identified in the affected members of the three-generation KC family.[44]

ZNF469

Mutations in the *ZNF469* gene cause brittle cornea syndrome (BCS), an autosomal recessive disorder associated with extreme corneal thinning and a high risk of corneal rupture.[45] Multiple studies by various research groups identified significant enrichment of potentially pathogenic *ZNF469* alleles in KC patients of different ethnicities.[46–48] However, recent sequencing analysis of *ZNF469* in Polish patients with KC found no significant enrichment of any sequence variants in

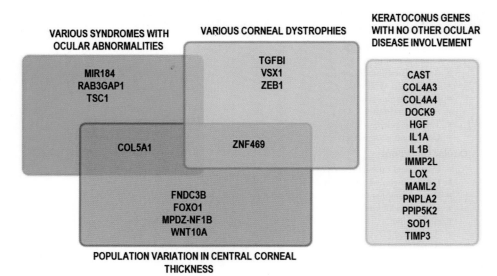

Fig. 4.3 Keratoconus genes and their involvement in other ocular diseases. (Adapted from Bykhovskaya Y, Margines B, Rabinowitz YS. Genetics in keratoconus: where are we? *Eye Vis (Lond)*. 2016;3:16.)

ZNF469.[80] Based on these results, together with the lack of evidence for the functional impact of the variants, its involvement remains contentious at this time.

TGFBI

TGFBI gene mutations have been identified frequently in patients with corneal epithelial-stromal dystrophies, a group of heterogeneous conditions that are characterized by progressive loss of corneal transparency.[49] TGF beta-induced protein (TGFBIP) is an important corneal extracellular protein that mediates cell adhesion to collagen and proteoglycans known to activate the TGFB signaling pathway in KC[50] and has been identified in corneal stromal amyloid deposits in KC patients.[51] *TGFBI* expression has been significantly elevated in corneas from KC patients.[52] Multiple studies identified found various polymorphisms in the *TGFBI* gene thus further confirming its probable involvement.[53]

Genome-Wide Association Studies

WHAT ARE GENOME-WIDE ASSOCIATION STUDIES (GWAS)?

Genome-wide association studies (GWAS) have evolved into a powerful tool for investigating the genetic architecture of human genetic diseases, especially complex and common genetic traits. Analytical methods used for GWAS are based on interrogating SNPs, single base-pair changes in the DNA sequence that were found to occur with high frequency in the human genome.[19] SNPs are by far the most abundant and common form of genetic variation in the human genome. Many SNPs are present in a large proportion of human populations.[54] A SNP with allele frequency significantly altered between the case and the control group is considered to be associated with the trait. Minimizing the false-positive rate is the most important consideration for GWAS. Thus a genome-wide significance threshold of a nominal P value $< 5 \times 10^{-8}$ has been established.[55] Well-designed GWAS would also include a replication and analyses with consideration of the joint, as well as the individual, discovery and replication datasets.

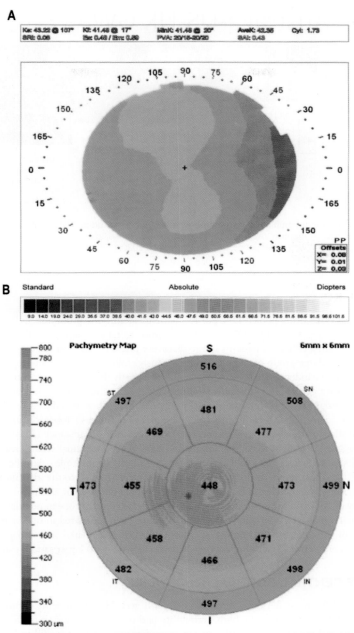

Fig. 4.4 (A) Videokeratography of an 18-year-old male with a family history of keratoconus (two cousins on maternal side). Topography illustrates with the rule astigmatism and no evidence of "forme fruste" keratoconus. (B) Optical coherence tomography pachymetry of the same eye demonstrating low central corneal thickness measurements with diffuse corneal thinning and no evidence of focal ectasia. (Adapted from Li X, Bykhovskaya Y, Canedo AL, et al. Genetic association of COL5A1 variants in keratoconus patients suggests a complex connection between corneal thinning and keratoconus. *Invest Ophthalmol Vis Sci.* 2013;54(4):2696–2704.)

Australia-US-UK GWAS

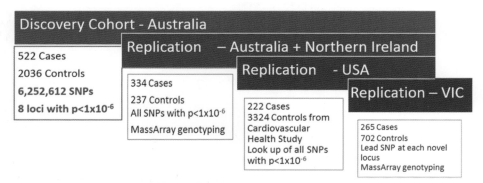

Fig. 4.5 Design of recent multinational genome-wide association studies *(GWAS)* of keratoconus. *SNP,* Single nucleotide polymorphism. (Adapted from McComish BJ, Sahebjada S, Bykhovskaya Y, et al. Association of genetic variation with keratoconus. *JAMA Ophthalmol.* 2020;138(2):174–181.)

GWAS OF KC

The first KC GWAS using pooled DNA of KC patients identifying promoter SNP rs3735520 in the *HGF* gene was published in 2011.[56] It was designed to take advantage of the genotyping of pooled DNA from a cohort of patients in the discovery phase (to save on the cost of genotyping while surveying a large group of samples simultaneously) followed by the two-step confirmation procedure using two independent case-control cohorts. Shortly thereafter, a more powerful GWAS based on extensive genotyping of hundreds of individual KC patients was published in 2012 and identified the variant rs4954218 in the *Rab3Gap1* gene.[57] Since then, two dozen KC susceptibility loci have been identified and confirmed (see Table 4.1,[21] updated October 2020). Some of the variants that did not reach the level of genome-wide statistical significance (P value $< 5 \times 10^{-8}$, a crucial statistical threshold to limit spurious findings) in the individual studies reached it after meta-analysis (a statistical analysis that combines the results of multiple scientific studies) was performed.[58] The most recent multinational KC GWAS (Fig. 4.5) led to the identification of two more genes, *PNPLA2* and *MAML2,*[59] which were already confirmed in an independent study.[60] The majority of KC risk variants identified by GWAS came from European populations of Caucasian ethnicity; however, a number of KC variants have been replicated in one or more patient populations of different ethnic origins.[61,62] The number of KC-related loci and pathways will increase after completion of additional more-powerful GWAS with larger samples sizes.

GWAS OF CENTRAL CORNEAL THICKNESS

CCT is one of the most heritable human traits, with very high heritability estimates ranging from 0.68 to 0.95.[63] Owing to the high heritability and normal distribution of this quantitative trait in the general population, several association studies were very successful in identifying the genetic network behind CCT variation. The first high-powered meta-analysis performed in 2013 on >20,000 individuals in European and Asian populations identified 16 new loci associated with CCT at genome-wide significance.[40] Another CCT meta-analysis completed in 2019 identified 44 GWAS significant SNPs and explained 8.5% of CCT variance,[64] only to be followed by another CCT meta-analysis identifying 98 genomic loci (41 novel) that now explain 14.2% of the population CCT variance.[63] Although CCT is a common heritable trait, variation in CCT exists between ethnic groups.[65] Interestingly, much lower powered population-specific GWAS confirmed some genes identified in multiethnic panels and also revealed novel CCT genes specific to certain populations such as *LOC100506532* in the Hispanic population[66] and *STON2* gene in the Japanese population.[67]

OVERLAP OF CENTRAL CORNEAL THICKNESS LOCI WITH KERATOCONUS

CCT GWAS gradually increased the number of KC-associated loci as the studies became more powerful. The first meta-analysis showed 6 CCT-associated loci to be associated with KC,[40] followed by 17 out of 36,[64] and finally by 20 out of 98 CCT-associated genomic loci.[63] *STON2* gene identified in the Japanese population is also thought to be involved in KC in this population.[67] Additionally, all CCT studies have consistently identified collagen and extracellular matrix (ECM) regulation as main pathways in both CCT regulation and KC susceptibility and have found genetic overlap with corneal dystrophies and Mendelian connective tissue disorders.[40,63,64]

In contrast, the potential contribution of genes involved in the regulation of corneal biomechanical properties—corneal hysteresis (CH) and corneal resistance factor (CRF)—to KC susceptibility does not seem to be nearly as great. Several studies have reported that CH and CRF are lower in KC patients than in control individuals.[68] However, others have found them to be poor parameters for discriminating between mild KC and normal corneas,[69] making discovery of meaningful associations less likely. Of the 200+ loci identified in the latest GWAS of CH and CRF, only four, *FNDC3B*, *ZNF469*, *MPDZ*, and *FOXO1* (Table 4.1), were also significantly associated with KC.[70] Notably, all four were also associated with CCT variation.

Transcriptomic and Expression Studies
WHAT ARE GENE EXPRESSION STUDIES?

Analysis of gene expression (or transcription) is a study of the functional products of genes present in the specific cell types and tissues of the body. Originally such studies were limited to protein-coding RNAs using microarray-based methods or by analyzing gene products individually by reverse transcription polymerase chain reaction (RT-PCR), which allows the use of RNA as a template. Now they have been extended to the nonprotein coding genes (coding for functional RNA molecules) using recently developed high-throughput RNA sequencing (RNA-Seq). RNA-Seq reveals the presence and quantity of RNA (similar to expression microarrays) using powerful NGS methodology.[71] Transcriptomic and gene expression studies have been a valuable source of information about functional genes and pathways important for KC pathogenesis.[72]

EXPRESSION OF CODING MRNA IN KERATOCONUS CORNEAS AND CORNEAL CELLS

Recent expression studies of corneal tissue from KC patients provided additional support to the functional importance of already identified KC genes. Targeted expression analysis of 45 candidate genes previously found to be involved in KC etiology found that 35 genes (including *LOX*, *SPARC*, *ZNF469*, and *TGFBI*) exhibited differential expression between KC and non-KC corneas.[73] Widespread decrease in the expression levels of multiple collagen genes and increase in the expression level of *TGFBI* gene were identified in another study of KC corneas.[52] Decrease in the expression levels of genes belonging to the collagen synthesis and maturation networks responsible for proper corneal organization and regulation of corneal ECM remodeling was identified in another study.[74] Similarly designed recent RNA-Seq studies found that most of the differentially expressed genes between KC and non-KC corneal tissue and cells were enriched for cell migration, ECM, adherence junction, and signaling pathways important for corneal functions.[75,76]

IDENTIFICATION OF NONCODING RNA (LNCRNAS AND MIRNAS) INVOLVED IN KERATOCONUS

Protein-coding genes have been studied much more extensively. However, only 1% to 2% of the human genome encodes proteins (coding RNA) leaving the rest of the RNAs act as cellular regulators without encoding proteins (noncoding RNA) making the vast world of RNAs without coding potential (noncoding RNAs) the majority of RNA.[77] Multiple roles for noncoding RNA have been described. In addition to the modulation of expression levels of protein-coding genes, noncoding RNAs, such as miRNAs and long noncoding RNAs (lncRNAs), have been shown to be regulators with significant involvement in the control of gene expression affecting multiple biological processes.[78] Recent studies aimed to look at the potential role of noncoding RNAs in corneal metabolism and development of KC.

Long Noncoding RNAs

lncRNAs, defined as transcripts longer than 200 nucleotides that do not code for proteins, might play a role as modulators of KC susceptibility. A recent survey of lncRNA catalogs showed that there might be >200,000 lncRNA transcripts in the human genome, although only a very small fraction of them have been characterized functionally.[79] Two studies performed to date resulted in recognition of a number of lncRNAs possibly regulating genes and biological pathways with known or plausible links to KC.[76,80]

MicroRNAs

Small noncoding RNAs between 18 and 25 nucleotides have been increasingly studied for their involvement in eye diseases.[81] First insights into their involvement in KC found that certain biological pathways such as cell junction, cell division, and motor activity are overrepresented among miRNA target genes in the corneal epithelia of KC patients.[82] Bioinformatic study of KC-associated genomic regions found nonrandom distribution of miRNAs genes and SNPs to the regions containing KC linkage loci.[83] Further investigation on both genomic and expression levels may open new avenues for using miRNAs as potential therapeutic targets and diagnostic biomarkers for KC.

Implementation of Genetic Insights in Clinical Practice

CORRELATION BETWEEN EXPRESSION LEVELS OF *LOX* GENE AND CORNEAL CROSS-LINKING OUTCOMES

The corneal collagen cross-linking (CXL) procedure results in major changes in corneal tissue with a notable difference between normal and KC-affected specimens. Recent studies documented major effects on the metabolites in corneal fibroblasts from healthy donors and KC patients,[84] and on the ECM organization in a three-dimensional (3D) in vitro cellular model.[85] Furthermore, a small study of KC patients undergoing CXL found procedure outcomes to be correlated with cone epithelium–specific expression levels of *LOX*—a confirmed KC gene.[86] However, another study that looked at the expression of LOX and other ectasia-related genes found no correlation with the outcomes of accelerated CXL.[87] In addition, detrimental changes in the extracellular proteins of the corneal stroma after Intacs have been documented.[88]

POTENTIAL GENETIC PREDISPOSITION TO THE ADVERSE EFFECTS

KC treatments such as CXL and intrastromal corneal ring segments generally have been shown to be safe treatment options for KC,[89-94] but adverse effects, such as corneal opacity (haze), punctate keratitis, corneal striae, corneal epithelial defects, eye pain, reduced sharpness of vision, blurred vision, corneal melting, and perforation, still occur. Recent work uncovered potentially pathogenic missense variants in KC gene *ZNF469* in a patient with atypical KC who developed spontaneous bilateral corneal perforation after CXL procedure.[95] Potentially, these discoveries can be applied to predict the potential occurrence of such adverse effects and to tailor clinical management of individual patients based on their genomic profiles.

POLYGENIC RISK SCORE FOR KERATOCONUS RISK AND RESPONSE TO THERAPIES

Clinicians are entering a new era of using polygenic risk scores (PRS) to predict diagnosis and progression of complex genetic diseases and traits. PRS has been successfully used to predict disease progression in complex genetic disorders of vision such as glaucoma and age-related macular degeneration (AMD),[96,97] but not in myopia.[98,99] PRS indicators can also be used to predict outcomes of therapies such as aflibercept in exudative AMD.[100] Continuous advancements in this field are powered by a great increase in samples available for GWAS and meta-analyses, including biobank and repository data.

Conclusion

Systematic well-powered studies at the genomic and transcriptomic levels using the most advanced technologies have identified multiple genetic factors that play a key role in KC development and affect KC treatments. Understanding the genetic susceptibility to KC can assist with better KC diagnosis, identifying new treatment targets, and improving the outcomes of already-developed treatments.

Abbreviations

GWAS	genome-wide association studies
GWLS	genome-wide linkage studies
CCT	central corneal thickness
CH	corneal hysteresis
CRF	corneal resistance factor
CXL	corneal collagen cross-linking
ECM	extracellular matrix
Intacs	type of intrastromal corneal ring segment device
KC	keratoconus
lncRNA	long noncoding RNA
MA	meta-analysis
miRNA	microRNA
NGS	next-generation sequencing
PRS	polygenic risk score
RNA-Seq	RNA sequencing
SNP	single nucleotide polymorphism
WES	whole exome sequencing
WGS	whole genome sequencing

References

1. Rabinowitz YS. Keratoconus. *Surv Ophthalmol*. 1998;42(4):297–319.
2. Kennedy RH, Bourne WM, Dyer JA. A 48-year clinical and epidemiologic study of keratoconus. *Am J Ophthalmol*. 1986;101(3):267–273.
3. Bak-Nielsen S, Ramlau-Hansen CH, Ivarsen A, Plana-Ripoll O, Hjortdal J. Incidence and prevalence of keratoconus in Denmark. *Acta Ophthalmol Scand*. 2007;85(8):890–892.
4. Jonas JB, et al. Prevalence and associations of keratoconus in rural Maharashtra in central India: the central India eye and medical study. *Am J Ophthalmol*. 2009;148(5):760–765.
5. Bak-Nielsen S, et al. A nationwide population-based study of social demographic factors, associated diseases and mortality of keratoconus patients in Denmark from 1977 to 2015. *Acta Ophthalmol*. 2019;97(5):497–504.
6. Barbaro V, et al. Expression of VSX1 in human corneal keratocytes during differentiation into myofibroblasts in response to wound healing. *Invest Ophthalmol Vis Sci*. 2006;47(12):5243–5250.
7. Godefrooij DA, et al. Age-specific incidence and prevalence of keratoconus: a nationwide registration study. *Am J Ophthalmol*. 2017;175:169–172.
8. Torres Netto EA, et al. Prevalence of keratoconus in paediatric patients in Riyadh, Saudi Arabia. *Br J Ophthalmol*. 2018;102(10):1436–1441.
9. Hashemi H, et al. The prevalence and risk factors for keratoconus: a systematic review and meta-analysis. *Cornea*. 2020;39(2):263–270.
10. Lapeyre G, et al. Keratoconus prevalence in families: a French study. *Cornea*. 2020;39(12):1473–1479.
11. Wang Y, et al. Genetic epidemiological study of keratoconus: evidence for major gene determination. *Am J Med Genet*. 2000;93(5):403–409.
12. Tuft SJ, et al. Keratoconus in 18 pairs of twins. *Acta Ophthalmol*. 2012;90(6):e482–e486.
13. Jamali H, Beigi V, Sadeghi-Sarvestani A. Consanguineous marriage as a risk factor for developing keratoconus. *Med Hypothesis Discov Innov Ophthalmol*. 2018;7(1):17–21.
14. Kriszt A, et al. Segregation analysis suggests that keratoconus is a complex non-Mendelian disease. *Acta Ophthalmol*. 2014;92(7):e562–e568.
15. Shneor E, et al. The prevalence of corneal abnormalities in first-degree relatives of patients with keratoconus: a prospective case-control study. *Ophthalmic Physiol Opt*. 2020;40(4):442–451.
16. Rabinowitz YS, Garbus J, McDonnell PJ. Computer-assisted corneal topography in family members of patients with keratoconus. *Arch Ophthalmol*. 1990;108(3):365–371.
17. Li X, Yang H, Rabinowitz YS. Longitudinal study of keratoconus progression. *Exp Eye Res*. 2007;85(4):502–507.
18. Altshuler D, Daly MJ, Lander ES. Genetic mapping in human disease. *Science*. 2008;322(5903):881–888.
19. Genomes Project C, et al. A map of human genome variation from population-scale sequencing. *Nature*. 2010;467(7319):1061–1073.
20. Kruglyak L, et al. Parametric and nonparametric linkage analysis: a unified multipoint approach. *Am J Hum Genet*. 1996;58(6):1347–1363.
21. Bykhovskaya Y, Margines B, Rabinowitz YS. Genetics in keratoconus: Where are we? *Eye Vis (Lond)*. 2016;3:16.
22. Li X, et al. Two-stage genome-wide linkage scan in keratoconus sib pair families. *Invest Ophthalmol Vis Sci*. 2006;47(9):3791–3795.
23. Bykhovskaya Y, et al. Variation in the lysyl oxidase (LOX) gene is associated with keratoconus in family-based and case-control studies. *Invest Ophthalmol Vis Sci*. 2012;53(7):4152–4157.
24. Hamalainen ER, et al. Molecular cloning of human lysyl oxidase and assignment of the gene to chromosome 5q23.3-31.2. *Genomics*. 1991;11(3):508–516.
25. Shetty R, et al. Attenuation of lysyl oxidase and collagen gene expression in keratoconus patient corneal epithelium corresponds to disease severity. *Mol Vis*. 2015;21:12–25.
26. Dudakova L, et al. Changes in lysyl oxidase (LOX) distribution and its decreased activity in keratoconus corneas. *Exp Eye Res*. 2012;104:74–81.
27. Czugala M, et al. Novel mutation and three other sequence variants segregating with phenotype at keratoconus 13q32 susceptibility locus. *Eur J Hum Genet*. 2012;20(4):389–397.
28. Karolak JA, et al. Variant c.2262A>C in DOCK9 leads to exon skipping in keratoconus family. *Invest Ophthalmol Vis Sci*. 2015;56(13):7687–7690.

29. Rabinowitz YS, et al. Molecular genetic analysis in autosomal dominant keratoconus. *Cornea*. 1992;11(4):302–308.

30. Bykhovskaya Y, et al. Linkage analysis of high-density SNPs confirms keratoconus locus at 5q chromosomal region. *Ophthalmic Genet*. 2016;37(1):109–110.

31. Khaled ML, et al. *PPIP5K2* and *PCSK1* are candidate genetic contributors to familial keratoconus. *Sci Rep*. 2019;9(1):19406.

32. Kloosterman WP, Plasterk RH. The diverse functions of microRNAs in animal development and disease. *Dev Cell*. 2006;11(4):441–450.

33. Hughes AE, et al. Mutation altering the miR-184 seed region causes familial keratoconus with cataract. *Am J Hum Genet*. 2011;89(5):628–633.

34. Bykhovskaya Y, et al. C.57 C >T mutation in MIR 184 is responsible for congenital cataracts and corneal abnormalities in a five-generation family from Galicia, Spain. *Ophthalmic Genet*. 2015;36(3):244–247.

35. Iliff BW, Riazuddin SA, Gottsch JD. A single-base substitution in the seed region of miR-184 causes EDICT syndrome. *Invest Ophthalmol Vis Sci*. 2012;53(1):348–353.

36. Luo Y, Liu S, Yao K. Transcriptome-wide investigation of mRNA/circRNA in miR-184 and its r.57c >u mutant type treatment of human lens epithelial cells. *Mol Ther Nucleic Acids*. 2017;7:71–80.

37. Mathan JJ, et al. Topographic screening reveals keratoconus to be extremely common in Down syndrome. *Clin Exp Ophthalmol*. 2020;48(9):1160–1167.

38. Loukovitis E, et al. Genetic aspects of keratoconus: a literature review exploring potential genetic contributions and possible genetic relationships with comorbidities. *Ophthalmol Ther*. 2018;7(2):263–292.

39. Malfait F, De Paepe A. Molecular genetics in classic Ehlers-Danlos syndrome. *Am J Med Genet C Semin Med Genet*. 2005;139C(1):17–23.

40. Lu Y, et al. Genome-wide association analyses identify multiple loci associated with central corneal thickness and keratoconus. *Nat Genet*. 2013;45(2):155–163.

41. Vithana EN, et al. Collagen-related genes influence the glaucoma risk factor, central corneal thickness. *Hum Mol Genet*. 2011;20(4):649–658.

42. Vitart V, et al. New loci associated with central cornea thickness include *COL5A1*, *AKAP13* and *AVGR8*. *Hum Mol Genet*. 2010;19(21):4304–4311.

43. Li X, et al. Genetic association of *COL5A1* variants in keratoconus patients suggests a complex connection between corneal thinning and keratoconus. *Invest Ophthalmol Vis Sci*. 2013;54(4):2696–2704.

44. Lin Q, et al. A novel splice-site variation in *COL5A1* causes keratoconus in an Indian family. *J Ophthalmol*. 2019;2019:2851380.

45. Rohrbach M, et al. ZNF469 frequently mutated in the brittle cornea syndrome (BCS) is a single exon gene possibly regulating the expression of several extracellular matrix components. *Mol Genet Metab*. 2013;109(3):289–295.

46. Davidson AE, et al. Brittle cornea syndrome *ZNF469* mutation carrier phenotype and segregation analysis of rare *ZNF469* variants in familial keratoconus. *Invest Ophthalmol Vis Sci*. 2015;56(1):578–586.

47. De Baere E. Heterozygous coding *ZNF469* variants enriched in New Zealand patients with isolated keratoconus. *Invest Ophthalmol Vis Sci*. 2014;55(9):5636.

48. Lechner J, et al. Enrichment of pathogenic alleles in the brittle cornea gene, *ZNF469*, in keratoconus. *Hum Mol Genet*. 2014;23(20):5527–5535.

49. Weiss JS, et al. IC3D classification of corneal dystrophies—edition 2. *Cornea*. 2015;34(2):117–159.

50. Engler C, et al. Transforming growth factor-beta signaling pathway activation in keratoconus. *Am J Ophthalmol*. 2011;151(5):752–759. e2.

51. Tai TY, et al. Keratoconus associated with corneal stromal amyloid deposition containing TGFBIp. *Cornea*. 2009;28(5):589–593.

52. Bykhovskaya Y, et al. Abnormal regulation of extracellular matrix and adhesion molecules in corneas of patients with keratoconus. *Int J Keratoconus Ectatic Corneal Dis*. 2016;5(2):63–70.

53. Burdon KP, Vincent AL. Insights into keratoconus from a genetic perspective. *Clin Exp Optom*. 2013;96(2):146–154.

54. International HapMap 3 Consortium; Altshuler DM, Gibbs RA, Peltonen L, et al. Integrating common and rare genetic variation in diverse human populations. *Nature*. 2010;467(7311):52–58.

55. Pe'er I, et al. Estimation of the multiple testing burden for genome-wide association studies of nearly all common variants. *Genet Epidemiol*. 2008;32(4):381–385.

56. Burdon KP, et al. Association of polymorphisms in the hepatocyte growth factor gene promoter with keratoconus. *Invest Ophthalmol Vis Sci.* 2011;52(11):8514–8519.
57. Li X, et al. A genome-wide association study identifies a potential novel gene locus for keratoconus, one of the commonest causes for corneal transplantation in developed countries. *Hum Mol Genet.* 2012;21(2):421–429.
58. Rong SS, et al. Genetic associations for keratoconus: a systematic review and meta-analysis. *Sci Rep.* 2017;7(1):4620.
59. McComish BJ, Sahebjada S, Bykhovskaya Y, et al. Association of genetic variation with keratoconus. *JAMA Ophthalmol.* 2020;138(2):174–181.
60. Zhang J, et al. Replication of the association between keratoconus and polymorphisms in *PNPLA2* and *MAML2* in a Han Chinese population. *Front Genet.* 2020;11:827.
61. Liskova P, et al. Replication of SNP associations with keratoconus in a Czech cohort. *PLoS One.* 2017;12(2):e0172365.
62. Hao X-D, et al. Evaluating the association between keratoconus and reported genetic loci in a Han Chinese population. *Ophthalmic Genet.* 2015;36(2):132–136.
63. Choquet H, et al. A multiethnic genome-wide analysis of 44,039 individuals identifies 41 new loci associated with central corneal thickness. *Commun Biol.* 2020;3(1):301.
64. Iglesias AI, et al. Cross-ancestry genome-wide association analysis of corneal thickness strengthens link between complex and Mendelian eye diseases. *Nat Commun.* 2018;9(1):1864.
65. Dimasi DP, Burdon KP, Craig JE. The genetics of central corneal thickness. *Br J Ophthalmol.* 2010;94(8):971–976.
66. Gao X, et al. A genome-wide association study of central corneal thickness in Latinos. *Invest Ophthalmol Vis Sci.* 2013;54(4):2435–2443.
67. Hosoda Y, et al. Keratoconus-susceptibility gene identification by corneal thickness genome-wide association study and artificial intelligence IBM Watson. *Commun Biol.* 2020;3(1):410.
68. Khawaja AP, et al. Genetic variants associated with corneal biomechanical properties and potentially conferring susceptibility to keratoconus in a genome-wide association study. *JAMA Ophthalmol.* 2019;137(9):1005–1012.
69. Fontes BM, et al. Ocular response analyzer measurements in keratoconus with normal central corneal thickness compared with matched normal control eyes. *J Refract Surg.* 2011;27(3):209–215.
70. Simcoe MJ, et al. Genome-wide association study of corneal biomechanical properties identifies over 200 loci providing insight into the genetic aetiology of ocular diseases. *Hum Mol Genet.* 2020;29(18):3154–3164.
71. Wang Z, Gerstein M, Snyder M. RNA-Seq: a revolutionary tool for transcriptomics. *Nat Rev Genet.* 2009;10(1):57–63.
72. Ghosh A, et al. Proteomic and gene expression patterns of keratoconus. *Indian J Ophthalmol.* 2013;61(8):389–391.
73. Karolak JA, et al. Further evaluation of differential expression of keratoconus candidate genes in human corneas. *PeerJ.* 2020;8:e9793.
74. Kabza M, et al. Collagen synthesis disruption and downregulation of core elements of TGF-beta, Hippo, and Wnt pathways in keratoconus corneas. *Eur J Hum Genet.* 2017;25(5):582–590.
75. Sharif R, et al. Transcriptional profiling of corneal stromal cells derived from patients with keratoconus. *Sci Rep.* 2019;9(1):12567.
76. Khaled ML, et al. Differential expression of coding and long noncoding RNAs in keratoconus-affected corneas. *Invest Ophthalmol Vis Sci.* 2018;59(7):2717–2728.
77. Consortium EP. An integrated encyclopedia of DNA elements in the human genome. *Nature.* 2012;489(7414):57–74.
78. Beermann J, et al. Non-coding RNAs in development and disease: background, mechanisms, and therapeutic approaches. *Physiol Rev.* 2016;96(4):1297–1325.
79. Xu J, et al. A comprehensive overview of lncRNA annotation resources. *Brief Bioinform.* 2017;18(2):236–249.
80. Szczesniak MW, et al. KTCNlncDB-a first platform to investigate lncRNAs expressed in human keratoconus and non-keratoconus corneas. *Database (Oxford).* 2017;2017:baw168.
81. Raghunath A, Perumal E. Micro-RNAs and their roles in eye disorders. *Ophthalmic Res.* 2015;53(4):169–186.

82. Wang YM, et al. Histological and microRNA signatures of corneal epithelium in keratoconus. *J Refract Surg*. 2018;34(3):201–211.
83. Nowak DM, Gajecka M. Nonrandom distribution of miRNAs genes and single nucleotide variants in keratoconus loci. *PLoS One*. 2015;10(7):e0132143.
84. Sharif R, et al. Effects of collagen cross-linking on the keratoconus metabolic network. *Eye (Lond)*. 2018;32(7):1271–1281.
85. Sharif R, Fowler B, Karamichos D. Collagen cross-linking impact on keratoconus extracellular matrix. *PLoS One*. 2018;13(7):e0200704.
86. Shetty R, et al. Outcomes of corneal cross-linking correlate with cone-specific lysyl oxidase expression in patients with keratoconus. *Cornea*. 2018;37(3):369–374.
87. Pahuja N, et al. Correlation of clinical and biomechanical outcomes of accelerated crosslinking (9 mW/cm(2) in 10 minutes) in keratoconus with molecular expression of ectasia-related genes. *Curr Eye Res*. 2016;41(11):1419–1423.
88. Maguen E, et al. Alterations of extracellular matrix components and proteinases in human corneal buttons with INTACS for post-laser in situ keratomileusis keratectasia and keratoconus. *Cornea*. 2008;27(5):565–573.
89. Seiler T. The paradigm change in keratoconus therapy. *Indian J Ophthalmol*. 2013;61(8):381.
90. Shetty R. Keratoconus and corneal collagen cross-linking. *Indian J Ophthalmol*. 2013;61(8):380.
91. Grisevic S, et al. Keratoconus progression classification one year after performed crosslinking method based on ABCD keratoconus grading system. *Acta Inform Med*. 2020;28(1):18–23.
92. O'Brart DPS. Corneal collagen crosslinking for corneal ectasias: a review. *Eur J Ophthalmol*. 2017;27(3):253–269.
93. Lim L, Lim EWL. A review of corneal collagen cross-linking—current trends in practice applications. *Open Ophthalmol J*. 2018;12:181–213.
94. Perez-Straziota C, Gaster RN, Rabinowitz YS. Corneal cross-linking for pediatric keratoconus review. *Cornea*. 2018;37(6):802–809.
95. Zhang W, et al. Corneal perforation after corneal cross-linking in keratoconus associated with potentially pathogenic *ZNF469* mutations. *Cornea*. 2019;38(8):1033–1039.
96. Cooke Bailey JN, et al. The application of genetic risk scores in age-related macular degeneration: a review. *J Clin Med*. 2016;5(3):31.
97. Craig JE, et al. Multitrait analysis of glaucoma identifies new risk loci and enables polygenic prediction of disease susceptibility and progression. *Nat Genet*. 2020;52(2):160–166.
98. Gao XR, Huang H, Kim H. Polygenic risk score is associated with intraocular pressure and improves glaucoma prediction in the UK biobank cohort. *Transl Vis Sci Technol*. 2019;8(2):10.
99. Ghorbani Mojarrad N, et al. Association between polygenic risk score and risk of myopia. *JAMA Ophthalmology*. 2019;138(1):7–13.
100. Shijo T, et al. Association between polygenic risk score and one-year outcomes following as-needed aflibercept therapy for exudative age-related macular degeneration. *Pharmaceuticals (Basel)*. 2020;13(9):257.
101. Li X, et al. An association between the calpastatin (CAST) gene and keratoconus. *Cornea*. 2013;32(5):696–701.
102. Stabuc-Silih M, et al. Polymorphisms in *COL4A3* and *COL4A4* genes associated with keratoconus. *Mol Vis*. 2009;15:2848–2860.
103. Saravani R, et al. Evaluation of possible relationship between *COL4A4* gene polymorphisms and risk of keratoconus. *Cornea*. 2015;34(3):318–322.
104. Xu X, et al. Three novel variants identified within ECM-related genes in Chinese Han keratoconus patients. *Sci Rep*. 2020;10(1):5844.
105. Gao X, et al. Genome-wide association study identifies WNT7B as a novel locus for central corneal thickness in Latinos. *Hum Mol Genet*. 2016;25(22):5035–5045.
106. Sahebjada S, et al. Association of the hepatocyte growth factor gene with keratoconus in an Australian population. *PLoS One*. 2014;9(1):e84067.
107. Dudakova L, et al. Validation of rs2956540:G>C and rs3735520:G>A association with keratoconus in a population of European descent. *Eur J Hum Genet*. 2015;23(11):1581–1583.
108. Nowak DM, et al. Substitution at *IL1RN* and deletion at *SLC4A11* segregating with phenotype in familial keratoconus. *Invest Ophthalmol Vis Sci*. 2013;54(3):2207–2215.

109. Wang Y, et al. Common single nucleotide polymorphisms and keratoconus in the Han Chinese population. *Ophthalmic Genet*. 2013;34(3):160–166.
110. Wang Y, et al. Association of interleukin-1 gene single nucleotide polymorphisms with keratoconus in Chinese Han population. *Curr Eye Res*. 2016;41(5):630–635.
111. Kim S-H, et al. Association of -31T>C and -511 C>T polymorphisms in the interleukin 1 beta (IL1B) promoter in Korean keratoconus patients. *Mol Vis*. 2008;14:2109–2116.
112. Mikami T, et al. Interleukin 1 beta promoter polymorphism is associated with keratoconus in a Japanese population. *Mol Vis*. 2013;19:845–851.
113. Hasanian-Langroudi F, et al. Association of lysyl oxidase (LOX) polymorphisms with the risk of keratoconus in an Iranian population. *Ophthalmic Genet*. 2015;36(4):309–314.
114. Gadelha DNB, et al. Screening for novel LOX and SOD1 variants in keratoconus patients from Brazil. *J Ophthalmic Vis Res*. 2020;15(2):138–148.
115. Zhang J, et al. Association of common variants in LOX with keratoconus: a meta-analysis. *PLoS One*. 2015;10(12):e0145815.
116. Sahebjada S, et al. Evaluating the association between keratoconus and the corneal thickness genes in an independent Australian population. *Invest Ophthalmol Vis Sci*. 2013;54(13):8224–8228.
117. Wang YM, et al. Analysis of multiple genetic loci reveals MPDZ-NF1B rs1324183 as a putative genetic marker for keratoconus. *Br J Ophthalmol*. 2018;102(12):1736–1741.
118. Bae HA, et al. Replication and meta-analysis of candidate loci identified variation at RAB3GAP1 associated with keratoconus. *Invest Ophthalmol Vis Sci*. 2013;54(7):5132–5135.
119. Udar N, et al. SOD1: a candidate gene for keratoconus. *Invest Ophthalmol Vis Sci*. 2006;47(8):3345–3351.
120. Guan T, et al. The point mutation and polymorphism in keratoconus candidate gene *TGFBI* in Chinese population. *Gene*. 2012;503(1):137–139.
121. Bykhovskaya Y, et al. *TSC1* mutations in keratoconus patients with or without tuberous sclerosis. *Invest Ophthalmol Vis Sci*. 2017;58(14):6462–6469.
122. Heon E, et al. *VSX1*: a gene for posterior polymorphous dystrophy and keratoconus. *Hum Mol Genet*. 2002;11(9):1029–1036.
123. Jeoung JW, et al. *VSX1* gene and keratoconus: genetic analysis in Korean patients. *Cornea*. 2012;31(7):746–750.
124. Saee-Rad S, et al. Mutation analysis of VSX1 and SOD1 in Iranian patients with keratoconus. *Mol Vis*. 2011;17:3128–3136.
125. Tang YG, et al. Three *VSX1* gene mutations, L159M, R166W, and H244R, are not associated with keratoconus. *Cornea*. 2008;27(2):189–192.
126. Tanwar M, et al. *VSX1* gene analysis in keratoconus. *Mol Vis*. 2010;16:2395–2401.
127. Cuellar-Partida G, et al. *WNT10A* exonic variant increases the risk of keratoconus by decreasing corneal thickness. *Hum Mol Genet*. 2015;24(17):5060–5068.
128. Lechner J, et al. Mutational spectrum of the *ZEB1* gene in corneal dystrophies supports a genotype–phenotype correlation. *Invest Ophthalmol Vis Sci*. 2013;54(5):3215–3223.
129. Mazzotta C, et al. First identification of a triple corneal dystrophy association: keratoconus, epithelial basement membrane corneal dystrophy and Fuchs' endothelial corneal dystrophy. *Case Rep Ophthalmol*. 2014;5(3):281–288.
130. Yu X, et al. Identification of seven novel *ZNF469* mutations in keratoconus patients in a Han Chinese population. *Mol Vis*. 2017;23:296–305.

CHAPTER 5

Pathophysiology of Keratoconus

Harminder S. Dua ▓ Darren S. J. Ting ▓ Mouhamed Al-Aqaba ▓ Dalia G. Said

KEY CONCEPTS

- Keratoconus is described as a "multifactorial" condition, implying that many factors contribute to its causation, structural alterations, and progression.
- The most important etiological association in keratoconus is believed to be eye rubbing; pressure on the eye, as seen with floppy eyelid syndrome and some lid and orbital tumors, is also a factor in the etiology of keratoconus.
- Atopic conditions are associated with 30% to 50% of cases of keratoconus and include vernal keratoconjunctivitis, atopic keratoconjunctivitis, atopic dermatitis (eczema), hay fever, and asthma.
- Connective tissue disorders and several syndromes with gene disorders are also important associations of keratoconus.
- Elastin degradation in the pre-Descemet (Dua's) layer has recently been recognized in the pathophysiology of keratoconus.

Introduction

Most diseases fall into one of these categories: degeneration, dystrophy, inflammation, trauma, or neoplasia. The pathogenesis of keratoconus (KC), the commonest ectatic disorder of the cornea, involves all of these except neoplasia. It is described as a "multifactorial" condition, implying that many factors contribute to its causation, structural alterations, and progression, some better understood than others. Despite a plethora of alterations and associations identified with KC, the cause-and-effect relationship remains unclear. Every structure of the cornea, from epithelium to endothelium, is affected at some point during the natural course of the disease.

In this chapter the etiopathophysiology of KC will be considered under the subheadings of causation and associations; clinical pathology, structural and histopathology, and the clinic-pathological correlation; biochemistry; and biomechanics. The evidence will then be synthesized to provide an understanding of the pathogenesis of manifest KC.

Causation and Associations

EYE RUBBING OR OCULAR MASSAGE

The single most important etiological association in KC is believed to be eye rubbing, which can be a factor in up to two-thirds of cases.[1] Several studies have confirmed this association and the fact that other associations like allergic disease and Down syndrome in turn have eye rubbing as a clinical feature. Contact lens (CL) wear is also a form of "eye rubbing"[2-8] and wearers have a greater incidence of KC.[9]

Analogous to eye rubbing, pressure on the eye, as seen with floppy eyelid syndrome and some lid and orbital tumors, is also a factor in the etiology KC. Unilateral lesions have been shown to be related to KC in the affected eye. This observation has also been reported with eye rubbing and unilateral atopic eye disease, in which the affected and most rubbed eye develops KC.

CONTACT LENS WEAR

The etiological relationship between KC and CL wear is uncertain. Given the early onset of myopia and astigmatism in KC, it is the case that many of these individuals will wear CLs. Similarly, many individuals in the general population also wear CLs and some of these wearers may have subclinical KC. CL wear can induce topographic changes in the cornea, rigid gas permeable CLs more so than soft lenses, with the former inducing early KC-like topography, which in the early stages is reversible on discontinuation of CL wear.

ATOPY AND ALLERGY

Atopy represents an inherent (genetic) predisposition to developing allergic eye disease. It is an enhanced type 1, immunoglobulin E (IgE)-mediated immune response to environmental allergens (antigens), especially those inhaled, ingested, or that make direct contact with the ocular surface. Allergy refers to any immune response; hence, all atopic reactions will be covered under the term allergy but not all allergic responses are atopy. Atopic conditions are associated with 30% to 50% of cases of KC and include vernal keratoconjunctivitis (VKC), atopic keratoconjunctivitis (AKC), atopic dermatitis (eczema), hay fever, and asthma.[3,8,10–12] Serum IgE levels are significantly elevated in 50% or more of patients with KC and are even higher in those with atopy.[13,14] All these conditions are present in a higher proportion in patients with KC compared with the general population.

CONNECTIVE TISSUE DISORDERS

Many connective tissue disorders have KC as a manifestation of their clinical spectrum of signs, suggesting that the corneal collagen changes leading to KC are a manifestation of systemic disorders of collagen metabolism. In the overall scheme of things, the disorders are rare and the number of cases of KC with these associations is therefore small. However, the association with diseases such as mitral valve prolapse, Ehlers-Danlos syndrome, pseudoxanthoma elasticum, osteogenesis imperfecta, and others does point to a fundamental affection of collagen metabolism. Other seemingly unrelated associations are also important, particularly systemic and ocular conditions with a genetic basis such as Apert, Bardet-Biedl, Crouzon, Down, and Turner syndromes; Leber congenital amaurosis; retinitis pigmentosa; Avellino and granular dystrophies; and endocrine dysfunction such as in the thyroid and sex hormone glands. KC is also significantly associated with learning disability, as part of one of the aforementioned genetic disorders or from other causes.

Histocompatibility antigens HLA B5 and B15 are increased in KC and HLAb7 is found with reduced frequency in KC, compared with controls.

Clinical Pathology

Pathological changes seen in KC relate to the underlying, usually bilateral but asymmetric, thinning and ectasia of the cornea. This results in increased curvature of the cornea inducing a change in the refraction of the optical system of the eye causing myopia and myopic astigmatism, with the latter becoming irregular as the disease advances. Myopia is also secondary to an increase in the axial length of the eye. The vitreous cavity length of KC eyes is reported to be longer by a mean of 0.55 mm compared with emmetropic controls. The anterior chamber depth and axial length too are significantly greater.[15] The corneal thickness and radius of curvature of the cornea are decreased in KC. The characteristic cone can be small and round, central "nipple cone," or oval shaped, and predominantly inferonasal or an inferotemporal "oval cone."[16]

Histopathology and In Vivo Confocal Microscopy

EPITHELIUM

The corneal epithelial cells are irregular in shape and show degradation of cell membrane, with an epithelial layer of irregular thickness. Epithelial abnormalities such as blebbing, thinning, and degeneration are noted early in KC. Ferritin molecules accumulate in basal intercellular spaces and in intracytoplasmic vacuoles, especially at the base of the cone, resulting in the clinical sign of Fleischer ring seen in 30% of cases.[17] Epithelial changes are postulated to initiate KC by inducing release of proteolytic chemicals leading to the fragmentation of Bowman's layer.[18] The basement membrane of the epithelium is thickened and disrupted. Fibrillar debris is seen accumulated beneath the basement membrane. Reduced basal epithelial cell density, preceded by degenerative changes in the form of enlargement and irregular arrangement of the basal epithelial cells, is also demonstrated by in vivo confocal microscopy (IVCM).[19–23]

BOWMAN'S LAYER

Fragmentation of Bowman's layer is a common feature seen in 70% of cases, especially those with oval cones.[24,25] The breaks in Bowman's layer are filled with abnormal collagen derived from underlying keratocytes, fibroblasts, and overlying epithelium. Epithelial cells in Bowman's layer breaks expressing the integrin α3β1 are seen just outside the cone. Linear scars so produced extend across Bowman's layer to the anterior stroma and are responsible for the clinical sign of anterior white lines. Ultrastructure examination demonstrates infiltration of the Bowman's layer with fine cellular processes and fragments that stain positive for vimentin, suggesting that they originate from keratocytes.[26]

STROMA

The most marked changes in KC are seen in the corneal stroma, especially in the region of the cone. These changes include a reduction in collagen fibers, thinning of the lamellae, and redistribution of the lamellae such that there are fewer lamellae in the cone with a more compact arrangement. With progression, the lamellae become wider, thinner, and disorganized, with loss of normal architecture.[27] A reduction in interlamellar adhesions and interlacing of the lamellae at the apex of the cone with reduced number of lamellar insertions in the Bowman's layer have been described.

Corneal stromal cells, the keratocytes, show reduced density, especially in the anterior stroma (Fig. 5.1). Keratocytes also show morphological changes in the form of pseudopodia, excessive cytoplasmic organelles and vacuolation, and nuclear changes. Some keratocytes are surrounded by fibrillogranular material and intercellular debris.[28,29] The reduction of keratocyte density, attributed to accelerated keratocyte apoptosis,[19–22,30] is also seen as a consistent feature on IVCM.

VOGT'S STRIAE

These fine vertical lines are present in the deep stroma and the Descemet membrane (DM). These are reported to be due to the unraveling of stromal lamellae along their lengths with opening of their bifurcations, which lead to the formation of undulations or wrinkles in the collagen lamellae. The striae are mainly formed of collagen VI fibrils bound together with glycosaminoglycans (GAGs), lumican, and keratocan.[31] Keratoconic eyes with Vogt striae are at greater risk of acute

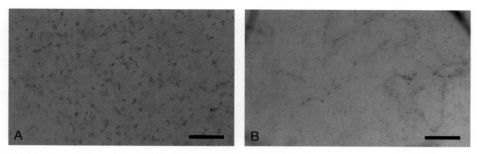

Fig. 5.1 Corneal stromal keratocytes in keratoconus compared with a normal cornea. NanoZoomer digital pathology photomicrographs of whole-mount acetylcholinesterase-stained corneas from a normal subject (A) and a keratoconic patient (B). In the normal cornea, enface sections of the anterior stroma show the abundance of keratocyte nuclei (A), whereas the density of the keratocyte nuclei in the keratoconic cornea is markedly reduced. Scale bar = 100 μm.

hydrops. On IVCM in acute corneal hydrops, the presence of certain unusual cell phenotypes within the epithelium and in the stroma can predict the formation of new blood vessels and subsequent development of corneal neovascularization.[32]

DESCEMET MEMBRANE AND ENDOTHELIUM

The DM shows variation in thickness, nodularity, and folds in 8% of cases, and endothelial changes such as pleomorphism and polymegathism, which may be secondary to mechanical stress and hypoxia from CL wear.[33,34] On IVCM, endothelial cell density (ECD) shows a positive correlation with pachymetric parameters and significant negative correlation with keratometric and elevation parameters, suggesting that ECD is associated with the progression of KC.[35]

CORNEAL NERVES IN KC

Increased visibility and prominence of stroma nerves on slit-lamp examination are an early sign of KC.[24] IVCM and whole-mount staining techniques have demonstrated a range of significant changes in corneal nerves, throughout their course, in all stages of KC (Fig. 5.2).[36] There is a significant decrease in the morphometric parameters of subbasal nerves including central corneal nerve branch density, nerve fiber length, total branch density, and nerve fiber area.[37–40] Some structural-functional disconnect is present, as a reduction in corneal sensation has been demonstrated only among CL-wearing KC patients.[38] IVCM and immune-histological studies on KC tissue obtained during corneal transplant surgery have revealed abnormal subbasal nerve architecture with loss of the normal radiating and central whorl pattern. This is replaced by a tortuous, coiled network of nerve fiber bundles, some terminating in closed loops, within the region of the cone.[39,41] Subbasal nerves fibers at the base of the cone present as concentric rings that follow the contour of the base. The bulb-like termination of stromal nerves anterior to the Bowman's layer is thickened in KC corneas.[41,42]

Stromal nerve bundles are thicker than normal, especially within the area of the cone, explaining why prominent corneal nerves are often seen on clinical examination.[43] Some authors have linked these nerve changes to progression of the disease.[44] On histology, stromal nerves within the conical region show a series of alterations of varying severity and have been classified into three grades based on the extent and severity of the morphologic changes. In grade 1, mild looping and coiling of the central stromal nerve bundles is seen. In grade 3, an excessive sprouting of tortuous nerves forms a very complex network within the central cornea, sparing the peripheral

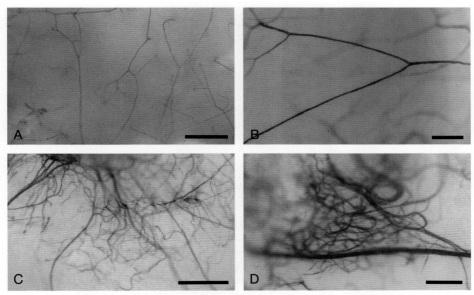

Fig. 5.2   Corneal nerves in keratoconus compared with a normal cornea. NanoZoomer digital pathology photomicrographs of whole-mount acetylcholinesterase-stained corneas from normal eyes (A and B) and keratoconic patients (C and D). (A) In the normal cornea, nerves enter at the middle third of the stroma in a series of large, radially oriented nerve bundles and run centripetally and anteriorly in a radial fashion toward the central area, giving rise to branches that innervate the anterior and mid stroma. (B) The large stromal nerve bundles divide dichotomously or trichotomously into thinner nerve branches. (C) In the keratoconic cornea, the anterior stromal nerves show excessive looping and coiling in the region of the cone. (D) Sprouting of small, tortuous nerves from a thickened stromal trunk is observed at the central keratoconic cornea. Scale bars: A = 500 μm, B = 250 μm, C = 500 μm, D = 250 μm.

innervation, and suggests a pathologic stimulus that is predominantly confined to the cone. Changes in the subbasal nerve orientation are likely to be due to the loss or disturbance of subbasal nerve-epithelial cell interaction. In addition, bulging of the central cornea and subsequent mechanical stretching of the subbasal nerves would distort the orientation and disrupt the normal whorl orientation.[41,45]

Whether nerve alterations in KC are associated causally or result from the overall metabolic derangement remains unclear. Nevertheless, these findings provide evidence of the involvement of corneal nerves in KC and indicate that neurodegeneration is likely to play a role in the pathophysiology of the disease and its progression.[41,46]

ACUTE HYDROPS

In acute hydrops, the DM and Dua's layer (DL; pre-Descemet layer) both rupture, and the broken ends curl with the endothelial cells outside. A break in DM alone does not lead to acute hydrops.[47–49] Breaks in both layers can be seen separately on optical coherence tomography (OCT) and are associated with adjacent DM and DL detachment over a variable area.[50] The stromal thickness of stromal lamellae increases and the space between them widens with accumulation of fluid lacunae. The collection of fluid is due to a direct passive ingress of aqueous humor. When acute hydrops is associated with hyphema, for example, after blunt trauma to a keratoconic eye, red blood cells can be seen in the stromal fluid lacunae. The overlying Bowman's layer may rarely break, causing epithelial edema and a positive Seidel's sign.[51] Acute hydrops resolves by the regeneration of a very thin DM and fibrosis along the torn edges of DM and DL. The relatively acellular DL shows infiltration with keratocyte-derived cells in chronic cases.[50] Subepithelial scarring may also occur and extend into the anterior stroma.

Biochemical Pathology

The morphological changes noted in KC are related to a plethora of biochemical changes that occur in the tear film, all layers of the cornea, and the aqueous humor and beyond, manifesting in the circulatory system.[52,53] These biochemical phenomena are primarily attributable to the three underlying processes[53]: (1) alteration of extracellular matrix (ECM) composition and enzymatic degradation of the cornea; (2) inflammation; and (3) oxidative stress.

ALTERATION OF EXTRACELLULAR MATRIX COMPOSITION AND ENZYMATIC DEGRADATION OF THE CORNEA

Collagen and proteoglycans, including keratan sulfate (e.g., lumican, keratocan, and osteoglycin) and chondroitin sulfate (e.g., biglycan and decorin), represent the main constituents of the ECM of cornea.[54] Type I, III, V, VI, and XII collagens, which are normally present in the corneal stroma, are shown to be reduced in KC,[53,55] suggesting a generalized loss of the ECM. Similarly, a reduction in type I, VI, VII, XII, and XIII collagens has also been reported in the corneal epithelium.[53] The loss of collagen content in the cornea has also been indicated by a reduction in hydroxyproline content[56] and prolyl-4-hydroxylase,[57] which is an enzyme essential for hydroxylation of proline residues of collagen.

Alteration of GAGs and proteoglycans, including keratan sulfate and chondroitin sulfate, is similarly observed in KC.[55,58] Studies have shown that the amount and gene expressions of major structural proteins, including lumican, keratocan, biglycan, and/or decorin, are significantly reduced in the corneal stroma of keratoconic eyes.[55,58] These proteoglycans are involved in the regulation of collagen fibrils, matrix assembly, and corneal transparency,[59,60] and reduction of these structural proteins may lead to corneal instability and contribute to the development of corneal thinning and ectasia. Transforming growth factor beta (TGFß) signaling, which regulates the production of ECM by keratocytes, is shown to be affected in KC.[61] In addition, dysregulated expressions of a number of genes coding for ECM proteins have been reported, including the upregulation of TGFBI and downregulation of THBS1, ADAMTS1, and SPP1, among others.[62]

Progressive stromal thinning in KC has been attributed to the enzymatic degradation of the cornea secondary to a dysregulated balance between proteases (e.g., matrix metalloproteinases [MMPs]) and proteases inhibitors (e.g., tissue inhibitors of metalloproteinases [TIMP]).[53,63] MMPs, particularly MMP-1 and MMP-9 (or gelatinase B), have been shown to be upregulated in the tears and corneas of patients with KC.[63–65] The level of MMP-9 in keratoconic eyes could increase as much as 10-fold when compared with normal eyes and subclinical keratoconic eyes,[66] and it might correlate with the severity of KC.[64] Interestingly, Shetty et al. observed that the progression of KC was arrested when MMP-9 level was reduced by topical ciclosporin treatment.[65] The role and expression of other types of MMPs, such as MMP-2 (or gelatinase A), MMP-3, MMP-7, and MMP-13, in KC have also been investigated but results were somewhat variable and conflicting at times.[63,67] Increased levels of other types of degradative enzymes such as cathepsin-B, cathepsin-G, and cathepsin-V/L2, phosphatases, and esterases are also demonstrated in KC.[53]

In addition to the increased MMP-driven proteolytic activity, downregulation of protease inhibitors, particularly TIMPs (the main inhibitors of MMPs), alpha-1 proteinase inhibitor, and alpha-2 macroglobulin, has been observed in keratoconic eyes, contributing to corneal stromal lysis and development of KC.[63,68,69]

INFLAMMATION

Although KC is traditionally regarded as a non-inflammatory corneal disease, emerging evidence suggests that inflammation plays a key role in the etiopathogenesis of KC.[9,52] At the ocular surface (particularly the tears and the corneal epithelium), a range of inflammatory cytokines, including interleukin (IL)-4,[70] IL-5,[70] IL-6,[64-66] IL-8,[70] and tumor necrosis factor (TNF)-α,[64-66,70] are shown to be upregulated. Moreover, Pahuja et al. observed that the corneal epithelium obtained from the cone apex of keratoconic eyes expressed a significantly higher level of inflammatory cytokines (e.g., IL-6 and TNF-α) and MMP-9 when compared with the peripheral corneal epithelium.[71] This phenomenon may explain the focal structural weakness observed in KC.

In addition, KC is strongly linked to eye rubbing and atopic diseases.[52] Studies have shown that trauma induced by eye rubbing could promote ocular surface inflammation and proteolytic activity in both keratoconic and healthy eyes, evidenced by the increased level of proinflammatory mediators and MMPs in tears.[9,72] Therefore, patients with KC must be advised against eye rubbing, to reduce the inflammatory drive and the risk of disease progression. Independent of the effect of eye rubbing, a significantly higher level of inflammatory cytokines (e.g., IL-1ß, IL-4, IL-5, IL-6, and IL-10, and TNF-α) has been shown to be expressed in tears during the active phase of atopic diseases such as VKC and AKC.[73] These inflammatory responses may account for the increased severity of KC observed in patients with VKC.[74]

OXIDATIVE STRESS

Oxidative stress, a phenomenon related to the disrupted balance between reactive oxygen species (ROS) and antioxidants,[75] has been postulated to be another key mechanism in the pathogenesis of KC.[61,63] Superoxide dismutase (SOD), catalase, and glutathione peroxidase represent the most important first-line defense antioxidant enzymes in the human body.[76] Behndig et al. observed that the extracellular activity of SOD in central corneas was only half in KC compared with normal corneas, potentially contributing to an increased oxidative stress.[77] More compellingly, examination of the previously transplanted corneas in patients with an original diagnosis of KC similarly revealed a reduction in extracellular SOD, suggesting that the cause of reduced SOD level was related to reduced host cellular activity.[77]

Kenney et al. observed a significantly upregulated messenger RNA (mRNA) level of degradative enzymes such as cathepsins-B, -G, and V/L2 in keratoconic eyes,[78] which could stimulate the production of hydrogen peroxide and upregulate the expression of catalase as a compensatory host antioxidative response. The increase in endoplasmic reticular stress and oxidative stress in the corneal epithelium and stroma of keratoconic eyes was further supported by a comprehensive proteomic study.[55]

Proteomic analysis of the aqueous humor obtained from keratoconic eyes has revealed a dysregulated expression of the proteins that participate in proteolytic regulation and oxidative stress response.[79] Furthermore, the plasma concentration of homocysteine has been shown to be significantly higher in patients with KC compared with healthy subjects.[80] Homocysteine is known to increase oxidative stress via the activation of protease-activated receptor (PAR)-4, which enhances the production of ROS.[81] Hence, a higher level of homocysteine indicates the mechanistic role of oxidative stress in KC.

Genetics of Keratoconus

Although KC often presents as an isolated clinical entity, the implication of genetics in the development of KC has been supported by various observations and studies such as history of familial inheritance (5%–20%), twin studies, candidate gene analysis, genome-wide linkage studies (GWLS), and genome-wide association studies (GWAS).[52,82]

GWLS are comprehensive genetic analyses used to map the relevant genetic markers of a particular disease across the genome of the affected families. GWAS is another powerful genetic tool used to analyze the genetic variations across the genomes, particularly single nucleotide polymorphisms (SNPs), of a population to determine genotype-phenotype associations.[83] To date, GWLS have been used to map out a range of genetic markers and changes in KC, including *LOX* gene at the 5q23.2 chromosomal region (which encodes for lysyl oxidase—a collagen cross-linking enzyme), *CAST* gene at the 5q15 region (which encodes for calpastatin—a protease inhibitor), and *DOCK9* gene at 13q32.3 region (dedicator of cytokinesis 9), among others.[84] In addition, GWAS have successfully identified several genetic mutations in patients with KC, including *HGF* SNP rs3735520, *RAB-3GAP1* SNP rs4954218, *PNPLA2* gene, *TGFBI* gene, *VSX1* gene, and others.[84,85] A meta-analysis of around 7000 participants also revealed that mutation in central corneal thickness (CCT)-associated loci, namely FOXO1 and FNDC3B, could significantly increase the risk of KC.[86]

Clinically, the spectrum of myopia, myopic astigmatism, KC, pellucid marginal degeneration, and keratoglobus are seen in family members and in the two eyes of the same individual, suggesting a phenotype spectrum of an underlying common etiopathogenic mechanism.[87–89]

Biomechanics in the Pathophysiology of Keratoconus

Biomechanics is defined as "the development, extension, and application of mechanics for a better understanding of physiology and physiopathology and consequently for a better diagnosis and treatment of disease and injury."[90] Understanding of certain terms used to describe physical properties helps in the understanding of biomechanics.

Stress refers to the tension, force, or pressure exerted on the cornea.

Strain refers to the amount by which the cornea is stretched or deformed in response to stress. Strain is the response to stress.

Shear refers to the strain (change in shape) induced by the sliding or lateral shifting of the lamellae in relation to one another, caused by stress (pressure) in the substance of the cornea.

Shear stress is the stress (pressure or sliding force) that causes the change in shape (strain) without a change in volume of the cornea.

Viscosity is the resistance of a liquid to flow, which is determined by the frictional forces within the fluid. Viscosity measures the consistency of a fluid. The greater the viscosity the greater the inability to flow. Corneal constituents can be regarded as fluid of high viscosity.

Elasticity is the ability of the corneal tissue to resume its normal shape after being stretched or compressed. In other words, it is the ability of the deformed cornea to return to its original shape and size when the forces causing the deformation are removed.

Viscoelasticity refers to a substance that has both viscosity and elasticity. The cornea is viscoelastic. Any stress applied to the cornea results in immediate elastic strain and a slightly delayed viscous strain dependent on duration of the stress.

Corneal hysteresis refers to the measure of the amount of stress (energy of the pressure or force applied) that can be absorbed or distributed within the stroma. Hysteresis of a substance creates a lag between the application of stress and the deformation of the substance and conversely between the cessation of the applied stress and the recovery. For example, when one lies on a mattress, the mattress is first compressed (energy distributed within the mattress—hysteresis) before it assumes a degree of concavity. Corneal hysteresis is calculated by measuring the difference between the pressure at which the cornea bends inward during an air jet applanation and the pressure at which it bends out again. This is determined by an infrared laser during an intraocular pressure measurement.[91]

The *corneal resistance factor* is a measurement provided by an instrument called the Ocular Response Analyzer (Reichert, Buffalo, NY). It is a measure of the overresistance of the cornea and determined largely by the elasticity of the cornea.[1]

The cornea is a viscoelastic tissue[92] that displays all the biomechanical properties described earlier, enabling it to function as a biological mechanotransducer of stress.[93] The corneal stroma accounts for most of the corneal strength.[94] The contributions of the epithelium, DM, and endothelium are generally weak, and the contribution of Bowman's layer is still debatable. The anterior 40% of the corneal stroma is the strongest region, whereas the posterior 60% of the stroma is at least 50% weaker according to tensile strength studies in human donor corneas.[95] The impact of the recently discovered pre-Descemet layer or DL on the posterior corneal biomechanics and its implications in corneal disease and during corneal surgeries are being investigated.[96]

Alterations in corneal biomechanical properties are believed to precede corneal tomographical changes in KC.[97] Reduced mechanical stability has been attributed to many factors such as apoptosis and subsequent reduction in keratocyte density, loss of stromal fibrils, altered architecture and orientation of collagen fibers, and reduced number of cross-links.[36] Therefore in vivo characterizations of corneal biomechanical parameters may enable the early diagnosis of subclinical (forme fruste) KC. Although both corneal hysteresis and corneal resistance factor describe uncertain viscoelastic properties, corneal hysteresis (viscous damping) is produced by the viscous GAGs, proteoglycans, and ECM interactions.[98] Both corneal hysteresis and corneal resistance have been reported to be significantly weak in keratoconic corneas compared with healthy ones.[99] The results lack specificity and sensitivity.

Another device, the Corvis ST, utilizes a noncontact air puff tonometer, combined with a high-speed Scheimpflug camera (4330 frames per second) to image a cross-section of the cornea during deformation. The device records 8.0-mm wide horizontal sections of the cornea and analyzes the deformation pattern. The software provides a range of measurements for different corneal biomechanical properties.[100] Deformation amplitude (DA), which is the displacement from original position at highest concavity, is significantly larger in keratoconic corneas (1.2531–1.3230 mm) compared with healthy corneas.[36] The sensitivity of DA is poor and, therefore, it cannot be used clinically to differentiate between normal and keratoconic corneas.

There is no doubt that significant biomechanical changes occur in the cornea in KC. These are likely to be secondary to the biochemical and cellular changes but in turn can affect cell behavior and contribute to the progression of KC.

The wide range of conditions that are associated with KC in a cause-and-effect, consequential, or coincidental relationship suggest that KC might be a common manifestation of different pathogenetic processes. Some environmental factors such as atopy and allergy, eye rubbing, and CL wear seem to be more important and common than others. Of several disorders with underlying genetic predisposition, Down syndrome stands out. However, the numerous other, though rare, associations and the well-documented racial and familial clusters of KC together with other ectatic corneal disorders such as keratoglobus and pellucid in different family members and also in the two eyes of the same individual strongly indicate a genetic basis. The bilateral but significantly asymmetrical nature of KC and forme fruste KC confound the pathogenetic hypotheses. Structural changes, namely thinning of the cornea, rearrangement of collagen lamellae, disruption of the Bowman's layer, and stretching of the cornea causing anterior protrusion, are fairly consistent features of KC, but here too are inconsistencies as seen with the different locations of the cone and the primary affection of the posterior cornea in posterior KC.

Putting all the evidence together in one coherent sequence of events that can translate into the pathogenesis of KC is difficult despite, or perhaps because of, the vast number of studies and the data generated from them. Primarily environmental factors, on the background of a genetic predisposition in some individuals, are likely to be the initiating stimulus. Induced cellular changes, primarily in the stromal keratocytes but not excluding the epithelium and the endothelium, lead to biochemical changes and physiological stress. The enormity of nerve changes demonstrated in KC suggests that neurons, although distantly located, must be included in any theory on the pathogenesis of KC. Oxidative stress, enzymatic degradation, and inflammation join forces to

alter the stromal matrix, ground substance, collagen, and elastin, leading to thinning. These alterations can be a consequence of insufficient or defective formation and degradation and destruction
of normally formed elements of the matrix. The resultant stroma loses its physical structure and
biochemical resilience. Elements of corneal biomechanics then come into play and alter the shape
of the cornea, producing a conical protrusion that clinicians call KC.

The simplistic sequence described earlier does not imply that when one event leads to the
other, the preceding event ceases. The whole process persists in a relentless cycle with perpetuation
of the pathology and clinical progression. To illustrate, if atopy and eye rubbing were the initiating
events, they will continue to influence the process when cellular and subcellular events are occurring in the stroma; alterations in corneal biomechanics will continue to be influenced by physiological biomechanical forces of blinking and corneal pulsation with heartbeats, compounded by
eye rubbing. Thus, what is described as a linear process is in reality a complex maze of actions,
counteractions, and interactions. Understanding of pathophysiology is crucial to developing treatment strategies. We are beginning to learn how to influence the process but are far away from a
cure. KC remains an enigma.[101]

References

1. Gritz DC, McDonnell PJ. Keratoconus and ocular massage. *Am J Ophthalmol*. 1988;106(6):757–758.
2. Ben-Eli H, Erdinest N, Solomon A. Pathogenesis and complications of chronic eye rubbing in ocular
   allergy. *Curr Opin Allergy Clin Immunol*. 2019;19(5):526–534.
3. Weed KH, MacEwen CJ, Giles T, Low J, McGhee CN. The Dundee University Scottish Keratoconus
   study: demographics, corneal signs, associated diseases, and eye rubbing. *Eye (Lond)*. 2008;22(4):534–541.
4. Ozcan AA, Ersoz TR. Severe acute corneal hydrops in a patient with Down syndrome and persistent eye
   rubbing. *Ann Ophthalmol (Skokie)*. 2007;39(2):158–160.
5. Shapiro MB, France TD. The ocular features of Down's syndrome. *Am J Ophthalmol*. 1985;99(6):659–663.
6. Sharma N, et al. Ocular allergy and keratoconus. *Indian J Ophthalmol*. 2013;61(8):407–409.
7. Hashemi H, et al. The prevalence and risk factors for keratoconus: a systematic review and meta-analysis.
   Cornea. 2020;39(2):263–270.
8. Lema I, et al. Inflammatory response to contact lenses in patients with keratoconus compared with myopic subjects. *Cornea*. 2008;27(7):758–763.
9. McMonnies CW. Inflammation and keratoconus. *Optom Vis Sci*. 2015;92(2):e35–e41.
10. Grunauer-Kloevekorn C, Duncker GI. Keratoconus: epidemiology, risk factors and diagnosis. *Klin Monbl
    Augenheilkd*. 2006;223(6):493–502.
11. Davidson AE, et al. The pathogenesis of keratoconus. *Eye (Lond)*. 2014;28(2):189–195.
12. Gordon-Shaag A, et al. The genetic and environmental factors for keratoconus. *Biomed Res Int*.
    2015;2015:795738.
13. Rahi A, et al. Keratoconus and coexisting atopic disease. *Br J Ophthalmol*. 1977;61(12):761–764.
14. Kemp EG, Lewis CJ. Immunoglobulin patterns in keratoconus with particular reference to total and
    specific IgE levels. *Br J Ophthalmol*. 1982;66(11):717–720.
15. Messina M, et al. Vitreous cavity length in keratoconus: implications for keratoplasty. *Eye (Lond)*.
    2018;32(2):359–363.
16. Rabinowitz YS. Keratoconus. *Surv Ophthalmol*. 1998;42(4):297–319.
17. Fernandes BF, et al. Histopathological study of 49 cases of keratoconus. *Pathology*. 2008;40(6):623–626.
18. Tsubota K, et al. Corneal epithelium in keratoconus. *Cornea*. 1995;14(1):77–83.
19. Yeniad B, Yilmaz S, Bilgin LK. Evaluation of the microstructure of cornea by in vivo confocal micros-
    copy in contact lens wearing and non-contact lens wearing keratoconus patients. *Cont Lens Anterior Eye*.
    2010;33(4):167–170.
20. Ku JY, et al. Laser scanning in vivo confocal analysis of keratocyte density in keratoconus. *Ophthalmology*.
    2008;115(5):845–850.
21. Niederer RL, et al. Laser scanning in vivo confocal microscopy reveals reduced innervation and reduction
    in cell density in all layers of the keratoconic cornea. *Invest Ophthalmol Vis Sci*. 2008;49(7):2964–2970.
22. Ucakhan OO, et al. In vivo confocal microscopy findings in keratoconus. *Eye Contact Lens*. 2006;
    32(4):183–191.

23. Bitirgen G, et al. In vivo corneal confocal microscopic analysis in patients with keratoconus. *Int J Ophthalmol.* 2015;8(3):534–539.
24. Krachmer JH, Feder RS, Belin MW. Keratoconus and related noninflammatory corneal thinning disorders. *Surv Ophthalmol.* 1984;28(4):293–322.
25. Ting DS, et al. Deep anterior lamellar keratoplasty: challenges in histopathological examination. *Br J Ophthalmol.* 2012;96(12):1510–1512.
26. Sherwin T, et al. Cellular incursion into Bowman's membrane in the peripheral cone of the keratoconic cornea. *Exp Eye Res.* 2002;74(4):473–482.
27. Takahashi A, et al. [Quantitative analysis of collagen fiber in keratoconus]. *Nippon Ganka Gakkai Zasshi.* 1990;94(11):1068–1073.
28. Bron AJ. Keratoconus. *Cornea.* 1988;7(3):163–169.
29. Morishige N, et al. Second-harmonic imaging microscopy of normal human and keratoconus cornea. *Invest Ophthalmol Vis Sci.* 2007;48(3):1087–1094.
30. Kaldawy RM, et al. Evidence of apoptotic cell death in keratoconus. *Cornea.* 2002;21(2):206–209.
31. Grieve K, et al. Stromal striae: a new insight into corneal physiology and mechanics. *Sci Rep.* 2017;7(1):13584.
32. Lockington D, et al. A prospective study of acute corneal hydrops by in vivo confocal microscopy in a New Zealand population with keratoconus. *Br J Ophthalmol.* 2014;98(9):1296–1302.
33. Singhal D, et al. Descemet membrane detachment. *Surv Ophthalmol.* 2020;65(3):279–293.
34. Sturbaum CW, Peiffer RL Jr. Pathology of corneal endothelium in keratoconus. *Ophthalmologica.* 1993;206(4):192–208.
35. Bozkurt B, et al. Correlation of corneal endothelial cell density with corneal tomographic parameters in eyes with keratoconus. *Turk J Ophthalmol.* 2017;47(5):255–260.
36. Gokul A, Vellara HR, Patel DV. Advanced anterior segment imaging in keratoconus: a review. *Clin Exp Ophthalmol.* 2018;46(2):122–132.
37. Alvani A, et al. Post-LASIK ectasia versus keratoconus: an in vivo confocal microscopy study. *Cornea.* 2020;39(8):1006–1012.
38. Patel DV, et al. Laser scanning in vivo confocal microscopy and quantitative aesthesiometry reveal decreased corneal innervation and sensation in keratoconus. *Eye (Lond).* 2009;23(3):586–592.
39. Patel DV, McGhee CN. Mapping the corneal sub-basal nerve plexus in keratoconus by in vivo laser scanning confocal microscopy. *Invest Ophthalmol Vis Sci.* 2006;47(4):1348–1351.
40. Simo Mannion L, Tromans C, O'Donnell C. An evaluation of corneal nerve morphology and function in moderate keratoconus. *Cont Lens Anterior Eye.* 2005;28(4):185–192.
41. Al-Aqaba MA, et al. The morphologic characteristics of corneal nerves in advanced keratoconus as evaluated by acetylcholinesterase technique. *Am J Ophthalmol.* 2011;152(3):364–376.e1.
42. Al-Aqaba MA, et al. Architecture and distribution of human corneal nerves. *Br J Ophthalmol.* 2010;94(6):784–789.
43. Mannion LS, Tromans C, O'Donnell C. Corneal nerve structure and function in keratoconus: a case report. *Eye Contact Lens.* 2007;33(2):106–108.
44. Brookes NH, et al. Involvement of corneal nerves in the progression of keratoconus. *Exp Eye Res.* 2003;77(4):515–524.
45. Al-Aqaba MA, et al. Corneal nerves in health and disease. *Prog Retin Eye Res.* 2019;73:100762.
46. Flockerzi E, Daas L, Seitz B. Structural changes in the corneal subbasal nerve plexus in keratoconus. *Acta Ophthalmol.* 2020;98(8):e928–e932.
47. Dua HS, Faraj LA, Said DG. Dua's layer: discovery, characteristics, clinical applications, controversy and potential relevance to glaucoma. *Expert Rev of Ophthalmol.* 2015;10(6):531–547.
48. Parker JS, et al. Are Descemet membrane ruptures the root cause of corneal hydrops in keratoconic eyes? *Am J Ophthalmol.* 2019;205:147–152.
49. Ting DSJ, Said DG, Dua HS. Are Descemet membrane ruptures the root cause of corneal hydrops in keratoconic eyes? *Am J Ophthalmol.* 2019;205:204.
50. Dua HS, et al. "Descemet membrane detachment" a novel concept in diagnosis and classification. *Am J Ophthalmol.* 2020;218:84–98.
51. McMonnies CW. Mechanisms for acute corneal hydrops and perforation. *Eye Contact Lens.* 2014;40(4):257–264.

52. Ferrari G, Rama P. The keratoconus enigma: a review with emphasis on pathogenesis. *Ocul Surf.* 2020;18(3):363–373.
53. Wojcik KA, et al. Role of biochemical factors in the pathogenesis of keratoconus. *Acta Biochim Pol.* 2014;61(1):55–62.
54. Meek KM. Corneal collagen-its role in maintaining corneal shape and transparency. *Biophys Rev.* 2009;1(2):83–93.
55. Chaerkady R, et al. The keratoconus corneal proteome: loss of epithelial integrity and stromal degeneration. *J Proteomics.* 2013;87:122–131.
56. Critchfield JW, et al. Keratoconus: I. Biochemical studies. *Exp Eye Res.* 1988;46(6):953–963.
57. Panjwani N, et al. Protein-related abnormalities in keratoconus. *Invest Ophthalmol Vis Sci.* 1989;30(12):2481–2487.
58. García B, et al. Differential expression of proteoglycans by corneal stromal cells in keratoconus. *Invest Ophthalmol Vis Sci.* 2016;57(6):2618–2628.
59. Zhang G, et al. Genetic evidence for the coordinated regulation of collagen fibrillogenesis in the cornea by decorin and biglycan. *J Biol Chem.* 2009;284(13):8888–8897.
60. Chakravarti S, et al. Lumican regulates collagen fibril assembly: skin fragility and corneal opacity in the absence of lumican. *J Cell Biol.* 1998;141(5):1277–1286.
61. Soiberman U, et al. Pathophysiology of keratoconus: what do we know today. *Open Ophthalmol J.* 2017;11:252–261.
62. Bykhovskaya Y, et al. Abnormal regulation of extracellular matrix and adhesion molecules in corneas of patients with keratoconus. *Int J Keratoconus Ectatic Corneal Dis.* 2016;5(2):63–70.
63. di Martino E, Ali M, Inglehearn CF. Matrix metalloproteinases in keratoconus—too much of a good thing? *Exp Eye Res.* 2019;182:137–143.
64. Lema I, Durán JA. Inflammatory molecules in the tears of patients with keratoconus. *Ophthalmology.* 2005;112(4):654–659.
65. Shetty R, et al. Elevated expression of matrix metalloproteinase-9 and inflammatory cytokines in keratoconus patients is inhibited by cyclosporine A. *Invest Ophthalmol Vis Sci.* 2015;56(2):738–750.
66. Lema I, et al. Subclinical keratoconus and inflammatory molecules from tears. *Br J Ophthalmol.* 2009;93(6):820–824.
67. Smith VA, et al. Keratoconus: matrix metalloproteinase-2 activation and TIMP modulation. *Biochim Biophys Acta.* 2006;1762(4):431–439.
68. Sawaguchi S, et al. Alpha-1 proteinase inhibitor levels in keratoconus. *Exp Eye Res.* 1990;50(5):549–554.
69. Sawaguchi S, et al. Alpha 2-macroglobulin levels in normal human and keratoconus corneas. *Invest Ophthalmol Vis Sci.* 1994;35(12):4008–4014.
70. Balasubramanian SA, et al. Proteases, proteolysis and inflammatory molecules in the tears of people with keratoconus. *Acta Ophthalmol.* 2012;90(4):e303–e309.
71. Pahuja N, et al. Differential molecular expression of extracellular matrix and inflammatory genes at the corneal cone apex drives focal weakening in keratoconus. *Invest Ophthalmol Vis Sci.* 2016;57(13):5372–5382.
72. Balasubramanian SA, Pye DC, Willcox MD. Effects of eye rubbing on the levels of protease, protease activity and cytokines in tears: relevance in keratoconus. *Clin Exp Optom.* 2013;96(2):214–218.
73. Cook EB. Tear cytokines in acute and chronic ocular allergic inflammation. *Curr Opin Allergy Clin Immunol.* 2004;4(5):441–445.
74. Naderan M, et al. Effect of allergic diseases on keratoconus severity. *Ocul Immunol Inflamm.* 2017; 25(3):418–423.
75. Pizzino G, et al. Oxidative stress: harms and benefits for human health. *Oxid Med Cell Longev.* 2017;2017:8416763.
76. Ighodaro OM, Akinloye OA. First line defence antioxidants-superoxide dismutase (SOD), catalase (CAT) and glutathione peroxidase (GPX): their fundamental role in the entire antioxidant defence grid. *Alexandria J Med.* 2018;54(4):293–298.
77. Behndig A, et al. Superoxide dismutase isoenzymes in the normal and diseased human cornea. *Invest Ophthalmol Vis Sci.* 2001;42(10):2293–2296.
78. Kenney MC, et al. Increased levels of catalase and cathepsin V/L2 but decreased TIMP-1 in keratoconus corneas: evidence that oxidative stress plays a role in this disorder. *Invest Ophthalmol Vis Sci.* 2005;46(3):823–832.

79. Soria J, et al. Label-free LC-MS/MS quantitative analysis of aqueous humor from keratoconic and normal eyes. *Mol Vis.* 2015;21:451–460.
80. Yilmaz M, Arikan S, Türkön H. Plasma homocysteine levels in patients with keratoconus. *Clin Exp Optom.* 2020;103(6):804–807.
81. Tyagi N, et al. Mechanisms of homocysteine-induced oxidative stress. *Am J Physiol Heart Circ Physiol.* 2005;289(6):H2649–H2656.
82. Chang HY, Chodosh J. The genetics of keratoconus. *Semin Ophthalmol.* 2013;28(5-6):275–280.
83. Tam V, et al. Benefits and limitations of genome-wide association studies. *Nat Rev Genet.* 2019;20(8):467–484.
84. Bykhovskaya Y, Margines B, Rabinowitz YS. Genetics in keratoconus: where are we? *Eye Vis (Lond).* 2016;3:16.
85. McComish BJ, et al. Association of genetic variation with keratoconus. *JAMA Ophthalmol.* 2019;138(2):174–181.
86. Lu Y, et al. Genome-wide association analyses identify multiple loci associated with central corneal thickness and keratoconus. *Nat Genet.* 2013;45(2):155–163.
87. Belin MW, et al. What's in a name: keratoconus, pellucid marginal degeneration, and related thinning disorders. *Am J Ophthalmol.* 2011;152(2):157–162.e1.
88. Ernst BJ, Hsu HY. Keratoconus association with axial myopia: a prospective biometric study. *Eye Contact Lens.* 2011;37(1):2–5.
89. Szentmary N. Keratoconus, keratoglobus, keratotorus and pellucid marginal degeneration. *Acta Ophthalmologica.* 2016;94:S256.
90. Pinero DP, Alcon N. Corneal biomechanics: a review. *Clin Exp Optom.* 2015;98(2):107–116.
91. Deol M, Taylor DA, Radcliffe NM. Corneal hysteresis and its relevance to glaucoma. *Curr Opin Ophthalmol.* 2015;26(2):96–102.
92. Dupps WJ Jr, Wilson SE. Biomechanics and wound healing in the cornea. *Exp Eye Res.* 2006;83(4):709–720.
93. Edmund C. Corneal elasticity and ocular rigidity in normal and keratoconic eyes. *Acta Ophthalmol (Copenh).* 1988;66(2):134–140.
94. Ma J, et al. Biomechanics and structure of the cornea: implications and association with corneal disorders. *Surv Ophthalmol.* 2018;63(6):851–861.
95. Esporcatte LPG, et al. Biomechanical diagnostics of the cornea. *Eye Vis (Lond).* 2020;7:9.
96. Dua HS, et al. Human corneal anatomy redefined: a novel pre-Descemet's layer (Dua's layer). *Ophthalmology.* 2013;120(9):1778–1785.
97. Roberts CJ, Dupps Jr WJ. Biomechanics of corneal ectasia and biomechanical treatments. *J Cataract Refract Surg.* 2014;40(6):991–998.
98. Dupps WJ Jr. Hysteresis: new mechanospeak for the ophthalmologist. *J Cataract Refract Surg.* 2007;33(9):1499–1501.
99. Shah S, et al. Assessment of the biomechanical properties of the cornea with the ocular response analyzer in normal and keratoconic eyes. *Invest Ophthalmol Vis Sci.* 2007;48(7):3026–3031.
100. Ali NQ, Patel DV, McGhee CN. Biomechanical responses of healthy and keratoconic corneas measured using a noncontact Scheimpflug-based tonometer. *Invest Ophthalmol Vis Sci.* 2014;55(6):3651–3659.
101. Dua HS. Keratoconus: still behind the cone. *J Eucornea.* 2020;7(11):23–24.

CHAPTER 6

Biomechanics of Keratoconus

Renato Ambrósio Jr. ■ Louise Pellegrino Gomes Esporcatte ■
Marcella Salomão ■ Nelson Baptiste Sena ■ Cynthia J. Roberts

KEY CONCEPTS

- Moderate and advanced stages of keratoconus are readily recognized, but the identification of milder or subclinical forms of this disease sometimes remains challenging.
- The advent of refractive surgery and the development of new treatment modalities for patients with corneal ectasia increased the need for the diagnosis and characterization of ectatic corneal diseases.
- Multimodal refractive imaging including Placido-disk based corneal topography, Scheimpflug corneal tomography, segmental tomography with epithelial thickness, and Bowman's layer characterization with optical coherence tomography (OCT) and very-high-frequency ultrasound (VHF-US) enhances the characterization of corneal shape and structure.
- Clinical corneal biomechanical assessment further augments the ability to diagnose keratoconus and ectatic corneal diseases.
- Artificial intelligence has been used to develop new indices that improve the diagnostics for ectatic corneal disorders.
- The quest for diagnosis evolved to the characterization of the intrinsic susceptibility for corneal ectasia development and progression.

Introduction

Corneal biomechanics has emerged as an important topic for research and development in ophthalmology because of the many potential applications.[1,2] The need to enhance diagnosis to recognize milder forms of the keratoconus (KC) and ectatic corneal diseases (ECDs) and identify the intrinsic predisposition for ectasia progression has gained significance because of refractive surgery and the development of new treatment modalities.[3]

There has been a paradigm change associated with the management of ECDs, which was restricted to spectacles, rigid contact lenses, or penetrating keratoplasty.[4] The advent of novel treatment modalities, such as corneal collagen cross-linking (CXL) and intrastromal corneal ring segments (ICRS), both with an underlying biomechanical mechanism, has established diverging situations on when, why, and how to proceed with surgery on these patients. Such considerations demonstrate the requirement for individualized treatment planning, which should comprise a precise evaluation of patient needs, advanced imaging with advanced geometric characterization, biomechanical assessment, and environmental factors such eye rubbing.[5]

Clinical Applications of Corneal Biomechanics

Knowledge of corneal biomechanics provides a substantial contribution to the diagnosis, staging, and prognosis of KC and other corneal ectatic conditions.[3,6,7] It has also become important for the detection of earlier stages of ectatic disease (subclinical KC), boosted by the development of new treatment modalities such as CXL and ICRS. In the setting of refractive surgery, the investigation of corneal biomechanical properties has become a critical part of the screening process to recognize patients at higher risk of developing iatrogenic ectasia after laser vision correction (LVC), along with improving the predictability and efficacy of these elective procedures.[8-11]

Biomechanical principles have been applied in several other clinical conditions,[1] including correcting intraocular pressure (IOP) measurements,[12,13] planning and following up corneal collagen CXL treatments,[14-17] and other treatment modalities such as ICRS, which can be combined in different approaches to manage KC patients.[4,18,19]

The introduction of Placido-disk based corneal topography increased the ability to identify ECD in earlier stages, even before the development of clinical signs or visual symptoms.[20,21] However, the limitations of this technology are shown by the occurrence of post-refractive keratectasia despite normal anterior curvature maps and cases with suspicious topographic patterns that proceeded with LCV, based on advanced corneal imaging, resulting in documented stable outcomes.[3]

Further developments in corneal diagnostic imaging technologies allowed for segmental or layered tomographic three-dimensional (3D) characterization with epithelial[22,23] and Bowman's layer regularity characterization and thickness mapping.[24] While corneal epithelial thickness was initially assessed by digital very-high-frequency ultrasound (VHF-US),[25] advances in corneal and anterior segment optical coherence tomography (OCT) allowed for such evaluation in a rapid examination without the necessity of a water bath. The assessment of the corneal surface evolved into 3D corneal tomography, with 3D reconstruction of front and back corneal surfaces with a full-thickness map.[26] Studies have demonstrated higher sensitivity of the tomographic approach to identify subclinical (or fruste) disorder in eyes with relatively normal topographic maps from patients with the fellow eye showing clinical ectatic disease.[27,28] The association with ocular biometry and ocular wavefront measurements can further improve the detection ability.

The current understanding is that the pathophysiology of ectatic diseases is related to a primary biomechanical abnormality, with architecture and morphologic instability as secondary events.[29,30] Beyond shape analysis, clinical biomechanical assessment has been promising as the ultimate tool (before genetic analysis is available) for enhancing the overall accuracy for identifying mild forms of ECDs.[31,32]

Corneal imaging should evolve further to integrate devices such as Scheimpflug tomography, OCT segmental tomography, ocular wavefront and biometry, and corneal biomechanical assessment. Considering the vast amount of generated data, the conscious use of artificial intelligence plays a major role in taking greater advantage of such information for clinical decisions.[5]

Chronic Biomechanical Failure of the Cornea (Keratectasia)

Chronic biomechanical failure occurs when a tissue fatigues over time due to chronic low-grade stress. Susceptibility to fatigue is a common phenomenon in biological tissues, which may fail in response to stress loads in a time-dependent fashion. However, a healthy balance exists in the cornea between extracellular matrix damage and subsequent wound repair, which prevents chronic biomechanical failure of the stroma proper via keratocyte-directed repair processes.[33]

In composite structures, two types of chronic biomechanical failure occur during fatigue: delamination and interfiber fracture. Delamination is the separation of two adjacent plies (lamellae) from each other, whereas the interfiber split is the development of a full-thickness interfibrillar matrix crack in a single ply. When this chronic biomechanical failure process progresses, the structure usually thins to measurable or detectable levels, and fibril fracture—defined as a direct, acute full-thickness breakage of collagen fibrils in a ply—may occur in Bowman's layer and also in the Descemet membrane.[33,34] Bulging or protrusion usually occurs after thinning has already started but may progress in severity; this is particularly important for identification of the earliest changes related to ectasia.[33]

Keratectasia therefore is an outcome of a nonspecific chronic biomechanical failure response by the cornea to various stresses. Some degree of slippage related to delamination and interfiber fracture can occur as part of a partial biomechanical response, but may not proceed to full-blown keratectasia. Each cornea has a unique ability to withstand internal stress, but it may be overwhelmed by additional stressors, such as eye rubbing, increasing IOP level, corneal-weakening procedures (Laser-Assisted in Situ Keratomileusis (LASIK) or photorefractive keratectomy surgery), and, possibly, external nocturnal eye pressure, as occurs with face-down positioning in sleep apnea. If progressive chronic biomechanical failure ensues, structural failure of the cornea may develop, with loss of shape. Loss of corneal shape ultimately may lead to reduced refractive function and reduced optical clarity.[33]

KC is the most common ECD. By definition, KC is a bilateral (but typically asymmetric) and progressive corneal dystrophy.[3] The most accepted hypothesis is that it occurs as a combination of a genetic predilection and environmental influences, such as eye rubbing and ocular trauma.[29,35] There is a consensus that KC is indeed a bilateral disease, but also that secondary ectasia may be caused by a purely mechanical process, such as after refractive surgery with tissue removal or due to excessive eye rubbing, and this may occur in only one eye.[29]

Ocular Response Analyzer

In vivo evaluation of corneal biomechanical response first became accessible with the launch of the Ocular Response Analyzer (ORA; Reichert Ophthalmic Instruments, Buffalo, NY) in 2005.[36,37] The ORA is a noncontact tonometer (NCT) with a collimated air puff to indent a central 3 to 6 mm area of the apical cornea. A sophisticated electro-optical system monitors the bidirectional movement of the cornea across its reflection of an infrared beam.[36,38,39] After the air pulse is triggered, the cornea deforms in an inward direction (ingoing phase), passing through a first applanation instant when the pressure (P1) is recorded. At first applanation, the air pump obtains a signal to shut off; the inertia in the piston permits the pressure to continue to grow so that the air pulse has a Gaussian configuration. The peak of the air pressure pulse is influenced by P1, making it a key parameter for each ORA measurement. As the air pressure continues to grow, the cornea adopts a concave shape. The outgoing phase is initiated as the air pressure declines, permitting the cornea to return to its original shape progressively. During the outgoing phase, the cornea passes through a second applanation, when the pressure of the air pulse (P2) is recorded. The pressure-derived parameters generated by the standard ORA software are corneal hysteresis (CH) and corneal resistance factor (CRF; Fig. 6.1). CH is the difference between the P1 and P2 values, whereas CRF is calculated according to the formula:

$$a[P1 - 0.7P2] + d$$

where a and d are calibration and regression constants, and the P2 coefficient of 0.7 was empirically determined to maximize correlation with central corneal thickness.[36,40]

Although studies have reported CH and CRF to be lower in KC compared with healthy corneas,[41] a substantial overlap in the distributions of both parameters was detected so that the sensitivity and specificity for KC diagnosis are quite weak.[42–44] Additional research found more precise ectasia identification when examining the ORA waveform signal and using new parameters related to the deformation response of the cornea during the NCT measurement.[44–48] Fig. 6.2 demonstrates the importance of evaluating the waveform signal when examining corneal properties in a 51-year-old patient who underwent bilateral LASIK. These properties were determined with the ORA, and it detects a nonectatic post-LASIK right eye and an ectatic post-LASIK left eye. It is important to note that both eyes had similar hysteresis but dramatically different signal characteristics.[48]

More recently, the integration of these new parameters with tomographic data demonstrated improved accuracy in the detection of mild or early ectatic disease.[49] Moreover, the

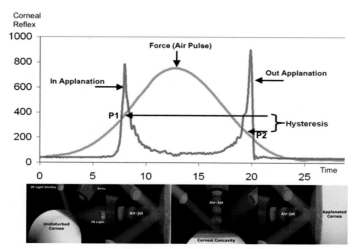

Fig. 6.1 Ocular response analyzer (ORA) measurements showing the air pulse deforming the cornea (ingoing phase) and registering corneal signal (x-axis) through time (y-axis) in milliseconds, in which P1 is the first applanation moment. The Gaussian configuration is from when the air pulse signal is shut off. With the continuing increase in the magnitude of the air pulse due to inertia in the piston, the cornea assumes a concave configuration. In the outgoing phase (air pressure decreases), the cornea passes through a second applanation, when the pressure of the air pulse (P2) is again registered. The pressure-derived parameters generated are corneal hysteresis (CH) and corneal resistance factor (CRF).

waveform-derived parameters were found to document corneal biomechanical changes after CXL procedures in KC, while CH and CRF did not detect significant differences.[49–51]

The Corvis ST

The Corvis ST (Oculus, Wetzlar, Germany) is also an NCT[52] that includes an ultra-high-speed (UHS) Scheimpflug camera for pachymetry and biomechanical assessment of the cornea. During measurement, similar to what happens in the ORA examination, the cornea deforms inward and outward while passing through two applanation moments. Nevertheless, the Corvis ST has two essential differences from the ORA. First, in place of using the reflection of the infrared beam to monitor the distortion of the cornea, it utilizes a UHS Scheimpflug camera that acquires 140 horizontal 8-mm frames throughout 33 ms. This approach allows a more comprehensive assessment of the deformation process in two dimensions. Also, unlike the ORA, the Corvis ST yields a fixed maximal peak pressure for the air puff in every examination.

The Corvis ST calculates corneal deformation parameters based on the dynamic inspection of the corneal response (Table 6.1).[2] By way of air pressure, the cornea begins to deform in the backward direction. Whole eye motion is instantaneously initiated with a slow linear increase in the same backward direction and then increases just after the cornea reaches maximum deformation. Dynamic corneal response (DCR) parameters thereby either include or subtract the whole eye motion. The parameters described as "deformation" are those in which entire eye motion is included, while the "deflection" parameters take into account and subtract the backward motion of the eye. The deformation amplitude (DA) indicates the displacement of the corneal apex in the anterior-posterior direction, and the maximum value is determined at the highest concavity (HC) instant. The DA ratio 1 or 2 mm is the central deformation divided by an average of the deformation 1 to 2 mm at either side of the center, with a maximum value near the first applanation. Applanation lengths (AL) and corneal velocities (CVel) are recorded during ingoing and outgoing phases. The radius of curvature at the

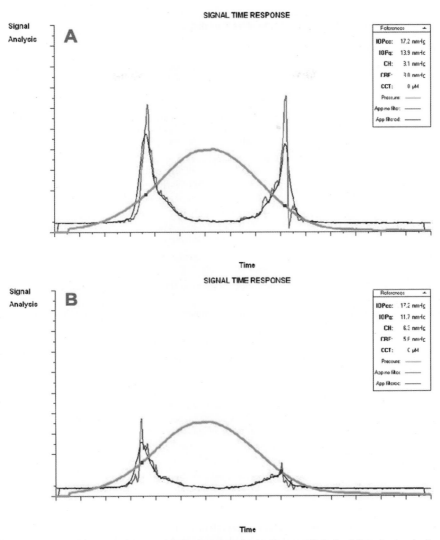

Fig. 6.2 (A) Nonectatic post-LASIK eye showing large amplitude, sharp peaks in the infrared curve *(red)*, and a higher magnitude *green* pressure curve. (B) Ectatic post-LASIK eye showing small-amplitude infrared peaks, indicating weakness, and blunted green pressure curve. Note that both eyes had similar hysteresis, but dramatically different signal characteristics. *CH,* Corneal hysteresis; *CRF,* corneal resistance factor; *IOP,* intraocular pressure; *CCT,* central corneal thickness; *IOPcc,* corneal compensated intraocular pressure; *IOPg,* gold standard, Goldmann correlated Intraocular pressure.

highest concavity (curvature radius HC) is also documented, and the integrated inverse radius is the reciprocal of the radius (analogous to curvature) during the concave state of the cornea. It should be noted that a greater concave radius (lower concave curvature) is associated with higher resistance to deform or a stiffer cornea. Thus the higher the integrated inverse radius and maximum inverse radius (greater concave curvature), the less resistance to deformation and lower corneal stiffness. Corneal thickness, the standard "Goldmann-correlated" IOP, and a biomechanically corrected IOP (bIOP) are recorded as well.[53,54]

TABLE 6.1 ■ Corneal Deformation Parameters Provided by the Corvis ST

Corvis ST Parameters

First applanation	The first applanation of the cornea during the air puff (in milliseconds). The length of the applanation at this instant is shown in parenthesis (in millimeters).
Highest concavity	The moment that the cornea assumes its maximum concavity during the air puff (in milliseconds). The length of the distance between the two peaks of the cornea at this instant appears in parenthesis (in millimeters).
Second applanation	The second applanation of the cornea during the air puff (in milliseconds). The length of the applanation at this moment appears in parenthesis (in millimeters).
Maximum deformation	The amount (in millimeters) of the maximum cornea deformation during the air puff.
Wing distance	The length of the distance between the two peaks of the cornea at this moment (in millimeters).
Maximum velocity (in)	Maximum velocity during the ingoing phase (in meters per second).
Maximum velocity (out)	The maximum velocity during the outgoing phase (in meters per second).
Curvature radius, normal	The cornea in its natural-state radius of curvature (in millimeters).
Curvature radius, highest concavity	The cornea radius of curvature at the time of maximum concavity during the air puff (in millimeters).
Cornea thickness	Measurement of the corneal thickness (in millimeters).
Integrated inverse radius	The inverse of the radius of curvature during the concave phase of the deformation.
Deformation amplitude ratio 1 or 2 mm	The central deformation divided by an average of the deformation 1 or 2 mm at either side of the center with a maximum value just prior to first applanation.
IOP	Measurement of the intraocular pressure (in millimeters of mercury [mmHg]).
bIOP	Biomechanically corrected IOP.

The initial generation measurement parameters of the Corvis ST offered a performance analogous to that obtained by the pressure-derived ORA data for discriminating healthy and KC eyes.[55,56] However, the more substantial details of the DCR from the Scheimpflug camera enabled the development of new parameters that are less influenced by IOP than the original DCR parameters, which revealed a greater capacity to detect the onset of ectatic disease.[57–60] The parameters which are indicative of corneal stiffness relate to the *shape* of the deformation, rather than the depth.

In 2014 a multicenter international investigation group was created to increase knowledge about Corvis ST technology with a distinct focus on the examination of ECD.[7,61,62] One of the outcomes of this collaborative work was the Vinciguerra screening report, which provides correlations of normative values and bIOP. It was established throughout a limited-element parametric study that uses central cornea thickness and age in addition to deformation response parameters to decrease the effect of stiffness on IOP estimates.[63,64] Fig. 6.3 shows the Vinciguerra screening report and Fig. 6.4 shows DCR of a 16-year-old patient with forme fruste of KC (FFKC).

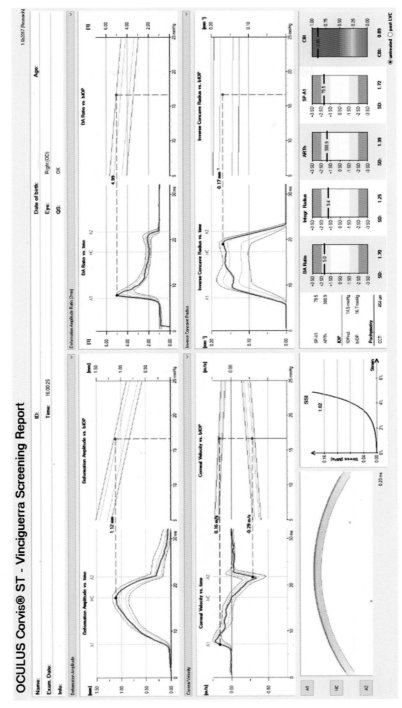

Fig. 6.3 Corvis ST Vinciguerra screening report of a 16-year-old patient with forme fruste keratoconus.

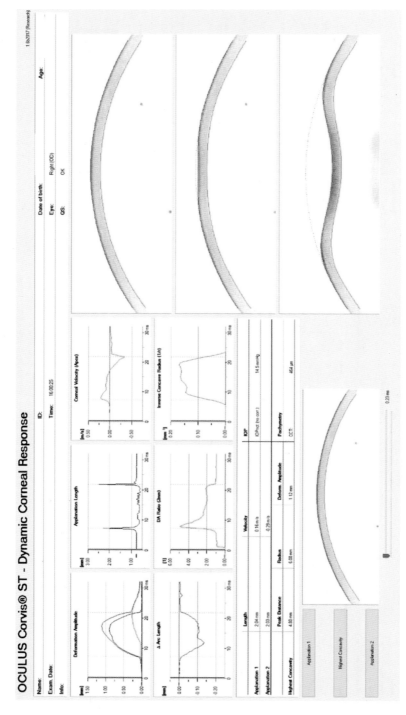

Fig. 6.4 The dynamic corneal response of the same patient with forme fruste keratoconus (see Fig. 6.3).

The horizontal Scheimpflug image of the undisturbed cornea also provides data for evaluating the profile or the proportion of increase of corneal thickness from the apex toward the nasal and temporal sides. The characterization of the thickness data on the horizontal Scheimpflug image (the division between corneal thickness at the thinnest point and the pachymetric progression index) enabled the calculation of the Ambrósio relational thickness over the horizontal meridian (ARTh).[2,65] Subsequently the investigators used linear regression analysis to combine ARTh with corneal deformation parameters to generate the corneal biomechanical index (CBI).[66] Vinciguerra and coworkers verified that a cut-off value of 0.5 CBI was able to correctly identify 98.2% of KC cases among normal cases with very high specificity.[66] As with any artificial intelligence approach, further optimization is possible and expected. Ambrósio and coworkers expanded the multicenter study to augment the training/testing databases in order to improve ectasia detection with new algorithms combining tomographic and biomechanical data—the optimized version, the tomographic biomechanical index (TBI).[7,11]

THE CORNEAL/CORVIS BIOMECHANICAL INDEX

In a retrospective study, one eye randomly selected from 227 healthy and 102 KC patients from the Rio de Janeiro Corneal Tomography and Biomechanics Study Group, Rio de Janeiro, Brazil (Database 1) and from 251 healthy and 78 KC patients from the Vincieye Clinic in Milan, Italy (Database 2) were enrolled. Sixteen different DCR parameters were evaluated, including the speed of corneal apex at first applanation (A1 velocity), the speed of corneal apex at second applanation (A2 velocity), the distance between the two bending peaks on the cornea at the maximum concavity state (peak distance), the radius of the central cornea at the maximum concavity state based on a parabolic fit (HC radius), the DA (the greatest displacement of corneal apex in the anterior-posterior course at the instant of HC), deflection amplitude (deflection from the cornea's original state minus whole eye motion), deflection area ("displaced" part of the cornea in the examined horizontal sectional plane), inverse concave radius, central-peripheral DA ratio, deflection amplitude ratio, Delta Arclength, ARTh, SP-A1 (resultant pressure divided by deflection amplitude at A1), bIOP, corneal thickness, and SD-deformation amplitude, among others.

The optimal combination of each index was determined by logistic regression analysis for the elaboration of the corneal biomechanical index (CBI). These parameters included pachymetry (central corneal thickness), bIOP, DA, SD-DA, A1 velocity, peak distance, HCdArclength, HC deflection area, DA ratio 2 mm, DA ratio 1 mm, deflection amplitude, inverse concave radius, radius HC, stiffness parameter-A1, and ARTh. The training dataset was calculated using Database 1, and the best cut-off point was obtained from the receiver operating characteristic (ROC) curves for an accurate separation between healthy and keratoconic eyes. Subsequently, to prevent overfitting and independently validate the developed parameter, CBI was verified in a validation dataset (Database 2). Using a cut-off of 0.5, 98.2% of the cases were properly classified in the training dataset (Dataset 1), with 100% specificity and 94.1% sensitivity, and an area under the curve (AUC) of 0.983. Then, in the validation dataset (Dataset 2), the same cut-off value correctly classified 98.8% of cases, with 98.4% specificity and 100% sensitivity and an AUC of 0.999.[66] At the beginning of the 2020s, a new algorithm has applied artificial intelligence to develop a new CBI-LVC index to distinguish ectatic eyes from stable post-LVC cases.[67]

THE TOMOGRAPHIC BIOMECHANICAL INDEX

The second retrospective study, including patients from Instituto de Olhos Renato Ambrósio in Rio de Janeiro, Brazil and the Vincieye Clinic in Milan, Italy, intended to develop an associate index for the Pentacam and Corvis ST. TBI was developed to characterize the inherent susceptibility to progression of ectasia. Also, the normal eyes (group 1) and KC eyes (group 2) in this study included unoperated ectatic eyes from patients with very asymmetric ectasia—VAE-E (group 3) who presented fellow eyes with normal topographic maps—VAE-NT (group 4). For groups 1 and 2, only one eye per patient was selected randomly for inclusion in the study, to avoid the bias of the relation between eyes. Data from Pentacam HR and Corvis ST were transferred to a custom spreadsheet using special research software, which is currently available on the instrument.

Distinctive artificial intelligence methods were tested, involving logistic regression analysis with forwarding stepwise inclusion, support vector machine, and random forest, which were applied to analyze and combine data from corneal deformation response, including CBI, with tomographic data, including Belin/Ambrosio Display (BAD-D); to optimize our ability to distinguish normal and altered eyes. The best cut-off point was acquired from the ROC curves for a precise split among healthy and KC eyes. With a cut-off value of 0.79, TBI had 100% sensitivity and specificity to discriminate frank ectasia cases (AUC = 1.0 in groups 2 and 3). However, for the exact classification of eyes with standard topography having no conclusive signs of ectasia from patients with clinical ectatic disease in the fellow eye, an optimization of cut-off value was required, and a value of 0.29 gave 90.4% sensitivity with 4% false-positive results (96% specificity; AUC = 0.985). The AUC of the TBI was statistically greater than all other surveyed parameters, including the CBI.[11]

Posterior external validation studies were conducted and proved the capacity of this new index to identify ectatic disease, even in milder forms of ectasia (Table 6.2).[2,8,57,67–69] Although some of these studies have found a moderately lower sensitivity for the VAE-NT eyes (some with normal topography and tomography [NTT]), it is important to note that some of these cases may be truly unilateral ectasia due to mechanical trauma.[70]

The importance of TBI is shown in the case of 16-year-old fraternal twins. Twin one has asymmetric KC with advanced KC in the right eye and mild in the left eye, distance-corrected visual acuity (DCVA) 20/100, and 20/20, respectively (Fig. 6.5). His brother has FFKC with best corrected visual acuity (BCVA) 20/20 in both eyes (Fig. 6.6). Both of the twins have an ocular allergy, but the one with asymmetric KC admits more eye rubbing than the other.

CORNEAL STIFFNESS AND STRESS-STRAIN INDEX

The Corvis ST provides a parameter that serves as a biomarker for corneal stiffness, called the SP-A1. It is the result of the division of the load (air pressure minus bIOP) on the cornea by the timing and position of the corneal apex at the first applanation moment. The SP-A1 value in KC eyes was reported to be lower in thinner corneas than in normal ones.[66] Interestingly, SP-A1 has a negative correlation with the corneal back-scattering (referred to as densitometry) values. This implies that, among patients with KC, increased corneal densitometry values, which are associated with higher scatter, may indicate compromised corneal stiffness.[71,72]

Studies have been performed to combine multiple parameters to evaluate and compare corneal biomechanical response between healthy and KC eyes, as one that applied a logistic regression equation to combine several Corvis ST parameters (A1 velocity, DA, DA Ratio Max 1 mm, Max Inverse Radius, and SP-A1) and found high sensitivity and specificity for differentiating healthy and KC eyes.[73] Another study investigated changes in corneal stiffness parameters (SP-A1) 2 years after accelerated collagen cross-linking (CXL) using Corvis ST. The authors demonstrated in vivo biomechanical increase in corneal stiffness following CXL treatment.[15]

The stress-strain index (SSI) algorithm is generated based on predictions of corneal behavior using finite element models simulating the effects of IOP and the Corvis ST air puff. It was the first standard mechanical metric that could be derived in vivo, allowing building of the entire stress-strain curve of corneal tissue. Besides the detection of patients with higher risk or susceptibility for ectasia development or progression after refractive surgery, the SSI may provide clinical documentation for the biomechanical changes after cross-linking procedures.[64]

TABLE 6.2 ■ Tomographic Biomechanical Index (TBI) Clinical Studies[2]

Author / Reference	NE (n)	Clinical Ectasia (n)	Cut-Off	Sensitivity (%)	Specificity (%)	AUC	VAE NT (n)	Cut-Off	Sensitivity (%)	Specificity (%)	AUC	Observation
Steinberg et al.[68]	105	96	–	98.00	100	0.998	32	0.11	72.00	71.00	0.825	VAE NTT: 18 eyes Sensitivity: 67% Specificity: 65% AUC: 0.732
Kataria et al.[67]	100	100	>0.63	99.00	100	0.995	100	>0.09	82.00	78.00	0.793	–
Ferreira-Mendes et al.[8]	312	118	0.335	94.40	94.90	0.988	57	0.295	89.50	91.00	0.96	–
Chan et al.[79]	37	23	–	–	–	–	–	0.16	84.4	82.4	0.925	–
Sedaghat et al.[57]	137	145	>0.49	100	100	1.000	–	–	–	–	–	–
Koc et al.[80]	35	–	–	–	–	–	21	0.29	67.00	86.00	0.790	–
Koh et al.[81]	70	–	–	–	–	–	23	>0.259	52.17	88.57	0.751	–

AUC, Area under the receiver operating characteristics curve; NE, normal eyes; NTT, eyes with normal topography and tomography; VAE-NT, very asymmetric eyes with normal topography.

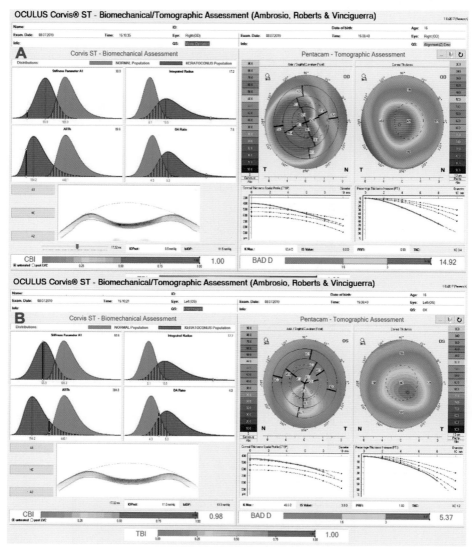

Fig. 6.5   Corvis ST/Pentacam integrated display of the right eye (A) and left eye (B) of a 16-year-old (twin one) with asymmetric keratoconus (KC). He has advanced KC in the right eye and mild in the left eye, distance-corrected visual acuity (DCVA) 20/100 and 20/20, respectively.

Some parameters measured by the Corvis ST are valuable to discriminate healthy from keratoconic corneas, and also cross-linked from non-cross-linked keratoconic corneas. These parameters include the applanation velocity 2 (A2V), which is the velocity of corneal apex during the second applanation, and the second applanation length (A2L), which measures the cord length of A2. The difference between the first applanation length (A1L; the cord length of A1) and A2L could consistently discriminate cross-linked from non-cross-linked and healthy corneas, which illustrates the potential of the Corvis ST in monitoring corneal changes after cross-linking treatment.[74]

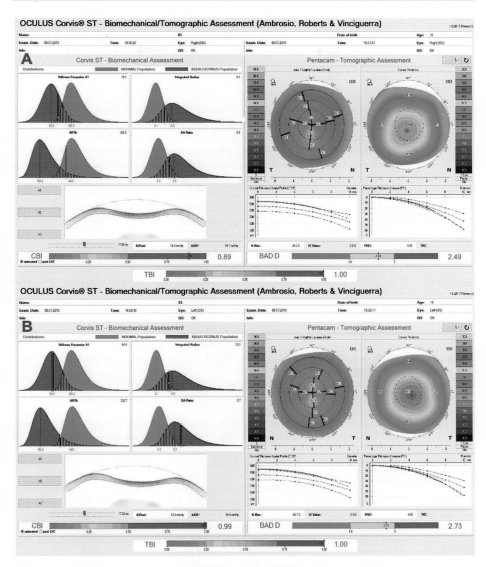

Fig. 6.6 Corvis ST/Pentacam integrated display of the right (A) and left eye (B) of a 16-year-old (twin two; brother of the patient in Figs. 6.3 and 6.4). Considering the tomographic biomechanical index, he has a forme fruste keratoconus (DCVA 20/20 in both eyes).

Brillouin Optical Microscopy

Brillouin optical microscopy was introduced to measure corneal biomechanics in vivo through the study of light scatter and mapping of the biomechanical state of the cornea with 3D capability. This technique can determine intrinsic viscoelastic properties decoupled from structural information and applied pressure.[75,76]

The cornea has nonlinear stress-strain behavior, which corroborates that the tissue does not have a constant modulus. The tangent modulus increases gradually with stress or applied pressure.[77]

Although the accuracy of the first reported findings is relatively weak, Seiler and coworkers demonstrated the impact of age on corneal stiffness findings by Brillouin spectroscopy and found statistically significant differences when comparing normal and keratoconic corneas.[79]

Conclusion

Advances in biomechanical assessment should be considered in combination with multimodal corneal and refractive imaging, incorporating Placido-disk based corneal topography, Scheimpflug corneal tomography, spectral-domain optical coherence tomography (SD-OCT), anterior segment tomography, VHF-US, ocular biometry, and ocular wavefront measurements.[2]

The incorporation of tomographic and biomechanical data into artificial intelligence systems has demonstrated the capacity to increase precision in detecting ectatic disease and characterize the inherent susceptibility for biomechanical failure and ectasia progression, which is a severe complication after LVC.[2] Furthermore, potential developments in the ability for genetic screening and molecular biological testing are promising, and these technologies have the potential to revolutionize diagnostic capabilities in ectatic disorders.[3]

References

1. Roberts CJ, Dupps WJ Jr. Biomechanics of corneal ectasia and biomechanical treatments. *J Cataract Refract Surg.* 2014;40:991–998.
2. Esporcatte LPG, Salomao MQ, Lopes BT, et al. Biomechanical diagnostics of the cornea. *Eye Vis (Lond).* 2020;7:9.
3. Salomão M, Hoffling-Lima AL, Lopes B, et al. Recent developments in keratoconus diagnosis. *Expert Rev Ophthalmol.* 2018;13:329–341.
4. Ambrósio R Jr, Lopes B, Amaral J, et al. Ceratocone: Quebra de paradigmas e contradições de uma nova subespecialidade. *Rev Bras Oftalmol.* 2019;78:81–85.
5. Ambrosio R Jr, Faria-Correia F, Silva-Lopes I, Azevedo-Wagner A, Tanos F, Lopes B. Paradigms, paradoxes, and controversies on keratoconus and corneal ectatic diseases. *Int J Kerat Ectatic Corneal Dis.* 2018;7:35–49.
6. Sedaghat MR, Ostadi-Moghadam H, Jabbarvand M, Askarizadeh F, Momeni-Moghaddam H, Narooie-Noori F. Corneal hysteresis and corneal resistance factor in pellucid marginal degeneration. *J Curr Ophthalmol.* 2018;30:42–47.
7. Ambrosio R Jr, Correia FF, Lopes B, et al. Corneal biomechanics in ectatic diseases: refractive surgery implications. *Open Ophthalmol J.* 2017;11:176–193.
8. Ferreira-Mendes J, Lopes BT, Faria-Correia F, Salomão MQ, Rodrigues-Barros S, Ambrósio R Jr. Enhanced ectasia detection using corneal tomography and biomechanics. *Am J Ophthalmol.* 2019;197:7–16.
9. Vinciguerra R, Rehman S, Vallabh NA, et al. Corneal biomechanics and biomechanically corrected intraocular pressure in primary open-angle glaucoma, ocular hypertension and controls. *Br J Ophthalmol.* 2019.
10. Bao F, Geraghty B, Wang Q, Elsheikh A. Consideration of corneal biomechanics in the diagnosis and management of keratoconus: is it important? *Eye Vis.* 2016;3:18.
11. Ambrosio R Jr, Lopes BT, Faria-Correia F, et al. Integration of Scheimpflug-based corneal tomography and biomechanical assessments for enhancing ectasia detection. *J Refract Surg.* 2017;33:434–443.
12. Ogbuehi KC, Osuagwu UL. Corneal biomechanical properties: precision and influence on tonometry. *Cont Lens Anterior Eye.* 2014;37:124–131.
13. Liu J, Roberts CJ. Influence of corneal biomechanical properties on intraocular pressure measurement: quantitative analysis. *J Cataract Refract Surg.* 2005;31:146–155.
14. Blackburn BJ, Jenkins MW, Rollins AM, Dupps WJ. A review of structural and biomechanical changes in the cornea in aging, disease, and photochemical crosslinking. *Front Bioeng Biotechnol.* 2019;7:66.
15. Hashemi H, Ambrosio R Jr, Vinciguerra R, et al. Two-year changes in corneal stiffness parameters after accelerated corneal cross-linking. *J Biomech.* 2019;93:209–212.
16. Vinciguerra R, Romano V, Arbabi EM, et al. In vivo early corneal biomechanical changes after corneal cross-linking in patients with progressive keratoconus. *J Refract Surg.* 2017;33:840–846.

17. Vinciguerra R, Tzamalis A, Romano V, Arbabi EM, Batterbury M, Kaye SB. Assessment of the association between in vivo corneal biomechanical changes after corneal cross-linking and depth of demarcation line. *J Refract Surg*. 2019;35:202–206.
18. Wollensak G, Spoerl E, Seiler T. Riboflavin/ultraviolet-A-induced collagen crosslinking for the treatment of keratoconus. *Am J Ophthalmol*. 2003;135:620–627.
19. da Paz AC, Bersanetti PA, Salomao MQ, Ambrosio R Jr, Schor P. Theoretical basis, laboratory evidence, and clinical research of chemical surgery of the cornea: cross-linking. *J Ophthalmol*. 2014;2014:890823.
20. Wilson SE, Ambrosio R. Computerized corneal topography and its importance to wavefront technology. *Cornea*. 2001;20:441–454.
21. Maeda N, Klyce SD, Tano Y. Detection and classification of mild irregular astigmatism in patients with good visual acuity. *Surv Ophthalmol*. 1998;43:53–58.
22. Li Y, Tan O, Brass R, Weiss JL, Huang D. Corneal epithelial thickness mapping by Fourier-domain optical coherence tomography in normal and keratoconic eyes. *Ophthalmology*. 2012;119:2425–2433.
23. Reinstein DZ, Gobbe M, Archer TJ, Silverman RH, Coleman DJ. Epithelial, stromal, and total corneal thickness in keratoconus: three-dimensional display with artemis very-high frequency digital ultrasound. *J Refract Surg*. 2010;26:259–271.
24. Pahuja N, Shroff R, Pahanpate P, et al. Application of high resolution OCT to evaluate irregularity of Bowman's layer in asymmetric keratoconus. *J Biophotonics*. 2017;10:701–707.
25. Reinstein DZ, Archer TJ, Gobbe M. Corneal epithelial thickness profile in the diagnosis of keratoconus. *J Refract Surg*. 2009;25:604–610.
26. Ambrosio R Jr, Belin MW. Imaging of the cornea: topography vs tomography. *J Refract Surg*. 2010;26:847–849.
27. Ambrosio R Jr, Valbon BF, Faria-Correia F, Ramos I, Luz A. Scheimpflug imaging for laser refractive surgery. *Curr Opin Ophthalmol*. 2013;24:310–320.
28. Smadja D, Touboul D, Cohen A, et al. Detection of subclinical keratoconus using an automated decision tree classification. *Am J Ophthalmol*. 2013;156:237–246. e1.
29. Gomes JA, Tan D, Rapuano CJ, et al. Global consensus on keratoconus and ectatic diseases. *Cornea*. 2015;34:359–369.
30. Ambrosio R Jr, Randleman JB. Screening for ectasia risk: what are we screening for and how should we screen for it? *J Refract Surg*. 2013;29:230–232.
31. Ambrósio R, Dawson DG, Salomão M, Guerra FP, Caiado ALC, Belin MW. Corneal ectasia after LASIK despite low preoperative risk: tomographic and biomechanical findings in the unoperated, stable, fellow eye. *J Refract Surg*. 2010;26:906–911.
32. Ambrósio R Jr, Nogueira LP, Caldas DL, et al. Evaluation of corneal shape and biomechanics before LASIK. *Int Ophthalmol Clin*. 2011;51:11–38.
33. Dawson DG, Ambrosio RJ, Lee WB. Corneal biomechanics: basic science and clinical applications. *Focal Point*. 2016;XXXIV:3–8.
34. Dawson DG, Randleman JB, Grossniklaus HE, et al. Corneal ectasia after excimer laser keratorefractive surgery: histopathology, ultrastructure, and pathophysiology. *Ophthalmology*. 2008;115:2181–2191 e1.
35. McGhee CN, Kim BZ, Wilson PJ. Contemporary treatment paradigms in keratoconus. *Cornea*. 2015;34(suppl 10):S16–S23.
36. Luce DA. Determining in vivo biomechanical properties of the cornea with an ocular response analyzer. *J Cataract Refract Surg*. 2005;31:156–162.
37. Luz A, Faria-Correia F, Salomão MQ, Lopes BT, Ambrósio R Jr. Corneal biomechanics: where are we? *J Curr Ophthalmol*. 2016;28:97.
38. Roberts CJ. Concepts and misconceptions in corneal biomechanics. *J Cataract Refract Surg*. 2014;40:862–869.
39. Pinero DP, Alcon N. In vivo characterization of corneal biomechanics. *J Cataract Refract Surg*. 2014;40:870–887.
40. Terai N, Raiskup F, Haustein M, Pillunat LE, Spoerl E. Identification of biomechanical properties of the cornea: the ocular response analyzer. *Curr Eye Res*. 2012;37:553–562.
41. Shah S, Laiquzzaman M, Bhojwani R, Mantry S, Cunliffe I. Assessment of the biomechanical properties of the cornea with the ocular response analyzer in normal and keratoconic eyes. *Invest Ophthalmol Vis Sci*. 2007;48:3026–3031.

42. Fontes BM, Ambrosio Junior R, Jardim D, Velarde GC, Nose W. Ability of corneal biomechanical metrics and anterior segment data in the differentiation of keratoconus and healthy corneas. *Arq Bras Oftalmol.* 2010;73:333–337.
43. Fontes BM, Ambrosio R Jr, Jardim D, Velarde GC, Nose W. Corneal biomechanical metrics and anterior segment parameters in mild keratoconus. *Ophthalmology.* 2010;117:673–679.
44. Luz A, Fontes BM, Lopes B, Ramos I, Schor P, Ambrosio R Jr. ORA waveform-derived biomechanical parameters to distinguish normal from keratoconic eyes. *Arq Bras Oftalmol.* 2013;76:111–117.
45. Galletti JD, Ruisenor Vazquez PR, Fuentes Bonthoux F, Pfortner T, Galletti JG. Multivariate analysis of the ocular response analyzer's corneal deformation response curve for early keratoconus detection. *J Ophthalmol.* 2015;2015:496382.
46. Hallahan KM, Sinha Roy A, Ambrosio R Jr, Salomao M, Dupps WJ Jr. Discriminant value of custom ocular response analyzer waveform derivatives in keratoconus. *Ophthalmology.* 2014;121:459–468.
47. Ventura BV, Machado AP, Ambrosio R Jr, et al. Analysis of waveform-derived ORA parameters in early forms of keratoconus and normal corneas. *J Refract Surg.* 2013;29:637–643.
48. Kerautret J, Colin J, Touboul D, Roberts C. Biomechanical characteristics of the ectatic cornea. *J Cataract Refract Surg.* 2008;34:510–513.
49. Luz A, Lopes B, Hallahan KM, et al. Enhanced combined tomography and biomechanics data for distinguishing forme fruste keratoconus. *J Refract Surg.* 2016;32:479–494.
50. Spoerl E, Terai N, Scholz F, Raiskup F, Pillunat LE. Detection of biomechanical changes after corneal cross-linking using Ocular Response Analyzer software. *J Refract Surg.* 2011;27:452–457.
51. Vinciguerra P, Albe E, Mahmoud AM, Trazza S, Hafezi F, Roberts CJ. Intra- and postoperative variation in ocular response analyzer parameters in keratoconic eyes after corneal cross-linking. *J Refract Surg.* 2010;26:669–676.
52. Ambrósio R Jr, Ramos I, Luz A, et al. Dynamic ultra high speed Scheimpflug imaging for assessing corneal biomechanical properties. *Rev Bras Oftalmol.* 2013;72:99–102.
53. Roberts CJ, Vinciguerra R, Vinciguerra P, et al. Biomechanical assessment with the Corvis ST integration with tomography. *Oculus Special Supplement.* 2016:2.
54. Salomao MQ, Hofling-Lima AL, Faria-Correia F, et al. Dynamic corneal deformation response and integrated corneal tomography. *Indian J Ophthalmol.* 2018;66:373–382.
55. Ali NQ, Patel DV, McGhee CN. Biomechanical responses of healthy and keratoconic corneas measured using a noncontact Scheimpflug-based tonometer. *Invest Ophthalmol Vis Sci.* 2014;55:3651–3659.
56. Steinberg J, Katz T, Lucke K, Frings A, Druchkiv V, Linke SJ. Screening for keratoconus with new dynamic biomechanical in vivo Scheimpflug analyses. *Cornea.* 2015;34:1404–1412.
57. Sedaghat M-R, Momeni-Moghaddam H, Ambrósio R Jr, et al. Diagnostic ability of corneal shape and biomechanical parameters for detecting frank keratoconus. *Cornea.* 2018;37:1025–1034.
58. Kataria P, Padmanabhan P, Gopalakrishnan A, Padmanaban V, Mahadik S, Ambrosio R Jr. Accuracy of Scheimpflug-derived corneal biomechanical and tomographic indices for detecting subclinical and mild keratectasia in a South Asian population. *J Cataract Refract Surg.* 2019;45:328–336.
59. Tian L, Huang Y-F, Wang L-Q, et al. Corneal biomechanical assessment using corneal visualization Scheimpflug technology in keratoconic and normal eyes. *J Ophthalmol 2014.* 2014.
60. Peña-García P, Peris-Martínez C, Abbouda A, Ruiz-Moreno JM. Detection of subclinical keratoconus through non-contact tonometry and the use of discriminant biomechanical functions. *J Biomech.* 2016;49:353–363.
61. Roberts CJ, Mahmoud AM, Bons JP, et al. Introduction of two novel stiffness parameters and interpretation of air puff–induced biomechanical deformation parameters with a dynamic Scheimpflug analyzer. *J Refract Surg.* 2017;33:266–273.
62. Vinciguerra R, Ambròsio R, Elsheikh A, et al. Analysis of corneal biomechanics using ultra high-speed Scheimpflug imaging to distinguish normal from keratoconic patients. *Invest Ophthalmol Vis Sci.* 2015;56:1130.
63. Joda AA, Shervin MM, Kook D, Elsheikh A. Development and validation of a correction equation for Corvis tonometry. *Comput Methods Biomech Biomed Engin.* 2016;19:943–953.
64. Eliasy A, Chen K-J, Vinciguerra R, et al. Determination of corneal biomechanical behavior in-vivo for healthy eyes using CorVis ST tonometry: stress-strain index. *Front Bioeng Biotechnol.* 2019;7.
65. Lopes BT, Ramos IdC, Salomão MQ, Canedo ALC, Ambrósio R Jr. Perfil paquimétrico horizontal para a detecção do ceratocone. *Rev Bras Oftalmol.* 2015;74:382–385.

66. Vinciguerra R, Ambrosio R Jr, Elsheikh A, et al. Detection of keratoconus with a new biomechanical index. *J Refract Surg*. 2016;32:803–810.
67. Vinciguerra R, Ambrósio R Jr, Elsheikh A, et al. Detection of postlaser vision correction ectasia with a new combined biomechanical index. *Journal of Cataract & Refractive Surgery*. 2021;47:1314–1318.
68. Steinberg J, Siebert M, Katz T, et al. Tomographic and biomechanical Scheimpflug imaging for keratoconus characterization: a validation of current indices. *J Refract Surg*. 2018;34:840–847.
69. Sedaghat MR, Momeni-Moghaddam H, Ambrosio R Jr, et al. Long-term evaluation of corneal biomechanical properties after corneal cross-linking for keratoconus: a 4-year longitudinal study. *J Refract Surg*. 2018;34:849–856.
70. Valbon BF, Ambrosio Jr R, Glicéria J, Santos R, Luz A, Alves MR. Unilateral corneal ectasia after bilateral LASIK: the thick flap counts. *Int J Keratoconus Ectatic Corneal Dis*. 2013;2:79.
71. Shen Y, Han T, Jhanji V, et al. Correlation between corneal topographic, densitometry, and biomechanical parameters in keratoconus eyes. *Transl Vis Sci Technol*. 2019;8:12.
72. Lopes B, Ramos I, Ambrosio R Jr. Corneal densitometry in keratoconus. *Cornea*. 2014;33:1282–1286.
73. Mercer RN, Waring GO, Roberts CJ, et al. Comparison of corneal deformation parameters in keratoconic and normal eyes using a non-contact tonometer with a dynamic ultra-high-speed Scheimpflug camera. *J Refract Surg*. 2017;33:625–631.
74. Fuchsluger TA, Brettl S, Geerling G, Kaisers W, Zeitz PF. Biomechanical assessment of healthy and keratoconic corneas (with/without crosslinking) using dynamic ultrahigh-speed Scheimpflug technology and the relevance of the parameter (A1L– A2L). *Br J Ophthalmol*. 2019;103:558–564.
75. Scarcelli G, Pineda R, Yun SH. Brillouin optical microscopy for corneal biomechanics. *Invest Ophthalmol Vis Sci*. 2012;53:185–190.
76. Scarcelli G, Yun SH. In vivo Brillouin optical microscopy of the human eye. *Opt Express*. 2012;20:9197–9202.
77. Scarcelli G, Kling S, Quijano E, Pineda R, Marcos S, Yun SH. Brillouin microscopy of collagen crosslinking: noncontact depth-dependent analysis of corneal elastic modulus. *Invest Ophthalmol Vis Sci*. 2013;54:1418–1425.
78. Seiler TG, Shao P, Eltony A, Seiler T, Yun SH. Brillouin spectroscopy of normal and keratoconus corneas. *Am J Ophthalmol*. 2019;202:118–125.
79. Chan TC, Wang YM, Yu M, Jhanji V. Comparison of corneal tomography and a new combined tomographic biomechanical index in subclinical keratoconus. *J Refract Surg*. 2018;34:616–621.
80. Koc M, Aydemir E, Tekin K, Inanc M, Kosekahya P, Kiziltoprak H. Biomechanical analysis of subclinical keratoconus with normal topographic, topometric, and tomographic findings. *J Refract Surg*. 2019;35:247–252.
81. Koh S, Ambrósio R, Inoue R, Maeda N, Miki A, Nishida K. Detection of subclinical corneal ectasia using corneal tomographic and biomechanical assessments in a Japanese population. *J Refract Surg*. 2019;35:383–390.

Clinical Classification
and Course

CHAPTER 7

Keratoconus Classification Systems

Ilyse D. Haberman ■ Claudia E. Perez-Straziota ■ J. Bradley Randleman

Introduction

As advances in diagnosis and treatment of keratoconus emerge, classification and staging become essential to monitor progression of the disease and response to treatment. There is currently no consensus on classification systems for keratoconus,[1] and several classification systems have been proposed. Although cone morphology remains the simplest descriptive classification, other more complex classifications systems related to disease severity and risk for progression are more commonly used in clinical decision-making.

The scope of this chapter is the review of the different classification systems to provide the reader with various approaches when making decisions on treatment and assessing results.

Cone Morphology

A simple way to approach classification is based on cone morphology. This approach is relevant in contact lens fittings and potential surgical planning.[2,3] Cone morphology can be evaluated on the tangential anterior curvature map. The types of cones include round *(nipple)* and *oval* cones. Nipple cones are typically smaller in diameter, and central or paracentral, often located inferonasally (Fig. 7.1), whereas oval cones are ellipsoid in shape and usually located in the inferotemporal meridian (Fig. 7.2A,B). Although morphology has relevance, this classification does little to impart significant understanding of the severity of current disease or future prognosis.

Keratoconus Disease Severity Classification Systems

Many systems have been proposed (Table 7.1); the most commonly referred to are the Amsler-Krumeich classification,[4] the Collaborative Longitudinal Evaluation of Keratoconus (CLEK) study classification,[5,6] and the more recent Belin ABCD classification.[7] Other less utilized proposed systems include the Keratoconus Severity Score,[8] the Alió-Shabayek classification,[9] and the anterior segment optical coherence tomography (AS-OCT) classification.[10]

AMSLER-KRUMEICH CLASSIFICATION (1938, MODIFIED 1998)

The Amsler-Krumeich (Table 7.2) is the oldest and most commonly used classification system. Corneas are graded according to severity of ectatic disease, ranging from stage 1 to 4, with 4 being the most severe. This system utilizes apex anterior corneal curvature, apex corneal thickness, manifest refraction, and presence or absence of corneal scarring.[4]

The main limitations of this system are that it predates many of the current imaging modalities currently used to diagnosis keratoconus, relies on subjective clinical judgment as diseased

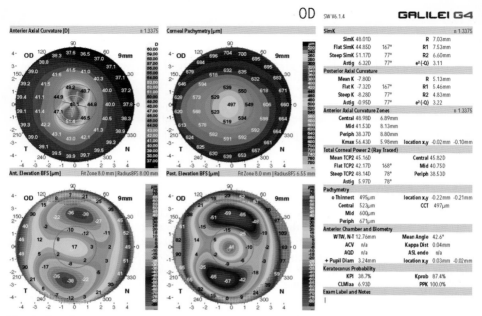

Fig. 7.1 Dual Scheimpflug/Placido map showing the morphology of a round (nipple) cone, with a focal central steepening, thinning, and increased elevations.

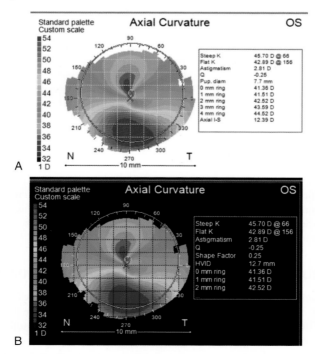

Fig. 7.2 Placido topography showing the morphology of an oval cone, with a broader base of steepening located inferiorly.

TABLE 7.1 ■ **Keratoconus Classification Systems**

System Name	Date Instituted	Primary Variables	Technology Used
Amsler-Krumeich[4,11]	1938, modified 1998	K_m, corneal thickness, manifest refraction, scarring	Manual keratometry
CLEK study[5,6]	1996	K_m	Manual keratometry
Alió-Shabayek[9]	2006	K_m, thickness, RMS HOA, scarring	Placido-disk videokeratography
Keratoconus Severity Score[8]	2006	Slit-lamp findings, topographic pattern, corneal power, RMS HOA	Placido-disk topography
AS-OCT[10]	2013	Corneal thickness, opacity	Fourier-domain optical coherence tomography
Belin ABCD[7]	2016	ARC, PRC, thickness, CDVA, scarring	Scheimpflug tomography

ARC, Anterior radius of curvature; *AS-OCT,* anterior segment optical coherence tomography; *CDVA,* corrected distance visual acuity; *CLEK,* Collaborative Longitudinal Evaluation of Keratoconus study; K_m, mean keratometry; *PRC,* posterior radius of curvature; *RMS HOA,* root mean square higher-order aberrations.

TABLE 7.2 ■ **Amsler-Krumeich Classification of Keratoconus[4]**

Severity	K_m (sim k, D)	Thickness (µm)	Myopia and Astigmatism (D)	Cornea
1	<48	>500	<5.00	Eccentric steepening, no central scars
2	48–53	400–500	5.00 to <8.00	No central scars
3	54–55	200–400	8.00 – 10.00	No central scars
4	>55	<200	Not measurable	Central scars

K_m, Mean keratometry; *sim k,* simulated keratometry; *µm,* microns.

corneas may fit into more than one stage, and does not provide easy monitoring of progression across stages.

Most importantly, as measurements are taken at the apical surface, they may not reflect the severity of the cone, which in the majority of cases is displaced.

CLEK STUDY CLASSIFICATION (1996)

The CLEK study was an observational study undertaken to identify risk for severity and progression of keratoconus. Based on keratometric readings, patients were classified as mild (steep keratometry [K] < 45 diopters [D]), moderate (steep K between 45 D and 52 D), or severe (steep K >52 D) (Figs. 7.3–7.5).[5,6] Other factors that were recorded were high- and low-contrast visual acuity, manifest refraction, fluorescein patterns in habitual contacts lens users, and slit-lamp biomicroscopic changes, most importantly related to scarring (Table 7.3, Figs. 7.6–7.8), first definite apical clearance contact lens (FDACL; the flattest rigid contact lens that demonstrated apical clearance), and patient-reported quality of life.[5,6]

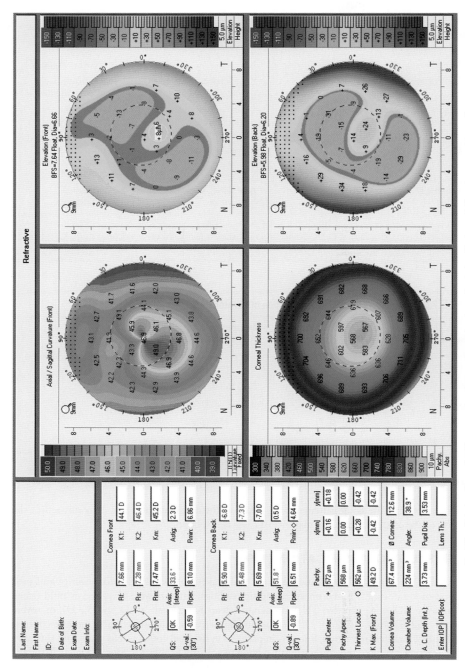

Fig. 7.3 Scheimpflug refractive map showing an example of a patient classified as mild keratoconus (stage 1).

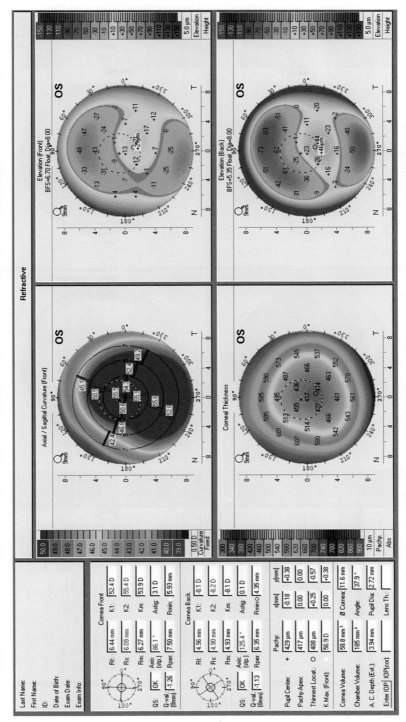

Fig. 7.4 Scheimpflug refractive map showing an example of a patient classified as moderate keratoconus (stages 2–3).

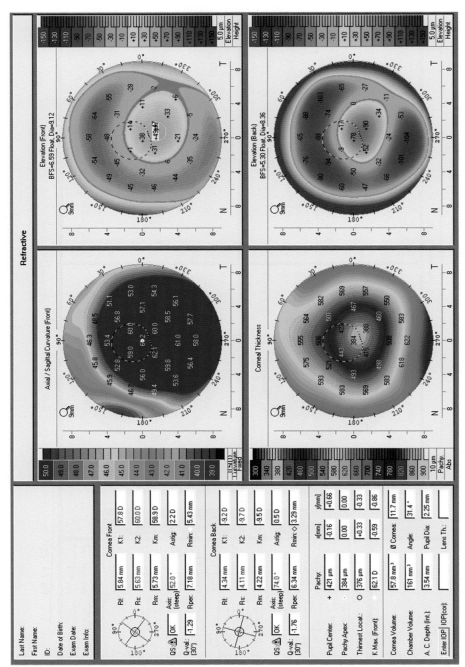

Fig. 7.5 Scheimpflug refractive map showing an example of a patient classified as severe keratoconus (stages 3–4).

TABLE 7.3 ■ **Grade of Corneal Scarring in the CLEK Study[8]**

Grade	Overall Scarring
1.0	Trace and not on line of sight, <1.5 mm total size
2.0	Easily noticeable and approaching line of sight, 1.5–2.5 mm total size
3.0	Dense but translucent and impinging on line of sight, total size 2.5 mm or greater
4.0	Opaque and on line of sight, size 2.5 mm or greater

CLEK, Collaborative Longitudinal Evaluation of Keratoconus study.

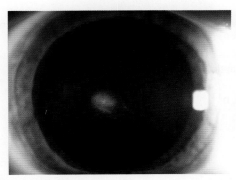

Fig. 7.6   Slit-lamp imaging showing a patient with keratoconus with mild scarring just at the edge of the visual axis. The scarring in this case was minimally symptomatic.

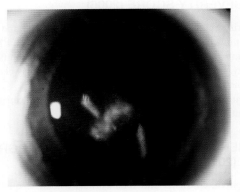

Fig. 7.7   Slit-lamp imaging showing a patient with keratoconus with moderate scarring within the visual axis. The scarring in this case was moderately symptomatic.

ALIÓ-SHABAYEK CLASSIFICATION (2006)

With the adoption of newer technology, higher-order aberrations were incorporated into a classification system using Placido-disk topography to measure Zernike coefficients.[9] The increase in higher-order aberrations in keratoconic corneas is mainly due to coma-like aberrations.[12,13] In this classification system, the root mean square value of coma-like aberrations is added to mean keratometry, corneal thickness, and biomicroscopic evidence of corneal scarring (Table 7.4).

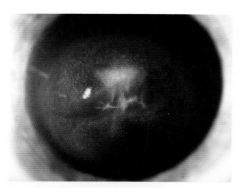

Fig. 7.8   Slit-lamp imaging showing a patient with keratoconus with more advanced scarring within the visual axis. The scarring in this case significantly limited visual acuity.

TABLE 7.4   ■   **Alió-Shabayek Classification[9]**

Severity	K_m (sim k, D)	Thickness (μm)	RMS of Coma-Like Aberrations (μm)	Cornea
1	<48		1.50–2.50	No central scars
2	48–53	>400	2.50–3.50	No central scars
3	53–55	300–400	3.50–4.50	No central scars
4	>55	200–300	>4.50	Central scars

K_m, Mean keratometry; *RMS,* root mean square; *sim k,* simulated keratometry; *μm,* microns.

KERATOCONUS SEVERITY SCORE (2006)

The Keratoconus Severity Score (Table 7.5) was published in 2006 and similarly included slit-lamp findings, topography characteristics, average corneal power (ACP), and higher-order first corneal surface wavefront root mean square error (HORMSE),[8] which is considered to correlate with corneal irregularity.[13-15] In this classification, corneal scarring is classified according to the CLEK criteria (see Table 7.5).

When additional features are assessed, the "worst" of the features carries the greater weight (as long as the required features are met).

ANTERIOR SEGMENT OCULAR COHERENCE TOMOGRAPHY CLASSIFICATION (2013)

In this classification system, epithelial and total corneal thickness qualitative and quantitative measurements are obtained at the cone, classifying corneas into stages 1 through 5. The severity of these structural changes has been correlated with the severity of visual acuity loss, higher-order aberrations, and corneal topographic and biomechanical changes (Figs. 7.9–7.11).[10,14]

AS-OCT stages are classified as follows[10]:
- Stage 1: thinning of epithelial and stromal layers at the conus
- Stage 2: hyperreflective anomalies occurring at the Bowman's layer level (varying from a barely visible hyperreflective line to a hypertrophic scar) and epithelial thickening at the conus
  - 2a: clear stroma
  - 2b: stromal opacities

TABLE 7.5 ■ Keratoconus Severity Score[8]

Severity	Scarring Typical for KCN	Slit-Lamp Findings for KCN	Axial Pattern	ACP (D)	HORMSE (μm)
0 Unaffected	None[a]	None[a]	Typical[a]	<47.75[a]	<0.65[a]
1 Unaffected—atypical topography	None[a]	None[a]	Atypical (irregular pattern, asymmetric bowtie, or inferior or superior steepening no more than 3 D steeper than ACP)[a]	<48[a]	<1.00[a]
2 Suspect	None[a]	None[a]	Isolated area of steepening[a]	<49[b]	1.0–1.50[b]
3 Affected—mild disease	None[a]	May have[a]	Pattern consistent with KCN[a]	<52[b]	1.50–3.50[b]
4 Affected—moderate disease	Up to grade 3.0[c]	Must have[a]	Pattern consistent with KCN[a]	52–56[b]	3.50–5.75[b]
5 Affected—severe disease	Grade 3.5 or greater[c]	Must have[a]	Pattern consistent with KCN[a]	>56[b]	>5.75[b]

[a]Required features.
[b]Additional features.
[c]Corneal scarring CLEK grade.
ACP, Average corneal power; CLEK, Collaborative Longitudinal Evaluation of Keratoconus; HORMSE, higher-order first corneal surface wavefront root mean square error; KCN, keratoconus.

- Stage 3: posterior displacement of the hyperreflective structures occurring at the Bowman's layer level with increased epithelial thickening and stromal thinning
  - 3a: clear stroma
  - 3b: stromal opacities
- Stage 4: pan-stromal scar
- Stage 5: acute form of keratoconus (hydrops)
  - 5a: acute onset, characterized by the rupture of Descemet membrane with dilacerations of collagen lamellae, large fluid-filled intrastromal cysts, and the formation of epithelial edema
  - 5b: healing stage, pan-stromal scarring with a remaining aspect of Descemet membrane rupture.

BELIN ABCD CLASSIFICATION (2016)

Newer imaging modalities provide more specific data points, which allows further classification and assessment of progression of ectatic corneas. The Belin ABCD classification system (Table 7.6) grades each criterion individually, and takes into account:

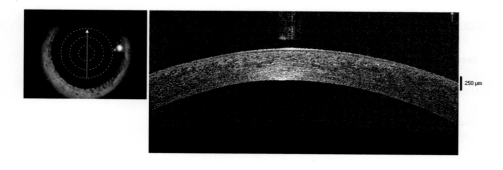

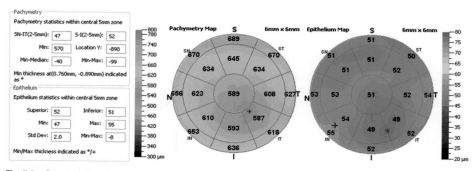

Fig. 7.9 Spectral domain optical coherence tomography image showing an example of a patient with mild keratoconus. Total thickness is 570 μm in the thinnest location, and there is focal epithelial thinning and no obvious alterations in terms of scarring or major corneal irregularity, as shown in the upper cross-sectional imaging.

A: anterior radius of curvature, measured in the 3-mm zone surrounding the thinnest point.
B: posterior radius of curvature, measured in the 3-mm zone surrounding the thinnest point.
C: thinnest corneal pachymetry, measured at the thinnest point rather than the apex.
D: best-corrected distance vision and scarring.

For the anterior radius of curvature parameter (expressed in millimeters), stages 1 to 4 use the equivalent keratometries (expressed in D) of the anterior classification in the Amsler-Krumeich system, with stage 0 approximating a normal cornea (Figs. 7.12 and 7.13).[7]

Classifying Keratoconus Progression

With the introduction of corneal cross-linking (CXL) into the treatment strategies for keratoconus, determining whether the disease is in a progressive phase that would benefit from CXL to halt progression has become critical. The first proposed metric to assess progression of keratoconus, and the metric used for most initial trials, was increase of K_{max}[16] by at least 1 D in a 24-month period.[17] It is important to distinguish K_{max}, which is the steepest K throughout the whole anterior surface, from steepest K, which is the steepest K measured within the central 3-mm diameter, as the central 3 mm of the cornea may not contain the steepest point in a displaced cone.

The use of K_{max} in isolation to determine progression is limited owing to its high intertest variation[18–20] and its true ability to accurately reflect the extent of the cone. Additionally, the use of only one anterior surface metric makes it difficult to evaluate progression in early keratoconus cases, as imaging early cones reproducibly is challenging, and there may be other metrics that are altered earlier than K_{max}.[21–23] For the US Food and Drug Administration (FDA) clinical trials, in

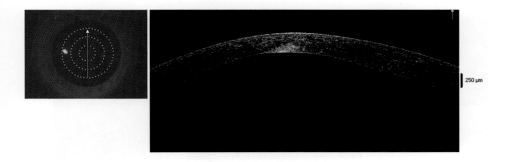

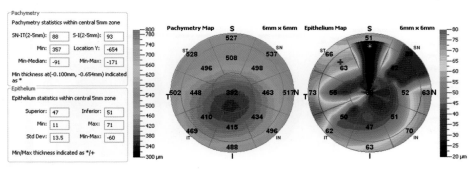

Fig. 7.10 Spectral domain optical coherence tomography image showing an example of a patient with more advanced keratoconus. Total thickness is 357 μm in the thinnest location; there is significant epithelial thinning and irregularity, and mild stromal hyperreflectivity indicating mild scarring is shown in the upper cross-sectional imaging.

addition to change in K_{max}, progressive keratoconus or ectasia was defined as one or more of the following changes over a period of 24 months: an increase of 1.00 D or more in the steepest K measurement, an increase of 1.00 D or more in manifest cylinder, or an increase of 0.50 D or more in manifest refraction spherical equivalent (MRSE).

The use of difference maps with Scheimpflug and Placido imaging provides a better visual representation of the K changes across the cornea, which may show progression of values outside of K_{max} (Fig. 7.14).

Other metrics have been explored to assess early changes and response to CXL treatments. No individual metrics appear to capture the changes better, especially in early keratoconic corneas, than the combination of different metrics from different technologies.[24–26]

The ABCD classification system also monitors progression and/or response to treatment over time using the four variables described earlier. For comparison of measurements over time, the OCULUS Pentacam ABCD Progression Display allows up to eight examination timepoints to be shown in a bar graph as well as numerical display (Figs. 7.15 and 7.16). The stage of each parameter is mapped with the associated confidence interval for normal and keratoconic eyes. This visual representation simplifies the assessment of progression over time.[27]

Conclusion

Keratoconus can manifest in various and very different severities with different prognoses and responses to treatment. There is currently no unified consensus on classification of disease or definition of progression. Innovations in technology have allowed classification systems to evolve

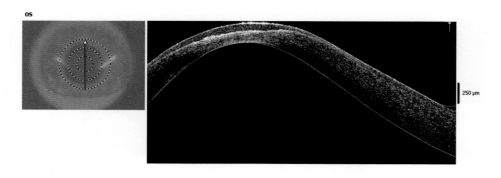

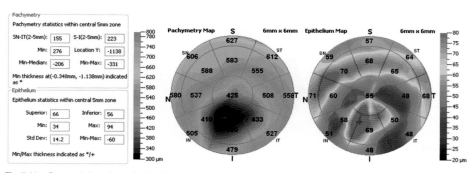

Fig. 7.11 Spectral domain optical coherence tomography image showing an example of a patient with severe keratoconus. Total thickness is 276 μm in the thinnest location; there is significant epithelial thinning and irregularity with focal epithelial hypertrophy, and significant stromal hyperreflectivity indicating scarring is shown in the upper cross-sectional imaging.

TABLE 7.6 ■ Belin ABCD Classification[7]

ABCD Criteria	A: ARC at 3-mm Zone (mm, D)	B: PRC at 3-mm Zone (mm, D)	C: Thinnest Pachymetry (μm)	D: CDVA	Scarring[a]
Stage 0	>7.25 (<46.5 D)	>5.90 (<57.25 D)	>490	≥20/20	–
Stage I	>7.05 (<48.0 D)	>5.7 (<59.25 D)	>450	<20/20	–/+/++
Stage II	>6.35 (<53 D)	>5.15 (<65.5 D)	>400	<20/40	–/+/++
Stage III	>6.15 (<55 D)	>4.95 (<68.5 D)	>300	<20/100	–/+/++
Stage IV	<6.15 (>55 D)	<4.95 (>68.5 D)	≤300	<20/400	–/+/++

[a]Scarring classified into (–) no scarring, (+) scarring that does not obscure iris details, or (++) scarring that obscures iris details.
ARC, Anterior radius of curvature; *CDVA,* corrected distance visual acuity; *PRC,* posterior radius of curvature; *μm,* microns.

from relying on manual K measurement to analyzing higher-order aberrations, and anterior and posterior curvatures. The most important feature of a classification system is the ability to detect early progression to make well-informed treatment decisions and treatment response predictions.

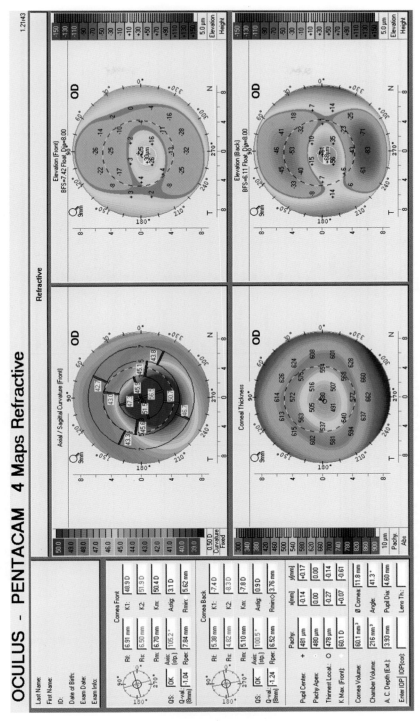

Fig. 7.12 Scheimpflug refractive map showing a patient with moderate keratoconus.

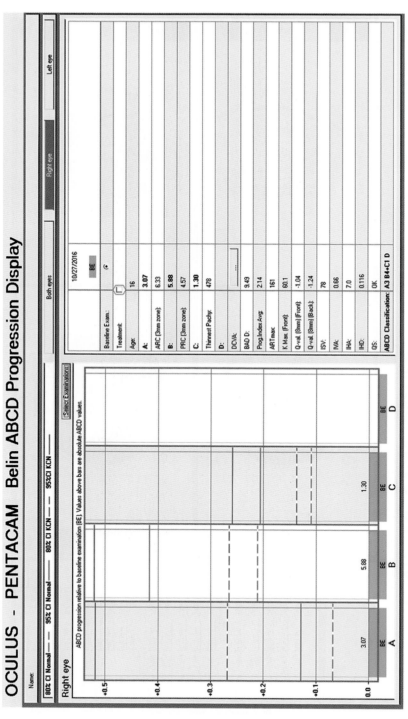

Fig. 7.13 Belin ABCD Progression Display for the same eye showing the baseline values for each category.

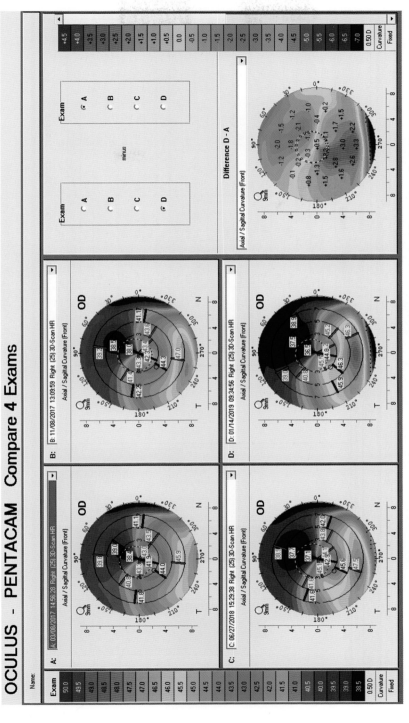

Fig. 7.14 Scheimpflug difference map showing change in anterior curvature for the right eye of a patient with keratoconus showing progression of disease based on steepening anterior curvature over four visits. The lower right image shows the total difference in anterior curvature over the course of 2 years.

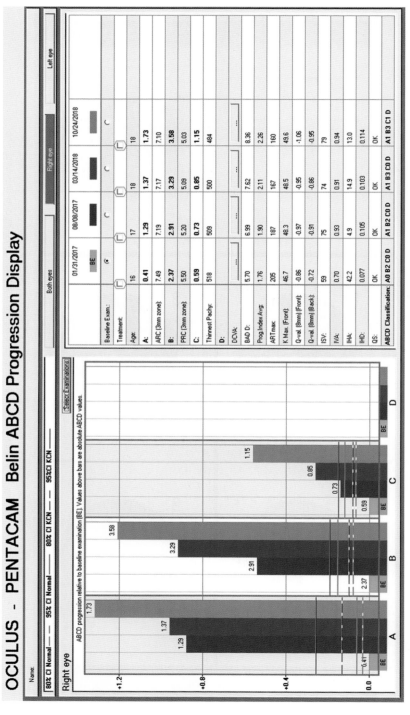

Fig. 7.15 Belin ABCD Progression Display for a patient with stable keratoconus. Over the course of 2 years there have been some fluctuations in values but no net change and ultimately no disease progression.

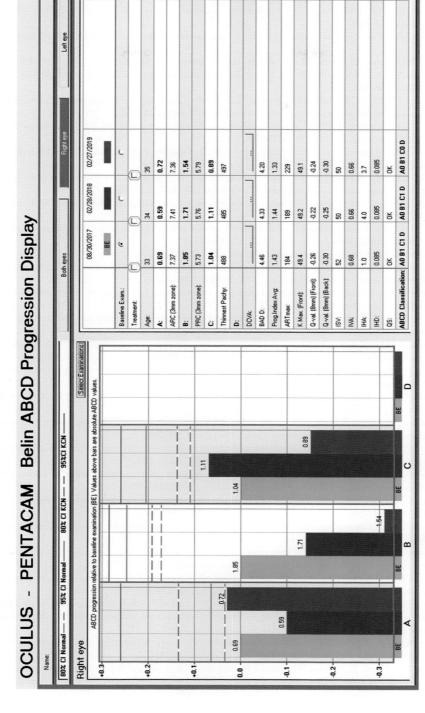

Fig. 7.16 Belin ABCD Progression Display for a different patient with progressive keratoconus. Over the course of 18 months there has been clear worsening in every category, confirming disease progression.

References

1. Gomes JA, Tan D, Rapuano CJ, et al. Global consensus on keratoconus and ectatic diseases. *Cornea.* 2015;34(4):359–369.
2. Sinjab MM. *Quick Guide to the Management of Keratoconus and Keratectasia.* Berlin, Heidelberg: Springer; 2012.
3. Perry HD, Buxton JN, Fine BS. Round and oval cones in keratoconus. *Ophthalmology.* 1980;87(9):905–909.
4. Krumeich JH, Daniel J, Knülle A. Live-epikeratophakia for keratoconus. *J Cataract Refract Surg.* 1998;24(4):456–463.
5. Wagner H, Barr JT, Zadnik K. Collaborative Longitudinal Evaluation of Keratoconus (CLEK) study: methods and findings to date. *Cont Lens Anterior Eye.* 2007;30(4):223–232.
6. Zadnik K. Baseline findings in the collaborative longitudinal evaluation of keratoconus study. *Invest Ophthalmol Vis Sci.* 1998;39:2537–2546.
7. Belin MW, Duncan JK. Keratoconus: the ABCD Grading System. *Klin Monbl Augenheilkd.* 2016;233(6):701–707.
8. McMahon TT, Szczotka-Flynn L, Barr JT, et al. CLEK study group. A new method for grading the severity of keratoconus: the Keratoconus Severity Score (KSS). *Cornea.* 2006;25(7):794–800.
9. Alió JL, Shabayek MH. Corneal higher order aberrations: a method to grade keratoconus. *J Refract Surg.* 2006;22(6):539–545.
10. Sandali O, et al. Fourier-domain optical coherence tomography imaging in keratoconus: a corneal structural classification. *Ophthalmology.* 2013;120(12):2403–2412.
11. Amsler M. Le kératocône fruste au Javal. *Ophthalmologica.* 1938;96:77–83.
12. Maeda N, Fujikado T, Kuroda T, et al. Wavefront aberrations measured with Hartmann-Shack sensor in patients with keratoconus. *Ophthalmology.* 2002;109(11):1996–2003.
13. Gobbe M, Guillon M. Corneal wavefront aberration measurements to detect keratoconus patients. *Cont Lens Anterior Eye.* 2005;28(2):57–66.
14. Pinero DP, et al. Corneal biomechanics, refraction, and corneal aberrometry in keratoconus: an integrated study. *Invest Ophthalmol Vis Sci.* 2010;51(4):1948–1955.
15. Piccinini AL, et al. Corneal higher-order aberrations measurements: Comparison between Scheimpflug and dual Scheimpflug-Placido technology in keratoconic eyes. *J Cataract Refract Surg.* 2019;45(7):985–991.
16. Wollensak G, Spoerl E, Seiler T. Riboflavin/ultraviolet-A-induced collagen crosslinking for the treatment of keratoconus. *Am J Ophthalmo.* 2003;135(5):620–627.
17. Hersh PS, et al. United States Multicenter Clinical Trial of corneal collagen crosslinking for keratoconus treatment. *Ophthalmology.* 2017;124(9):1259–1270.
18. Vianna LM, Muñoz B, Hwang FS, Gupta A, Jun AS. Variability in Oculus Pentacam tomographer measurements in patients with keratoconus. *Cornea.* 2015;34(3):285–289.
19. Meyer JJ, et al. Repeatability and agreement of Orbscan II, Pentacam HR, and Galilei tomography systems in corneas with keratoconus. *Am J Ophthalmol.* 2017;175:122–128.
20. Hashemi H, Yekta A, Khabazkhoob M. Effect of keratoconus grades on repeatability of keratometry readings: comparison of 5 devices. *J Cataract Refract Surg.* 2015;41(5):1065–1072.
21. Shajari M, et al. Early tomographic changes in the eyes of patients with keratoconus. *J Refract Surg.* 2018;34(4):254–259.
22. Bae GH, et al. Corneal topographic and tomographic analysis of fellow eyes in unilateral keratoconus patients using Pentacam. *Am J Ophthalmol.* 2014;157(1):103–109. e1.
23. Reinstein DZ, et al. Detection of keratoconus in clinically and algorithmically topographically normal fellow eyes using epithelial thickness analysis. *J Refract Surg.* 2015;31(11):736–744.
24. Lang PZ, et al. Comparing change in anterior curvature after corneal cross-linking using scanning-slit and Scheimpflug technology. *Am J Ophthalmol.* 2018;191:129–134.
25. Lang PZ, Hafezi NL, Khandelwal SS, Torres-Netto EA, Hafezi F, Randleman JB. Comparative functional outcomes after corneal crosslinking using standard, accelerated, and accelerated with higher total fluence protocols. *Cornea.* 2019;38(4):433–441.
26. Savini G, et al. Repeatability of automatic measurements by a new Scheimpflug camera combined with Placido topography. *J Cataract Refract Surg.* 2011;37(10):1809–1816.
27. Belin BW, Meyer JJ, Duncan JK, Gelman R, Borgstrom M, Ambrósio R Jr. Assessing progression of keratoconus and cross-linking efficacy: the Belin ABCD Progression Display. *Int J Keratoconus Ectatic Corneal Dis.* 2017;6(1):1–10.

CHAPTER 8

Clinical Course and Progression of Keratoconus

David Smadja ■ Mark Krauthammer

KEY CONCEPTS

- The progression of keratoconus is variable and is linked to environmental factors and eye-rubbing habits, as well as to multiple genes.
- To date, there is no consensus on criteria or cutoff values to define progression in keratoconus. The use of multiple parameters may help to better identify patients who might benefit from cross-linking treatments.
- Caution should be taken when assessing progression on a single parameter, as measurement predictability drops as the severity of keratoconus increases.

Clinical Course and Progression of Keratoconus: Current State of the Art

NATURAL CLINICAL COURSE

Keratoconus (KC) is defined as a bilateral and asymmetric progressive corneal ectasia with onset typically during the second decade of life.[1] Although KC may rarely manifest at a later age, progression is uncommon.[2] The average age at diagnosis reported in the literature stands between 25 and 27 years.[3-11] However, with increased awareness by ophthalmologists and optometrists, studies published over the past 10 years have reported an average age at diagnosis to be less than 20 years.[12-15] Although KC patients can be of any ethnic or geographic background,[16] worldwide, younger patients at diagnosis are frequently from the Middle East or Asia[17,18] and tend to present initially with more severe KC.

The manifestation and progression of the disease are highly variable and are most often asymmetric between the two eyes of the same patient. It is widely accepted that there is no truly unilateral KC. Even when no clinical signs of the disease can be seen in the fellow eye, it is still considered that KC has simply not yet manifested in that eye. This condition is also known in the literature as "subclinical keratoconus," and it has already been reported that approximately 50% of clinically normal fellow eyes of patients with a unilateral KC progress to KC within 16 years, with a greater risk during the first 6 years of onset.[19] A meta-analysis that reviewed the natural progression of 11,529 untreated KC eyes identified the population below 17 years old with steeper corneas at presentation (above 55 diopters [D] of maximum keratometry (K_{max})) has increased risk of progression.[20] However, a complex relationship exists between the natural course of the disease and the kinetics of its progression, and patient behaviors such as eye rubbing.[21] More recently, a study of KC in a pediatric population has raised the question of the possible impact of the awareness of the patient and their family about eye rubbing and the potential of this awareness to slow or halt disease progression. In this study, the second eye of the patient, left untreated, remained stable over a 5-year period after cross-linking of the first eye.[15] Although not investigated in a randomized comparative study, the authors hypothesized that the reduction or discontinuation of eye rubbing after cross-linking treatment of the first eye might have contributed to slowing the progression of the second eye.

DEFINITION OF A PROGRESSIVE STATE

Progression of ectatic disease remains challenging to define and therefore explains the diversity of indices presented in the literature that indicate progression. A summary of the current indices is shown in Table 8.1. The Global Delphi Panel on Keratoconus and Ectatic Disease recognized that there was no clear definition of ectasia progression. The panel suggested that it should be defined by a reliable change for the worse in two or three of the following parameters: radius of the anterior corneal curvature; radius of the posterior corneal curvature and central corneal thickness; or increase in the rate of change of pachymetry from the periphery to the thinnest point.[10] The panel of experts considered that although KC progression frequently leads to a worsening in corrected distance visual acuity (CDVA), a change in both uncorrected distance visual acuity (UCDVA) and CDVA was not required for documenting progression. In addition, they agreed that specific quantitative data were lacking to determine progression and that such data would most probably be specific to a given device. Interestingly, although multiple diagnostic grading systems for ectatic disease have been proposed over the past years, there is still no true correlation or association between those grading systems and the criteria used to monitor disease progression. The oldest grading system, the Amsler-Krumeich scale, which is still the most commonly used, grades the disease from early (grade 1) to severe (grade 4) KC, and is based only on anterior keratometric and corneal thickness measurements, together with refraction and clinical assessment.[22] More recent scales, such as those proposed by Alió and Shabayek[23] and the RET-ICS classification,[24] have added the measurement of coma aberrations, which reflects the level of corneal asymmetry. However, none of these have been applied to monitoring disease progression The Belin ABCD Classification/Staging display and the Belin ABCD Progression display—both based on information from minimal corneal thickness, the anterior and posterior radius of curvature, and best spectacle distance visual acuity—represent a promising way of being able to establish the relationship between the diagnosis/classification and the progression of the ectasia.

One of the most important studies, which contributed to the United States Food and Drug Administration (FDA) approval of collagen cross-linking treatment, was performed on behalf of the United States Crosslinking Study Group and published in 2017. KC progression or ectasia in this study was defined as one or more of the following changes over a period of 24 months: an increase of 1.00 D or more in the steepest keratometry measurement, an increase of 1.00 D or more in manifest cylinder, or an increase of 0.50 D or more in manifest refraction spherical equivalent.[25] As illustrated in Table 8.1, the challenge of defining progression of ectatic disease remains incomplete and requires further study to designate widely acceptable monitoring guidelines. Significant problems are the disparity of diagnostic tools for measuring corneal properties and a lack of knowledge of the kinetics of disease progression. Further understanding may lead to an optimization of monitoring and to guidelines on the frequency of monitoring. To date, it seems reasonable to follow a KC patient before their third decade every 6 months unless risk factors such as younger age, pregnancy, or even warning signs such as recent isolated progression of the coma or posterior steepening are identified, which would require closer monitoring (every 3 months or more frequently depending on the case).

IDENTIFIED RISK FACTORS OF PROGRESSION

Several risk factors have been identified for KC and its progression and are summarized in Table 8.2. Some of these risk factors, especially eye rubbing, are preventable.

TABLE 8.1 ■ Diversity of the Criteria Used in the Literature for Defining the Progressive State of Ectatic Disease (in Chronological Order)

Publication	Year	K_{max} Ant	Corneal Thickness	Cylinder	Visual Acuity	MRSE	Other Criteria
Raiskup-Wolf et al.[49]	2008	>1 D in 1 year			Subjective loss of BCVA		
Wittig-Silva et al.[50]	2008	>1 D over 6–12 months				SE >0.5 D in 6–12 months	
Vinciguerra et al.[51]	2009	>1.5 D in 6 months	Thinning TP >5% in 6 months	>3 D in 6 months		Myopia >3 D in 6 months	
Hersh et al.[52]	2011	>1 D in 2 years		>1 D in 2 years		SE >0.5 D in 2 years	
O'Brart et al.[53]	2011	>0.75 D in 18 months		>0.75 D in 18 months	Worsening >1 line in 18 months		
Choi and Kim[6]	2012	>1.5 D in 1 year					
Chatzis and Hafezi[54]	2012	>1 D in 1 year					
Hashemi et al.[55]	2013	>1 D in 1 year		>1 D in 1 year		SE >1 D in 1 year	
Mazzotta et al.[56]	2014	>1 D in 6 months	Thinning TP >10 μm in 6 months		Worsening >0.5 line UDVA/CDVA in 6 months	SE >0.5 D in 6 months	SAI or IS >0.5 D in 6 months
Stojanovic et al.[57]	2014	>1.5 D in 12 months		>1 D in 12 months		Myopia >1 D in 12 months	
Shetty et al.[58]	2015	>1 D in 6 months	Thinning TP >5% in 6 months			SE >1 D in 6 months	
Poli et al.[59]	2015	>0.7 5 D in 6 months	Thinning TP >10 μm in 6 months		Worsening >1 line UDVA/CDVA in 6 months	SE >0.5 D in 6 months	
Godefrooij et al.[60]	2016	>1 D in 6–12 months					
Hersh et al.[25]	2017	≥1 D in 24 months		≥1 D in 24 months		SE > -0.5 D in 24 months	

AntK, Anterior keratometry; *BCVA,* best corrected visual acuity; *CDVA,* corrected distance visual acuity; *D,* diopters; *IS,* inferior-superior index; *Kmax,* Maximum Keratometry; *MRSE,* manifest refractive spherical equivalent; *OZ,* optical zone; *SAI,* surface asymmetry index; *SE,* spherical equivalent; *TP,* thinnest point; *UDVA,* uncorrected distance visual acuity.

TABLE 8.2 ■ Risk Factors for Ectatic Corneal Disease and Keratoconus Progression and Their Preventability

	Risk Factors	
Mechanical factors	Surgically induced weakening (LASIK or PRK) in subclinical or early keratoconus	P
	Surgically induced weakening in normal preoperative topographies with PTA >40%	P
	Persistent and forceful eye rubbing	P
Genetic factors	Relative with KC in the family (first degree at higher risk)	N
	Connective tissue disorders (Ehlers-Danlos syndrome)	N
	Down syndrome	N
	Leber congenital amaurosis	N
Age	Younger age: children and adolescent	N
Corneal features	Advanced KC: AntK >50 D; TP <450 µm; MPE >50 µm; Cyl >1.9 D	N
	"Unilateral" keratoconus diagnosed implies FFKC in the CL eye	N
	Progression of corneal vertical coma over three successive examinations	N
	Progression of posterior Ks over three successive examinations	N
Biological and hormonal factors	Pregnancy	P
	Low vitamin D levels	NA

AntK, Anterior keratometry; *CL,* contralateral; *Cyl, Cylinder; D,* diopters; *FFKC,* forme fruste keratoconus; *K,* keratometry; *KC,* keratoconus; *MPE,* maximal posterior elevation; *N,* nonpreventable; *NA,* not available; *P,* preventable; *PRK,* photorefractive keratectomy; *PTA,* percentage tissue altered; *TP,* thinning point.

Mechanical Factors

A well-recognized risk factor for corneal weakening is eye rubbing (and the diseases that are associated with eye rubbing, such as chronic inflammation of the ocular surface, ocular allergy, and atopy).[26] Eye rubbing has been shown to increase the level of inflammatory mediators in tears (matrix metalloproteinase 13 [MMP-13], interleukin [IL]-6, and tumor necrosis factor [TNF]-α) in a population of normal subjects. This increase in protease activity and inflammatory mediators in the tears may be exacerbated during the persistent and forceful eye rubbing seen in the KC population and may contribute to the progression of the disease.[27] More recently a case-control study has demonstrated a strong correlation between the type of eye-rubbing habits and sleep position and KC. Surgical weakening by LASIK or even photorefractive keratectomy (PRK) is another well-known risk factor for the decompensation of ectatic disease,[28] although it has been shown that this could occur in preoperative normal corneas that undergo a surgical procedure that may weaken its structure beyond its natural threshold of resistance.[29] Indeed, our group has recently demonstrated that a percentage of tissue altered by surgery above 40% of the preoperative corneal thickness was considered the strongest risk factor for ectasia and therefore should be carefully taken into account during preoperative screening for laser vision correction.[29]

Genetic Factors

Although the precise etiology of KC remains unknown, several studies suggest that genetic background plays a significant role in the pathogenesis of the disorder.[30] KC has been associated with a wide range of genetic diseases, including Down syndrome, connective tissue disorders (Ehlers-Danlos syndrome), and Leber congenital amaurosis, implying that genetics may have a key role in the development of KC or that these genetic disorders favor a "two-hit" phenomenon.[30] Genetic predisposition has also been well characterized, with high prevalence in families with one affected individual and high concordance among monozygotic twins.[31] In the literature the prevalence of familial KC varies from 6% to 53%.[30,32] The most recent reports by Kymionis et al. found that 53% of clinically unaffected relatives presented with abnormal corneal patterns in at least one eye, further indicating an increased frequency of abnormal corneal topographic patterns in relatives of KC patients.[32]

Age

Age has been well documented as a critical risk factor for KC progression, as the disease may appear very early in life.[33] As age increases, corneal collagen fibrils become thicker, and naturally occurring cross-linking increases stiffness of the tissue (determined by a parameter called the Young's modulus). These natural changes might explain why when KC presents earlier in life, the patient has a higher risk of progression and progresses until the third to fourth decades of life, when it typically halts. Therefore children and adolescents diagnosed with KC are considered at higher risk of faster KC progression than adults.

Corneal Features

Advanced KC with higher corneal curvature (Anterior Keratometry) and high corneal cylinder over 1.9 D has been shown in several studies to be associated with more rapid progression.[10] Similar findings were recently confirmed in pediatric KC, where eyes with the thinnest point inferior to 450 μm, anterior keratometry above 50 D, and posterior elevation above 50 μm at presentation demonstrated higher rates of progressive corneal thinning.[34] More recently our group has demonstrated the relevance of other key parameters in the monitoring of KC progression, such as the steepest posterior keratometry and the vertical corneal coma. Progression in these parameters may occur months before the increase in anterior keratometry, which is the most classic parameter used today for monitoring KC progression. Therefore progression observed in such parameters can be considered as potential warning signs of KC progression.[5] This finding has been supported recently by another group monitoring KC progression using anterior segment optical coherence tomography.[8]

A major unaddressed issue concerning the monitoring of ectatic disease is the repeatability of measurements. This becomes more apparent as the disease progresses, and with greater maximum keratometry (K_{max}) values (≥ 50 D), where the reliability of all imaging systems significantly drops.[35] The ability to recognize true progression of KC, by maximizing the repeatability of K_{max}, is of crucial importance, as it is a decisive factor in the decision to treat the patient with corneal collagen cross-linking. Therefore the parameters used for monitoring the disease progression should have a clinically adequate repeatability limit. If we consider that most clinicians use the threshold of 1 D increase in the K_{max} as evidence of disease progression, then the repeatability limit of such a parameter should be lower than this cutoff value that defines progression. Recently, Asroui et al. have suggested using zone average instead of single point measurement to overcome this repeatability issue in advanced KC. They reported that instantaneous curvature zone average centered on K_{max} could significantly improve repeatability in eyes with K_{max} over 50 D.[36]

Biological and Hormonal Factors

Hormonal changes during pregnancy have been reported to affect corneal biomechanics negatively and may be considered a potential risk factor for progression of KC.[37] More recently a surge of interest has emerged regarding a possible association with serum hydroxyvitamin D levels in

KC patients with severe disease. In a study from Akkaya and Ulusoy,[38] although a decreasing serum vitamin D level was not significantly associated with increasing severity of KC, patients with KC had an overall lower serum vitamin D level than those of age- and sex-matched healthy controls.

Keratoconus Progression Monitoring: New Insights

PROGRESSION GRADING SCORES

To overcome the challenge of unreliable monitoring due to poor repeatability in advanced KC corneas, the idea of considering multiple parameters for defining KC progression has emerged. In this context, the relatively recent ABCD KC grading system has been proposed to assess disease progression.[39] This system combines several corneal parameters, including the central 3-mm average anterior and posterior radius of axial curvature, centered on the point of thinnest corneal pachymetry. Although the repeatability of the parameters of this grading system should be evaluated further, this monitoring system shows promise for characterizing ectatic disease progression. In a similar way, the Dutch Crosslinking for Keratoconus (DUCK) score has been proposed, which combines five clinical parameters that are routinely assessed: age, visual acuity, refraction error, keratometry, and subjective patient experience.[40] The DUCK score is derived by scoring 0 to 2 points per item and has been shown to outperform the conventional maximum keratometry criterion of more than 1.0 D for selecting which patients should benefit from cross-linking treatment.

CONCEPT OF SUSPECT PROGRESSIVE KERATOCONUS: MONITORING FREQUENCY ADJUSTMENT

Anterior segment imaging technologies have vastly improved over the last 10 years, thus providing a thorough analysis of the characteristics of the cornea, including posterior surface and thickness distribution profiles, corneal total power, and corneal wavefront. These parameters have been studied extensively with several different systems and are very useful for improving the sensitivity of early KC detection.[41-44] Although the current leading hypothesis is that KC may be first detectable at the posterior surface,[45,46] interestingly, this finding still has not impacted the way ectatic disease is monitored. Indeed, most of the parameters used for the definition of a progressive KC and ultimately for indicating when a cross-linking procedure should be recommended or not are still based on modifications of the anterior surface (anterior keratometry and corneal astigmatism) and corneal thinning.[47,48] However, in view of these recent findings, it seemed reasonable to question the use of anterior corneal parameters alone as a gold standard in monitoring the ectatic process and to track the earliest signs of progression. In an attempt to evaluate the kinetics of these various corneal parameters in a progressive KC cohort, our group has recently reported the relevance of tracking changes to the posterior surface and vertical coma, as they were found to be modified significantly earlier than anterior keratometry readings[5] (Fig. 8.1). This finding is consistent with the generally accepted approach for detecting KC in the earliest stages, which includes the analysis of the posterior surface and corneal coma. Therefore these parameters may be relevant warning signs when monitoring progressive KC. Cutoff values of posterior surface changes and corneal coma, as well as the factors predicting progression, have yet to be determined through additional studies with larger progressive KC cohorts. However, the consistency of findings in early KC detection and progressive KC, along with improvements in anterior imaging technology, challenge our current approach to monitoring the disease and our definition of progressive KC.

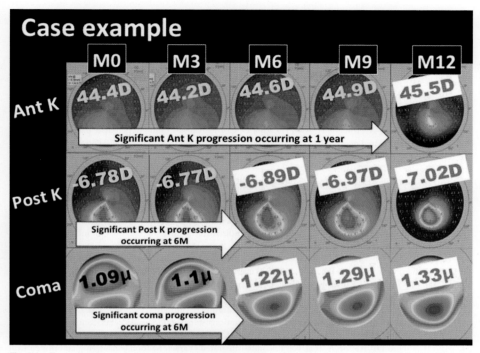

Fig. 8.1 Example of a patient with keratoconus progression. Change of coma and posterior keratometry detected prior to anterior keratometry modifications. *AntK,* Anterior keratometry; *D,* diopter; *M,* month; *Post K,* posterior keratometry.

References

1. Olivares Jiménez JL, Guerrero Jurado JC, Bermudez Rodriguez FJ, Serrano Laborda D. Keratoconus: age of onset and natural history. *Optom Vis Sci.* 1997;74(3):147–151.
2. Naderan M, Jahanrad A. Topographic, tomographic and biomechanical corneal changes during pregnancy in patients with keratoconus: a cohort study. *Acta Ophthalmol.* 2017;95(4):e291–e296.
3. Musch DC, Farjo AA, Meyer RF, Waldo MN, Janz NK. Assessment of health-related quality of life after corneal transplantation. *Am J Ophthalmol.* 1997;124(1):1–8.
4. Li X, Liu L, Qiu L. Early diagnosis of keratoconus with Orbscan-II anterior system. *J Huazhong Univ Sci Technolog Med Sci.* 2002;22(4):369–370.
5. Tellouck J, Touboul D, Santhiago MR, Tellouck L, Paya C, Smadja D. Evolution profiles of different corneal parameters in progressive keratoconus. *Cornea.* 2016;35(6):807–813.
6. Choi JA, Kim MS. Progression of keratoconus by longitudinal assessment with corneal topography. *Invest Ophthalmol Vis Sci.* 2012;53(2):927–935.
7. McMahon TT, Edrington TB, Szczotka-Flynn L, et al. Longitudinal changes in corneal curvature in keratoconus. *Cornea.* 2006;25(3):296–305.
8. Fujimoto H, Maeda N, Shintani A, et al. Quantitative evaluation of the natural progression of keratoconus using three-dimensional optical coherence tomography. *Invest Ophthalmol Vis Sci.* 2016;57(9):169–175.
9. Mazzotta C, Balestrazzi A, Traversi C, et al. Treatment of progressive keratoconus by riboflavin-UVA-induced cross-linking of corneal collagen: ultrastructural analysis by Heidelberg retinal tomograph II in vivo confocal microscopy in humans. *Cornea.* 2007;26(4):390–397.
10. Gomes JA, Rapuano CJ, Belin MW, Ambrósio R Jr. Group of Panelists for the Global Delphi Panel of Keratoconus and Ectatic Diseases. Global consensus on keratoconus diagnosis. *Cornea.* 2015;34(12):e38–e39.

11. Craig JA, Mahon J, Yellowlees A, et al. Epithelium-off photochemical corneal collagen cross-linkage using riboflavin and ultraviolet a for keratoconus and keratectasia: a systematic review and meta-analysis. *Ocul Surf.* 2014;12(3):202–214.

12. Salman AG. Transepithelial corneal collagen crosslinking for progressive keratoconus in a pediatric age group. *J Cataract Refract Surg.* 2013;39(8):1164–1170.

13. Sidky MK, Hassanein DH, Eissa SA, Salah YM, Lotfy NM. Prevalence of subclinical keratoconus among pediatric Egyptian population with astigmatism. *Clin Ophthalmol.* 2020;14:905–913.

14. El-Khoury S, Abdelmassih Y, Hamade A, et al. Pediatric keratoconus in a tertiary referral center: incidence, presentation, risk factors, and treatment. *J Refract Surg.* 2016;32(8):534–541.

15. Or L, Rozenberg A, Abulafia A, Avni I, Zadok D. Corneal cross-linking in pediatric patients: evaluating treated and untreated eyes—5-year follow-up results. *Cornea.* 2018;37(8):1013–1017.

16. Gordon-Shaag A, Millodot M, Shneor E, Liu Y. The genetic and environmental factors for keratoconus. *Biomed Res Int.* 2015;2015:795738.

17. Tuft SJ, Moodaley LC, Gregory WM, Davison CR, Buckley RJ. Prognostic factors for the progression of keratoconus. *Ophthalmology.* 1994;101(3):439–447.

18. Pearson AR, Soneji B, Sarvananthan N, Sanford-Smith JH. Does ethnic origin influence the incidence or severity of keratoconus? *Eye.* 2000;14(4):625–628.

19. Li X, Rabinowitz YS, Rasheed K, Yang H. Longitudinal study of the normal eyes in unilateral keratoconus patients. *Ophthalmology.* 2004;111(3):440–446.

20. Ferdi AC, Nguyen V, Gore DM, Allan BD, Rozema JJ, Watson SL. Keratoconus natural progression: a systematic review and meta-analysis of 11 529 eyes. *Ophthalmology.* 2019;126(7):935–945.

21. Moran S, Gomez L, Zuber K, Gatinel D. A case-control study of keratoconus risk factors. *Cornea.* 2020;39(6):697–701.

22. Amsler M. Keratocone classique et keratocone fruste, arguments unitaires. *Oftalmologica.* 1946;111:96–101.

23. Alió JL, Shabayek MH. Corneal higher order aberrations: a method to grade keratoconus. *J Refract Surg.* 2006;22(6):539–546.

24. Alió JL, Piñero DP, Alesón A, et al. Keratoconus-integrated characterization considering anterior corneal aberrations, internal astigmatism, and corneal biomechanics. *J Cataract Refract Surg.* 2011;37(3):552–568.

25. Hersh PS, Stulting RD, Muller D, et al. United States multicenter clinical trial of corneal collagen cross-linking for keratoconus treatment. *Ophthalmology.* 2017;124(9):1259–1270.

26. Galvis V, Sherwin T, Tello A, Merayo-Lloves J, Barrera R, Acera A. Keratoconus: an inflammatory disorder? *Eye (Lond).* 2015;29(7):843–859.

27. Shetty R, Sureka S, Kusumgar P, Sethu S, Sainani K. Allergen-specific exposure associated with high immunoglobulin E and eye rubbing predisposes to progression of keratoconus. *Indian J Ophthalmol.* 2017;65(5):399–402.

28. Randleman JB, Woodward M, Lynn MJ, Stulting RD. Risk assessment for ectasia after corneal refractive surgery. *Ophthalmology.* 2008;115(1):37–50.

29. Santhiago MR, Smadja D, Gomes BAF, et al. Association between the percent tissue altered and post-laser in situ keratomileusis ectasia in eyes with normal preoperative topography. *Am J Ophthalmol.* 2014;158(1):87–95.

30. Nielsen K, Hjortdal JØ, Pihlmann M, Corydon T. Update on keratoconus genetics. *Acta Ophthalmol.* 2013;91(2):106–113.

31. Tuft SJ, Hashemi H, George S, Frazer D, Willoughby C, Liskova P. Keratoconus in 18 pairs of twins. *Acta Ophthalmol.* 2012;90(6):482–486.

32. Kymionis GD, Blazaki S, Tsoulnaras K, Giarmoukakis A, Grentzelos M, Tsilimbaris M. Corneal imaging abnormalities in familial keratoconus. *J Refract Surg.* 2017;33(1):62–63.

33. Zadnik K, Barr JT, Edrington TB, et al. Baseline findings in the Collaborative Longitudinal Evaluation of Keratoconus (CLEK) study. *Invest Ophthalmol Vis Sci.* 1998;39:2537–2546.

34. Hamilton A, Wong S, Carley F, Chaudhry N, Biswas S. Tomographic indices as possible risk factors for progression in pediatric keratoconus. *J AAPOS.* 2016;20(6):523–526.

35. Flynn TH, Sharma DP, Bunce C, Wilkins MR. Differential precision of corneal Pentacam HR measurements in early and advanced keratoconus. *Br J Ophthalmol.* 2016;100(9):1183–1187.

36. Asroui L, Mehanna CJ, Salloum A, Chalhoub R, Roberts CJ, Awwad ST. Repeatability of zone averages compared to single point measurements of maximal curvature in keratoconus. *Am J Ophthalmol.* 2021;221:226–234.

37. Bligihan K, Hondur A, Sul S, Ozturk S. Pregnancy-induced progression of keratoconus. *Cornea.* 2011;30(9):991–994.

38. Akkaya S, Ulusoy DM. Serum vitamin D levels in patients with keratoconus. *Ocul Immunol Inflamm.* 2020;28(3):348–353.

39. Duncan JK, Belin MW, Borgstrom M. Assessing progression of keratoconus: novel tomographic determinants. *Eye Vis.* 2016;3(1):6.

40. Wisse RPL, Simons RWP, van der Vossen MJB, et al. Clinical evaluation and validation of the Dutch crosslinking for keratoconus score. *JAMA Ophthalmol.* 2019;137(6):610.

41. Smadja D, Touboul D, Cohen A, et al. Detection of subclinical keratoconus using an automated decision tree classification. *Am J Ophthalmol.* 2013;156(2):237–246.

42. Saad A, Gatinel D. Topographic and tomographic properties of forme fruste keratoconus corneas. *Invest Ophthalmol Vis Sci.* 2010;51(11):5546–5555.

43. Ambrósio R Jr, Caiado AL, Guerra FP, et al. Novel pachymetric parameters based on corneal tomography for diagnosing keratoconus. *J Refract Surg.* 2011;27(10):753–758.

44. Bühren J, Kook D, Yoon G, Kohnen T. Detection of subclinical keratoconus by using corneal anterior and posterior surface aberrations and thickness spatial profiles. *Invest Ophthalmol Vis Sci.* 2010;51(7):3424–3432.

45. Smadja D, Santhiago MR, Mello GR, Krueger RR, Colin J, Touboul D. Influence of the reference surface shape for discriminating between normal corneas, subclinical keratoconus and keratoconus. *J Refract Surg.* 2013;29(4):274–281.

46. Khachikian SS, Belin MW. Posterior elevation in keratoconus. *Ophthalmology.* 2009;116(4):816–817.

47. Belin MW. Tomographic parameters for the detection of keratoconus: suggestions for screening and treatment parameters. *Eye Contact Lens.* 2014;40(6):326–330.

48. Brown SE, Simmasalam R, Antonova N, Gadaria N, Asbell PA. Progression in keratoconus and the effect of corneal cross-linking on progression. *Eye Contact Lens.* 2014;40(6):331–338.

49. Raiskup-Wolf F, Hoyer A, Spoerl E, Pillunat LE. Collagen crosslinking with riboflavin and ultraviolet-A light in keratoconus: long-term results. *J Cataract Refract Surg.* 2008;34(5):796–801.

50. Wittig-Silva C, Whiting M, Lamoureux E, Lindsay RG, Sullivan LJ, Snibson GR. A randomized controlled trial of corneal collagen cross-linking in progressive keratoconus: preliminary results. *J Refract Surg.* 2008;24(7):S720–S725.

51. Vinciguerra P, Albè E, Trazza S, Seiler T, Epstein D. Intraoperative and postoperative effects of corneal collagen cross-linking on progressive keratoconus. *Arch Ophthalmol.* 2009;127(10):1258–1265.

52. Hersh PS, Greenstein SA, Fry KL. Corneal collagen crosslinking for keratoconus and corneal ectasia: one-year results. *J Cataract Refract Surg.* 2011;37:149–160.

53. O'Brart DPS, Chan E, Samaras K, Patel P, Shah SP. A randomised, prospective study to investigate the efficacy of riboflavin/ultraviolet A (370 nm) corneal collagen cross-linkage to halt the progression of keratoconus. *Br J Ophthalmol.* 2011;95(11):1519–1524.

54. Chatzis N, Hafezi F. Progression of keratoconus and efficacy of corneal collagen cross-linking in children and adolescents. *J Refract Surg.* 2012;28(11):753–758.

55. Hashemi H, Seyedian MA, Miraftab M, Fotouhi A, Asgari S. Corneal collagen cross-linking with riboflavin and ultraviolet a irradiation for keratoconus: long-term results. *Ophthalmology.* 2013;120(8):1515–1520.

56. Mazzotta C, Traversi C, Paradiso AL, Latronico ME, Rechichi M. Pulsed light accelerated crosslinking versus continuous light accelerated crosslinking: one-year results. *J Ophthalmol.* 2014;2014:604–731.

57. Stojanovic A, Zhou W, Utheim TP. Corneal collagen cross-linking with and without epithelial removal: a contralateral study with 0.5% hypotonic riboflavin solution. *Biomed Res Int.* 2014;2014:619398.

58. Shetty R, Pahuja NK, Nuijts RM, et al. Current protocols of corneal collagen cross-linking: visual, refractive, and tomographic outcomes. *Am J Ophthalmol.* 2015;160(2):243–249.

59. Poli M, Lefevre A, Auxenfans C, Burillon C. Corneal collagen cross-linking for the treatment of progressive corneal ectasia: 6-year prospective outcome in a French population. *Am J Ophthalmol.* 2015;160(4):654–662. e1.

60. Godefrooij DA, Soeters N, Imhof SM, Wisse RP. Corneal cross-linking for pediatric keratoconus: long-term results. *Cornea.* 2016;35(7):954–958.

Diagnosis and Associated Disorders

CHAPTER 9

Differential Diagnosis of Keratoconus

Victoria Grace C. Dimacali ▪ Jodhbir S. Mehta

KEY CONCEPTS

- Pertinent medical (systemic and ocular) and family history must be elicited.
- Many conditions can mimic keratoconus. These can be classified as ectatic and nonectatic disorders.
- Other ectatic disorders include pellucid marginal degeneration, keratoglobus, and postrefractive surgery ectasia.
- Nonectatic conditions to consider include corneal warpage, measurement artifacts, corneal scars, asymmetric and irregular astigmatism, and tear film instability and dry eye.
- Tomographic maps of both eyes must always be analyzed in relation to each other. In suspicious cases, repeat scanning may be done to confirm results.
- Newer imaging with biomechanics can help differentiate tomographic normal cases.
- Patients with equivocal findings must be followed up regularly with repeat corneal imaging.

Introduction

Keratoconus must be differentiated from other forms of keratectasia and other causes of irregular or asymmetric corneal astigmatism, because the management and prognosis are specific for each condition. Identifying underlying ectatic disease is also critical when screening candidates for laser refractive surgery, to avoid inadvertent acceleration of any underlying ectasia.[1] An accurate diagnosis can often be made after consideration of corneal findings on slit lamp biomicroscopy, corneal tomography, and respectively generated keratoconus indices in relation to the ocular history, including details of contact lens wear and any prior corneal ablative or incisional procedure. The presence of other ocular and systemic comorbidities such as vernal keratoconjunctivitis, atopy, and connective tissue disease are also important to establish. Any family history of keratoconus or other corneal and ocular conditions must also be elicited. Newer diagnostics such as epithelial thickness mapping, corneal aberrometry, and corneal biomechanical measurement such as with the Corvis ST (Oculus Optikgeräte GmbH, Wetzlar, Germany) may help detect early ectatic disease. Hence, the differential diagnoses of keratoconus can be classified into other corneal ectatic diseases, and nonectatic conditions mimicking keratoconus.

Ectatic Disorders

The most important conditions to consider are the other ectatic disorders. These include pellucid marginal degeneration (PMD), keratoglobus, and postrefractive surgical ectasia. The latter is easily identifiable once a history of laser vision correction (LVC) is obtained.

PELLUCID MARGINAL DEGENERATION

Like keratoconus, PMD is a degenerative disorder characterized by progressive corneal thinning and ectasia.[2–4] Both are typically bilateral and asymmetric at presentation, although unilateral PMD has been reported.[5–8] PMD is often misdiagnosed as keratoconus, because they may closely resemble each other in clinical presentation.[1] Patients with PMD, however, typically present later, between the second to the fifth decades of life, compared with keratoconus, wherein patients present from puberty to the third decade of life.[2] PMD is also less commonly seen than keratoconus, with incidence depending on the geographic location, ranging from 0.0003% in Russia to 2.3% in Central India.[9,10] Tummanapalli and colleagues, in a large study of 1133 patients with corneal ectasia, documented keratoconus in 97% of patients and PMD in 3%.[1]

PMD is characterized by a clear, narrow band of peripheral corneal thinning, classically located concentric to the limbus inferiorly from 4 to 8 o'clock and best demonstrated by a full-coverage 12-mm pachymetric map.[11] Superior, nasal, and temporal quadrant involvement have also been reported.[1,4,9] Between the area of thinning and the limbus often lies 1 to 2 mm of unaffected cornea.[9] There is central or paracentral corneal protrusion, most prominent above the area of thinning, but central corneal thickness (CCT) usually remains unaffected.[9] Keratoconus, on the other hand, usually shows corneal thinning in the paracentral region, with central or inferior steepening and asymmetric bowtie astigmatism on corneal tomography.[11]

The exact etiology and incidence of PMD is still not known.[2] Some authors have suggested that keratoconus, PMD, and keratoglobus may be phenotypic variations of the same underlying corneal disorder.[3,12–14] Another hypothesis is that PMD is a peripheral form of keratoconus.[11,15–19] Reports have also been made of PMD and keratoconus concomitantly occurring in the same eye or in fellow eye.[4,20,21]

Patients with PMD tend to present later than those with keratoconus, typically with decreased vision caused by a progressive increase in irregular, against-the-rule astigmatism.[1,4] Rarely, patients may experience acute scleral injection, eye pain, or sudden blurring of vision and photophobia from acute hydrops or corneal perforation.[4,9] In the largest review of PMD patients to date, Sridhar and colleagues documented hydrops in 7 out of 116 eyes (6.0%),[4] while a more recent study reported hydrops in as much as 11.5% of patients.[22] Most cases of hydrops seen are associated with keratoconus because of its prevalence, but the incidence of hydrops in keratoconus is actually lower than in PMD, with previous clinical estimates at 2.4% to 2.8%.[22–24] In both conditions, hydrops presents with acute corneal edema and a break in the Descemet membrane secondary to progressive corneal thinning. Corneal vascularization and scarring may be seen after acute hydrops in both keratoconus and PMD.[9] Sridhar and colleagues in their review reported that among seven PMD patients who experienced acute hydrops, the breaks in the Descemet membrane occurred above the area of thinning.[4]

Moderate cases of PMD may be easily identified on biomicroscopic examination because of the classic location of inferior thinning with protrusion above the thinnest area, in contrast to keratoconus in which the thinnest area coincides with the most ectatic region.[11,25] A "beer-belly" contour of the central and inferior cornea may be observed when the eye is viewed from the side, compared to a conical profile in keratoconus.[9,11] Early cases, however, may look unremarkable, and severe cases may resemble keratoconus if the corneal thinning extensively involves the inferior cornea.[25] A Fleischer ring, apical corneal scarring or vascularization, lipid deposition, Rizutti's phenomenon, and Munson's sign do not develop in PMD.[4,9] Descemet folds may be seen concentric with the inferior limbus. These folds disappear when pressure is applied to the cornea.[3,9,26]

Corneal Tomography

Corneal tomography is the gold standard for distinguishing between the two conditions.[9,25] Early PMD may show a topographic pattern of mild to moderate against-the-rule astigmatism, normal keratometric values, and normal CCT (Fig. 9.1).[1] A "crab-claw" pattern, also known as "butterfly,"

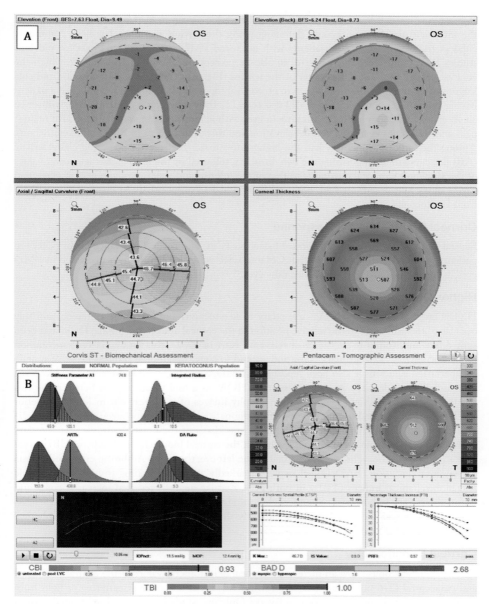

Fig. 9.1 (A) Pentacam tomography of an eye of a patient with early pellucid marginal degeneration who had undergone penetrating keratoplasty in the other eye with more advanced disease. This eye had against-the-rule regular asymmetric bowtie astigmatism of 1.8D. Note the mild elevation on anterior and posterior maps. (B) Belin-Ambrósio enhanced ectasia display total deviation *(BAD-D)* was high, Corvis biomechanical analysis showed high corneal biomechanical index *(CBI)* and tomographic and biomechanical index *(TBI)* values.

"lobster," or "kissing doves" sign, on the sagittal anterior curvature map, signifying steepening of the inferior corneal periphery and flattening along the vertical meridian, has been commonly cited as the classic finding in patients with advanced PMD (Fig. 9.2).[1,2,11] However, previous studies have shown that this pattern can also be present in inferior keratoconus, in which the cone is located away from the center of the cornea (Fig. 9.3).[9,11,27,28] In a study by Koc and colleagues of 47 eyes with crab-claw pattern on corneal topography, a higher probability of a patient having inferior keratoconus than PMD was found.[11] The pachymetric map, however, will reveal an absence of inferior crescentic thinning in eyes with keratoconus. In another study, Tummanapalli and colleagues evaluated corneal elevation and thickness indices in PMD and keratoconus. Among the indices, asphericity had the highest area under the receiver operating characteristic (AROC) curve in distinguishing the two disorders, followed by the ratio of average power values of the nasal and temporal quadrants to that of the inferior and superior quadrants.[1] A generated PMD index by the authors had 90% sensitivity and 93.7% specificity in distinguishing PMD from keratoconus.

Corneal Biomechanical Response

Several studies have investigated corneal hysteresis (CH) and corneal resistance factor (CRF) in patients with PMD. These showed that CH and CRF were also significantly decreased in PMD eyes, as in keratoconus, compared to healthy eyes.[29–31]

Higher Order Aberrations

Higher order aberrations (HOAs) secondary to keratoconus and PMD are different, probably because of the difference in the relative position of the corneal apex to the pupil.[2] Trefoil has been shown in some studies to be the most relevant HOA in PMD; this finding is very uncommon in keratoconus.[32,33] Less primary coma and a trend to larger magnitude and less negative spherical aberration values have also been reported in PMD, compared with keratoconus.[2,33] However, no compelling evidence is available to support HOAs as a tool to distinguish between the two conditions.[2] Fig. 9.4 shows Pentacam tomography images of a 27-year-old male with superior PMD who had bilateral asymmetric bowtie astigmatism with superior steepening and associated corneal thinning. No angling of the hemi-meridians of the bowtie patterns was seen and posterior elevation maps were normal. Although the corneal biomechanical indices (CBIs) were only suspicious in the right eye and normal in the left eye, the Belin-Ambrósio enhanced ectasia display total deviation (BAD-D) values were markedly abnormal, leading to high tomographic and biomechanical indices (TBIs) in both eyes. Zernike analysis revealed increased coma and trefoil aberrations in both eyes. Spherical aberration was +0.733 μm on the right eye and –0.203 μm on the left eye. The case in Fig. 9.2 similarly showed increased coma, trefoil, and spherical aberrations (+0.753 μm).

Corneal Densitometry

Eyes with keratoconus show an increase in corneal densitometry values at the central (0–2 mm) and paracentral (2–6 mm) regions of the cornea. This is because of backscattering of light from disruption of the epithelial and stromal layers.[2] Only one study to date has investigated corneal densitometry in PMD. Koc and colleagues evaluated densitometric, topographic, and tomographic properties of eyes with PMD and inferior keratoconus who had crab-claw patterns on sagittal topography and compared them with control eyes.[11] Densitometry values were shown to be significantly higher in PMD compared with normal eyes in all corneal zones and layers. These were also significantly higher in PMD than in inferior keratoconus at the 6- to 10-mm and 10- to 12-mm zones. More studies are needed to determine if these values can be used to help distinguish PMD from keratoconus.

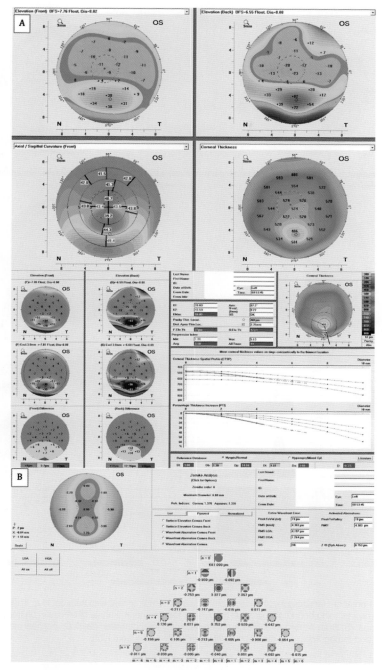

Fig. 9.2 (A) Pentacam tomography showing a crab-claw pattern of corneal steepening causing against-the-rule astigmatism in an eye with more advanced pellucid marginal degeneration. Note the inferior bands of anterior and posterior elevation and thinning sparing the peripheral cornea. (B) Zernike analysis revealed increased coma, trefoil, and spherical aberrations in both eyes.

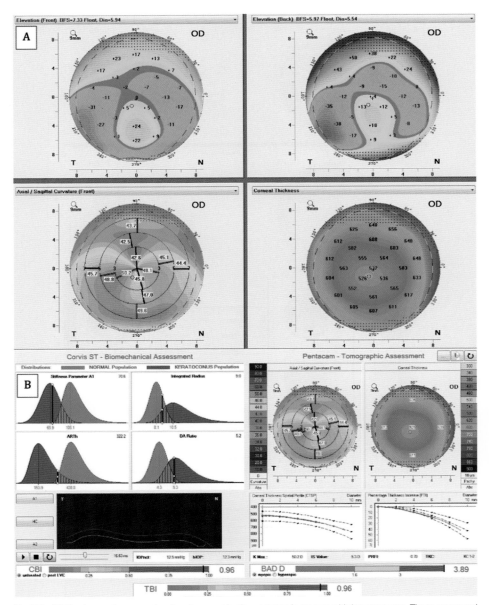

Fig. 9.3 (A) Pentacam tomography showing a crab-claw pattern in an eye with keratoconus. There appeared to be no corneal thinning on the pachymetric map. Note the paracentral areas of elevation on front and back elevation maps. (B) Belin-Ambrósio enhanced ectasia display total deviation *(BAD-D)*, corneal biomechanical index *(CBI)*, and tomographic and biomechanical index *(TBI)* values were high.

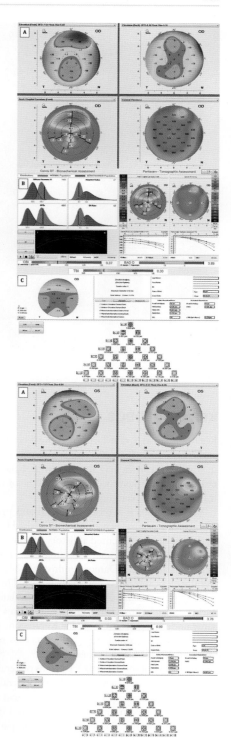

Fig. 9.4 (A) Pentacam tomography of atypical pellucid marginal degeneration demonstrating bilateral asymmetric bowtie astigmatism with superior steepening and associated corneal thinning. Posterior elevation maps were unremarkable. (B) Whereas corneal biomechanical index *(CBI)* values were only suspicious in the right eye and normal in the left eye, Belin-Ambrósio enhanced ectasia display total deviation *(BAD-D)* values were markedly abnormal, leading to increased tomographic and biomechanical index *(TBI)* values in both eyes. (C) Zernike analysis revealed increased coma, trefoil, and spherical aberrations in both eyes. *OD*, Right eye; *OS*, left eye.

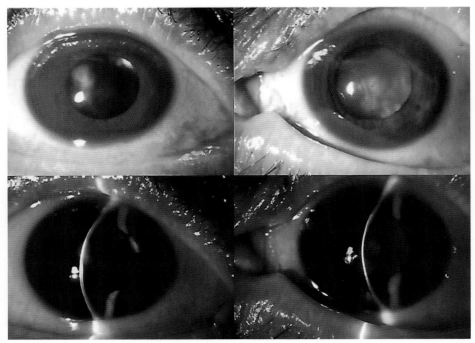

Fig. 9.5   Slit lamp anterior segment photographs of a patient with keratoglobus. Note bilateral apical scarring, diffuse corneal thinning, and generalized corneal protrusion.

KERATOGLOBUS

Keratoglobus is a rare form of corneal ectasia in which globular protrusion results from diffuse corneal thinning (Figs. 9.5 and 9.6).[25,34,35] It may be confused with cases of advanced keratoconus, in which the cornea may also appear globular and thin. However, a small area of the superior cornea in advanced keratoconus may still be of relatively normal thickness as opposed to the diffuse thinning seen in keratoglobus.[25]

Keratoglobus is typically bilateral and present at birth; inheritance has been assumed to be autosomal recessive as previously described by Pouliquen and colleagues.[34,36] Rathi and colleagues in their series documented a history of consanguinity in 3 out of 21 pediatric patients, 2 of whom had blue sclera syndrome.[35] Keratoglobus may be associated with certain connective tissue disorders such as Ehlers-Danlos syndrome,[37] Marfan syndrome,[38] and Rubinstein-Taybi syndrome.[39] Similar clinical features have been reported in association with vernal keratoconjunctivitis, chronic marginal blepharitis, idiopathic orbital inflammation, and thyroid eye disease.[34,35] As mentioned earlier, keratoconus, PMD, and keratoglobus are believed by some to represent a spectrum of the same underlying ectatic disorder. Keratoconus and keratoglobus have been found among different members of the same family.[40] Reports of keratoglobus occurring in eyes with keratoconus and in eyes with PMD have also been made.[4,35,36,41] Some authors hypothesize that "acquired" keratoglobus represents a severe, advanced form of keratoconus,[36,37] whereas others believe it may be a result of circumferential extension of the peripheral gutter in PMD.[41] Corneal thinning in keratoconus is localized centrally or paracentrally, whereas the thinning in keratoglobus extends from limbus to limbus and is maximal at the periphery (see Fig. 9.6).[25,34,40] Associated scleral thinning in keratoglobus has also been reported.[42] Central and paracentral elevation and steepening are demonstrated

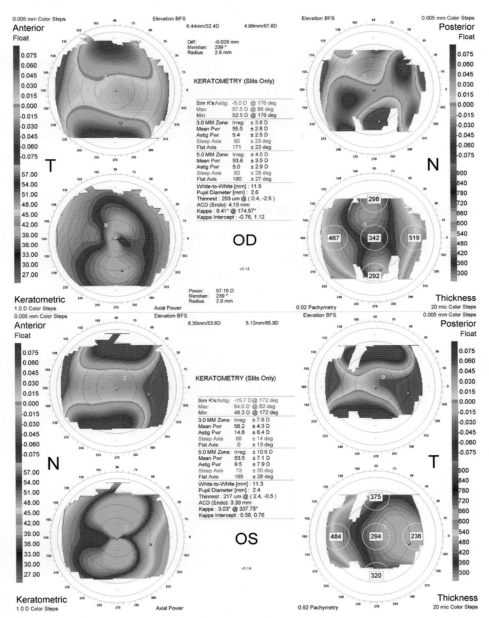

Fig. 9.6 Orbscan topography of the patient in Fig. 9.5. Bilateral diffuse corneal steepening and thinning were evident. Sagittal maps showed with-the-rule asymmetric bowtie astigmatism. Flattest simulated keratometry readings were 52.5D and 48.3D in the right and left eyes, respectively. Both eyes had maximal corneal thinning at the periphery. *K*, Angle kappa intercept; *OD*, right eye; *OS*, left eye; *red circle,* thinnest corneal thickness.

on corneal tomography.[40] Although disease progression is absent to minimal, patients have poor vision owing to high myopia and irregular astigmatism.[34,40]

Keratoglobus corneas are typically clear at presentation unless they develop hydrops and subsequent scarring. Unlike in keratoconus, Vogt striae and Fleischer rings are not seen.[34] The incidence of acute hydrops in keratoglobus and PMD is higher than in keratoconus. In the largest series to date, Rathi and colleagues documented 13.2% of 53 eyes with keratoglobus to have presented with acute hydrops and another 13.2% showed scars consistent with healed hydrops.[35] Other series have reported the incidence of hydrops in keratoglobus to range from 11.0%[22] to as high as 90.48%.[37] Compared to those with keratoconus, patients with keratoglobus are more prone to experiencing corneal perforation, either occurring spontaneously or after mild eye trauma, as the thinning can progress to as much as to 20% of normal corneal thickness.[25,34,40] Hard contact lenses are thus contraindicated and protective eyewear encouraged in these patients.[25]

CORNEAL ECTASIA AFTER REFRACTIVE SURGERY

Corneal ectasia should be suspected in patients who have had any prior ablative or incisional refractive procedure, especially myopic laser in-situ keratomileusis (LASIK).[43–45] Ectasia in this population can develop because of postsurgical biomechanical instability of the cornea with or without unrecognized preexisting keratoconus, subclinical keratoconus, or PMD, or by chance secondary to other intrinsic factors such as eye rubbing and subclinical atopy.[46–48] Similar to keratoconus, post-LASIK ectasia manifests as progressive central or inferior corneal steepening and thinning (Figs. 9.7 and 9.8) leading to increased myopia, irregular astigmatism, decreased uncorrected and best corrected visual acuity, and optical phenomena including glare and halos.[46,47] The epithelium is also significantly thinner over the corneal apex in both keratoconus and postoperative corneal ectasia when compared with normal eyes.[49] Corneal tomography in post-LASIK ectasia may show signs of posterior corneal elevation alone without an increase in the maximum keratometry (K_{max}) or a decrease in uncorrected visual acuity.[47]

Although less common, ectasia has also been documented after radial and hexagonal keratotomy (Fig. 9.9),[50,51] photorefractive keratectomy (PRK),[52–54] and more recently, small-incision lenticule extraction (SMILE).[55,56] Some patients may not recall having had LVC, so a careful search for a LASIK flap or a SMILE incision, which may not be obvious on cursory examination with broad beam illumination, must be undertaken to avoid a misdiagnosis of keratoconus. Post-PRK patients do not have corneal flaps or incisions; thus evaluation of curvature and pachymetry maps of both eyes must be analyzed in relation to each other. An ablation pattern seen on sagittal and pachymetric maps in the uninvolved eye will reveal prior LVC. Recurrence of ectasia has also been described following penetrating keratoplasty[57,58] and deep anterior lamellar keratoplasty for keratoconus.[59,60] Some controversy still exists as to whether keratoconus pathology reemerges by migration of the disease from host to donor cornea, or from incomplete excision of the cone.[61] Latency for recurrence following penetrating keratoplasty is long (mean 19 years; range 3–40 years).[58]

Non-ectatic Disorders

Corneas without frank ectasia may be misdiagnosed as keratoconus when an abnormal topographic pattern is detected. A wide variety of pseudokeratoconus conditions exist that may also demonstrate focal corneal steepening, high astigmatism and posterior corneal elevation, significant negative corneal asphericity, and increased anterior and posterior corneal aberrations.[62] Stein and Salim reviewed 1000 consecutive patients who were referred for corneal cross-linking, topography-guided PRK, and intrastromal corneal rings for presumed keratoconus, PMD, or ectasia after LVC. They found 26 eyes without ectasia in 20 patients. Among these were, in order

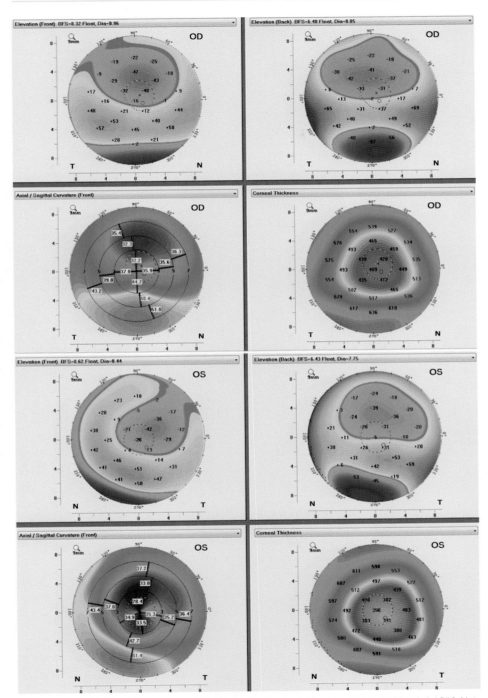

Fig. 9.7 Pentacam tomography of bilateral corneal ectasia after myopic laser in-situ keratomileusis (LASIK). Note bilateral inferior corneal steepening, advanced corneal thinning, and anterior and posterior bands of elevation.

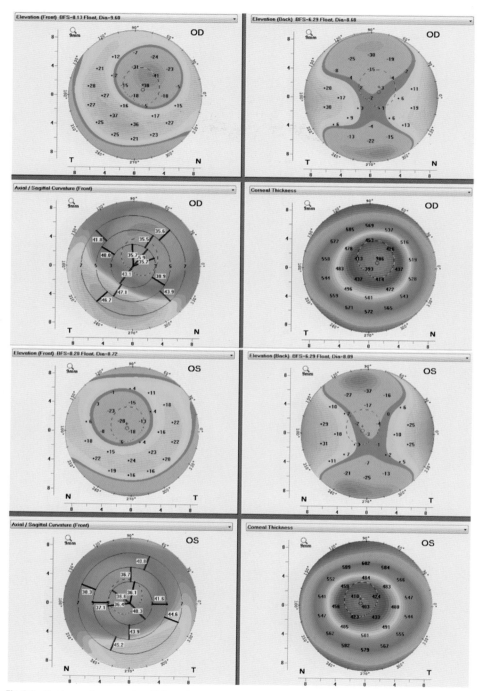

Fig. 9.8 Pentacam tomography of bilateral corneal ectasia after myopic epithelial laser in-situ keratomileusis (epi-LASIK). Note inferior corneal steepening and advanced corneal thinning. Back elevation maps appeared unremarkable although front elevation maps show crescentic paracentral elevation.

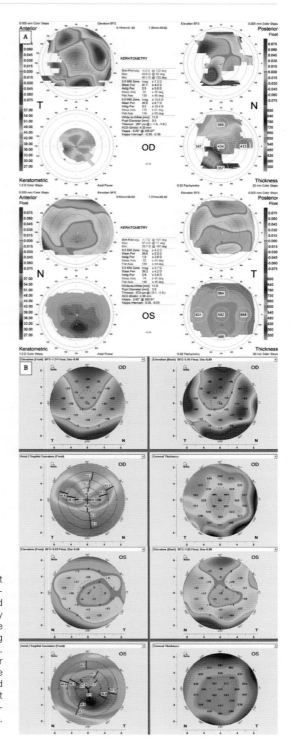

Fig. 9.9 (A) Orbscan topography of a patient who had undergone bilateral radial keratotomy. The right eye developed ectasia and underwent deep anterior lamellar keratoplasty (DALK) more than 20 years later. Note the area of inferotemporal thinning corresponding to an island of increased posterior elevation. (B) Pentacam tomography done 2 years after undergoing DALK, on the right eye. Despite high residual astigmatism, the best corrected visual acuity with rigid gas-permeable contact lenses was 6/9 for the right eye. The tomographic profile of the left eye remained stable. *OD,* Right eye; *OS,* left eye.

of decreasing frequency, epithelial basement membrane dystrophy, superficial punctate keratitis, amblyopia secondary to high astigmatism, whorl-like keratopathy, corneal warpage secondary to contact lenses, measurement error with topography, and corneal scars.[63] An integrated analysis of corneal biomicroscopic findings, tomographic and epithelial maps, and biomechanical properties is needed to differentiate ectatic from nonectatic disease, thus avoiding unnecessary or contraindicated treatments such as PRK and LASIK in the former and cross-linking and intrastromal corneal ring segment implantation in the latter.[63]

CONTACT LENS–INDUCED CORNEAL WARPAGE

Chronic wear of contact lenses, especially rigid gas-permeable and soft toric lenses, may lead to reversible alterations in the anterior corneal topographic pattern.[62,64] This warpage may be due either to a direct mechanical effect or to a combination of mechanical and metabolic changes related to the corneal epithelium.[65] As many LVC candidates wear contact lenses, differentiation between warpage and keratoconus is crucial for the proper selection of patients for refractive surgery and for the identification of patients with ectasia who could benefit from collagen cross-linking.[64,66] Clinical signs of corneal warpage include changes in refractive error, a reduction in corrected visual acuity, and absence of progressive corneal thinning.[65] Patients suspected of having corneal warpage may be instructed to discontinue hard lenses for at least 1 month or soft lenses for at least 1 week.[63] Regular follow-ups with serial corneal topography are then used to monitor for partial or complete reversal of findings typically seen with corneal warpage, to arrive at a definite diagnosis.[65,67] The time required for significant stabilization varies among individuals and contact lens type.[65] A long waiting period that may reach several months may not be acceptable to patients who lead a spectacle-free lifestyle and have planned for LVC at a specific time.[67]

Corneal warpage can also result in focal topographic steepening. It may mimic the topography seen in ectasia, especially when the steepening is located inferiorly or inferotemporally, but is not progressive.[66] Fig. 9.10A shows superior corneal steepening without associated thinning or increased corneal elevation on Orbscan imaging of a patient who was a chronic soft contact lens user. Repeat imaging showed the same pattern. After 2 months of discontinuation of soft contact lens use, resolution of the corneal warpage was seen with restoration of normal symmetric bow-tie astigmatism (see Fig. 9.10B). Fig. 9.11 shows Pentacam images of a patient who was using orthokeratology lenses in both eyes. Corneal warpage was indicated by unusual evenness across the entire corneas on curvature maps. Small central islands of depression secondary to orthokeratology lens wear were also seen on anterior elevation maps, whereas posterior elevation maps were unremarkable.

Fourier-domain optical coherence tomography (OCT) such as the RTVue system (Optovue, Fremont, CA) can produce corneal epithelial maps that are useful for detecting focal changes in epithelial thickness patterns.[66] Although keratoconus is associated with focal epithelial thinning, in corneal warpage an opposite association of focal epithelial thickening is seen, typically in the same or adjacent sector as the location of maximum topographic steepening.[66] Schallhorn and colleagues in their case series demonstrated perfect agreement of the locations of maximum epithelial thickness with maximum mean power in all corneal warpage eyes.[66] Pachymetry maps will also reveal corresponding focal corneal thinning in keratoconus, which is absent in corneal warpage.[64,66] It must be kept in mind that keratoconus and corneal warpage can occur simultaneously in the same eye. Contact lens use with the changes in early subclinical keratoconus in patients wearing contact lenses could be misclassified as warpage; contact lens cessation is, therefore, necessary for accurate diagnosis in these cases.[64]

Alipour and colleagues compared the corneal biomechanical findings of the Ocular Response Analyzer in normal eyes and in those with contact lens–induced corneal warpage and keratoconus.

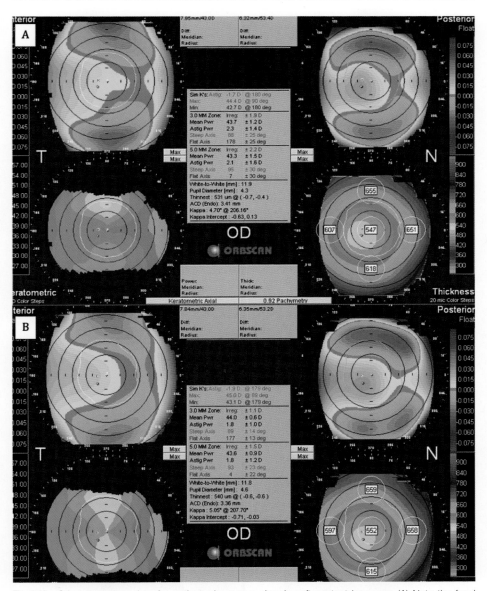

Fig. 9.10 Orbscan topography of a patient who was a chronic soft contact lens user. (A) Note the focal superior steepening on the curvature map. After contact lens use was stopped for 2 months, repeat imaging (B) revealed regular symmetric bowtie astigmatism indicating resolved corneal warpage. *K,* Angle kappa intercept; *red circle,* thinnest corneal thickness.

CH, CRF, and CCT values were highest in eyes with corneal warpage.[67] All measurements were found to be similar when compared with normal eyes, but were significantly different when compared with keratoconus eyes. The authors proposed that corneal biomechanics could be used for differentiating corneal warpage from keratoconus eyes.

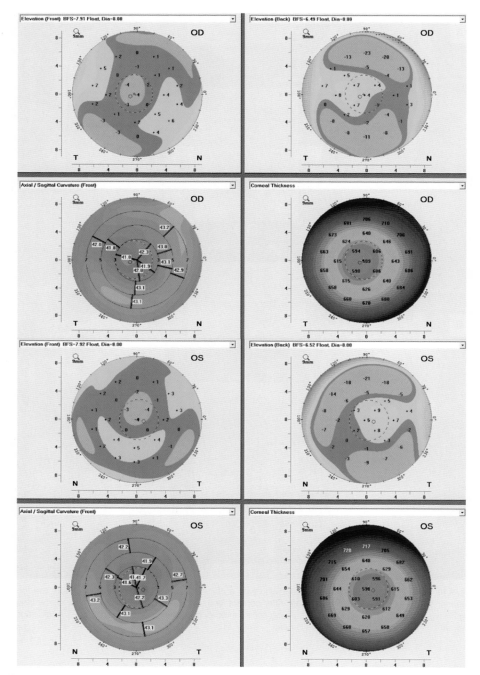

Fig. 9.11   Pentacam tomography of a patient who was using orthokeratology lenses. At first glance, the maps might seem unremarkable but corneal warpage was present, indicated by unusual evenness across the entire corneas on curvature maps. The anterior elevation maps also showed small central islands of depression showing the effect of the orthokeratology lenses.

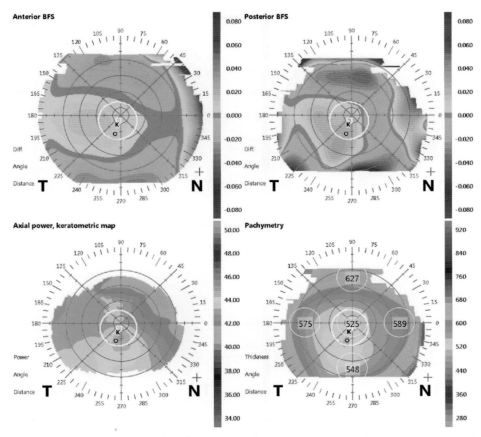

Fig. 9.12 Pseudokeratoconus pattern secondary to misalignment in Orbscan. Mild inferior deviation of fixation from the central axis was observed during the test. examination. Note asymmetric bowtie astigmatism with thinnest corneal thickness decentered inferiorly. An area of suspicious posterior elevation on best-fit-sphere *(BFS)* map was also noted. A closer look reveals that the pupil *(white circle)* is decentered inferiorly. *K,* Angle kappa intercept; *white square,* center of pupil; *yellow circle,* thinnest corneal thickness.

MEASUREMENT ARTIFACTS

Measurement errors when performing corneal topography or tomography may result in falsely ectatic patterns.[63,68] Misalignment of the visual axis by as little as 5 degrees below from the central axis of the videokeratoscope was found by Hubbe and Foulks to induce a significant increase in the inferior-superior (I-S) value proportional to the amount of deviation.[69] Anterior elevation maps will show displacement of the corneal apex in the direction of eye movement and an increase in the apex elevation.[70] An asymmetric bowtie or pseudokeratoconus pattern may also be reflected on anterior curvature maps. Fig. 9.12 shows Orbscan images of a normal eye with improper fixation. Mild inferior deviation of fixation from the central axis resulted in a pseudokeratoconus pattern of inferior steepening, suspicious posterior elevation, and inferiorly decentered thinnest corneal thickness. Proper alignment of the visual axis resulted in normalization of the topography maps (Fig. 9.13).

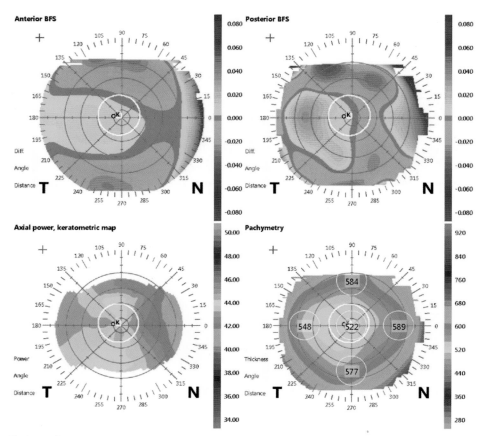

Fig. 9.13 Orbscan topography of the same patient as in Fig. 9.12 with normal alignment of the eye. Note symmetric bowtie astigmatism, center central thinnest corneal thickness, and normal posterior elevation. The pupil *(white circle)* is seen to be centered on the topographic maps. *BFS,* Best-fit-sphere; *K,* angle kappa intercept; *white square,* center of pupil; *yellow circle,* thinnest corneal thickness.

Improper fixation may result from the patient's lack of concentration or misunderstanding of instructions.[70] A high level of suspicion should also be maintained in patients with low vision such as aphakes, who may not be able to fixate well on the target.[69] In such cases, analysis of pupil position will reveal the center of the pupil to be inferiorly displaced from the center of the topographic map. (see Fig. 9.12)[63] Results may also be verified by comparing them with the other eye. Fig. 9.14 shows tomographic maps of a patient who had symmetric astigmatism in the right eye and asymmetric superior astigmatism in the left eye. Reexamination of the patient showed residual ophthalmic gel on the left cornea, which created the artifactual steepening. Removal of the gel and repeat tomography revealed regular symmetric astigmatism of the left eye (see Fig. 9.14B).

When confronted with cases suspected of misalignment and in those where a keratoconus-like pattern or inter-eye asymmetry is seen, topography should be repeated with clear instructions to the patient to remain still and concentrate on the central fixation target during the examination or to use the other eye for fixation in the case of poor vision in the eye being examined.[70] Repeat scanning using a machine with a different mechanism of imaging may also be done if available.

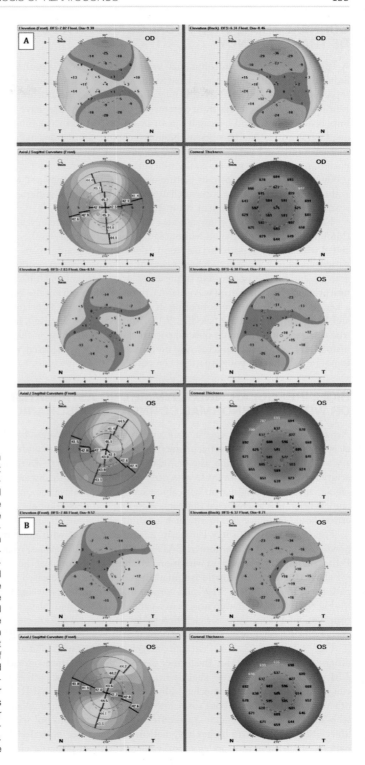

Fig. 9.14 (A) Pentacam tomography of a patient showing inter-eye asymmetry. The right eye had regular symmetric bowtie astigmatism, whereas the left eye showed asymmetric bowtie astigmatism with superior keratoconus-like steepening. Posterior elevation values and corneal thicknesses were normal in both eyes. The patient was reexamined and was found to have residual ophthalmic gel on the left cornea. (B) Repeat Pentacam tomography of the left eye was performed after removal of the residual gel from the ocular surface. Astigmatism was then seen to be regular and symmetric, reestablishing inter-eye symmetry. *OD*, Right eye; *OS*, left eye

CORNEAL AREAS WITH FOCAL SCARS OR A LOSS OF TRANSPARENCY

A false diagnosis of keratoconus may be made in cases of corneal scars or leukomas, in which induced local flattening is associated with subsequent steepening of adjacent areas.[62] Corneal topography of postinfected corneas may also demonstrate keratoconus-like protrusion patterns.[71] Distinguishing these scars from keratoconus, which may also have associated corneal scars, is important.[63] Hanet and colleagues described a case of recurrent interstitial keratitis that developed keratoconus-like changes on biomicroscopic examination, such as Vogt striae, incomplete Fleischer ring, and paracentral stromal thinning, 1 year after disease onset.[72] Maximal anterior, posterior, and true net powers had significantly increased and thinnest corneal thickness decreased, producing a pseudokeratoconus picture on corneal tomography and anterior segment OCT. The authors proposed that the corneal changes arose from initial stiffening of the cornea due to the scarring process and subsequent stromal melting.

Figs. 9.15A and 9.16 show anterior segment photographs revealing focal posterior stromal thinning in a patient with and without keratoconus, respectively. The areas of thinning were associated with increased posterior elevation values on tomography maps (Figs. 9.15C and 9.17). The patient in Figs. 9.16 and 9.17 had recurrent keratouveitis that resulted in dense central stromal scarring and further progression of posterior stromal thinning. Unlike the patient with keratoconus, protrusion of the cornea was absent. Corneal tomography of the keratouveitis patient revealed a keratoconus-like pattern consisting of inferior steepening associated with posterior elevation and focal corneal thinning (see Fig. 9.17). This posterior elevation, however, does not represent true ectasia, as it is the result of focal posterior stromal thinning in the area of the scar. The ocular history and slit lamp biomicroscopy findings should be considered when interpreting a corneal tomographic map showing a pattern compatible with keratoconus.[62]

HIGH, IRREGULAR, AND ASYMMETRIC ASTIGMATISM WITH OR WITHOUT ABNORMAL CORNEAL BIOMECHANICS

Astigmatic eyes without ectasia may display pseudokeratoconus patterns of localized corneal steepening, asymmetric bowtie, or irregular astigmatism on curvature maps. Amblyopia secondary to high astigmatism may also be mistaken for keratoconus.[63] In these patients, pinhole visual acuity is reduced, unlike in those with early to moderate ectatic disease. These cases will also show regular and stable astigmatism with absence of posterior elevation on corneal tomography. Other clinical tests such as epithelial thickness mapping and evaluation of corneal biomechanical properties should be performed to establish a definitive diagnosis.[62]

Figs. 9.18 and 9.19 show Pentacam images of patients with nonectatic bilateral asymmetric bowtie astigmatism. Note normal BAD-D values and CBI values, respectively. Fig. 9.20 shows Pentacam imaging of a patient with more advanced keratoconus of the right eye. Although the left eye showed asymmetric bowtie astigmatism and absence of increased posterior elevation as in the patients in Figs. 9.18 and 9.19, mild corneal thinning was present and CBI was high.

Fig. 9.21 shows Pentacam images of a patient who had mild bilateral irregular superior astigmatism without ectasia. Posterior elevation values and corneal thicknesses were normal in both eyes. Although CBI values were high on the right and suspicious on the left, TBI values were both normal.

Figs. 9.22 and 9.23 show Pentacam images of patients with bilateral regular symmetric bowtie astigmatism without ectasia. The former shows high symmetric astigmatism with normal CBI and TBI values. The latter shows slightly irregular astigmatism in both eyes. The left eye had suspicious CBI, indicating a biomechanically weak cornea, but normal BAD-D and TBI values. The other eye had normal CBI but suspicious TBI. In contrast, Fig. 9.24 shows a keratoconus patient who also had bilateral regular symmetric bowtie astigmatism but with very asymmetric ectasia. The right eye, which had higher astigmatism, had increased posterior elevation in a regular ridge pattern. The left eye was topographically normal without posterior elevation or corneal thinning.

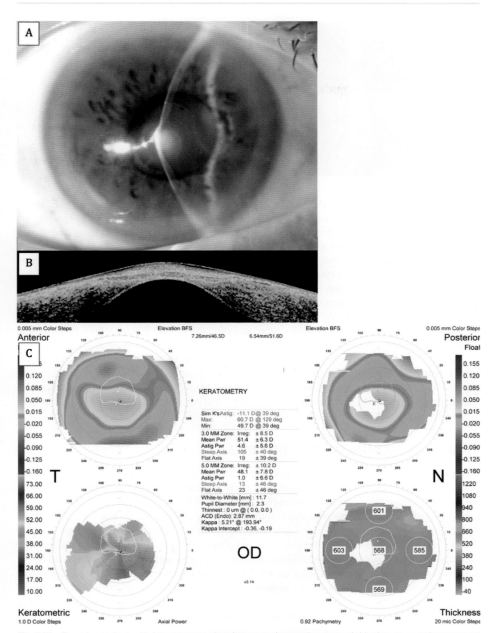

Fig. 9.15 Eye of a patient with keratoconus showing central posterior stromal thinning on anterior segment photograph (A) and anterior segment optical coherence tomography (B). (A) Note the central protrusion involving the anterior and posterior corneal surfaces. A Kayser-Fleischer ring surrounding the area of subepithelial and stromal scarring can be seen as hyperreflective areas in (B). (C) Orbscan topography showed high irregular astigmatism on the curvature map. White areas on posterior elevation and pachymetric maps reflect the areas of dense scarring that precluded measurement. *K,* Angle kappa intercept; *red circle,* thinnest corneal thickness.

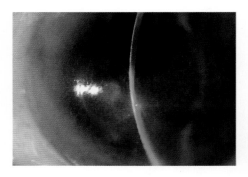

Fig. 9.16 Anterior segment photograph of a patient with recurrent keratouveitis and epithelial herpetic keratitis. Note the central posterior stromal thinning. However, unlike the patient in Fig. 9.15, no protrusion of the overlying cornea was present.

Both eyes had abnormal CBI values, but TBI was 1.00 on the right and 0.00 on the left. Inter-eye asymmetry in terms of clinical signs, corneal curvature, and tomographic findings in patients with keratoconus has been well documented.[73,74] Henriquez and colleagues in their study using Scheimpflug imaging were also able to demonstrate greater inter-eye asymmetry in eyes with very early keratoconus (VEKC) compared to high ametropic eyes with respect to all of the parameters evaluated, including keratometric, pachymetric, and anterior and posterior corneal elevation variables.[75] Consistent with previous studies, their results confirmed that the best parameter distinguishing VEKC eyes from normal eyes in unilateral analysis was the final D value from the BAD. Employing a mixed model using the nonasymmetry parameter final D and the asymmetry values increased the area under the ROC curve analysis value from 0.975 to 0.9957, showing that bilateral/asymmetry evaluation would help in the diagnosis of early keratoconus.[75]

Patients with equivocal tomographic findings should also be advised to follow up regularly with repeat corneal imaging. Fig. 9.25 shows Pentacam tomography of a patient with bilateral superior asymmetric bowtie astigmatism who was regularly followed over 3 years. Refraction and imaging remained stable, and Corvis biomechanical analysis revealed normal TBI despite high CBI in both eyes.

TEAR FILM INSTABILITY AND DRY EYE

Chronic desiccation from reduced aqueous tear production and tear film instability can lead to alterations of the corneal surface.[62,76] Epitheliopathies can cause corneal surface irregularity and artifacts on corneal topographic examination that resemble keratoconus.[76] Fig. 9.26A shows the Orbscan topography of a patient with dry eye who had asymmetric bowtie astigmatism on the left eye and symmetric bowtie astigmatism on the right. After treatment with lubricants for 1 month, repeat imaging showed regularization of the anterior curvature (see Fig.9.26B). De Paiva and colleagues reported on a series of dry eye patients who had inferior corneal steepening with keratoconus predicted by the Klyce software.[76] Among patients being screened at a refractive surgery clinic, El Wardani and colleagues demonstrated keratoconus-like topographic changes in six patients due to inferior inhomogenous epithelial thickening on anterior segment OCT mapping.[77] These patients were postulated to have risk factors such as dry eyes and exposure, tear film abnormality, or contact lens warpage.

OTHER CAUSES OF PSEUDOKERATOCONUS

Hyperopic LASIK and PRK can lead to corneal steepening and topographic pseudokeratectasia, especially if the area of ablation is decentered.[63,78] Other less common conditions that have been reported to produce tomographic patterns mimicking keratoconus include ocular rosacea,[79,80] vernal keratoconjunctivitis and associated eye rubbing,[81] and blepharoptosis.[82,83] These cases, however, will show absence of posterior corneal elevation on corneal tomography.

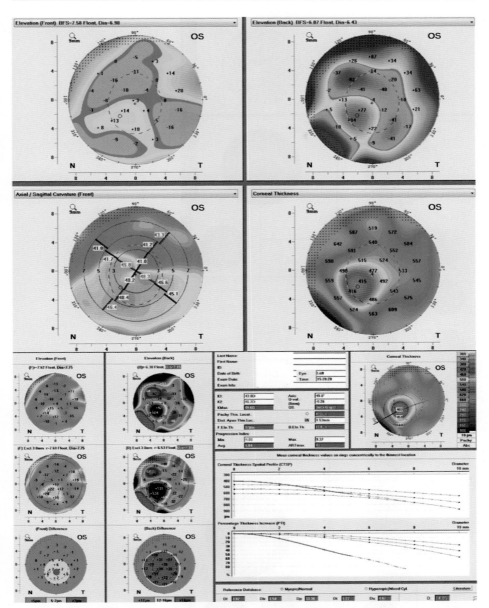

Fig. 9.17 Pentacam tomography of the patient from Fig. 9.16 2 years later showing false corneal ectasia. This patient developed dense central stromal scarring and further progression of posterior stromal thinning from recurrent keratouveitis. Note inferior steepening associated with increased posterior elevation and paracentral corneal thinning.

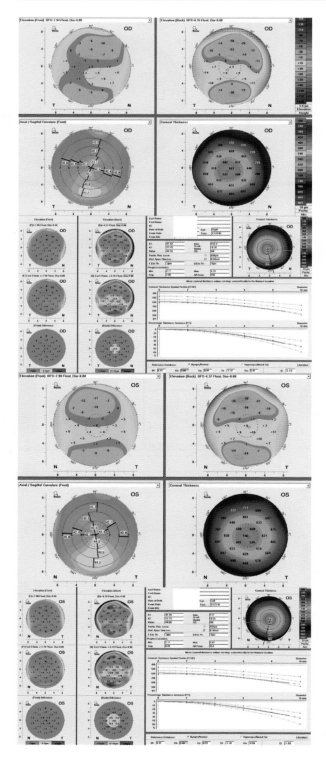

Fig. 9.18 Pentacam tomography of a patient who had bilateral asymmetric bowtie astigmatism. Although deviation of back elevation difference map (Db) values were suspicious in both eyes, Belin-Ambrósio enhanced ectasia display total deviation values were both normal.

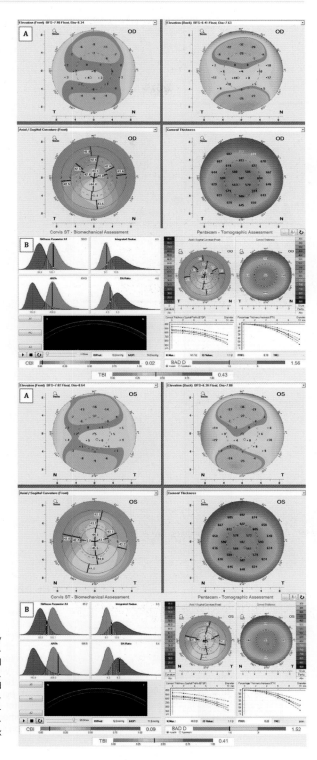

Fig. 9.19 Pentacam tomography (A) and Corvis biomechanical analysis (B) of a patient who had bilateral asymmetric bowtie astigmatism. Although Belin-Ambrósio enhanced ectasia display total deviation (BAD-D) and tomographic and biomechanical index (TBI) values were suspicious, corneal biomechanical index (CBI) was normal in both eyes.

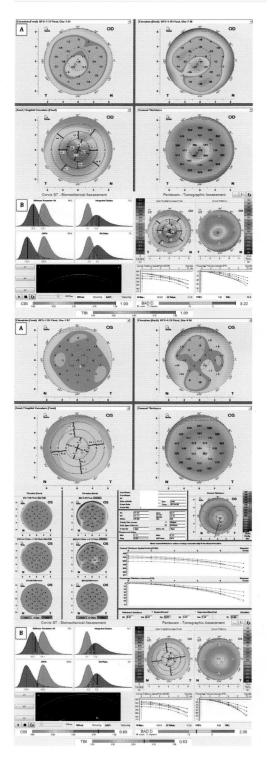

Fig. 9.20 Pentacam tomography (A) and Corvis biomechanical analysis (B) of a patient with keratoconus. The right eye had more advanced disease with central steepening associated with corneal thinning and anterior and posterior islands of elevation. The left eye had oblique asymmetric bowtie astigmatism and mild corneal thinning without posterior elevation. Whereas corneal biomechanical indices *(CBIs)* were high in both eyes, Belin-Ambrósio enhanced ectasia display total deviation *(BAD-D)* and tomographic and biomechanical index *(TBI)* values were only suspicious for the left eye. *OD,* Right eye; *OS,* left eye.

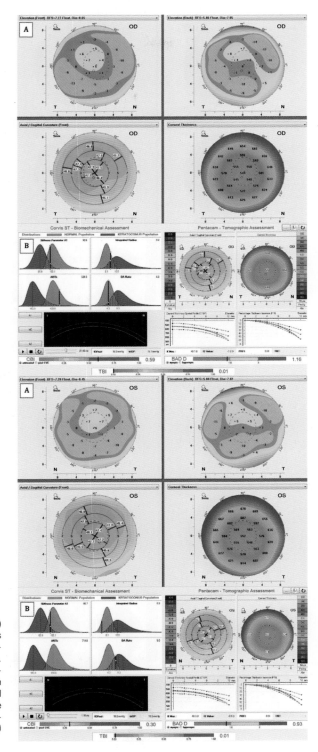

Fig. 9.21 Pentacam tomography (A) and Corvis biomechanical analysis (B) of a patient who had mild bilateral irregular superior astigmatism. Note normal posterior elevation values and corneal thicknesses in both eyes. Although corneal biomechanical index *(CBI)* values were high on the right and suspicious on the left, tomographic and biomechanical index *(TBI)* values were both normal.

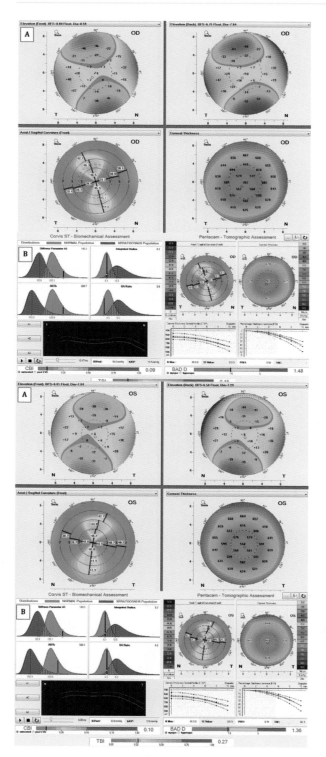

Fig. 9.22 Pentacam tomography (A) and Corvis biomechanical analysis (B) of a patient who had bilaterally high regular symmetric bowtie astigmatism with intereye symmetry. Note normal posterior elevation values and absence of corneal thinning. Belin-Ambrósio enhanced ectasia display total deviation *(BAD-D)*, corneal biomechanical index *(CBI)*, and tomographic and biomechanical index *(TBI)* values were normal in both eyes.

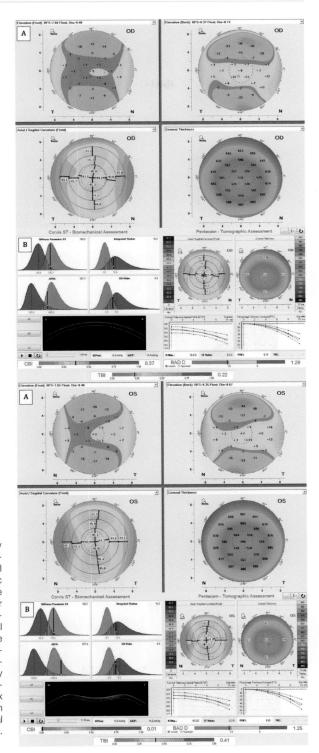

Fig. 9.23 Pentacam tomography (A) and Corvis biomechanical analysis (B) of a patient with bilateral and slightly irregular but symmetric bowtie astigmatism with intereye symmetry. Note normal posterior elevation values and corneal thicknesses. The corneal biomechanical index *(CBI)* was suspicious for the right eye, indicating a biomechanically weak cornea, whereas Belin-Ambrósio enhanced ectasia display total deviation *(BAD-D)* and tomographic and biomechanical index *(TBI)* values were normal. Although CBI and BAD-D values were normal for the left eye, TBI was suspicious. *OD,* Right eye; *OS,* left eye.

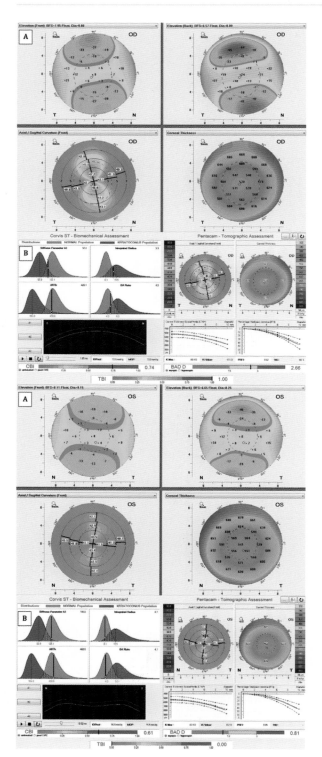

Fig. 9.24 Pentacam tomography (A) and Corvis biomechanical analysis (B) in a keratoconus patient who had higher astigmatism in the right eye than the left. Both eyes showed regular with-the-rule symmetric bowtie astigmatism. Note increased posterior elevation values and a thinner cornea on the right eye, with the left eye tomographically normal. Although corneal biomechanical index *(CBI)* values were high in both eyes, tomographic and biomechanical index *(TBI)* was 1.00 for the right eye and 0.00 for the left eye. *OD,* Right eye; *OS,* left eye.

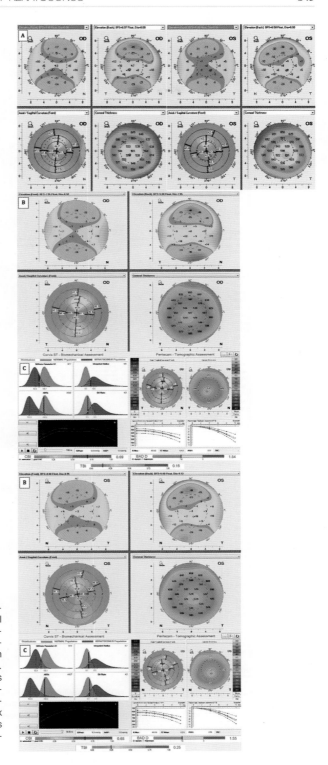

Fig. 9.25 (A) Pentacam tomography of a patient who had bilateral superior asymmetric bowtie astigmatism. (B) The tomographic profile and manifest refraction of both eyes remained stable over 3 years. (C) Corvis biomechanical analysis revealed high corneal biomechanical index *(CBI)* but normal tomographic and biomechanical index *(TBI)* in both eyes. The patient was listed for bilateral advanced surface ablation.

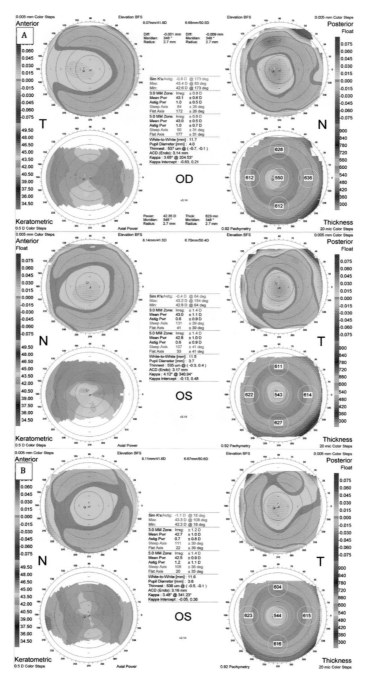

Fig. 9.26 Orbscan topography of a patient who underwent refractive surgery screening. (A) The right eye was unremarkable, whereas the left eye had asymmetric bowtie astigmatism without associated thinning or increased posterior elevation. The other maps were comparable between the two eyes. A diagnosis of dry eye was made and lubricants started. (B) One month later, the anterior curvature profile of the left eye became more regular, reestablishing inter-eye symmetry. *OD,* Right eye; *OS,* left eye.

References

1. Tummanapalli SS, Maseedupally V, Mandathara P, Rathi VM, Sangwan VS. Evaluation of corneal elevation and thickness indices in pellucid marginal degeneration and keratoconus. *J Cataract Refract Surg.* 2013;39(1):56–65.
2. Martínez-Abad A, Piñero DP. Pellucid marginal degeneration: detection, discrimination from other corneal ectatic disorders and progression. *Cont Lens Anterior Eye.* 2019;42(4):341–349.
3. Krachmer JH, Feder RS, Belin MW. Keratoconus and related noninflammatory corneal thinning disorders. *Surv Ophthalmol.* 1984;28(4):293–322.
4. Sridhar MS, Mahesh S, Bansal AK, Nutheti R, Rao GN. Pellucid marginal corneal degeneration. *Ophthalmology.* 2004;111(6):1102–1107.
5. Kaushik S, Jain AK, Saini JS. Unilateral pellucid marginal degeneration. *Eye (Lond).* 2003;17(2):246–248.
6. Basak SK, Hazra TK, Bhattacharya D, Sinha TK. Unilateral pellucid marginal degeneration. *Indian J Ophthalmol.* 2000;48(3):233–234
7. Biswas S, Brahma A, Tromans C, Ridgway A. Management of pellucid marginal corneal degeneration. *Eye (Lond).* 2000;14(Pt 4):629–634.
8. Wagenhorst BB. Unilateral pellucid marginal degeneration in an elderly patient. *Br J Ophthalmol.* 1996;80(10):927–928.
9. Jinabhai A, Radhakrishnan H, O'Donnell C. Pellucid corneal marginal degeneration: a review. *Cont Lens Anterior Eye.* 2011;34(2):56–63.
10. Gokhale NS. Epidemiology of keratoconus. *Indian J Ophthalmol.* 2013;61(8):382–383.
11. Koc M, Tekin K, Inanc M, Kosekahya P, Yilmazbas P. Crab claw pattern on corneal topography: pellucid marginal degeneration or inferior keratoconus? *Eye (Lond).* 2018;32(1):11–18.
12. Rumelt S, Rehany U. Surgically induced keratoglobus in pellucid marginal degeneration. *Eye (Lond).* 1998;12(Pt 1):156-158.
13. Robin JB, Schanzlin DJ, Verity SM, et al. Peripheral corneal disorders. *Surv Ophthalmol.* 1986;31(1):1–36.
14. Krachmer JH. Pellucid marginal corneal degeneration. *Arch Ophthalmol.* 1978;96(7):1217–1221.
15. Gomes JA, Tan D, Rapuano CJ, et al. Global consensus on keratoconus and ectatic diseases. *Cornea.* 2015;34(4):359–369.
16. Rodrigues MM, Newsome DA, Krachmer JH, Eiferman RA. Pellucid marginal corneal degeneration: a clinicopathologic study of two cases. *Exp Eye Res.* 1981;33(3):277–288.
17. Pouliquen Y, Chauvaud D, Lacombe E, Amiet F, Savoldelli M. [Marginal pellucid degeneration of the cornea, or marginal keratoconus (author's transl)]. *J Fr Ophtalmol.* 1980;3(2):109–114.
18. François J, Hanssens M, Stockmans L. [Pellucid marginal degeneration of the cornea]. *Ophthalmologica.* 1968;155(5):337–356.
19. Zucchini G. [On an unusual case of parenchymal hematoma of the cornea following caustic alkali burn]. *Ann Ottalmol Clin Ocul.* 1962;88:161–165.
20. Kayazawa F, Nishimura K, Kodama Y, Tsuji T, Itoi M. Keratoconus with pellucid marginal corneal degeneration. *Arch Ophthalmol.* 1984;102(6):895–896.
21. Varley GA, Macsai MS, Krachmer JH. The results of penetrating keratoplasty for pellucid marginal corneal degeneration. *Am J Ophthalmol.* 1990;110(2):149–152.
22. Basu S, Vaddavalli PK, Ramappa M, Shah S, Murthy SI, Sangwan VS. Intracameral perfluoropropane gas in the treatment of acute corneal hydrops. *Ophthalmology.* 2011;118(5):934–939.
23. Tuft SJ, Gregory WM, Buckley RJ. Acute corneal hydrops in keratoconus. *Ophthalmology.* 1994;101(10):1738–1744.
24. Amsler M. [Some data on the problem of keratoconus]. *Bull Soc Belge Ophtalmol.* 1961;129:331–354.
25. Rabinowitz YS. Keratoconus. *Surv Ophthalmol.* 1998;42(4):297–319.
26. Golubović S, Parunović A. Acute pellucid marginal corneal degeneration. *Cornea.* 1988;7(4):290–294.
27. Sinjab MM, Youssef LN. Pellucid-like keratoconus. *F1000Res.* 2012;1:48.
28. Lee BW, Jurkunas UV, Harissi-Dagher M, Poothullil AM, Tobaigy FM, Azar DT. Ectatic disorders associated with a claw-shaped pattern on corneal topography. *Am J Ophthalmol.* 2007;144(1):154–156.
29. Labiris G, Giarmoukakis A, Sideroudi H, et al. Diagnostic capacity of biomechanical indices from a dynamic bidirectional applanation device in pellucid marginal degeneration. *J Cataract Refract Surg.* 2014;40(6):1006–1012.
30. Lenk J, Haustein M, Terai N, Spoerl E, Raiskup F. Characterization of ocular biomechanics in pellucid marginal degeneration. *Cornea.* 2016;35(4):506–509.

31. Sedaghat MR, Ostadi-Moghadam H, Jabbarvand M, Askarizadeh F, Momeni-Moghaddam H, Narooie-Noori F. Corneal hysteresis and corneal resistance factor in pellucid marginal degeneration. *J Curr Ophthalmol*. 2018;30(1):42–47.
32. Saad A, Gatinel D. Evaluation of total and corneal wavefront high order aberrations for the detection of forme fruste keratoconus. *Invest Ophthalmol Vis Sci*. 2012;53(6):2978–2992.
33. Oie Y, Maeda N, Kosaki R, et al. Characteristics of ocular higher-order aberrations in patients with pellucid marginal corneal degeneration. *J Cataract Refract Surg*. 2008;34(11):1928–1934.
34. Wallang BS, Das S. Keratoglobus. *Eye (Lond)*. 2013;27(9):1004–1012.
35. Rathi VM, Murthy SI, Bagga B, Taneja M, Chaurasia S, Sangwan VS. Keratoglobus: an experience at a tertiary eye care center in India. *Indian J Ophthalmol*. 2015;63(3):233–238.
36. Pouliquen Y, Dhermy P, Espinasse MA, Savoldelli M. [Keratoglobus]. *J Fr Ophtalmol*. 1985;8(1):43–54.
37. Cameron JA. Keratoglobus. *Cornea*. 1993;12(2):124–130.
38. Reddy SC. Keratoglobus and complicated microphthalmos. *Indian J Ophthalmol*. 1978;26(3):23–26.
39. Nelson ME, Talbot JF. Keratoglobus in the Rubinstein-Taybi syndrome. *Br J Ophthalmol*. 1989;73(5):385–387.
40. Feder RS, Neems LC. Noninflammatory ectatic disorders. In: Mannis MJ, Holland EJ, eds. *Cornea: Fundamentals, Diagnosis and Management*. 4th ed. Edinburgh: Elsevier Inc; 2017:820–843.
41. Karabatsas CH, Cook SD. Topographic analysis in pellucid marginal corneal degeneration and keratoglobus. *Eye (Lond)*. 1996;10(Pt 4):451–455.
42. Biglan AW, Brown SI, Johnson BL. Keratoglobus and blue sclera. *Am J Ophthalmol*. 1977;83(2):225–233.
43. Randleman JB, Woodward M, Lynn MJ, Stulting RD. Risk assessment for ectasia after corneal refractive surgery. *Ophthalmology*. 2008;115(1):37–50.
44. Wolle MA, Randleman JB, Woodward MA. Complications of refractive surgery: ectasia after refractive surgery. *Int Ophthalmol Clin*. 2016;56(2):127–139.
45. Giri P, Azar DT. Risk profiles of ectasia after keratorefractive surgery. *Curr Opin Ophthalmol*. 2017;28(4):337–342.
46. Padmanabhan P, Rachapalle Reddi S, Sivakumar PD. Topographic, tomographic, and aberrometric characteristics of post-LASIK ectasia. *Optom Vis Sci*. 2016;93(11):1364–1370.
47. Bohac M, Koncarevic M, Pasalic A, et al. Incidence and clinical characteristics of post LASIK ectasia: a review of over 30,000 LASIK cases. *Semin Ophthalmol*. 2018;33(7-8):869–877.
48. Santhiago MR, Giacomin NT, Smadja D, Bechara SJ. Ectasia risk factors in refractive surgery. *Clin Ophthalmol*. 2016;10:713–720.
49. Rocha KM, Perez-Straziota CE, Stulting RD, Randleman JB. SD-OCT analysis of regional epithelial thickness profiles in keratoconus, postoperative corneal ectasia, and normal eyes. *J Refract Surg*. 2013;29(3):173–179.
50. Ferreira TB, Marques EF, Filipe HP. Combined corneal collagen crosslinking and secondary intraocular lens implantation for keratectasia after radial keratotomy. *J Cataract Refract Surg*. 2014;40(1):143–147.
51. Mehta P, Rathi VM, Murthy SI. Deep anterior lamellar keratoplasty for the management of iatrogenic keratectasia occurring after hexagonal keratotomy. *Indian J Ophthalmol*. 2012;60(2):139–141.
52. Roszkowska AM, Sommario MS, Urso M, Aragona P. Post photorefractive keratectomy corneal ectasia. *Int J Ophthalmol*. 2017;10(2):315–317.
53. Richoz O, Mavrakanas N, Pajic B, Hafezi F. Corneal collagen cross-linking for ectasia after LASIK and photorefractive keratectomy: long-term results. *Ophthalmology*. 2013;120(7):1354–1359.
54. Leccisotti A. Corneal ectasia after photorefractive keratectomy. *Graefes Arch Clin Exp Ophthalmol*. 2007;245(6):869–875.
55. Moshirfar M, Albarracin JC, Desautels JD, Birdsong OC, Linn SH, Hoopes PC Sr. Ectasia following small-incision lenticule extraction (SMILE): a review of the literature. *Clin Ophthalmol*. 2017;11:1683–1688.
56. Chiche A, Trinh L, Baudouin C, Denoyer A. [SMILE (Small Incision Lenticule Extraction) among the corneal refractive surgeries in 2018 (French translation of the article)]. *J Fr Ophtalmol*. 2018;41(7):650–658.
57. Yoshida J, Murata H, Miyai T, et al. Characteristics and risk factors of recurrent keratoconus over the long term after penetrating keratoplasty. *Graefes Arch Clin Exp Ophthalmol*. 2018;256(12):2377–2383.
58. Bergmanson JP, Goosey JD, Patel CK, Mathew JH. Recurrence or re-emergence of keratoconus—what is the evidence telling us? Literature review and two case reports. *Ocul Surf*. 2014;12(4):267–272.

59. Feizi S, Javadi MA, Rezaei Kanavi M. Recurrent keratoconus in a corneal graft after deep anterior lamellar keratoplasty. *J Ophthalmic Vis Res*. 2012;7(4):328–331.

60. Gatzioufas Z, Panos GD, Gkaragkani E, Georgoulas S, Angunawela R. Recurrence of keratoconus after deep anterior lamellar keratoplasty following pregnancy. *Int J Ophthalmol*. 2017;10(6):1011–1013.

61. Gatzioufas Z, Seitz B. Deep anterior lamellar keratoplasty for corneal opacification in Maroteaux-Lamy syndrome: is it the treatment of choice? *Cornea*. 2011;30(12):1519–1520.

62. Piñero DP. Misdiagnosing keratoconus. *Exp Rev Ophthalmol*. 2016;11(1):29–39.

63. Stein R, Salim G. False corneal ectasia in patients referred for corneal crosslinking, topography-guided photorefractive keratectomy, and intrastromal corneal rings. *Can J Ophthalmol*. 2019;54(3):374–381.

64. Tang M, Li Y, Chamberlain W, Louie DJ, Schallhorn JM, Huang D. Differentiating keratoconus and corneal warpage by analyzing focal change patterns in corneal topography, pachymetry, and epithelial thickness maps. *Invest Ophthalmol Vis Sci*. 2016;57(9):OCT544–OCT549.

65. Patrão LF, Canedo AL, Azevedo JL, Correa R, Ambrósio R Jr. Differentiation of mild keratoconus from corneal warpage according to topographic inferior steepening based on corneal tomography data. *Arq Bras Oftalmol*. 2016;79(4):264–267.

66. Schallhorn JM, Tang M, Li Y, Louie DJ, Chamberlain W, Huang D. Distinguishing between contact lens warpage and ectasia: usefulness of optical coherence tomography epithelial thickness mapping. *J Cataract Refract Surg*. 2017;43(1):60–66.

67. Alipour F, Letafatnejad M, Beheshtnejad AH, et al. Corneal biomechanical findings in contact lens induced corneal warpage. *J Ophthalmol*. 2016;2016:5603763.

68. Mandell RB, Chiang CS, Yee L. Asymmetric corneal toricity and pseudokeratoconus in videokeratography. *J Am Optom Assoc*. 1996;67(9):540–547.

69. Hubbe RE, Foulks GN. The effect of poor fixation on computer-assisted topographic corneal analysis. Pseudokeratoconus. *Ophthalmology*. 1994;101(10):1745–1748.

70. Hick S, Laliberté JF, Meunier J, Chagnon M, Brunette I. Effects of misalignment during corneal topography. *J Cataract Refract Surg*. 2007;33(9):1522–1529.

71. Shimizu E, Yamaguchi T, Yagi-Yaguchi Y, et al. Corneal higher-order aberrations in infectious keratitis. *Am J Ophthalmol*. 2017;175:148–158.

72. Hanet MS, Zimpfer A, Lepper S, Seitz B. Keratoconus-like tomographic changes in a case of recurrent interstitial keratitis. *J Ophthalmic Inflamm Infect*. 2018;8(1):4.

73. Dienes L, Kránitz K, Juhász E, et al. Evaluation of intereye corneal asymmetry in patients with keratoconus. A scheimpflug imaging study. *PLoS One*. 2014;9(10):e108882.

74. Galletti JD, Ruiseñor Vázquez PR, Minguez N, et al. Corneal asymmetry analysis by Pentacam Scheimpflug tomography for keratoconus diagnosis. *J Refract Surg*. 2015;31(2):116–123.

75. Henriquez MA, Izquierdo L Jr, Belin MW. Intereye asymmetry in eyes with keratoconus and high ammetropia: Scheimpflug imaging analysis. *Cornea*. 2015;34(Suppl 10):S57–S60.

76. De Paiva CS, Harris LD, Pflugfelder SC. Keratoconus-like topographic changes in keratoconjunctivitis sicca. *Cornea*. 2003;22(1):22–24.

77. El Wardani M, Hashemi K, Aliferis K, Kymionis G. Topographic changes simulating keratoconus in patients with irregular inferior epithelial thickening documented by anterior segment optical coherence tomography. *Clin Ophthalmol*. 2019;13:2103–2110.

78. Jin GJ, Lyle WA, Merkley KH. Laser in situ keratomileusis for primary hyperopia. *J Cataract Refract Surg*. 2005;31(4):776–784.

79. Stoesser F, Lévy D, Moalic S, Colin J. [Pseudokeratoconus and ocular rosacea]. *J Fr Ophtalmol*. 2004;27(3):278–284.

80. Dursun D, Piniella AM, Pflugfelder SC. Pseudokeratoconus caused by rosacea. *Cornea*. 2001;20(6):668–669.

81. Gautam V, Chaudhary M, Sharma AK, Shrestha GS, Rai PG. Topographic corneal changes in children with vernal keratoconjunctivitis: a report from Kathmandu, Nepal. *Cont Lens Anterior Eye*. 2015;38(6):461–465.

82. Zhu T, Ye X, Xu P, et al. Changes of corneal tomography in patients with congenital blepharoptosis. *Sci Rep*. 2017;7(1):6580.

83. Kim T, Khosla-Gupta B, Debacker C. Blepharoptosis-induced superior keratoconus. *Am J Ophthalmol*. 2000;130(2):232–234.

Further Reading

1. El Wardani Mohamad, Hashemi Kattayoon, Aliferis Konstantinos, Kymionis George Topographic changes simulating keratoconus in patients with irregular inferior epithelial thickening documented by anterior segment optical coherence tomography Clin Ophthalmol. 2019;13:2103–2110. 1177–5467. doi: https://doi.org/10.2147/OPTH.S208101.31802839.

CHAPTER 10

Keratoconus: Associated Systemic Diseases

Milad Modabber ■ Ivan R. Schwab

KEY CONCEPTS

- Numerous systemic conditions have been linked to development and progression of keratoconus.
- Eye rubbing may represent the common pathway in the progression of keratoconus across a range of conditions such as atopy, contact lens wear, or oculodigital stimulation secondary to Down syndrome or Leber congenital amaurosis.
- Keratoconus has been associated with noninflammatory connective tissue disorders, such as Marfan syndrome, Ehlers-Danlos syndrome, osteogenesis imperfecta, and mitral valve prolapse.
- It may reflect both a decrease in collagen content and localized dysfunction in corneal collagen elasticity owing to altered enzymatic metabolism.
- A range of chromosomal abnormalities have been associated with keratoconus, most commonly Down syndrome and Turner syndrome.

Introduction

Keratoconus is a progressive ectatic disorder of the cornea, characterized by conical steepening and thinning. It typically manifests at puberty and is most commonly bilateral, albeit often asymmetric.[1] Although keratoconus has been extensively investigated, its precise cause remains elusive. It is clear, however, that this multifactorial disease is influenced by a complex interplay of genetic and environmental factors.[2] Although keratoconus is most commonly an isolated ocular abnormality, numerous systemic conditions have been linked to its development and progression. The majority of these systemic associations have generally been classified as conditions of atopy or eczema leading to eye rubbing, connective tissue disorders with abnormal collagen elasticity, and abnormal retinal function or altered mental status associated with oculodigital stimulation.[3]

ATOPY

Over the past half-century, much has been written linking keratoconus to atopic disease. The Dunedin University Scottish Keratoconus Study of 200 keratoconus patients found that the prevalence of asthma (23% of keratoconus vs. 6% controls) and hay fever (30% keratoconus vs. 16% controls) was higher than in the control cohort.[4] These results were further strengthened by the Collaborative Longitudinal Evaluation of Keratoconus (CLEK) study, which noted the prevalence of hay fever to be 53% among the over 1200 keratoconus patients studied.[5,6] Similarly, Rahi et al. found a significantly higher rate of atopy in keratoconus than seen in controls (35% vs. 12%).[7] A significant correlation in the severity of atopy and keratoconus has also been observed.[8,9] Notably,

Tuft et al. reported that severe allergic eye disease among keratoconus patients tended to reduce the time to penetrating keratoplasty (PKP) (*P* = 0.06).[10]

A recent meta-analysis of 29 studies encompassing over 50 million subjects by Hashemi et al. found allergy, asthma, and eczema to be significant risk factors for keratoconus with odds ratios (ORs) of 1.42 (95% confidence interval [CI]: 1.06–1.79), 1.94 (95% CI: 1.30–2.58), and 2.95 (95% CI: 1.30–4.59), respectively.[11] Although atopy was positively associated with keratoconus, the linkage was not statistically significant (OR: 1.12; 95% CI: 0.40–1.85).[11] It was postulated that inconsistent definition of "atopy" contributed to the conflicting results across the referenced reports.

Atopic disease likely contributes to keratoconus through eye rubbing associated with allergic symptoms and atopic pruritus.[12] Atopy is one of the primary causes of eye rubbing, which in turn is one of the most well-established environmental risk factors for the development and progression of keratoconus. It is even plausible that eye rubbing itself, and not the atopy, is the culprit.[3] However, it would be difficult to establish causality. Indeed, there are several reports of unilateral keratoconus secondary to chronic unilateral eye rubbing.[3,13,14]

The pathogenesis of eye rubbing in keratoconus is controversial. It likely serves as the second hit in a two-hit hypothesis in genetically susceptible individuals.[15] Chronic eye rubbing can cause mechanical wear on the cornea that leads to progressive ectasia.[14,16] Moreover, recurrent epithelial trauma because of eye rubbing can perpetuate a chronic inflammatory event.[3] In turn, this activates inflammatory mediators such as interleukin (IL)-6, tumor necrosis factor alpha (TNF-α), and matrix metalloproteinase-9 (MMP-9), which are overexpressed in the tears of keratoconus patients.[17,18] Eye rubbing in keratoconus induces IL-1-mediated apoptosis through the binding of Fas ligand by keratocytes.[19] Keratocytes in keratoconus patients have four times the density of IL-1 receptors compared with healthy controls.[20] Notably, keratoconic eyes have been observed to respond differently to eye rubbing than normal eyes, exhibiting higher degrees of posterior astigmatism, intraocular pressure change, and anterior chamber volume change.[21] Taken together, eye rubbing may represent the common pathway in the progression of keratoconus across a range of conditions such as atopy, contact lens wear, or oculodigital stimulation secondary to Down syndrome or Leber congenital amaurosis (LCA).

OBSTRUCTIVE SLEEP APNEA

Obstructive sleep apnea (OSA) is a clinical syndrome characterized by recurrent episodes of apnea and hypopnea during sleep and is often associated with daytime somnolence.[22] OSA is an independent risk factor for stroke and death.[22,23] Floppy eyelid syndrome (FES) typically presents with lax eyelids that evert with minimal traction and chronic papillary conjunctivitis of the upper palpebral conjunctiva. Virtually all patients with FES have OSA, but only a subset of OSA patients have FES.[22] The association between keratoconus and FES is well established, and laterality in both tends to coincide with sleeping side preference.[22] Frequent eye rubbing has also been suggested as a common causative factor in both conditions, as supported by asymmetric disease progression owing to same-side sleeping or asymmetric eye rubbing.[24]

Multiple studies have observed that keratoconus patients are more likely to suffer from sleep apnea or be at high risk for it based on the Berlin questionnaire.[25–27] Ezra et al. found a strong association between keratoconus and FES (OR: 19.3), and even more markedly so in patients with unilateral keratoconus (OR: 35.0).[26] Gupta et al. observed that of the patients who had undergone prior PKP for keratoconus but were not yet diagnosed with OSA, 69% scored as high risk for developing OSA on the Berlin questionnaire compared with only 21% of milder keratoconus patients who had not undergone surgery (OR: 8.6; 95% CI: 2.8–26.6).[27] Moreover, the average body mass index (BMI) of those postkeratoplasty patients was significantly higher than those who had not undergone PKP (33.9 vs. 26.4 kg/m²; *P* < 0.0001).[27]

Nocturnal eyelid eversion in FES is thought to result in chronic microtrauma to the cornea and conjunctiva, especially with pillow-ocular surface interface. Upregulation of MMP activity has been associated with both FES and keratoconus and may be the pathophysiologic link between the two conditions.[28,29] Immunohistochemistry studies in patients with keratoconus and FES have shown an increased immunoreactivity for MMP-7 and MMP-9 compared with controls, potentially pointing to a shared common pathway in perpetuating connective tissue degradation.[30]

Ophthalmologists should refer patients with FES for nocturnal polysomnography ("sleep study") to evaluate for occult OSA. Treatment of OSA with continuous positive airway pressure (CPAP) therapy or surgical uvulopalatoplasty has been shown to reduce the signs and symptoms of FES and reduce systemic sequelae.[22]

CONNECTIVE TISSUE DISORDERS

Keratoconus has long been associated with noninflammatory connective tissue disorders, such as Marfan syndrome,[31] Ehlers-Danlos syndrome,[32,33] osteogenesis imperfecta,[34] and mitral valve prolapse (MVP).[35-37] Robertson found the prevalence of hypermobility in joints to be 50% in 44 consecutive keratoconus patients.[33] Subsequent studies also observed increased joint hypermobility, particularly in the metacarpophalangeal and wrist joints.[38,39] However, more recent studies have failed to observe an association of joint hypermobility among keratoconus patients.[10,40]

Biochemically, keratoconus may reflect both a decrease in collagen content, as well as localized dysfunction in corneal collagen elasticity owing to altered enzymatic metabolism. It has been proposed that the corneal tissue of such individuals with a genetic predisposition is more easily weakened by oxidative corneal stress caused by sustained mechanical trauma, eventually leading to corneal ectasia.[41] In fact, studies on Marfan syndrome demonstrate a reduction in corneal hysteresis and progressive thinning.[42]

MVP is a connective tissue abnormality of the leaflets, chordate tendinea, and annulus of the mitral valve, diagnosed through cardiac echocardiography.[43] An increased prevalence (22.6%–58%) of MVP has been observed in keratoconus patients, with a positive correlation between disease severity and that of corneal disease.[35-37,44] In a case-control study, Rabbanikhah et al. found the prevalence of MVP in patients with corneal hydrops secondary to keratoconus to be 65.6% compared with 9% in controls, and the risk of developing MVP in corneal hydrops patients was also much higher (OR: 26.7; 95% CI: 9.5–75.2).[35] However, in a study of 95 keratoconus patients, Street et al. did not find a significant association between keratoconus, MVP, and joint hypermobility.[40] Moreover, a Danish national registry did not find a significant association between keratoconus and mitral valve disorder (OR: 1.00; 95% CI: 0.52–1.92).[45] Future prospective studies are thus warranted to better delineate this association.

IMMUNE DISORDERS

Keratoconus has historically been considered a non-inflammatory condition. However, more recently, the immune system has been implicated in its pathogenesis. The tears of keratoconus patients have been observed to exhibit an overexpression of inflammatory mediators, including IL-6, TNF-α, and MMP-9, when compared with healthy controls.[17,18] The increased activity of these intracorneal inflammatory mediators has been proposed as a possible mechanism for stromal degradation and reduced biomechanical stability in keratoconus.[18]

Rheumatoid arthritis (RA) is most commonly associated with keratoconjunctivitis sicca, anterior scleritis, or peripheral ulcerative keratitis (PUK). However, in a retrospective case-control study, Nemet et al. found an increased risk of keratoconus in RA patients (OR: 8.1; 95% CI: 1.5–44.2), although the numbers were so small that these findings need to be replicated in a larger study.[46] The chronic epitheliopathy secondary to the upregulation of inflammatory mediators in RA was proposed as the predisposing factor for the development of keratoconus.

Other immune disorders were also linked to keratoconus by Nemet et al., including ulcerative colitis (OR: 12.1; 95% CI: 1.3–116), autoimmune chronic active hepatitis (OR: 6; 95% CI: 1.01–36), Hashimoto thyroiditis (OR: 2.0; 95% CI: 1.2–3.3), and irritable bowel syndrome (OR: 5; 95% CI: 2.1–12.1).[46] Notably, Kahan et al. found an excess of thyroxin in tears of patients with keratoconus, independent of their thyroid function, at 2 to 50 times higher concentration than that of healthy subjects. It has been proposed that excess levels of thyroxin in tears may affect corneal metabolism and, in turn, corneal structural integrity.[47] These findings are still preliminary, however, and need to be replicated with larger numbers of participants.

DOWN SYNDROME

A range of chromosomal abnormalities have been associated with keratoconus, most commonly Down syndrome and Turner syndrome.[48–50] Most series have reported a 5.5% to 15% prevalence of keratoconus among people with Down syndrome.[48,51,52] A retrospective longitudinal cohort study by Woodward et al. also noted increased odds of keratoconus in patients with Down syndrome (OR: 6.22; 95% CI: 2.08–18.66).[12] Corneal hydrops in keratoconus patients has also been observed at higher rates in those with concomitant Down syndrome than in isolated keratoconus patients.[53]

The role of genetic abnormalities in trisomy 21, which may underlie the structural or biochemical changes of keratoconus, has been evaluated. The isoenzyme superoxide dismutase *SOD1* gene on chromosome 21, which plays a role in the oxidative stress response, demonstrated higher levels of expression in keratoconic corneas compared with healthy corneas.[2] An intronic sequence deletion was found to segregate with disease in two families with keratoconus.[54] However, owing to the overall rarity of this mutation in keratoconus patients, the existence and strength of a true pathogenic association is still unclear.[55–57]

Keratoconus also occurs with higher frequency among developmentally delayed individuals without Down syndrome.[54] In fact, the prevalence of unilateral disease is considerably higher in this group compared with the general population, plausibly because of oculodigital stimulation in low mentally functioning patients.[58]

DIABETES

The role of diabetes mellitus (DM) in the development and progression of keratoconus has been conflicting. Although most studies have found DM to be protective against keratoconus,[12,59–61] these findings have not been universal.[62] A retrospective longitudinal cohort study by Woodward et al. observed that patients with uncomplicated DM had 20% lower odds of keratoconus (OR: 0.80; 95% CI: 0.71–0.90), and patients with severe DM complicated by end-organ damage had 52% lower odds of having keratoconus (OR: 0.48; 95% CI: 0.40–0.58) in comparison with nondiabetic controls.[12] Seiler et al. found that the prevalence of DM was significantly less in keratoconus patients than in controls ($P = 0.037$).[59] Kuo et al. noted that although the incidence of keratoconus was not different between diabetic and control groups, the severity of keratoconus, as measured by best-corrected visual acuity (BCVA), was less severe in diabetic patients.[60] Conversely, a retrospective study by Kosker et al., which differentiated between type I and type II DM and stratified by age, observed a positive association in the presence and severity of keratoconus in type II DM, but not in type I.[62] This study found that the odds of developing keratoconus were 1.4 times higher in diabetic versus healthy subjects. Lastly, a meta-analysis of six studies (two reporting protective effects of diabetes, one reporting it as a risk factor, and three reporting a nonsignificant relationship) showed that the odds of developing keratoconus were 23% lower in patients with type II diabetes, albeit not statistically significant (95% CI: 0.50–1.21).[11]

The aforementioned studies have mostly been limited by the lack of differentiation between type I and type II DM, absent documentation of the duration and temporal relationship between keratoconus and DM, and the lack of an objective evaluation of the severity of both diabetes types, as measured by hemoglobin A1c (Hb A1c), and keratoconus, via corneal tomography. Furthermore, given that it would not be ethically possible to evaluate prospectively the effect of increasing glycosylation status and severity of diabetes in stabilizing keratoconus, all studies have been retrospective in nature. Therefore conclusions about the association of diabetes and keratoconus are not necessarily definitive.

Diabetes exerts histological changes on all layers of the human cornea.[63] It has been postulated that prolonged diabetes-mediated hyperglycemia leads to a cascade of non-enzymatic glycation reactions that result in the formation of advanced glycation end products (AGEs).[64,65] The uninhibited propagation of these chemical substances produces intermolecular cross-links in the ultrastructure of corneal collagen fibers, leading to corneal stiffening.[66] This non–age-related form of collagen cross-linking induced by DM is thought to have a protective effect on the development of keratoconus in humans. In fact, it has been shown that people with DM have increased central corneal thickness, corneal hysteresis, and corneal resistance factor (CRF), possibly reflecting the increased rigidity of diabetic corneas.[67] Animal models have also documented abnormally polymorphous collagen fibril aggregates in the corneal stroma of diabetic monkeys.[68] However, the impact of glucose concentration and duration of exposure in regulating the degree of cross-linking in the human corneal stroma have yet to be elucidated.

GENETIC OCULAR SYNDROMES

Another group of disorders associated with keratoconus include those with abnormal retinal function, leading to oculodigital stimulation. Such disorders include albinism, congenital rubella, Bardet-Biedl syndrome, LCA, neurofibromatosis, retinitis pigmentosa, Laurence-Moon-Bardet-Biedl syndrome, cone dystrophy, tapetoretinal degeneration, and Kurz syndrome.[3] Oculodigital stimulation has been proposed as the shared pathway for the development of keratoconus among these patients, but this remains theoretical.

Many genetically inherited corneal dystrophies have also been observed to occur in association with keratoconus, including lattice dystrophy,[69] granular dystrophy,[70] posterior polymorphous corneal dystrophy,[71] and Fuchs endothelial dystrophy.[72] The association of keratoconus with such a wide range of corneal dystrophies and ocular abnormalities may reflect either a shared underlying genetic defect or a tightly linked network of interacting proteins, with a final common developmental pathway.[2] Further prospective controlled studies are warranted in this area.

References

1. Krachmer JH, Feder RS, Belin MW. Keratoconus and related non-inflammatory corneal thinning disorders. *Surv Ophthalmol.* 1984;28:293–322.
2. Burdon KP, Vincent AL. Insights into keratoconus from a genetic perspective. *Clin Exp Optom.* 2013;96:146–154.
3. Sugar J, Macsai MS. What causes keratoconus? *Cornea.* 2012;31:716–719.
4. Weed KH, MacEwen CJ, Giles T, et al. The Dundee University Scottish Keratoconus study: demographics, corneal signs, associated diseases, and eye rubbing. *Eye (Lond).* 2008;22:534–541.
5. Wagner H, Barr JT, Zadnik K. Collaborative Longitudinal Evaluation of Keratoconus (CLEK) study: methods and findings to date. *Cont Lens Anterior Eye.* 2007;30:223–232.
6. Zadnik K, Barr JT, Edrington TB, et al. Baseline findings in the Collaborative Longitudinal Evaluation of Keratoconus (CLEK) study. *Invest Ophthalmol Vis Sci.* 1998;39:2537–2546.
7. Rahi A, Davies P, Ruben M, et al. Keratoconus and coexisting atopic disease. *Br J Ophthalmol.* 1977;61:761–764.

8. Millodot M, Shneor E, Albou S, et al. Prevalence and associated factors of keratoconus in Jerusalem: a cross-sectional study. *Ophthalmic Epidemiol*. 2011;18:91–97.
9. Mukhtar S, Ambati BK. Pediatric keratoconus: a review of the literature. *Int Ophthalmol*. 2018;38:2257–2266.
10. Tuft SJ, Moodaley LC, Gregory WM, Davison CR, Buckley RJ. Prognostic factors for the progression of keratoconus. *Ophthalmology*. 1994;101(3):439–447.
11. Hashemi H, Heydarian S, Hooshmand E, et al. The prevalence and risk factors for keratoconus: a systematic review and meta-analysis. *Cornea*. 2020;39(2):263–270.
12. Woodward MA, Blachley TS, Stein JD. The association between sociodemographic factors, common systemic diseases, and keratoconus: an analysis of a Nationwide Health Care Claims Database. *Ophthalmology*. 2016;123(3):457–465. e2.
13. Moran S, Gomez L, Zuber K, Gatinel D. A case-control study of keratoconus risk factors. *Cornea*. 2020;39(6):697–701.
14. Coyle JT. Keratoconus and eye rubbing. *Am J Ophthalmol*. 1984;97:527–528.
15. Jafri B, Lichter H, Stulting RD. Asymmetric keratoconus attributed to eye rubbing. *Cornea*. 2004;23:560–564.
16. Carlson AN. Expanding our understanding of eye rubbing and keratoconus. *Cornea*. 2010;29:245.
17. Lema I, Durán JA. Inflammatory molecules in the tears of patients with keratoconus. *Ophthalmology*. 2005;112:654–659.
18. Balasubramanian SA, Pye DC, Willcox MDP. Effects of eye rubbing on the levels of protease, protease activity and cytokines in tears: relevance in keratoconus. *Clin Exp Optom*. 2013;96:214–218.
19. Wilson SE, He YG, Weng J, et al. Epithelial injury induces keratocyte apoptosis: hypothesized role for the interleukin-1 (IL-1) system in the modulation of corneal tissue organization. *Exp Eye Res*. 1996;62:325–338.
20. Fabre EJ, Bureau J, Pouliquen Y, et al. Binding sites for human interleukin 1 alpha, gamma interferon and tumor necrosis factor on cultured fibroblasts of normal cornea and keratoconus. *Curr Eye Res*. 1991;10:585–592.
21. Henriquez MA, Cerrate M, Hadid MG, et al. Comparison of eye-rubbing effect in keratoconic eyes and healthy eyes using Scheimpflug analysis and a dynamic bidirectional applanation device. *J Cataract Refract Surg*. 2019;45:1156–1162.
22. Idowua OO, Ashrafa DC, Vagefia MR, Kerstena RC, Winna BJ. Floppy eyelid syndrome: ocular and systemic associations. *Curr Opin Ophthalmol*. 2019;30(6):513–524.
23. Ali LK, Avidan AY. Sleep-disordered breathing and stroke. *Rev Neurol Dis*. 2008;5:191–198.
24. Culbertson WW, Ostler HB. The floppy eyelid syndrome. *Am J Ophthalmol*. 1981;92:568–575.
25. Saidel MA, Paik JY, Garcia C, Russo P, Cao D, Bouchard C. Prevalence of sleep apnea syndrome and high-risk characteristics among keratoconus patients. *Cornea*. 2012;31:600–603.
26. Ezra DG, Beaconsfield M, Sira M, Bunce C, Wormald R, Collin R. The associations of floppy eyelid syndrome: a case control study. *Ophthalmology*. 2010;117(4):831–838.
27. Gupta PK, Stinnett SS, Carlson AN. Prevalence of sleep apnea in patients with keratoconus. *Cornea*. 2012;31:595–599.
28. Collier SA, Madigan MC, Penfold PL. Expression of membrane-type 1 matrix metalloproteinase (MT1-MMP) and MMP-2 in normal and keratoconus corneas. *Curr Eye Res*. 2000;21:662–668.
29. Tazaki T, Minoguchi K, Yokoe T, et al. Increased levels and activity of matrix metalloproteinase-9 in obstructive sleep apnea syndrome. *Am J Respir Crit Care Med*. 2004;170:1354–1359.
30. Schlötzer-Schrehardt U, Stojkovic M, Hofmann-Rummelt C, et al. The pathogenesis of floppy eyelid syndrome: involvement of matrix metalloproteinases in elastic fiber degradation. *Ophthalmology*. 2005;112:694–704.
31. Austin MG, Schaefer RF. Marfan's syndrome, with unusual blood vessel manifestations. *AMA Arch Pathol*. 1957;64:205–209.
32. Krachmer JH, Feder RS, Belin MW. Keratoconus and related noninflammatory corneal thinning disorders. *Surv Ophthalmol*. 1984;28:293–322.
33. Robertson I. Keratoconus and the Ehlers-Danlos syndrome: a new aspect of keratoconus. *Med J Aust*. 1975;1:571–573.
34. Beckh U, Schonherr U, Naumann GO. Autosomal dominant keratoconus as the chief ocular symptom in Lobstein osteogenesis imperfecta tarda. *Klin Monatsbl Augenheilkd*. 1995;206:268–272.

35. Rabbanikhah Z, Javadi MA, Rostami P, et al. Association between acute corneal hydrops in patients with keratoconus and mitral valve prolapse. *Cornea*. 2011;30:154–157.
36. Javadi MA, Saadat HA, Jafarinasab MR, et al. Association of keratoconus and mitral valve prolapse. *Iran J Ophthalmic Res*. 2007;2:15–18.
37. Beardsley TL, Foulks GN. An association of keratoconus and mitral valve prolapse. *Ophthalmology*. 1982;89:35–37.
38. Woodward EG, Morris MT. Joint hypermobility in keratoconus. *Ophthalmic Physiol Opt*. 1990;10(4):360–362.
39. Ihalainen A. Clinical and epidemiological features of keratoconus genetic and external factors in the pathogenesis of the disease. *Acta Ophthalmol Suppl*. 1986;178:1–64.
40. Street DA, Vinokur ET, Waring GO III, et al. Lack of association between keratoconus, mitral valve prolapse, and joint hypermobility. *Ophthalmology*. 1991;98:170–176.
41. Chwa M, Atilano SR, Hertzog D, et al. Hypersensitive response to oxidative stress in keratoconus corneal fibroblasts. *Invest Ophthalmol Vis Sci*. 2008;49:4361–4369.
42. Kara N, Bozkurt E, Baz O, et al. Corneal biomechanical properties and intraocular pressure measurement in Marfan patients. *J Cataract Refract Surg*. 2012;38:309–314.
43. Perloff JK, Child JS, Edwards JE. New guidelines for the clinical diagnosis of MVP. *Am J Cardiol*. 1986;7:1124.
44. Lichter H, Loya NEI, Sagie A. Keratoconus and mitral valve prolapse. *Am J Ophthalmol*. 2000;129:667–668.
45. Bak-Nielsen S, Ramlau-Hansen CH, Ivarsen A, Plana-Ripoll O, Hjortdal J. A nationwide population-based study of social demographic factors, associated diseases and mortality of keratoconus patients in Denmark from 1977 to 2015. *Acta Ophthalmol*. 2019;97:497–504.
46. Nemet AY, Vinker S, Bahar I, Kaiserman I. The association of keratoconus with immune disorders. *Cornea*. 2010;29:1261–1264.
47. Kahan IL, Varsanyi-Nagy M, Toth M, et al. The possible role of tear fluid thyroxine in keratoconus development. *Exp Eye Res*. 1990;50:339–343.
48. Shapiro MB, France TD. The ocular features of Down's syndrome. *Am J Ophthalmol*. 1985;99:659–663.
49. Macsai M, Maguen E, Nucci P. Keratoconus and Turner's syndrome. *Cornea*. 1997;16:534–536.
50. Mas Tur V, MacGregor C, Jayaswal R, O'Brart D, Maycock N. A review of keratoconus: diagnosis, pathophysiology, and genetics. *Survey Ophthalmol*. 2017;62:770–783.
51. Cullen JF, Butler HG. Mongolism (Down's syndrome) and keratoconus. *Br J Ophthalmol*. 1963;47(6):321–330.
52. Pierce K, Eustace P. Acute keratoconus in Mongols. *Br J Ophthalmol*. 1971;55:50–54.
53. Udar N, Atilano SR, Brown DJ, et al. *SOD1*: a candidate gene for keratoconus. *Invest Ophthalmol Vis Sci*. 2006;47:3345–3351.
54. Feder RS, Neems LC. Noninflammatory ectatic disorders. In: Mannis MJ, Holland EJ, eds. *Cornea: Fundamentals, Diagnosis and Management*. Elsevier Health Sciences; 2017:820–843.
55. Stabuc-Silih M, Strazisar M, Hawlina M, Glavac D. Absence of pathogenic mutations in *VSX1* and *SOD1* genes in patients with keratoconus. *Cornea*. 2010;29:172–176.
56. De Bonis P, Laborante A, Pizzicoli C, et al. Mutational screening of *VSX1*, *SPARC*, *SOD1*, *LOX*, and *TIMP3* in keratoconus. *Mol Vis*. 2011;17:2482–2894.
57. Saee-Rad S, Hashemi H, Miraftab M, et al. Mutation analysis of *VSX1* and *SOD1* in Iranian patients with keratoconus. *Mol Vis*. 2011;17:3128–3136.
58. Haugen OH. Keratoconus in the mentally retarded. *Acta Ophthalmol*. 1992;70(1):111–114.
59. Seiler T, Huhle S, Spoerl E, Kunath H. Manifest diabetes and keratoconus: a retrospective case-control study. *Graefes Arch Clin Exp Ophthalmol*. 2000;238(10):822–825.
60. Kuo IC, Broman A, Pirouzmanesh A, et al. Is there an association between diabetes and keratoconus? *Ophthalmology*. 2006;113:184–190.
61. Naderan M, Naderan M, Rezagholizadeh F, Zolfaghari M, Pahlevani R, Rajabi MT. Association between diabetes and keratoconus: a case-control study. *Cornea*. 2014;33:1271–1273.
62. Kosker M, Suri K, Hammersmith KM, Nassef AH, Nagra PK, Rapuano CJ. Another look at the association between diabetes and keratoconus. *Cornea*. 2014;33:774–779.
63. Lee JS, Oum BS, Choi HY, et al. Differences in corneal thickness and corneal endothelium related to duration in diabetes. *Eye (Lond)*. 2006;20:315–318.

64. Dyer DG, Dunn JA, Thorpe SR, et al. Accumulation of Maillard reaction products in skin collagen in diabetes and aging. *J Clin Invest*. 1993;91:2463–2469.
65. Sady C, Khosrof S, Nagaraj R. Advanced Maillard reaction and cross-linking of corneal collagen in diabetes. *Biochem Biophys Res Commun*. 1995;214:793–797.
66. Robert L, Menasche M, Robert AM, et al. Effect of high glucose concentration on corneal collagen biosynthesis. *Ophthalmologica*. 2006;220:317–322.
67. Goldich Y, Barkana Y, Gerber Y, et al. Effect of diabetes mellitus on biomechanical parameters of the cornea. *J Cataract Refract Surg*. 2009;35:715–719.
68. Zou C, Wang S, Huang F, et al. Advanced glycation end products and ultrastructural changes in corneas of long-term streptozotocin-induced diabetic monkeys. *Cornea*. 2012;31:1455–1459.
69. Sassani JW, Smith SG, Rabinowitz YS. Keratoconus and bilateral lattice-granular corneal dystrophies. *Cornea*. 1992;11:343–350.
70. Wollensak G, Green WR, Temprano J. Keratoconus associated with corneal granular dystrophy in a patient of Italian origin. *Cornea*. 2002;21:121–122.
71. Gasset AR, Zimmerman TJ. Posterior polymorphous dystrophy associated with keratoconus. *Am J Ophthalmol*. 1974;78:535–537.
72. Lipman RM, Rubenstein JB, Torczynski E. Keratoconus and Fuchs' corneal endothelial dystrophy in a patient and her family. *Arch Ophthalmol*. 1990;108:993–994.

CHAPTER 11

Inflammation in Keratoconus

Rohit Shetty ■ Pooja Khamar ■ Gairik Kundu ■ Arkasubhra Ghosh ■ Swaminathan Sethu

KEY CONCEPTS

- Inflammatory mediators are among the key contributing and modifiable factors in keratoconus (KC).
- A significant increase in the inflammatory factors and immune components in the corneal tissues, tear fluid, and/or blood of KC patients is observed.
- Endogenous inflammation dampeners such as vitamin D and vitamin D receptors are reduced in KC.
- KC is strongly associated with immune disorders such as atopy and allergy that are known to increase itch factors and subsequent eye rubbing, a key risk factor in KC pathogenesis.
- Topical anti-inflammatory treatments and management of atopy or allergic conditions have been shown to reduce the levels of inflammatory factors, along with stabilizing the disease in KC patients.

Introduction

The long adhered to definition of keratoconus (KC) has described it to be a noninflammatory corneal ectatic disease. KC is considered a noninflammatory condition, and the definition has remained so despite the growing evidence of altered inflammatory factors in the KC cornea. This is due to the lack of the "cardinal signs" of inflammation (redness, heat, pain swelling) expect for the loss of function in the majority of KC patients. Studies over the last two decades have demonstrated the relationship between KC and a variety of dysregulated inflammatory factors, both local (ocular surface, cornea) and systemic, along with the increase in prevalence of KC in subjects with immunological conditions, such as atopy and allergy. Management of inflammation and/or associated immune conditions has shown cessation or stabilization of disease progression, suggesting the pivotal role of inflammatory factors in the pathogenesis of KC. Therefore, it is apparent that the focal ectatic condition of the human cornea in KC is mediated by inflammatory factors. This chapter discusses the altered inflammatory factors in KC and their relevance in pathogenesis, and offers insights into dampening of the local inflammatory milieu in the management of KC.

Status of Inflammatory Factors in Keratoconus

Altered levels and expression of various inflammatory factors in the tear fluid, corneal tissues, cultured primary corneal cells, aqueous humor, serum, and/or saliva of KC patients have been reported. Fig. 11.1 summarizes the factors altered in the various types of sample in KC.

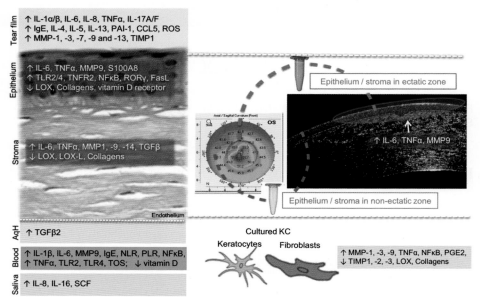

Fig. 11.1   Altered inflammatory factors in keratoconus (KC). Schematic summarizes changes in the proinflammatory factors, endogenous inflammation modulators, and extracellular matrix components in KC patients. Inflammatory factor classes such as cytokines, chemokines, IgE, and S100A proteins are increased in the tear fluid, corneal tissues, cultured corneal fibroblasts, aqueous humor, serum, and/or saliva of KC patients. Molecular mediators such as oxidative stress inducers (ROS), receptors (TLR2, TLR4, TNFR2), and transcription factors (NFκB, RORγ) that facilitate the increase in inflammatory factors are also higher in KC. Endogenous inflammation dampeners such as vitamin D and vitamin D receptors are reduced in KC. The altered levels of extracellular matrix component and remodeling factors such as collagen, endogenous cross-linking enzyme (LOX), proteolysis enzymes (MMPs), and their regulators (TIMP) in KC are also shown in the schematic. *CCL5,* Chemokine (C-C motif) ligand 5; *FasL,* Fas ligand; *IFN,* interferon; *IgE,* immunoglobulin E; *IL,* interleukin; *LOX,* lysyl oxidase; *MMP,* matrix metalloproteinase; *NFκB,* nuclear factor kappa-light-chain-enhancer of activated B cells; *PAI-1,* plasminogen activator inhibitor-1; *PGE2,* prostaglandin E2; *ROS,* reactive oxygen species; *RORγ,* RAR-related orphan receptor gamma; *TIMP,* tissue inhibitor of metalloproteinases; *TLR,* toll-like receptor; *TNF,* tumor necrosis factor; *TNFR,* tumor necrosis factor receptor.

TEAR FLUID

The levels of classical proinflammatory factors including interleukin (IL)-1α/β,[1–4] IL-6,[1,5–7] IL-8,[1,8,9] tumor necrosis factor alpha (TNF-α),[3] IL-17A,[2,10] C-C motif chemokine ligand 5 (CCL5),[11–13] and nerve growth factor (NGF)[11,14] have been found to be increased in the tear fluid of KC patients. Tear fluid immunoglobulin E (IgE)[15] and allergy-associated cytokines such as IL-4,[1–3] IL-5,[1,2] and IL-13[2] were also elevated in KC patients. A group of other inflammatory factors that were reported to be elevated in tear fluid of KC patient in at least one study include epidermal growth factor (EGF),[12] IL-2,[2] IL-3,[1] IL-21,[2] IL-23,[2] interferon alpha (IFN-α),[2] interferon gamma (IFN-γ),[13] monocyte chemoattractant protein-1 (MCP1),[2] macrophage inflammatory protein-1 alpha/beta (MIP1-α/β),[2] E-selectin,[2] soluble intercellular adhesion molecule 1 (sICAM1),[2] S100A6,[16] and plasminogen activator inhibitor type 1 (PAI-1).[12] An antiinflammatory factor, IL-10, was reported to be either increased[1–3] or decreased[10,11,17] in the tear fluid of KC patients. IL-11,[18] interferon γ-induced protein (IP-10),[2,11] secretory immunoglobulin A (sIgA),[19] and serum albumin[19] were lower in the tear fluid of KC patients compared with controls. The key matrix metalloproteinase, MMP-9,[1,5–7,9,11,12,16,20–22] was higher in the tear fluid of KC patients. The other MMPs that were also higher in tear fluid of KC patients include MMP-1,[1,18] MMP-2,[1] MMP-3,[1] MMP-7,[1] and MMP-13.[1,12–14] Importantly, the endogenous regulator of MMPs, tissue inhibitor of metalloproteinases 1 (TIMP1), was lower in the tear fluid of KC patients compared with controls.[8,11] More recently, altered immune cell proportions on the ocular surface of KC patients compared with normal controls were also reported.[23] These observations clearly indicate an increased inflammatory factor milieu on the ocular surface of KC patients.

CORNEAL TISSUES AND CULTURED CORNEAL FIBROBLASTS

Inflammatory cellular infiltrates were observed in the corneal tissue sections from a subset of KC patients.[24,25] In addition, elevated expressions of inflammatory factors such as IL-1α/β,[24,26] IL-6,[7,27] IL-17A,[28] TNF-α,[7,27] S100A8,[29] MMP-1,[30] MMP-2,[31] MMP-8,[32] and MMP-9,[7,33,34] with potential to modulate extracellular matrix (ECM) remodeling, were higher and TIMP1[35] was lower in the corneal epithelium and/or stroma of KC patients. The expressions of TNF-α, IL-6, and MMP-9 were higher in the epithelium/stroma from the ectatic region (cone) compared with the nonectatic region (periphery) of the KC cornea.[34] Further, the levels of IL-1α/β,[36] IL-6,[37] MMP-1,[37,38] MMP-2,[38,39] MMP-3,[38] and MMP-9[38,40] were also higher in cultured primary corneal fibroblasts/keratocytes from KC patients compared with non-KC controls. These findings corroborate the inflammatory milieu findings in the tear fluid of KC patients mentioned earlier.

Cell surface receptor expressions that are known to mediate inflammatory signaling such as toll-like receptors (TLR2, TLR4), TNF receptor 2 (TNFR2), EGF receptor, and hepatocyte growth factor (HGF) receptor-/c-Met[41] have been found to be higher in KC corneas. Transcription factors such as nuclear factor kappa-light-chain-enhancer of activated B cells (NFκB),[42] transcription factor p65 (RelA),[27] and RAR-related orphan receptor gamma (RORγ)[28] that regulate the production of proinflammatory cytokines such as IL-6, TNF-α, and IL-17A were also higher in KC epithelium. In addition, the endogenous negative modulator of inflammatory response, the vitamin D receptor, was decreased[43] in KC epithelium. A higher expression of Fas ligand (FasL)—apoptosis inducer or regulator of cell death—was also observed in KC cornea,[44] which may be related to decrease in keratocyte density in KC. These findings indicate an aberrant cellular inflammatory factor profile in the KC cornea.

BLOOD, SALIVA, AND AQUEOUS HUMOR

Systemic alteration in some of the inflammatory factors has also been reported in KC. IL-1β,[45] IL-6,[45] TNF-α,[27] MMP-9,[45] and IgE[46] were found to be higher in the serum of KC patients. Altered immune cell proportions in the blood such as neutrophil to lymphocyte ratio (NLR),[47,48] platelets to lymphocyte ratio (PLR),[49] and monocyte to high-density lipoprotein cholesterol ratio (MHR),[48] indicative of oxidative stress and systemic inflammation, were higher in the KC patients compared with controls. The expression of inflammatory signaling mediators such as TLR2, TLR4, and NFκB was raised in the peripheral blood leukocytes of KC patients. An increase in the systemic inflammatory status in KC patients has been observed with a decrease in serum vitamin D,[50] a major endogenous inflammatory modulator. IL-8, IL-16, and stem cell factor (SCF) were increased in the saliva[51] and transforming growth factor beta 2 (TGFβ2) was higher in the aqueous humor[52] of KC patients compared with controls.

GENETIC VARIATIONS

Genetic alterations such as single nucleotide polymorphisms (SNPs) in collagens and lysyl oxidase, and endogenous collagen cross-linking enzymes, have been implicated as predisposing factors in KC.[53,54] Genetic variants in inflammatory genes have also been associated with increased predisposition to KC. SNPs in *IL-1α* (rs2071376) and *IL-1β* (rs1143627, rs16944, rs16944, s1143627) genes were associated with an increased risk of development and severity of KC.[55–57] TNF-α promoter polymorphism rs1800629 was significantly associated with the development of KC with increased levels of TNF-α in the serum and expressions of TNF-α, TNFR2, RelA, and IL-6 in corneal tissues.[27] Polymorphism (rs763110) in FASL gene was associated with increased occurrence of KC.[58] A single nucleotide variation was also reported in *IL-17B* gene in the KC patients,[59] thus indicating a genetic basis for altered inflammatory factors in some KC patients.

Association Between Inflammatory Factors and Disease Characteristics

The association between the levels of certain altered inflammatory factors and KC-related corneal clinical indices suggests the plausibility of their role in KC pathogenesis. IL-1β has exhibited a positive correlation with disease severity and a negative correlation with central corneal thickness (CCT), corneal hysteresis (CH), and corneal resistance factor (CR).[3] A positive relationship between IL-6 levels and disease stage,[3,7] maximum curvature power on front of cornea (K_{max}),[3] and steep keratometric reading (K2),[5] along with a negative relationship with CCT,[3] CH,[3] and Klyce/Maeda KC index[14] was observed. Similarly, a positive association between TNF-α levels and the Belin/Ambrósio display enhanced ectasia total derivation value (BAD-D),[34] average curvature power on front of cornea (K_{mean}),[34] K2,[5] and deformation amplitude,[34] as well as a negative association with thinnest corneal thickness,[34] CH[3], and CR[3] was observed. IL-4 levels positively correlated with disease severity and negatively with CCT, CH, and CR.[3] IL-8 level positively correlated with BAD-D and negatively with corneal thickness at the thinnest point of the cornea.[60] IFN-γ levels associated with progression[13] exhibited a negative correlation with CCT, CH, and CR.[3] NGF correlated positively with K2 index.[14] CCL5 showed a positive association with disease stage and a negative association with CH and CCT.[3] The expression of TLR2 and TLR4 had a positive association with K2 and coma along with a negative association with minimum thickness point of cornea.[61] MMP-9 levels showed a positive relationship with severity of KC.[5,7,21,22,33] MMP-9 levels positively correlated with K2,[5,60] BAD-D,[60] and negatively with thinnest corneal thickness in KC.[6] In addition, the disease progression in KC patients was related to increased tear MMP-9 levels.[21] Similarly, MMP-13 was also associated with KC severity and progression.[1,12–14] Lysyl oxidase, a key enzyme that facilitates endogenous cross-linking between collagen and elastin fibrils, was reduced[62,63] in KC and demonstrated a decreasing trend with increasing grades of KC.[33] The increased expression of TNF-α, IL-6, and MMP-9 in the ectatic region also exhibited a decrease in the levels of collagen and lysyl oxidase compared with the nonectatic region KC cornea,[34] thus emphasizing the inverse relationship between inflammatory factors and ECM components in the KC cornea.

Inflammatory Factors and Keratoconus Pathogenesis

The KC cornea is characterized by biomechanical weakening and structural change in the form of steepening with consequent decrease in visual acuity. The key changes in the KC cornea are observed in the corneal epithelium, epithelial basement membrane, Bowman's layer, and stroma.[64] Ultrastructural changes in the KC cornea include reduced expression of ECM components such as collagens, altered lamellar organization, fibril features, proteoglycan profile, and fewer stromal keratocytes.[64,65] Although KC is an ectatic condition, fibrotic changes in the cornea have also been observed,[66,67] particularly in later stages of disease, owing to a compensatory response that contributes to KC pathology by causing scarring. This was supported by studies reporting higher levels of TGF-β—an antiinflammatory and profibrotic factor in KC.[2,26,68] Ectasia and fibrosis are conditions at the opposite ends of the spectrum of ECM-associated diseases affecting different organs. The dynamic and reparative nature of the ECM remodeling process and the factors influencing them need to be determined to understand disease pathogenesis.

Inflammatory mediators and immune cells are known as one of the major factors that contribute to dysregulation in ECM modeling by modulating cellular signaling pathways that regulate the key ECM component production such as collagens, proteoglycans, cross-linking enzymes, and proteolysis enzymes. Environmental insults including oxidative stress, atopic conditions, and eye rubbing can induce the production of inflammatory factors on the ocular surface that can compromise barrier function and alter cellular metabolism and signaling, which can further amplify the level of inflammatory mediators. Eye rubbing is considered as an important risk factor associated with KC. Itch sensations are also mediated by inflammatory or immune factors that stimulate release of itch factors. Studies have demonstrated an increase in IL-6, TNF-α, and MMP-13 levels in tear fluid following eye rubbing even in normal eyes,[69,70] suggesting an inflammatory factor–associated mechanism in KC. Inflammatory factors such as IL-1β and FasL that are increased in the KC cornea mediate corneal tissue organization by regulating keratocyte apoptosis.[44,71,72] Hence, increased activity of these factors may induce keratocyte apoptosis resulting in reduced keratocyte density and impacting ECM remodeling. TNF-α and/or IL-1β that are increased in KC are known to reduce collagen synthesis and lysyl oxidase expression.[73–75] Altered collagen and abnormal arrangement are also due to increase in proteolytic enzymes and decreased endogenous levels of protease inhibitors.[70] Inflammatory factors trigger tissue protease activity and progression in KC, which is supported by disease grade–dependent increase in the levels of MMP-9 in KC.[34,76] Interestingly, IL-17, a known inducer of MMP-9 and barrier function breakdown,[77,78] is also elevated in KC. These factors can collectively act on the stromal cells (keratocytes or fibroblasts) resulting in their altered function and density. The altered stromal cells affect the ECM remodeling processes with an increase in MMPs and decrease in collagens and endogenous cross-linking enzyme, thus causing structural weakening of the corneal stroma, KC initiation, and progression.

Inflammatory Factors Modulation and Keratoconus Management

The management of early stage KC includes glasses and rigid contact lenses for visual rehabilitation. Strategies such as intracorneal ring segments or topography-guided treatments are also available to prevent disease progression. More recently, collagen cross-linking has evolved as one of the effective ways to stabilize the progression of the disease. However, corneal transplants are required to manage advanced stage KC to restore vision. Therefore it would be clinically prudent to detect KC at its earliest form and manage it by treating the associated risk factors in the patient. It is becoming apparent that allergy, atopy, eye rubbing, and aberrant inflammatory factors are key modifiable risk factors that impact the prognosis and treatment outcomes of KC.

Ocular allergy and eye rubbing are major risk factors that contribute to initiation and progression of KC owing to the increase in associated inflammatory factors.[79,80] Hence, controlling local and systemic allergy would aid in the reduction of eye rubbing and the related surge in inflammatory factors at the ocular surface. Modulation of inflammatory and immune-mediated mechanisms underpins the management of atopy and allergy. It includes the topical and systemic use of steroids, antihistamines, and leukotriene receptor antagonists.[81] Targeting IgE, IL-4, and IL-13 by using monoclonal antibodies against these factors and mast cell stabilizing agents has been successful in the management of systemic allergy and atopic conditions. Since high IgE is associated with increasing severity of KC and progression,[15] controlling it is important in improving ocular allergy status and associated KC. Identifying the causal allergen, adhering to allergen avoidance measures, and using allergen-specific immunotherapy such as sublingual immunotherapy (SLIT) reduce the specific IgE load, eye rubbing, and associated ocular surface inflammatory factors.

SLIT shifts the T cell responses, that is, from Th2 to Th1, to facilitate the development of anergy or tolerance to the allergen.[82,83]

Cyclosporine is an immunomodulatory agent that acts by inhibiting the intracellular calcineurin-mediating signaling that is required for the production of inflammatory factors. Use of cyclosporine in the management of autoimmune diseases is well known. Topical cyclosporine is also used to manage ocular surface inflammation in dry eye disease. Modulating the ocular surface inflammatory factor milieu using topical cyclosporine in KC patients has shown promise with stabilization of the disease.[7] The use of cyclosporine also resulted in a significant reduction in the tear fluid MMP-9 levels in these patients.[7] Collagen cross-linking procedures that resulted in stabilization of KC progression also resulted in a decrease in tear fluid inflammatory factors, including MMPs.[12,16,38]

It is important to note that higher expression of lysyl oxidase, an endogenous collagen cross-linking agent in the ectatic zone, has shown a favorable relationship with collagen cross-linking outcome.[84] Hence, reducing the inflammatory factors that can reduce the levels of lysyl oxidase would be useful[73-75] to improve the stabilization of disease. Targeting inflammatory or molecular factors such as MMPs and their precursors (e.g., IL-17) that are significantly dysregulated in the KC cornea using previously approved drugs can be beneficial. For example, doxycycline, a derivative of tetracycline known to reduce expression and activity of MMP and other inflammatory factors,[85] is a potential agent. Similarly, batimastat, a hydroxamic acid–based MMP inhibitor,[86] is the other probable agent that might be explored. IL-17 blockade using RORγ inhibitors[87] can also be used. IL-17, reported to be higher in KC, is a known inducer of MMP-9 and corneal barrier function loss.[77,78] Finally, augmenting endogenous antiinflammatory mechanisms by vitamin D

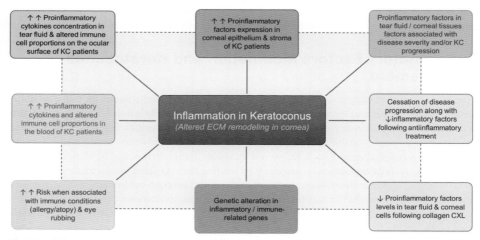

Fig. 11.2 Inflammatory facets in keratoconus *(KC)*. The figure shows the different aspects of inflammatory components that are associated with KC. The main factors are as follows: (1) A significant increase in the inflammatory factors and immune components in the corneal tissues, tear fluid, and/or blood of KC patients is observed. Some of these inflammatory factors have been shown to be unfavorably associated with clinical indices suggestive of disease severity and progression. (2) KC is strongly associated with immune disorders such as atopy and allergy that are known to increase itch factors and subsequent eye rubbing—a key risk factor in KC pathogenesis. Genetic alterations such as single nucleotide polymorphisms in the inflammatory genes have been shown in KC. (3) Topical antiinflammatory treatments have been shown to reduce the levels of inflammatory factors and proteolysis enzymes, along with stabilizing the disease in KC patients. Management of atopy and allergic conditions has also resulted in the stabilization of the disease. A reduction in some of the inflammatory factors in the tear fluid of KC patients following collagen cross-linking has been observed. These facets suggest the role of inflammatory factors in mediating aberrant extracellular matrix remodeling in KC and the potential for inflammatory factor modulation in the management of KC.

supplementation in KC patients deficient in vitamin D would be beneficial in prevention of disease progression.

Conclusion

Based on the mounting evidence regarding the multifaceted associations between inflammatory factors and KC (Fig. 11.2), it is apparent that inflammatory mediators are among the key contributing and modifiable factors in KC. Hence, monitoring and managing inflammatory milieu changes, including subclinical inflammation, would be clinically beneficial in stabilizing the disease and improving clinical outcomes.

References

1. Balasubramanian SA, Mohan S, Pye DC, Willcox MD. Proteases, proteolysis and inflammatory molecules in the tears of people with keratoconus. *Acta Ophthalmol*. 2012;90(4):e303–e309.
2. Shetty R, Deshmukh R, Ghosh A, Sethu S, Jayadev C. Altered tear inflammatory profile in Indian keratoconus patients—the 2015 Col Rangachari award paper. *Indian J Ophthalmol*. 2017;65(11):1105–1108.
3. Ionescu IC, Corbu CG, Tanase C, et al. Overexpression of tear inflammatory cytokines as additional finding in keratoconus patients and their first degree family members. *Mediators Inflamm*. 2018;2018:4285268.
4. Sorkhabi R, Ghorbanihaghjo A, Taheri N, Ahoor MH. Tear film inflammatory mediators in patients with keratoconus. *Int Ophthalmol*. 2015;35(4):467–472.
5. Lema I, Duran JA. Inflammatory molecules in the tears of patients with keratoconus. *Ophthalmology*. 2005;112(4):654–659.
6. Lema I, Sobrino T, Durán JA, Brea D, Díez-Feijoo E. Subclinical keratoconus and inflammatory molecules from tears. *Br J Ophthalmol*. 2009;93(6):820–824.
7. Shetty R, Ghosh A, Lim RR, et al. Elevated expression of matrix metalloproteinase-9 and inflammatory cytokines in keratoconus patients is inhibited by cyclosporine A. *Invest Ophthalmol Vis Sci*. 2015;56(2):738–750.
8. Fodor M, Kolozsvari BL, Petrovski G, et al. Effect of contact lens wear on the release of tear mediators in keratoconus. *Eye Contact Lens*. 2013;39(2):147–152.
9. Andrade FEC, Covre JL, Ramos L, et al. Evaluation of galectin-1 and galectin-3 as prospective biomarkers in keratoconus. *Br J Ophthalmol*. 2018;102(5):700–707.
10. Jun AS, Cope L, Speck C, et al. Subnormal cytokine profile in the tear fluid of keratoconus patients. *PLoS One*. 2011;6(1):e16437.
11. Pasztor D, Kolozsvari BL, Csutak A, et al. Tear mediators in corneal ectatic disorders. *PLoS One*. 2016;11(4):e0153186.
12. Kolozsvari BL, Berta A, Petrovski G, et al. Alterations of tear mediators in patients with keratoconus after corneal crosslinking associate with corneal changes. *PLoS One*. 2013;8(10):e76333.
13. Fodor M, Vitályos G, Losonczy G, et al. Tear mediators NGF along with IL-13 predict keratoconus progression. *Ocul Immunol Inflamm*. 2021;29(6):1090–1101.
14. Kolozsvari BL, Petrovski G, Gogolak P, et al. Association between mediators in the tear fluid and the severity of keratoconus. *Ophthalmic Res*. 2014;51(1):46–51.
15. Patel P, Shetty R, Ghosh A, et al. Ocular surface immune trafficking and eye rubbing in keratoconus, and its impact on treatment outcomes. International CXL Experts Meeting. Zurich, Switzerland; 2018.
16. Recalde JI, Duran JA, Rodriguez-Agirretxe I, et al. Changes in tear biomarker levels in keratoconus after corneal collagen crosslinking. *Mol Vis*. 2019;25:12–21.
17. Lema I, Duran JA, Ruiz C, et al. Inflammatory response to contact lenses in patients with keratoconus compared with myopic subjects. *Cornea*. 2008;27(7):758–763.
18. Pannebaker C, Chandler HL, Nichols JJ. Tear proteomics in keratoconus. *Mol Vis*. 2010;16:1949–1957.
19. Balasubramanian SA, Pye DC, Willcox MD. Levels of lactoferrin, secretory IgA and serum albumin in the tear film of people with keratoconus. *Exp Eye Res*. 2012;96(1):132–137.
20. Smith VA, Rishmawi H, Hussein H, Easty DL. Tear film MMP accumulation and corneal disease. *Br J Ophthalmol*. 2001;85(2):147–153.

21. Mazzotta C, Traversi C, Mellace P, et al. Keratoconus progression in patients with allergy and elevated surface matrix metalloproteinase 9 point-of-care test. *Eye Contact Lens*. 2018;44(suppl 2):S48–S53.
22. Mutlu M, Sarac O, Cagil N, Avcioglu G. Relationship between tear eotaxin-2 and MMP-9 with ocular allergy and corneal topography in keratoconus patients. *Int Ophthalmol*. 2020;40(1):51–57.
23. Sethu S, Nair AP, D'souza S, Rohit S, Ghosh A. Distinct immune cell subsets on the ocular surface of dry eye disease and keratoconus patients is associated with pathology. ARVO Annual Meeting. *Invest Ophthalmol Vis Sci*. 2019; 60.
24. Becker J, Salla S, Dohmen U, et al. Explorative study of interleukin levels in the human cornea. *Graefes Arch Clin Exp Ophthalmol*. 1995;233(12):766–771.
25. Fan Gaskin JC, Loh IP, McGhee CN, Sherwin T. An immunohistochemical study of inflammatory cell changes and matrix remodeling with and without acute hydrops in keratoconus. *Invest Ophthalmol Vis Sci*. 2015;56(10):5831–5837.
26. Zhou L, Yue BY, Twining SS, et al. Expression of wound healing and stress-related proteins in keratoconus corneas. *Curr Eye Res*. 1996;15(11):1124–1131.
27. Arbab M, Tahir S, Niazi MK, et al. TNF-alpha genetic predisposition and higher expression of inflammatory pathway components in keratoconus. *Invest Ophthalmol Vis Sci*. 2017;58(9):3481–3487.
28. Selot R, Naidu J, Kumar N, et al. Increased expression of retinoic acid-related orphan receptor gamma transcription factor and its products in keratoconus patients. ARVO Annual Meeting. *Invest Ophthalmol Vis Sci*. 2018; 59.
29. Chaerkady R, Shao H, Scott SG, et al. The keratoconus corneal proteome: loss of epithelial integrity and stromal degeneration. *J Proteomics*. 2013;87:122–131.
30. Seppala HP, Maatta M, Rautia M, et al. EMMPRIN and MMP-1 in keratoconus. *Cornea*. 2006;25(3):325–330.
31. Smith VA, Matthews FJ, Majid MA, Cook SD. Keratoconus: matrix metalloproteinase-2 activation and TIMP modulation. *Biochim Biophys Acta*. 2006;1762(4):431–439.
32. Rohini G, Murugeswari P, Prajna NV, et al. Matrix metalloproteinases (MMP-8, MMP-9) and the tissue inhibitors of metalloproteinases (TIMP-1, TIMP-2) in patients with fungal keratitis. *Cornea*. 2007;26(2):207–211.
33. Shetty R, Sathyanarayanamoorthy A, Ramachandra RA, et al. Attenuation of lysyl oxidase and collagen gene expression in keratoconus patient corneal epithelium corresponds to disease severity. *Mol Vis*. 2015;21:12–25.
34. Pahuja N, Kumar NR, Shroff R, et al. Differential molecular expression of extracellular matrix and inflammatory genes at the corneal cone apex drives focal weakening in keratoconus. *Invest Ophthalmol Vis Sci*. 2016;57(13):5372–5382.
35. Kenney MC, Chwa M, Atilano SR, et al. Increased levels of catalase and cathepsin V/L2 but decreased TIMP-1 in keratoconus corneas: evidence that oxidative stress plays a role in this disorder. *Invest Ophthalmol Vis Sci*. 2005;46(3):823–832.
36. Bureau J, Fabre EJ, Hecquet C, et al. Modification of prostaglandin E2 and collagen synthesis in keratoconus fibroblasts, associated with an increase of interleukin 1 alpha receptor number. *C R Acad Sci III*. 1993;316(4):425–430.
37. Du G, Liu C, Li X, et al. Induction of matrix metalloproteinase-1 by tumor necrosis factor-alpha is mediated by interleukin-6 in cultured fibroblasts of keratoconus. *Exp Biol Med (Maywood)*. 2016;241(18):2033–2041.
38. Sharif R, Fowler B, Karamichos D. Collagen cross-linking impact on keratoconus extracellular matrix. *PLoS One*. 2018;13(7):e0200704.
39. McKay TB, Hjortdal J, Priyadarsini S, Karamichos D. Acute hypoxia influences collagen and matrix metalloproteinase expression by human keratoconus cells in vitro. *PLoS One*. 2017;12(4):e0176017.
40. Soiberman US, Shehata AEM, Lu MX, et al. Small molecule modulation of the integrated stress response governs the keratoconic phenotype in vitro. *Invest Ophthalmol Vis Sci*. 2019;60(10):3422–3431.
41. You J, Wen L, Roufas A, et al. Expression of HGF and c-Met proteins in human keratoconus corneas. *J Ophthalmol*. 2015;2015:852986.
42. Stachon T, Latta L, Kolev K, Seitz B, Langenbucher A, Szentmáry N. Increased NF-κB and iNOS expression in keratoconus keratocytes—hints for an inflammatory component? *Klin Monbl Augenheilkd*. 2021;238(9):1010–1017.

43. Shivakumar S, Rohit S, Ghosh A, Jeyabalan N. Vitamin D enhances the autophagic lysosomal clearance in oxidatively stressed human corneal epithelial cells: a therapeutic intervention for keratoconus. ARVO Annual Meeting. *Invest Ophthalmol Vis Sci.* 2019; 60.

44. Hasby EA, Saad HA. Immunohistochemical expression of Fas ligand (FasL) and neprilysin (neutral endopeptidase/CD10) in keratoconus. *Int Ophthalmol.* 2013;33(2):125–131.

45. Sobrino T, Regueiro U, Malfeito M, et al. Higher expression of toll-like receptors 2 and 4 in blood cells of keratoconus patients. *Sci Rep.* 2017;7(1):12975.

46. Ahuja P, Dadachanji Z, Shetty R, et al. Relevance of IgE, allergy and eye rubbing in the pathogenesis and management of keratoconus. *Indian J Ophthalmol.* 2020;68(10):2067–2074.

47. Karaca EE, Ozmen MC, Ekici F, et al. Neutrophil-to-lymphocyte ratio may predict progression in patients with keratoconus. *Cornea.* 2014;33(11):1168–1173.

48. Katipoglu Z, Mirza E, Oltulu R, Katipoglu B. May monocyte/HDL cholesterol ratio (MHR) and neutrophil/lymphocyte ratio (NLR) be an indicator of inflammation and oxidative stress in patients with keratoconus? *Ocul Immunol Inflamm.* 2020;28(4):632–636.

49. Bozkurt E, Ucak T. Serum inflammation biomarkers in patients with keratoconus. *Ocul Immunol Inflamm.* 2021;29(6):1164–1167.

50. Zarei-Ghanavati S, Yahaghi B, Hassanzadeh S, et al. Serum 25-hydroxyvitamin D, selenium, zinc and copper in patients with keratoconus. *J Curr Ophthalmol.* 2020;32(1):26–31.

51. McKay TB, Hjortdal J, Sejersen H, et al. Endocrine and metabolic pathways linked to keratoconus: implications for the role of hormones in the stromal microenvironment. *Sci Rep.* 2016;6:25534.

52. Maier P, Broszinski A, Heizmann U, et al. Active transforming growth factor-beta2 is increased in the aqueous humor of keratoconus patients. *Mol Vis.* 2007;13:1198–1202.

53. Zhang J, Zhang L, Hong J, et al. Association of common variants in LOX with keratoconus: a meta-analysis. *PLoS One.* 2015;10(12):e0145815.

54. Li X, Bykhovskaya Y, Canedo AL, et al. Genetic association of COL5A1 variants in keratoconus patients suggests a complex connection between corneal thinning and keratoconus. *Invest Ophthalmol Vis Sci.* 2013;54(4):2696–2704.

55. Nabil KM, Elhady GM, Morsy H. The association between interleukin 1 beta promoter polymorphisms and keratoconus incidence and severity in an Egyptian population. *Clin Ophthalmol.* 2019;13:2217–2223.

56. Kim SH, Mok JW, Kim HS, Joo CK. Association of -31 T>C and -511 C>T polymorphisms in the interleukin 1 beta (IL1B) promoter in Korean keratoconus patients. *Mol Vis.* 2008;14:2109–2116.

57. Wang Y, Wei W, Zhang C, et al. Association of interleukin-1 gene single nucleotide polymorphisms with keratoconus in Chinese Han population. *Curr Eye Res.* 2016;41(5):630–635.

58. Synowiec E, Wojcik KA, Izdebska J, et al. Polymorphisms of the apoptosis-related FAS and FAS ligand genes in keratoconus and Fuchs endothelial corneal dystrophy. *Tohoku J Exp Med.* 2014;234(1):17–27.

59. Karolak JA, Gambin T, Pitarque JA, et al. Variants in SKP1, PROB1, and IL17B genes at keratoconus 5q31.1-q35.3 susceptibility locus identified by whole-exome sequencing. *Eur J Hum Genet.* 2016;25(1):73–78.

60. Pasztor D, Kolozsvari BL, Csutak A, et al. Scheimpflug imaging parameters associated with tear mediators and bronchial asthma in keratoconus. *J Ophthalmol.* 2016;2016:9392640.

61. Malfeito M, Regueiro U, Perez-Mato M, et al. Innate immunity biomarkers for early detection of keratoconus. *Ocul Immunol Inflamm.* 2019;27(6):942–948.

62. Dudakova L, Liskova P, Trojek T, et al. Changes in lysyl oxidase (LOX) distribution and its decreased activity in keratoconus corneas. *Exp Eye Res.* 2012;104:74–81.

63. Dudakova L, Sasaki T, Liskova P, et al. The presence of lysyl oxidase-like enzymes in human control and keratoconic corneas. *Histol Histopathol.* 2016;31(1):63–71.

64. Blackburn BJ, Jenkins MW, Rollins AM, Dupps WJ. A review of structural and biomechanical changes in the cornea in aging, disease, and photochemical crosslinking. *Front Bioeng Biotechnol.* 2019;7:66.

65. White TL, Lewis PN, Young RD, et al. Elastic microfibril distribution in the cornea: differences between normal and keratoconic stroma. *Exp Eye Res.* 2017;159:40–48.

66. Keratoconus Rabinowitz YS. *Surv Ophthalmol.* 1998;42(4):297–319.

67. Sherwin T, Brookes NH, Loh IP, et al. Cellular incursion into Bowman's membrane in the peripheral cone of the keratoconic cornea. *Exp Eye Res.* 2002;74(4):473–482.

68. Saee-Rad S, Raoofian R, Mahbod M, et al. Analysis of superoxide dismutase 1, dual-specificity phosphatase 1, and transforming growth factor, beta 1 genes expression in keratoconic and non-keratoconic corneas. *Mol Vis.* 2013;19:2501–2507.

69. Agrawal VB. Characteristics of keratoconus patients at a tertiary eye center in India. *J Ophthalmic Vis Res.* 2011;6(2):87–91.

70. Balasubramanian SA, Pye DC, Willcox MD. Effects of eye rubbing on the levels of protease, protease activity and cytokines in tears: relevance in keratoconus. *Clin Exp Optom.* 2013;96(2):214–218.

71. Kim WJ, Rabinowitz YS, Meisler DM, Wilson SE. Keratocyte apoptosis associated with keratoconus. *Exp Eye Res.* 1999;69(5):475–481.

72. Wojcik KA, Blasiak J, Szaflik J, Szaflik JP. Role of biochemical factors in the pathogenesis of keratoconus. *Acta Biochim Pol.* 2014;61(1):55–62.

73. Greenwel P, Tanaka S, Penkov D, et al. Tumor necrosis factor alpha inhibits type I collagen synthesis through repressive CCAAT/enhancer-binding proteins. *Mol Cell Biol.* 2000;20(3):912–918.

74. Rodriguez C, Alcudia JF, Martinez-Gonzalez J, et al. Lysyl oxidase (LOX) down-regulation by TNFalpha: a new mechanism underlying TNFalpha-induced endothelial dysfunction. *Atherosclerosis.* 2008;196(2):558–564.

75. Zhang Y, Jiang J, Xie J, et al. Combined effects of tumor necrosis factor-alpha and interleukin-1beta on lysyl oxidase and matrix metalloproteinase expression in human knee synovial fibroblasts in vitro. *Exp Ther Med.* 2017;14(6):5258–5266.

76. Kittaka H, Tominaga M. The molecular and cellular mechanisms of itch and the involvement of TRP channels in the peripheral sensory nervous system and skin. *Allergol Int.* 2017;66(1):22–30.

77. De Paiva CS, Chotikavanich S, Pangelinan SB, et al. IL-17 disrupts corneal barrier following desiccating stress. *Mucosal Immunol.* 2009;2(3):243–253.

78. Hou A, Tong L. Expression, regulation, and effects of interleukin-17f in the human ocular surface. *Ocul Immunol Inflamm.* 2018;26(7):1069–1077.

79. Sharma N, Rao K, Maharana PK, Vajpayee RB. Ocular allergy and keratoconus. *Indian J Ophthalmol.* 2013;61(8):407–409.

80. El Rami H, Chelala E, Dirani A, et al. An update on the safety and efficacy of corneal collagen cross-linking in pediatric keratoconus. *Biomed Res Int.* 2015;2015:257927.

81. Dhami S, Nurmatov U, Roberts G, et al. Allergen immunotherapy for allergic rhinoconjunctivitis: protocol for a systematic review. *Clin Transl Allergy.* 2016;6:12.

82. Frati F, Scurati S, Puccinelli P, et al. Development of a sublingual allergy vaccine for grass pollinosis. *Drug Des Devel Ther.* 2010;4:99–105.

83. Kari O, Saari KM. Updates in the treatment of ocular allergies. *J Asthma Allergy.* 2010;3:149–158.

84. Shetty R, Rajiv Kumar N, Pahuja N, et al. Outcomes of corneal cross-linking correlate with cone-specific lysyl oxidase expression in patients with keratoconus. *Cornea.* 2018;37(3):369–374.

85. Pflugfelder SC. Antiinflammatory therapy for dry eye. *Am J Ophthalmol.* 2004;137(2):337–342.

86. Zhou C, Petroll WM. MMP regulation of corneal keratocyte motility and mechanics in 3-D collagen matrices. *Exp Eye Res.* 2014;121:147–160.

87. Huh JR, Littman DR. Small molecule inhibitors of RORγt: targeting Th17 cells and other applications. *Eur J Immunol.* 2012;42(9):2232–2237.

CHAPTER 12

Psychology of Keratoconus

Madeline Yung ■ Mark J. Mannis

- Keratoconus can have a psychological impact due to its onset during the formative years of adolescence and a decrease in quality of life, even in the presence of good visual acuity.
- Although the anecdotal concept of a "keratoconic personality" exists, characterized by a highly anxious, diffident, and suspicious patient, studies have failed to substantiate a distinct personality profile.
- Patients with keratoconus tend to display maladaptive coping mechanisms that may interfere with a productive patient-provider relationship.
- Providers should anticipate the altered psyche, maladaptive behaviors, and high disease burden of keratoconus when counseling these patients.

Introduction

As a chronic progressive disease that develops during the formative adolescent years, keratoconus can have a significant impact on the psyche, so much so that many physicians characterize patients with keratoconus as having a distinct personality profile. The psychological effects of keratoconus, in turn, may influence patients' interactions with their healthcare providers and ultimately their treatment outcomes. Ophthalmologists should account for the altered psychology in keratoconic patients when tailoring their treatment approach. This chapter will review the existing literature on the association between keratoconus and personality traits, quality of life, and mental health.

Psychological Roots of Keratoconus

The psychological impact of keratoconus stems largely from its onset during adolescence and its severe impact on quality of life.[1]

ADOLESCENT ONSET

Keratoconus develops between the ages of 12 and 39 in 94% of patients and is a disease of adolescence and young adulthood.[2] Adolescence is the major life stage for the formation of self-image, social identity, and independence. The development of a chronic, progressive, and visually debilitating illness during adolescence can have a devastating emotional impact on young adults who are otherwise healthy and have little interaction with healthcare providers.[3] In addition, developing a disability during this crucial time of psychological maturation can fundamentally alter personality and behavioral traits.[4]

QUALITY OF LIFE IMPACT

Patients with keratoconus experience a significant decrease in quality of life on all fronts, on average scoring similar to patients with advanced age-related macular degeneration on validated question-naires.[5,6] This impact is independent of visual acuity. Keratoconic patients report a negative impact on their quality of life even if their best corrected acuity is 20/20.[7] This may be explained in part by the psychological burden of disease; many patients do not fully understand the good visual progno-sis of keratoconus with appropriate treatment and may harbor irrational fears of future blindness.[8]

Nevertheless, keratoconus can limit patient visual function, well-being, and work capacity. Patients with keratoconus have scored lower than controls on all visual function and well-being scales on the National Eye Institute Visual Function Questionnaire (NEI-VFQ) and reported elevated anxiety and frustration with their sight.[5] Almost all patients report that keratoconus has had some impact on their lives, with over a third characterizing the impact as moderate or severe.[8] Baseline data from the Collaborative Longitudinal Evaluation of Keratoconus (CLEK) study reveal that 1.4% of patients changed jobs, 2.1% received disability compensation, and 11.5% missed work due to keratoconus.[9] Quality of life continues to decline over time, especially with disease progression and continued visual decline.[10]

Definitive treatments such as corneal collagen cross-linking and corneal transplantation can diminish the psychological burden of possible disease progression and boost quality-of-life scores. Cross-linking and combination cross-linking photorefractive keratectomy treatments improve quality-of-life scores.[7,11] Along with improved visual function, patients who undergo cross-linking report improved general health and mental health, with decreased anxiety levels 1 year after the procedure.[12] Patients with keratoconus also report high satisfaction and improved quality of life after corneal transplantation, especially when delivered with comprehensive patient education.[13]

Keratoconus and Personality

Personality traits in keratoconus have been characterized by a small body of literature consisting primarily of physician surveys, case reports, and case-control studies.[1] Over the years, the altered psychology of patients with keratoconus has colored physician-patient interactions, leaving the impression of a "keratoconic personality" within the ophthalmology community.[4] The notional kera-toconic personality is generally characterized by high anxiety, low self-confidence, compulsion, and suspicion. Evidence on the existence of a distinct keratoconic personality is conflicting, and review of the literature largely fails to establish a clear association between keratoconus and personality.

PHYSICIAN SURVEYS

In attitudinal surveys, ophthalmologists well-versed with keratoconus have characterized patients as less self-confident, less friendly, and poorly adjusted.[4] A trend toward the additional descriptors of less insightful, less self-controlled, and more emotionally labile is seen.

CASE-CONTROL STUDIES—CONTROLS WITHOUT EYE DISEASE

Personality studies of keratoconus vary widely in the selection of control patients, the question-naire or assessment tool used, and their conclusions (Table 12.1). Control groups have ranged from healthy subjects without eye disease, to patients with chronic nonkeratoconus eye disease, to patients with high refractive error. Study results must be interpreted in the context of control group selection, to parse out personality traits associated specifically with keratoconus as opposed to with chronic eye disease in general.

In 1976, Karseras and Ruben conducted the first personality survey of 75 patients with kera-toconus compared with randomly selected outpatient controls but did not find any significant

TABLE 12.1 ■ Studies Correlating Keratoconus With Personality Traits

Authors	Personality Assessment Tool Used	Study Population	Summary of Findings
Mannis et al.[20]	Millon Clinical Multiaxial Inventory (MCMI)	52 patients with keratoconus, 35 patients with chronic eye disease, 32 patients without eye disease	Both patients with keratoconus and patients with chronic eye disease exhibited personality deviations compared with normal controls[a]
Cooke et al.[21]	Eysenck Personality Questionnaire, Maudsley Obsessive-Compulsive Inventory	118 patients with keratoconus, 75 patients with bilateral high myopia	No difference in personality dimensions or obsessionality
Gorskova et al.[16]	Brief Multifactorial Questionnaire for Personality Examination (BMQP)	84 patients with keratoconus, 63 normal controls[a]	Patients with keratoconus showed increased psychasthenia and schizophrenia
Swartz et al.[19]	Minnesota Multiphasic Personality Inventory (MMPI)	28 patients with keratoconus, 16 patients with HSV keratitis	Patients with keratoconus were more likely to have abnormal clinical scale elevations
García-Monlléo and Melgosa[18]	16 Personality Factor Questionnaire of the Institute for Personality and Ability Testing (16 PF)	22 patients with keratoconus, 19 patients with retinitis pigmentosa	Patients with keratoconus had abnormal scores for mental capacity, ego strength, guilt proneness, submissiveness, and praxernia
Moreira et al.[17]	Short Form 36 Health Survey (SF-36), Millon Index of Personality Styles Revised (MIPS)	68 patients with keratoconus, 52 normal controls[a]	Patients with keratoconus were more pessimistic, scores improved with successful contact lens wear
Giedd et al.[8]	Millon Behavioral Health Inventory (MBHI)	153 patients with keratoconus, 153 normal controls[a]	Patients with keratoconus scored lower on the respectful coping style scale

[a]Normal controls did not have eye disease.
HSV, Herpes simplex virus.

differences between groups.[14] In 1980, Besançon et al. reported the results of psychiatric interviews with 34 patients with keratoconus shortly prior to corneal transplantation, finding a higher incidence of "neurotic and psychosomatic traits" compared to reference normals, although no comparison with a control group was made.[15]

Gorskova et al. found that patients with keratoconus displayed increased levels of psychasthenia (characterized by phobias, obsessions, compulsions, and anxiety) and schizophrenia, as well as a higher risk for depression in female subjects, compared with normal controls.[16] Similarly, Moreira et al. found keratoconic patients to show increased pain avoidance, imaginative intuition, social withdrawal, and anxious hesitation compared with healthy controls without ocular disease.[17]

CASE-CONTROL STUDIES—CONTROLS WITH EYE DISEASE

García-Monlléo and Melgosa compared patients with keratoconus to patients with retinitis pigmentosa, another progressive and visually debilitating condition with an early onset.[18] Patients with keratoconus had abnormal scores in terms of lower mental capacity, lower ego strength, more guilt proneness, more submissiveness, and praxernia (practicality), whereas patients with retinitis pigmentosa were characterized as shrewder, more refined, experienced, and astute compared with normal controls. The authors concluded that keratoconus and retinitis pigmentosa are associated with distinct personality profiles independent of vision loss. However, retinitis pigmentosa typically preserves central vision until late in the disease course and requires infrequent follow up, whereas keratoconus has an early impact on visual function and often requires frequent healthcare visits for contact lens or corneal transplantation management. These differences in disease course and burden can make it difficult to compare keratoconus and retinitis pigmentosa.

Swartz et al. compared keratoconus patients with those with a history of herpes simplex keratitis. Patients with keratoconus were more likely to have an abnormal score on at least one psychological scale. However, there was considerable variability in abnormalities and the authors could not define a specific keratoconus personality profile.[19] Patients who had undergone penetrating keratoplasty were significantly less likely to have abnormal scale scores.

Two case-control studies did not find sufficient evidence to support a keratoconic personality distinct from patients with similar eye conditions. When compared with patients with other chronic eye disease, patients with keratoconus were found to have similar personality characteristics.[20] Mannis et al. found that both patients with keratoconus and patients with other chronic eye disease exhibited less conforming and more disorganized, passive-aggressive, paranoid, and hypomanic tendencies compared with normal controls.[20] Patients with chronic eye disease additionally displayed more avoidant, dependent, and borderline traits and scored higher on personality and psychotic scales compared with keratoconic patients.

Similarly, Cooke et al. found no differences in personality or obsessive-compulsive propensity between patients with keratoconus and those with high myopia, controlling for poor uncorrected visual acuity and contact lens use.[21]

Physician Interactions

MALADAPTIVE COPING MECHANISMS

Although no consensus has been established on a true keratoconic personality, patients with keratoconus can display maladaptive coping mechanisms when interfacing with healthcare services, leading to negative patient-provider interactions and the impression of an abnormal personality. Ophthalmologists who care for patients with keratoconus have noted an abnormal psychosocial profile and general disenchantment in these patients,[4] a perception that extends across geographic and cultural boundaries.[1]

Giedd et al. found that when interacting with healthcare providers, patients with keratoconus scored lower than normative controls on the respectful coping style scale of the Millon Behavioral Health Inventory and were described as having less self-control, being less cooperative, and less likely to follow treatment recommendations.[8] Women scored higher on the confident scale and were described as appearing calm and confident, but also as more likely to expect special treatment. Meanwhile, men were found to be more introverted, emotionally flat, and unconcerned with their problems.[8] Whether these coping mechanisms are specific to keratoconus or also seen in patients with nonkeratoconus eye disease is unclear. However, the disrespectful, confident, and introversive coping mechanisms used by keratoconic patients likely contribute to the clinical stereotype of an unusual personality.

DISEASE BURDEN PERCEPTION

The severe negative impact of keratoconus on quality of life may be underestimated by physicians and consequently undermine the patient-provider relationship. Patients report decreased quality of life even with mild disease and good visual acuity[7] and experience anxiety even when good vision is achieved with contact lenses. Whereas myopic controls reported increased satisfaction with appearance, career image, and self-confidence after starting contact lens wear, patients with keratoconus did not experience these changes and instead reported greater anxiety about potential worsening of their refractive error and ineffective treatment.[22]

Two-Hit Hypothesis

A popular theory is a "two-hit hypothesis" to explain the concept of the keratoconic personality.[23] The first "hit" arises from the insidious onset of decreased vision and knowledge of a progressive, potentially blinding disease during a vulnerable period in psychosocial development, which in turn engenders pathologic coping mechanisms. Patients with keratoconus tend to utilize a maladaptive and disrespectful coping style while interacting with healthcare providers. The second hit results from incongruous patient and physician expectations, where a dissonance in perception of disease burden strains the relationship and leaves physicians with the impression of a keratoconic personality.

Association With Mental Health Disorders

DEPRESSION

Evidence on the relationship between keratoconus and depression is conflicting. Keratoconus correlated with higher Patient Health Questionnaire-9 (PHQ-9) score and Zung Self-rating Depression Scale scores compared with healthy gender-matched controls, with older age and worse visual acuity being additional risk factors.[24] However, other high-powered studies found no significant association between keratoconus and depression.[25,26]

PERSONALITY DISORDERS

Keratoconus has been reported in patients with personality disorders, although no clear association or causality has been established. Two case reports link keratoconus with schizophreniform disorder[27] or schizophrenia.[28] The low incidence of these cases raises the possibility of a coincidental rather than causative relationship. Three additional case reports detail the development of keratoconus in patients with obsessive-compulsive eye rubbing.[29–31] However, although eye rubbing is a recognized physiologic risk factor for keratoconus, no clear association between keratoconus and obsessive-compulsive personality disorder has been found.

Modifications to Patient Counseling

When interacting with keratoconus patients, physicians must consider the altered psyche, maladaptive behaviors, and disease burden. Alves et al. found that patients with keratoconus were often dissatisfied with the diagnostic and prognostic counseling provided by their physicians.[32] Satisfaction rates increased with the degree of professional training, awareness of language and social representation of the disease, and consideration of the patient's socioeconomic and cultural status.

Patients may expect substantial attention and counseling proportional to the impact of keratoconus on their lives, although physicians may not fully appreciate the effects on quality of life, especially in patients with good corrected visual acuity. Physicians should anticipate patient anxiety and accommodate maladaptive behaviors during counseling. In addition, patients may view keratoconus as a blinding condition without recourse and require counseling on the good visual prognosis with appropriate treatment. With this nuanced approach, a healthy and productive patient-provider relationship can be achieved.

References

1. Mannis MJ, Ling JJ, Kyrillos R, Barnett M. Keratoconus and personality — a review. *Cornea*. 2018;37:400–404.
2. Kennedy RH, Bourne WM, Dyer JA. A 48-year clinical and epidemiologic study of keratoconus. *Am J Ophthalmol*. 1986;101:267–273.
3. Feldman HS, Lopez MA. *Developmental Psychology for the Health Care Professions. Part 2: Adulthood and Aging*. Boulder, CO: Westview Press; 1982.
4. Farge EJ, Baer PE, Adams GL, Paton D. Personality correlates of keratoconus. In:. *Phenomenology and Treatment of Psychophysiological Disorders*. Ed. Fann W.E., Karacan I., Pokorny A.D., Williams R.L. Dordrecht: Springer Netherlands; 1982.
5. Kymes SM, Walline JJ, Zadnik K, Gordon MO. Quality of life in keratoconus. *Am J Ophthalmol*. 2004;138:527–535.
6. Wagner H, Barr JT, Zadnik K. Collaborative Longitudinal Evaluation of Keratoconus (CLEK) study: methods and findings to date. *Cont Lens Anterior Eye*. 2007;30:223–232.
7. Tatematsu-Ogawa Y, Yamada M, Kawashima M, Yamazaki Y, Bryce T, Tsubota K. The disease burden of keratoconus in patients' lives: comparisons to a Japanese normative sample. *Eye Contact Lens*. 2008;34:13–16.
8. Giedd KK, Mannis MJ, Mitchell GL, Zadnik K. Personality in keratoconus in a sample of patients derived from the internet. *Cornea*. 2005;24:301–307.
9. Zadnik K, Barr JT, Edrington TB, et al. Baseline findings in the Collaborative Longitudinal Evaluation of Keratoconus (CLEK) study. *Invest Ophthalmol Vis Sci*. 1998;39:2537–2546.
10. Kymes SM, Walline JJ, Zadnik K, Sterling J, Gordon MO. Changes in the quality-of-life of people with keratoconus. *Am J Ophthalmol*. 2008;145:611–617.
11. Labiris G, Giarmoukakis A, Sideroudi H, Gkika M, Fanariotis M, Kozobolis V. Impact of keratoconus, cross-linking and cross-linking combined with photorefractive keratectomy on self-reported quality of life. *Cornea*. 2012;31:734–739.
12. Cingu AK, Bez Y, Cinar Y, et al. Impact of collagen cross-linking on psychological distress and vision and health-related quality of life in patients with keratoconus. *Eye Contact Lens*. 2015;41:349–353.
13. Uiters E, van den Borne B, van der Horst FG, Völker-Dieben HJ. Patient satisfaction after corneal transplantation. *Cornea*. 2001;20:687–694.
14. Karseras AG, Ruben M. Aetiology of keratoconus. *Br J Ophthalmol*. 1976;60:522–525.
15. Besançon G, Baikoff G, Deneux A, Mauvoisin M, Bergaud F. [Preliminary note on the psychological and mental status of patients with keratoconus]. *Bull Soc Ophtalmol Fr*. 1980;80:441–443.
16. Gorskova EN, Sevost'ianov EN, Baturin NA. [Results of psychological testing of patients with keratoconus]. *Vestn Oftalmol*. 1998;114:44–45.
17. Moreira LB, Alchieri JC, Belfort Jr R, Moreira H. [Psychological and social aspects of patients with keratoconus]. *Arquivos Brasileiros de Oftalmologia*. 2007;70:317–322.
18. García-Monlléo R., Melgosa J.M.R.M. Personality factors in patients with keratoconus or retinitis pigmentosa. *Atti Della Fondazione Giorgio Ronchi*. 2003;58(2):201–211.
19. Swartz NG, Cohen EJ, Scott DG, Genvert GI, Arentsen JJ, Laibson PR. Personality and keratoconus. *CLAO J*. 1990;16:62–64.
20. Mannis MJ, Morrison TL, Zadnik K, Holland EJ. Krachmer JH. Personality trends in keratoconus. an analysis. *Arch Ophthalmol*. 1987;105:798–800.
21. Cooke CA, Cooper C, Dowds E, Frazer DG, Jackson AJ. Keratoconus, myopia, and personality. *Cornea*. 2003;22:239–242.
22. Lee S, Jung G, Lee HK. Comparison of contact lens corrected quality of vision and life of keratoconus and myopic patients. *Korean J Ophthalmol*. 2017;31:489–496.
23. Vazirani J, Basu S. Keratoconus: current perspectives. *Clin Ophthalmol (Auckland, NZ)*. 2013;7:2019–2030.
24. Moschos MM, Gouliopoulos NS, Kalogeropoulos C, et al. Psychological aspects and depression in patients with symptomatic keratoconus. *J Ophthalmol*. 2018;2018:7314308.

25. Woodward MA, Blachley TS, Stein JD. The association between sociodemographic factors, common systemic diseases, and keratoconus: an analysis of a nationwide heath care claims database. *Ophthalmology.* 2016;123:457–465. e2.
26. Xu L, Wang YX, Guo Y, You QS, Jonas JB. Prevalence and associations of steep cornea/keratoconus in Greater Beijing. The Beijing Eye Study. *PloS One.* 2012;7:e39313.
27. Rudisch B, D'Orio B, Compton MT. Keratoconus and psychosis. *Am J Psychiatry.* 2003;160:1011.
28. Schürhoff F, Leboyer M, Szöke A. Comorbidity between schizophrenia and keratoconus. *Psychiatry Res.* 2017;247:315–316.
29. Scullica L. [Acute posttraumatic keratoconus caused by self-mutilation in a patient with obsessive psychoasthenia]. *Boll Ocul.* 1962;41:270–277.
30. Kandarakis A, Karampelas M, Soumplis V, et al. A case of bilateral self-induced keratoconus in a patient with tourette syndrome associated with compulsive eye rubbing: case report. *BMC Ophthalmol.* 2011;11:28.
31. Panikkar K, Manayath G, Rajaraman R, Saravanan V. Progressive keratoconus, retinal detachment, and intracorneal silicone oil with obsessive-compulsive eye rubbing. *Oman J Ophthalmol.* 2016;9:170–173.
32. Alves VL, Alves MR, Lane ST. [The diagnostic communication of keratoconus and its influence on the social representation that the patient has of his/her illness]. *Arquivos Brasileiros de Oftalmologia.* 2007;70:790–796.

CHAPTER 13

Artificial Intelligence in Keratoconus

Maria A. Henriquez ■ Gustavo Hernandez Sahagún ■ Diana Quintanilla Perez ■ Arthur Mauricio Delgadillo ■ David Mauricio ■ Luis Izquierdo Jr.

KEY CONCEPTS

- Machine learning models have been used effectively in the diagnosis of keratoconus.
- Machine learning models such as neural networks, decision trees, and support vector machines have shown excellent sensitivity and specificity in diagnosis.
- Data from topographers, Scheimpflug imaging analysis, and anterior segment optical coherence tomography devices can adequately feed machine learning models, producing excellent results in the diagnosis of keratoconus.

Introduction

The estimated prevalence of keratoconus (KC) has increased 5- to 10-fold over previously reported rates in population studies, and the increase is considered to be the result of a combination of earlier and more advanced tomography detection and comprehensive data collection.[1] An early diagnosis of KC is crucial because of its significant prevalence and the ability of early intervention to obviate the need for corneal transplantation. This is particularly important, as KC and ectatic diseases represent the most common indications for transplant in pediatric patients.[2]

Artificial intelligence (AI) is one of the major fields of computer science research. In particular, its subfield, machine learning (ML), is being applied in several industries ranging from product recommendation in e-commerce to various uses in medicine.[3] ML has been used in ophthalmology to diagnose eye conditions such as glaucoma and diabetic retinopathy.[4] At a very basic level, the goal is to build a concise distribution model of class labels in terms of predictive features. The resulting classifier can then be used to assign class labels in test cases where the values of the predictor features are known but that of the class label is unknown.[5] The defining characteristic of ML algorithms is the improvement in prediction quality with increasing experience; therefore, the more data we provide, the better the resultant prediction model.[6]

ML systems can be categorized into two types: supervised and unsupervised.

Supervised learning involves training a model with previously labeled training data, tuning the input weights to improve the accuracy of its predictions until they are optimized, and then mapping the test datasets as corresponding outputs. It may expedite the classification process and helps distinguish various clinical outcomes. In **unsupervised learning**, we train a model with unlabeled data (without a human-labeled process). There is no actual instructor or teacher in unsupervised learning, and the algorithm must learn to understand the data without any guide. This type of learning incorporates models that describe hidden structures that are usually invisible to humans and can lead to new discoveries.

In the unsupervised learning subtype, the most common method is deep learning (DL), also referred to as deep neural networks, which involves using an unsupervised method and multiple layers between the input and output, avoiding manual selection and segmenting the areas of study, speeding up the processes.[7]

The most important difference between DL and traditional ML is their performance while handling increasing amounts of data. DL algorithms do not perform well with small amounts of data, because they require a large amount of data for adequate analysis. DL is applied in various AI fields such as speech recognition, image recognition, natural language processing (NLP), robot navigation systems, and self-driving cars. Fig. 13.1 presents a schematic visualization of AI.

Models of Artificial Intelligence in Keratoconus

Several AI models have been used in the diagnosis of KC and its milder forms. The ML models most frequently used to discriminate between normal and KC eyes are neural networks, decision trees, and the support vector machine (SVM) model, followed by random forests and linear discriminant analysis. Table 13.1 shows the ML models used in different studies using AI for KC diagnosis. Studies have reported up to 100% accuracy, sensitivity, and specificity using neural networks,[16] random forests,[24] and Bayesian networks.[33]

ARTIFICIAL NEURAL NETWORK

An artificial neural network (ANN) is an ML model inspired by brain architecture. The central concept behind an ANN is the neuron, which is the computation unit that acquires knowledge during the training process (using a training algorithm). The neurons are organized and composed in layers that are organized in multiple ways, resulting in several ANN architectures.[35–38] Fig. 13.2 illustrates a basic example of an ANN used for KC diagnosis. The use of multiple successive layers for learning (several modern ANN architectures involve hundreds of layers) is called DL.[39]

DECISION TREES

Decision trees are structures that divide the data based on a series of questions. Each internal node represents a question based on a feature (e.g., is the inferior-superior asymmetry lower than

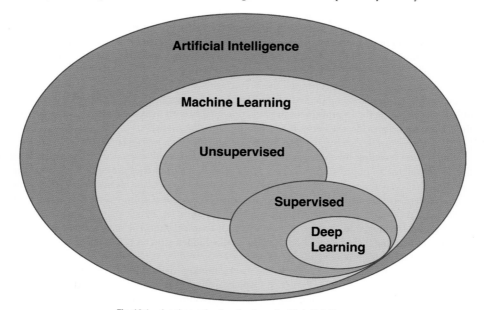

Fig. 13.1 A schematic visualization of artificial intelligence.

TABLE 13.1 ■ **Machine Learning Models in Various Studies Using Artificial Intelligence for Keratoconus Diagnosis**

Author, Year	Device Used for Keratoconus Diagnosis	Machine Learning Models Used
Kovács et al., 2016[8]	Pentacam HR, OCULUS Optikgeräte GmbH	Neural network
Twa et al., 2005[9]	Keratron corneal topographer (v3.49; Optikon 2000, Rome, Italy)	Decision tree
Chastang et al., 2000[10]	EyeSys System 2000	Decision tree
Maeda et al., 1994[11]	Computer-assisted videokeratoscope (TMS-1, Computed Anatomy, New York, NY)	Decision tree, linear discriminant
Karimi et al., 2018[12]	Corvis ST (software version 1.00r30), corneal topography (Allegro Topolyzer; WaveLight AG, Germany), corneal tomography (Pentacam)	Neural network
Chandapura et al., 2019[13]	OCT (RTVue, Optovue Inc., Irvine) and Scheimpflug (Pentacam, OCULUS Optikgeräte GmbH, Wetzlar, Germany)	Random forest
Maeda et al., 1995[14]	Videokeratoscope, points on rings 2, 3, and 4 from videokeratographs (TMS-1, Computed Anatomy Inc., New York, NY)	Decision tree, linear discriminant
Issarti et al., 2019[15]	Pentacam HR, OCULUS Optikgeräte GmbH	Neural network
Smolek and Klyce, 1997[16]	TMS-2 for Windows videokeratography system (software version W1.2)	Neural network
Smadja et al., 2013[17]	GALILEI system (software version 5.2.1)	Decision tree
Lopes et al., 2018[18]	Pentacam HR, OCULUS GmbH, Wetzlar, Germany software (version 1.20r118)	Random forest, SVM, neural network, regularized discriminant analysis, Naive Bayes
Silverman et al., 2014[19]	Artemis-1 (ArcScan, Inc., Morrison, CO) very high-frequency (VHF) digital ultrasound system; Procyon P2000 pupillometer (Haag-Streit, Bern, Switzerland). Tomography was assessed using the Orbscan II (Bausch & Lomb, Claremont, CA), and topography and simulated keratometry (K) were assessed using the Atlas corneal topography system (Carl Zeiss Meditec AG, Dublin, CA).	Neural network
Ruiz Hidalgo et al., 2016[20]	Pentacam HR, software version 1.20 r02 (Oculus, Wetzlar, Germany)	SVM
Souza et al., 2010[21]	Orbscan IITM (Bausch & Lomb)	SVM, neural network
Saika et al., 2013[22]	TMS-4 Advance Corneal Topographer (Tomey Corporation, Nagoya, Japan) corneal topographer (KR-9000PW, TOPCON, Tokyo, Japan)	kNN, linear discriminant, Mahalanobis distance (DIS), neural network
Lopes et al., 2015[23]	Pentacam HR, OCULUS GmbH, Wetzlar, Germany	SVM

(Continued)

TABLE 13.1 ■ Machine Learning Models in Various Studies Using Artificial Intelligence for
Keratoconus Diagnosis.—cont'd

Author, Year	Device Used for Keratoconus Diagnosis	Machine Learning Models Used
Ambrósio et al., 2017[24]	Pentacam HR and Corvis ST (OCULUS Optikgeräte GmbH, Wetzlar, Germany)	Random forest
Yousefi et al., 2018[25]	SS-1000 CASIA OCT Imaging Systems (Tomey, Japan)	Density-based clustering
Lavric and Valentin, 2019[26]	Not mentioned in the manuscript	Neural network
Maeda et al.,1995[27]	Videokeratocope (TMS-1, computed anatomy, NY)	Neural network
Accardo and Pensiero, 2003[28]	Videokeratoscope (EyeSys)	Neural network
Feizi et al., 2016[29]	Tomey, EM-3000, version 4.20, Nagoya, Japan	Decision tree
Carvalho, 2005[30]	EyeSys System 2000 (EyeSys Vision, Houston, TX)	Neural network
Arbelaez et al., 2012[31]	Sirius, software version 1.2, CSO, Firenze, Italy	SVM
Ruiz Hidalgo et al., 2017[32]	Pentacam HR (v1.20 r53; OCULUS GmbH, Wetzlar, Germany)	SVM
Castro-Luna et al., 2000[33]	CSO topography system (CSO, Firenze, Italy)	Bayesian network
Kamiya et al., 2019[34]	CASIA SS-1000 (Tomey, Aichi, Japan)	Deep learning

kNN, k-nearest neighbor algorithm; *SVM,* Support vector machine.

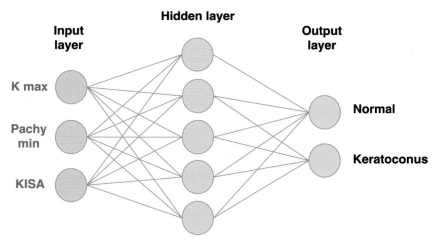

Fig. 13.2   A basic example of an artificial neural network used for keratoconus diagnosis.
K_{max}, Maximum keratometry; y*Pachy min*, thinnest pachymetry. KISA%: (K) X (I-S) X (AST)
X (SRAX) X 100 where *K*: keratometric value; *I-S*: inferior superior dioptric asymmetry;
AST index: degree of regular corneal astigmatism; *SRAX*: skewed radial axis.

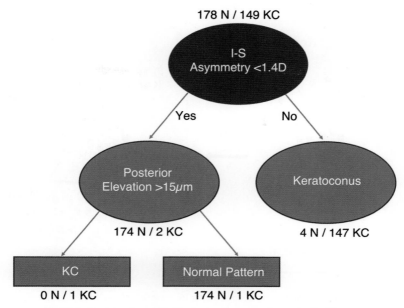

178 N / 149 KC

I-S
Asymmetry <1.4D

Yes   No

Posterior
Elevation >15μm   Keratoconus

174 N / 2 KC   4 N / 147 KC

KC   Normal Pattern

0 N / 1 KC   174 N / 1 KC

Fig. 13.3 Decision tree example for keratoconus diagnosis. *D*, Diopters; *I-S*, inferior-superior; *KC*, keratoconus; *N*, normal.

1.4 diopter [D]?). Each branch of the tree is the result of the internal nodes (e.g., the answer to the previous question can be yes/no), branching out to reach the leaf nodes (which are nodes that no longer give rise to other branches). The leaf nodes are the final result of the task (e.g., in KC diagnosis, they decide if a patient eye has the condition or not) (Fig. 13.3). For simplicity, imagine a tree where each branch is the product of a question until a final branch is reached that no longer divides. This last branch represents the final result that is sought (e.g., keratoconus or not). Decision trees can be created manually, but in ML, optimal decision trees are automatically generated from the data by employing algorithms.[40] An important characteristic of decision trees is their **interpretability** (only for small trees),[41] which is one of the main reasons why they are used in medical fields,[42] especially in KC diagnosis.

SUPPORT VECTOR MACHINE

SVMs aim to determine the parent class of provided sample data by finding an optimal decision boundary (the line that separates the data into two classes). The optimal decision boundary can achieve the maximum possible separation of the data (with a process called *large margin classification*), compared with other boundaries where the classes can remain close together (meaning that they would not perform as well on new instances).[36–39] To find this optimal decision boundary, the data (e.g., corneal parameters) are mapped to a new *high–dimensional* representation. To understand this model, imagine a dividing line that allows us to separate the data into two groups. The model seeks to create this line by graphing the data in dimensions (two-dimensional [2D], three-dimensional [3D], four-dimensional [4D] ... nD), which is necessary to achieve the best possible division. Fig. 13.4 shows a basic example of use of a SVM for KC diagnosis.

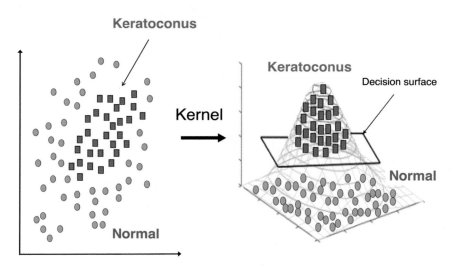

Fig. 13.4   A basic example of a support vector machine used for keratoconus diagnosis.

PARAMETERS AND DEVICES USED IN AI MODELS

The most frequently used AI devices mentioned in the literature for KC diagnosis are topographers, Scheimpflug imaging analysis, anterior segment optical coherence tomography, and devices related to corneal biomechanics (e.g., Corvis ST). Table 13.1 lists the devices used in studies of AI in KC diagnosis. The most frequently used parameters in ML models are the curvature map, corneal irregularity indices, anterior chamber parameters, and pachymetry.

SENSITIVITY AND SPECIFICITY

Three studies achieved 100% sensitivity and specificity in distinguishing normal from KC eyes: Smolek and Klyce,[16] using an ANN approach based on topographic parameters in 33 KC eyes; Ambrósio et al.,[24] using a random forest approach in a multicenter study combining data from corneal deformation response and tomography corneal data in 204 eyes; and Castro-Luna et al.,[33] using a Naive Bayes classifier based on Placido-disk indices in 30 eyes. However, the total sample sizes (including controls and KC eyes) used in these studies were different (300, 850, and 60, respectively), as were the number of classes used, affecting their results. For example, Smolek and Klyce included 11 classes, with 66 KC eyes, whereas Ambrósio et al. included 204 eyes and four classes. Table 13.2 shows the sensitivity, specificity, accuracy, and area under the receiving operating characteristic curve (AUROC) for each study analyzing normal and KC eyes.

Artificial Intelligence in Milder Forms of Keratoconus

Models that allow the diagnosis of milder forms of KC have also been reported. At least 14 studies have been published describing the diagnosis of forme fruste keratoconus (FFKC), subclinical keratoconus, suspicious keratoconus, and very asymmetric ectasia with normal topography (VAE-NT). However, comparisons among these studies are not possible because of differences in terminologies, sample sizes, and AI models.

TABLE 13.2 ■ Sensitivity, Specificity, and Accuracy in Each Study Analyzing Normal and Keratoconus Eyes

Author, Year	N (Total Eyes)	N (Keratoconus Eyes)	Sensitivity (%)	Specificity (%)	Accuracy (%)	AUROC (%)
Kovács et al., 2016[8]	135	60	100	98		100
Twa et al., 2005[9]	244	112	92	93	93	97
Chastang et al., 2000[10]	208	46	88.5	94.9		
Maeda et al., 1994[11]	200	50	89	99	96	
Karimi et al., 2018[12]	235	93			91.2	
Chandapura et al., 2019[13]	439	116	93.97	96.28	95.7	
			93.97	97.21	96.4	
Maeda et al., 1995[14]	176	44	98	99		
Issarti et al., 2019^[15]	838	229	99.91	99.90	99.6	
Smolek and Klyce, 1997[16]	300	66	100	100	100	
Smadja et al., 2013[17]	372	148	100	99.5		
Lopes et al., 2018[18]	3693	370	100	99.7		
Silverman et al., 2014[19]	204	74	94.6	99.2		
			98.9	99.5		
Ruiz Hidalgo et al., 2016[20]	860	454	99.1	98.5	98.9	99.8
			96.3	93.6		99
Souza et al., 2010[21]	318	46	100	98		99
Saika et al., 2013[22]	212	51	71.43	88.24	84.9	79.83
			71.43	88.24	84.9	79.83
			68.00	90.12	84.9	79.06
			63.15	98.52	85.8	80.84
Lopes et al., 2015[23]	560	335	96	98		99.1
Ambrósio et al., 2017[24]	850	204	100	100	100	100
Yousefi et al., 2018[25]	3156	796	97.7	94.1		
Lavric and Valentin, 2019[26]	3000	1500			99.3	
Maeda et al., 1995[27]	183	26	92	98	97	
Accardo and Pensiero, 2002[28]	396	120	100	98.6	99	
Feizi et al., 2016[29]	210	51	100	99.3	99.4	
Carvalho, 2005[30]	80	16	93.75	98.44	97.5	
Arbelaez et al., 2012[31]	3502	877	95.0	99.3	98.2	
Ruiz Hidalgo et al., 2017[32]	131	54	92.6	96.1	94.7	94.3
	131	51	98.0	96.3	96.9	97.1
Castro-Luna et al., 2020[33]	60	30	100	100	100	
Kamiya et al., 2019[34]	543	304	100	98.4	99.1	

AUROC, Area under the receiving operating characteristic.

Authors who evaluated eyes with a certain degree of abnormal topography against fellow eyes with KC (referred to as subclinical or suspicious KC) have found high sensitivity and specificity for its diagnosis using AI. Smolek and Klyce[16] reported 100% sensitivity and specificity in terms of AUROC. However, their sample size was small (six suspected KC eyes). By using dual Scheimpflug parameters as the inputs to a decision tree classifier, Feizi et al.[29] achieved 100% sensitivity and 91.3% specificity (95.65% in AUROC) in 23 eyes with subclinical KC. However, no validation technique was applied. Arbelaez et al.[31] used an SVM classifier trained on the curvature, thickness, pachymetry indices, and height data of both the anterior and posterior corneal surfaces with a 3502-eye dataset (a larger dataset of eyes than any previous study, which included 426 subclinical KC eyes), and achieved sensitivity and specificity of 92.0% and 97.7%, respectively.

Authors who evaluated eyes with normal topography compared with fellow eyes with KC (referred as FFKC or VAE-NT) also had excellent results in terms of sensitivity and specificity. Smadja et al.[17] analyzed 55 parameters from anterior and posterior corneal measurements and created two decision trees each for KC and FFKC detection, respectively. The large FFKC detection tree (based on just five parameters) achieved sensitivity and specificity of 93.6% and 97.2%, respectively (95.4% in AUROC). Ambrósio et al.[24] evaluated tomographic and biomechanical parameters with various ML models, reporting their maximum sensitivity and specificity in VAE-NT detection with values of 96.0% and 90.4%, respectively (93.2% in AUROC), using a random forest model and leave-one-out cross validation (LOO). Table 13.3 shows the sensitivity and specificity of studies in which milder forms of KC were evaluated using AI models.

TABLE 13.3 ■ Sensitivity and Specificity in Studies That Evaluated Milder Forms of Keratoconus Using Artificial Intelligence Models

Author, Year	N (Eyes)	N (Eyes With Milder Forms of Keratoconus)	Sensitivity (%)	Specificity (%)	Accuracy (%)	AUROC (%)
FFKC						
Kovács et al., 2016[8]	75	15	92	85		96
Chandapura et al., 2019[13]	293	72	59.72	93.73	88.2	
			72.22	95.64	91.8	
Ruiz Hidalgo et al., 2016[20]	261	67	79.1	97.9	93.1	92.2
			37.3	98.0		92.5
Subclinical KC						
Smadja et al., 2013[17]	224	47	93.6	97.2		
Saika et al., 2013[22]	111	46	46.66	82.42	77.4	64.54
			45.00	83.72	76.5	64.36
			63.63	83.15	81.1	73.39
			33.33	79.00	76.4	56.16
Feizi et al., 2016[29]	159	23	100	91.3	73.9	
Arbelaez et al., 2012[31]	1685	426	92.0	97.7	97.3	
Suspected KC						
Issarti et al., 2019[15]	389	77	97.78	95.56	96.6	
Karimi et al., 2018[12]	235	35			83.3	
Smolek and Klyce, 1997[16]	150	6	100	100	100	

TABLE 13.3 ■ Sensitivity and Specificity in Studies That Evaluated Milder Forms of Keratoconus Using Artificial Intelligence Models—(Continued)

Author, Year	N (Eyes)	N (Eyes With Milder Forms of Keratoconus)	Sensitivity (%)	Specificity (%)	Accuracy (%)	AUROC (%)
Ruiz Hidalgo et al., 2017[32]	131	23	60.8	75.0	72.5	67.9
	131	8	100	73.2	74.8	86.5
VAE-NT						
Chandapura et al., 2019[13]	251	30	6.67	98.29	92	
			0	99.02	92.3	
Lopes et al., 2018[18]	3693	188	85.2	96.6		96.8
Ambrósio et al., 2017[24]	574	94	90.4	96.0	93.2	98.5

AUROC, Area under the receiving operating characteristic curve; *FFKC,* forme fruste keratoconus; *KC,* keratoconus; *VAE-NT,* very asymmetric ectasia with normal topography.

Although several studies have demonstrated excellent results, creating standard data sets, such as those used in heart disease, diabetic retinopathy, and cancer diagnosis, with strict and globally accepted KC definitions will help in the evaluation and comparison of ML models. More importantly, if this is not achievable, existing data sets need to be publicly available and ML phases should be described in more detail to make the studies reproducible and create a base for future comparisons. Finally, AI is clearly here to stay and will represent one of the most effective diagnostic modalities for KC, both in general and for the subtle forms of this disease.

Acknowledgment

We would like to thank Josefina Mejias, for bibliographic research and Cristóbal Moctezuma, MD, for English grammar corrections.

References

1. Mas Tur V, MacGregor C, Jayaswal R, O'Brart D, Maycock N. A review of keratoconus: diagnosis, pathophysiology, and genetics. *Surv Ophthalmol.* 2017;62(6):770–783.
2. Zhu AY, Prescott CR. Recent surgical trends in pediatric corneal transplantation: a 13-year review. *Cornea.* 2019;38(5):546–552.
3. Géron A. *Hands-On Machine Learning With Scikit-Learn, Keras, and TensorFlow: Concepts, Tools, and Techniques to Build Intelligent Systems.* CA: O'Reilly Media; 2019.
4. Hogarty DT, Mackey DA, Hewitt AW. Current state and future prospects of artificial intelligence in ophthalmology: a review. *Clin Exp Ophthalmol.* 2019;47(1):128–139.
5. Kotsiantis SB, Zaharakis ID, Pintelas PE. Machine learning: a review of classification and combining techniques. *Artif Intell Rev.* 2006;26(3):159–190.
6. Lu W, Tong Y, Yu Y, Xing Y, Chen C, Shen Y. Applications of artificial intelligence in ophthalmology: general overview. *J Ophthalmol.* 2018;2018:5278196.
7. Balyen L, Peto T. Promising artificial intelligence-machine learning-deep learning algorithms in ophthalmology. *Asia Pac J Ophthalmol (Phila).* 2019;8(3):264–272.
8. Kovács I, Miháltz K, et al. Accuracy of machine learning classifiers using bilateral data from a Scheimpflug camera for identifying eyes with preclinical signs of keratoconus. *J Cataract Refract Surg.* 2016;42(2):275–283.
9. Twa MD, Parthasarathy S, Roberts C, et al. Automated decision tree classification of corneal shape. *Optom Vis Sci.* 2005;82(12):1038–1046.

10. Chastang PJ, Borderie VM, Carvajal-Gonzalez S, et al. Automated keratoconus detection using the Eye-Sys videokeratoscope. *J Cataract Refract Surg*. 2000;26(5):675–683.
11. Maeda N, Klyce SD, Smolek MK, et al. Automated keratoconus screening with corneal topography analysis. *Invest Ophthalmol*. 1994;35(6):9.
12. Karimi A, Meimani N, Razaghi R, et al. Biomechanics of the healthy and keratoconic corneas: a combination of the clinical data, finite element analysis, and artificial neural network. *Curr Pharm Des*. 2018;24(37):4474–4483.
13. Chandapura R, Salomão MQ, Jr Ambrósio R, et al. Bowman's topography for improved detection of early ectasia. *J Biophotonics [Internet]*. 2019;12(10):e201900126.
14. Maeda N, Klyce SD, Smolek MK. Comparison of methods for detecting keratoconus using videokeratography. *Arch Ophthal*. 1995;113(7):870–874.
15. Issarti I, Consejo A, Jiménez-García M, et al. Computer aided diagnosis for suspect keratoconus detection. *Comput Biol Med.*. 2019;109:33–42.
16. Smolek MK, Klyce SD. Current keratoconus detection methods compared with a neural network approach. *Invest Ophthalmol*. 1997;38(11):10.
17. Smadja D, Touboul D, Cohen A, et al. Detection of subclinical keratoconus using an automated decision tree classification. *Am J Ophthalmol*. 2013;156(2):237–246. e1.
18. Lopes BT, Ramos IC, Salomão MQ, et al. Enhanced tomographic assessment to detect corneal ectasia based on artificial intelligence. *Am J Ophthalmol*. 2018;195:223–232.
19. Silverman RH, Urs R, RoyChoudhury A, et al. Epithelial remodeling as basis for machine-based identification of keratoconus. *Invest Ophthalmol Vis Sci*. 2014;55(3):1580.
20. Ruiz Hidalgo I, Rodriguez P, Rozema JJ, et al. Evaluation of a machine-learning classifier for keratoconus detection based on Scheimpflug tomography. *Cornea*. 2016;35(6):827–832.
21. Souza MB, Medeiros FW, Souza DB, et al. Evaluation of machine learning classifiers in keratoconus detection from Orbscan II examinations. *Clinics*. 2010;65(12):1223–1228.
22. Saika M, Maeda N, Hirohara Y, et al. Four discriminant models for detecting keratoconus pattern using Zernike coefficients of corneal aberrations. *Jpn J Ophthalmol*. 2013;57(6):503–509.
23. Lopes B, Ramos I, Salomão MQ, et al. Horizontal pachymetric profile for the detection of keratoconus. *Rev Bras Oftalmol*. 2015;74(6):382–385.
24. Ambrósio R, Lopes BT, Faria-Correia F, et al. Integration of Scheimpflug-based corneal tomography and biomechanical assessments for enhancing ectasia detection. *J Refract Surg*. 2017;33(7):434–443.
25. Yousefi S, Yousefi E, Takahashi H, et al. Keratoconus severity identification using unsupervised machine learning. *PLoS One*. 2018;13(11):e0205998.
26. Lavric A, Valentin P. KeratoDetect: keratoconus detection algorithm using convolutional neural networks. *Comput Intell Neurosci*. 2019;2019:1–9.
27. Maeda N, Klyce SD, Smolek MK. Neural network classification of corneal topography. Preliminary demonstration [published correction appears in *Invest Ophthalmol* Vis Sci. 1995;36(10):1947–1948]. *Invest Ophthalmol Vis Sci*. 1995;36(7):1327–1335.
28. Accardo PA, Pensiero S. Neural network-based system for early keratoconus detection from corneal topography. *J Biomed Inform*. 2002;35(3):151–159.
29. Feizi S, Yaseri M, Kheiri B. Predictive ability of Galilei to distinguish subclinical keratoconus and keratoconus from normal corneas. *J Ophthalmic Vis Res*. 2016;11(1):8.
30. Carvalho LA. Preliminary results of neural networks and Zernike polynomials for classification of videokeratography maps. *Optom Vis Sci*. 2005;82(2):151–158.
31. Arbelaez MC, Versaci F, Vestri G, et al. Use of a support vector machine for keratoconus and subclinical keratoconus detection by topographic and tomographic data. *Ophthalmology*. 2012;119(11):2231–2238.
32. Ruiz Hidalgo I, Rozema JJ, Saad A, et al. Validation of an objective keratoconus detection system implemented in a Scheimpflug tomographer and comparison with other methods. *Cornea*. 2017;36(6):689–695.
33. Castro-Luna GM, Martínez-Finkelshtein A, Ramos-López D. Robust keratoconus detection with Bayesian network classifier for Placido-based corneal indices. *Cont Lens Anterior Eye*. 2020;43(4):366–372.
34. Kamiya K, Ayatsuka Y, Kato Y, et al. Keratoconus detection using deep learning of colour-coded maps with anterior segment optical coherence tomography: a diagnostic accuracy study. *BMJ Open*. 2019;9(9):e031313.

35. Raschka S. *Python Machine Learning.* Birmingham: Packt Publishing Ltd.; 2015.

36. Géron A. *Hands-On Machine Learning With Scikit-Learn, Keras, and TensorFlow: Concepts, Tools, and Techniques to Build Intelligent Systems.* CA: O'Reilly Media; 2019.

37. Haykin SS. *Neural Networks: A Comprehensive Foundation.* 2nd ed. Upper Saddle River, NJ: Prentice Hall; 1999.

38. Chollet F. *Deep Learning With Python.* New York: Manning Publications; 2017.

39. Breiman L, Friedman JH, Stone CJ, Olshen RA. *Classification and Regression Trees.* New York: CRC press; 1984:368.

40. Friedman J, Hastie T, Tibshirani R. The Elements of Statistical Learning (Springer Series in Statistics). Berlin: Springer; 2009

41. Lamy JB, Sekar B, Guezennec G, Bouaud J, Séroussi B. Explainable artificial intelligence for breast cancer: a visual case-based reasoning approach. *Artif Intell Med.* 2019;94:42–53.

42. Van De Schoot R, Winter SD, Ryan O, Zondervan-Zwijnenburg M, Depaoli S. A systematic review of Bayesian articles in psychology: the last 25 years. *Psychol Methods.* 2017;22(2):217.

Imaging

CHAPTER 14

Corneal Topography in Keratoconus

Marcony R. Santhiago

KEY CONCEPTS

- Corneal topography is an important tool for detecting corneal morphology, enabling both correct classification of keratoconus (KC) and detection of suspicious or initial patterns of the disease.
- Different color combinations can be used to help interpretation of corneal topographic maps and can increase or decrease the sensitivity for detecting deviations from normality.
- Qualitative information generated by the axial and tangential curvature maps of the anterior surface of the cornea is very useful in the screening of patients with suspected KC, especially for the experienced clinician.

Introduction

Keratoconus (KC) is defined as a progressive, non-inflammatory, bilateral, and asymmetric disease that leads to bulging and thinning of the cornea generating irregular astigmatism and visual impairment.[1-3] Early recognition and correct diagnosis of the disease are essential and allow prevention of complications. Alternatives to halt progression of the disease such as corneal collagen cross-linking potentially avoid corneal transplantation in many young patients.[4,5]

Anamnesis and a careful physical examination are sometimes insufficient for detecting KC, especially because in the early stages of the disease there may be no symptoms or loss of best-corrected visual acuity.[6-8] Corneal topography is an important tool for detecting corneal morphology, enabling both correct classification of KC and detection of suspicious or initial patterns of the disease.[8,9]

Corneal Topography

Videokeratoscopy, based on Placido disk topography, is based on the principle that the cornea behaves like a convex mirror, and the reflection of known white placid disks interspersed with black color disks directly on the surface of the cornea can be measured and analyzed.

The distance in millimeters between the disks is converted to diopters using a formula that uses the theoretical refractive index of the cornea. This information allows evaluation of thousands of data points both in the center and at the periphery of the cornea. Greater distances between the disks indicate flatter corneas and are represented by cooler (blue, violet, purple) colors, whereas smaller distances between disks reveal more curved or prolate corneas and are represented by warmer colors (yellow, orange, red). The shades of green, in general, represent measurements more compatible with the aspheric pattern of a normal cornea.[1,4]

To extract the maximum amount of information with adequate quality, direct observation of the Placido disk map also allows the examiner to observe if there is a lack of information or any

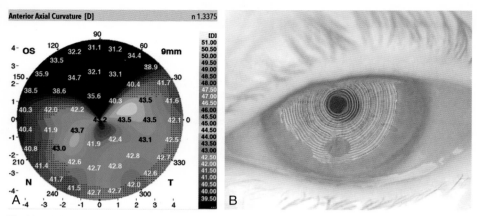

Fig. 14.1 (A) Anterior axial curvature map showing irregular astigmatism. (B) Correspondent Placido ring images showing irregular pattern, probably because of surface debris and tear film instability.

inaccuracy. Adequate exposure, centralization of the image, and avoidance of shadowing by the nose and lashes are important to preserve the complete image and linearity of the Placido disk. The quality and the integrity of the tear film and corneal surface may also interfere with the clarity and linearity of the image. Severe dry eye with debris and mucus in the tear film may create an artificially altered surface and generate a secondary irregular curvature (Fig. 14.1A,B). Treatment of the dry eye, allergies, and other ocular surface disease is important, and repeating the examination after treatment may be necessary in more severe cases.[10] Modern capture software has quality assessment tools with standard scores to assist the clinician in cases in which the capture is not of sufficient quality for an adequate interpretation of the examination.

In general, corneas with KC, when analyzed through corneal topography, exhibit greater complexity in the interpretation of measurements. This is primarily because keratoconic corneas are more prolate with higher keratometry values and are more irregular in shape. Together with the limitations of technology, this leads to low reproducibility between measurements and adds complexity in the evaluation, especially when comparing different topography and keratometry devices (Fig. 14.2A,B).[11]

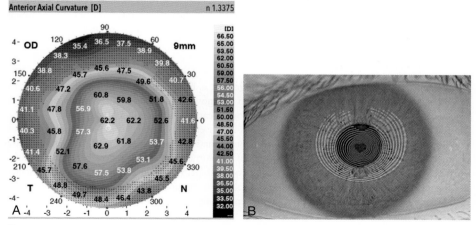

Fig. 14.2 (A) Anterior axial curvature of a hyperprolate keratoconic cornea. (B) Corresponding Placido ring images showing very irregular central pattern.

SCALES

Different color combinations can be used to help interpretation of corneal topographic maps and can increase or decrease the sensitivity for detecting deviations from normality. Absolute scales display fixed color values for each curvature regardless of the map analyzed. Although such scales may not be useful in cases of subtle curvature changes, they allow an appropriate comparison between the two eyes of the same patient, detecting asymmetries between them.[12,13]

Relative scales display the range of curvature calculated based on the specific map. A specific combination of colors can be used and different steps between colors (1.5 diopters [D], 1.0 D, 0.5 D, or 0.25 D) (Fig. 14.3A–C). Screening using small steps increases sensitivity and allows detection of subtle and initial KC patterns. These small steps are less interesting for moderate and advanced cases of KC, because those corneas usually have steeper keratometry and a wide variation of value from the apex to the periphery. This combination (small steps plus relative scales) provides quantitatively inaccurate values and generates noisy patterns with red color spreading over large areas of the axial map. Steps of 1.5 D can better locate the apex and the variation from the center to the periphery of the cone.[12,13]

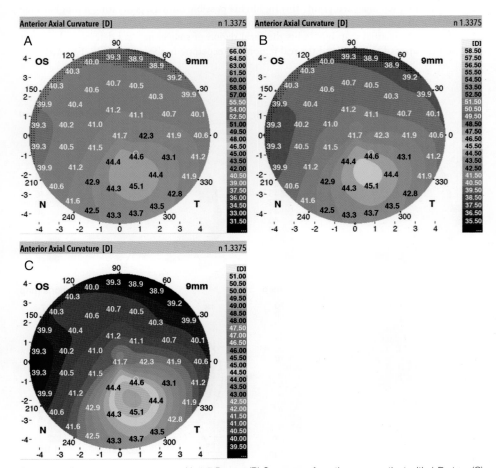

Fig. 14.3 (A) Anterior axial curvature with 1.5 D step. (B) Same map from the same patient with 1 D step. (C) Same map from the same patient with 0.5 D step.

It is important that the examiner chooses a scale that is sensitive enough to detect suspicious patterns but which is not noisy enough to lead to a misclassification of normal corneas as suspicious corneas or KC.

Axial Versus Tangential Map

The more important maps extracted from the Placido disk data are the anterior axial curvature map, the tangential map, the anterior elevation map, and the aberration map (high-order aberration) (Fig. 14.4A–D).

The *anterior axial curvature map* is the reconstruction of the corneal surface by an algorithm that measures the radius of curvature of the cornea centered on the optical axis. This strategy attempts to illustrate the aspherical geometry of the corneal surface. The transition from the center to the periphery on the axial curvature map is smoother, and there is a gradual transition of colors from the center to the periphery of a normal cornea.

In the *tangential curvature map*, the measurement of the radius of curvature is performed locally at each point of the cornea, generating more precise information about the real radius of curvature at the each analyzed point. This highlights possible outliers, generating a rougher map and showing the peripheral region with greater precision.

In KC, the tangential map highlights the focal region of steepening and detects with greater precision the apex of the cone and the real region of steepening in the cornea (Fig. 14.5A,B).

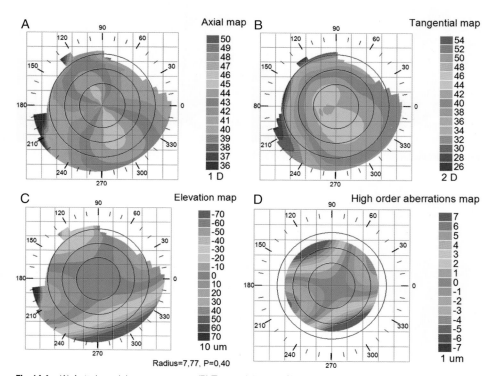

Fig. 14.4 (A) Anterior axial curvature map. (B) Tangential map. (C) Elevation map. (D) Aberrometry map (high-order aberration map).

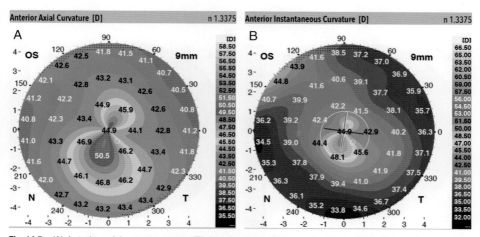

Fig. 14.5 (A) Anterior axial curvature map. (B) Anterior tangential curvature map. Note that on the tangential map, it is possible to better locate the cone apex and its relation to the periphery.

Corneal Topography in Suspected Keratoconus Cases

Definition of subclinical KC cornea or forme fruste KC varies in the literature. Henriquez et al. observed that the most common definition of subclinical KC refers to an eye with topographic signs of KC and/or suspicious topographic findings with a normal slit-lamp examination and KC in the fellow eye.[14]

The topographic signs classically described in suspect corneas are related to focal steepening, higher keratometry readings, and asymmetry in the inferior, infero-temporal, or inferonasal quadrants possibly extending to the central and paracentral regions of the cornea.

The region of focal steepening can appear as regular astigmatism with marked inferior asymmetry. A mild tendency to irregularity of the most curved meridian (skew) can also be present. The region of greater curvature usually is higher than 47 D and becomes progressively flatter toward the periphery of the cornea.

Red Flags

1. Steepening areas with dioptric values higher than 47.0 D (Fig. 14.6A)
2. With-the-rule (WTR) astigmatism with inferior-superior (I-S) asymmetry within the midperipheral cornea (see Fig. 14.6B)
3. Skewed meridian from 20 or 30 degrees in relation to the vertical meridian (see Fig. 14.6C)
4. Against-the-rule (ATR) astigmatism where the midperiphery of the steeper meridian starts to bend meeting downward (see Fig. 14.6D)
5. Oblique astigmatism with any kind of asymmetry.

When analyzing KC as a progressive disease, it is important to understand the disease as a continuum and to observe how a KC begins with a subtle inferior asymmetry and over time progresses to marked asymmetry with a truncated and irregular pattern (Fig. 14.7A,B and Fig. 14.8A,B).

PELLUCID MARGINAL DEGENERATION VERSUS KERATOCONUS

Pellucid marginal degeneration (PMD) is an uncommon and progressive type of ectasia in which there is peripheral inferior corneal thinning in a crescent-shaped pattern. This area of corneal

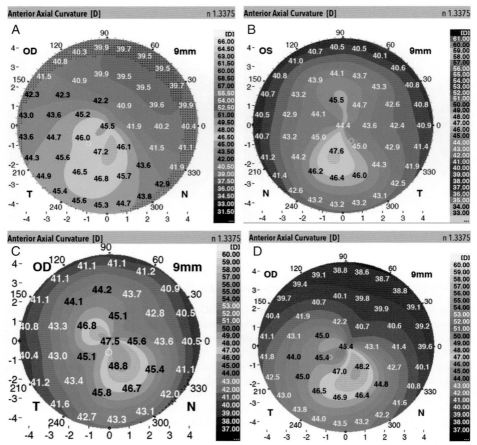

Fig. 14.6 (A) Steepening areas with dioptric values higher than 47.0 D. (B) With-the-rule astigmatism with inferior-superior asymmetry within the midperipheral cornea. (C) Skewed meridian from 20 or 30 degrees in relation to the vertical meridian. (D) Against-the-rule astigmatism where the midperiphery of the steeper meridian starts to inflect downward.

thinning is usually at least 1 mm away from the limbus. Corneal apical protrusion is observed above the thinned cornea.

The differential diagnosis between PMD and KC is complicated because corneal topographic patterns may be similar in early cases. A special feature that is more frequently observed in PMD is the crab claw pattern, and high ATR cylinder is observed in more advanced cases. Pachymetric maps are also useful in determining the thinned area related to the apical protrusion above.[15]

It is important to differentiate the two conditions. PMD generally begins later in life (third or fourth decade) and frequently continues to progress. Both conditions, in general, are treated in the same way, and PMD patients may be good candidates for corneal cross-linking in case of progression.

Indices

Qualitative information generated by the axial and tangential curvature maps of the anterior surface of the cornea is very useful in the screening of patients with suspected KC, especially for the

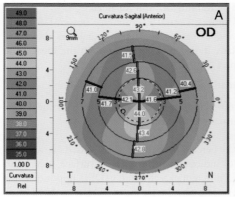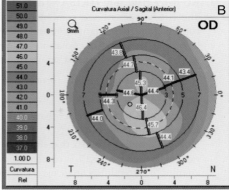

Fig. 14.7 (A) Inferior asymmetry of approximately 1 D. (B) Inferior asymmetry with subtle irregular astigmatism.

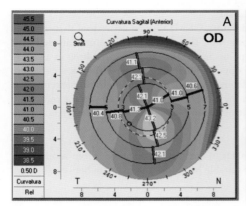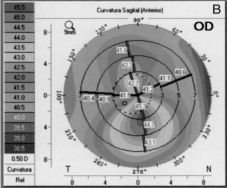

Fig. 14.8 (A) Inferior asymmetry of aproximately 0.5 D. (B) Inferior marked asymmetry of 2 D.

experienced clinician. In an attempt to standardize the diagnosis and to identify early patterns of KC suspects, quantitative information has been extracted from these maps through indices or quantitative descriptors.

Clinical studies have been performed to try to determine cut-off values and to distinguish between normal and pathologic corneas. Such indices are also useful for classifying the severity of KC. Single indices and the combination of several indices have been described in the literature, and here we list those that we consider the most important for analysis of suspected KC:

1. **I-S ratio described by Rabinowitz[16,19,20]**

   The I-S ratio compares the difference in five points of the inferior hemisphere of the cornea in the zone of 3 mm from the apex with five points of the superior hemisphere. The points are located at spatial intervals of 30 degrees. It is an index that describes asymmetry. Values greater than 1.4 D are suggestive of clinical KC.

2. **Asphericity coefficient (Q)**

   The Q coefficient describes the change in corneal curvature from the center to the periphery within a predetermined diameter of the cornea. Normal corneas have a Q value that ranges from approximately −0.3 to −0.15. The normal cornea is aspherical and slightly prolate when comparing the center to the periphery. More prolate corneas have more negative Q values and oblate corneas have more positive Q values.

3. **KC percentage index (KISA%) described by Rabinowitz and Rasheed**[17]

The KISA% describes a combination of indices: central keratometry power, I-S index, corneal simulated astigmatism, and relative skewing of the steepest radial axes above and below the horizontal meridian index (SRAX index) that corresponds to the most acute angle formed by the steepest semimeridians.

$$KISA\% = (K) \times (I\text{-}S) \times \text{corneal astigmatism (AST)} \times (SRAX) \times 100/300$$

Normal corneas have KISA% lower than 60%. Suspect cases are between 60% and 100%. Corneas with KISA% greater than 100% usually are considered KC cases.

4. **KC prediction index (KPI)**[18]

KPI is a compilation index that simulates the percent probability of KC based on the anterior surface analysis. KPI is combination of indices from the anterior surface, used in an attempt to better differentiate eyes with KC: differential sector index (DSI), opposite sector index (OSI), center/surround index (CSI), surface asymmetry index (SAI), simulated keratometry flat (SimKf), simulated keratometry steep (SimKs), irregular astigmatism index (IAI), and analyzed area (AA). Values of KPI greater than 20% are suggestive of KC.

5. **Cone location and magnitude index (CLMI)**[19]

Described by Cynthia Roberts and collaborators, CLMI uses an active tool that searches for the 2-mm steepest region in a zone of 8 mm. The average of all points outside this 2 mm is subtracted from the average of all points inside the same area, resulting in a curvature magnitude. The same is done in the opposite direction, also resulting in a curvature magnitude. CLMI is derived from the difference of those magnitudes. In simple terms, the software routine finds the steepest area on the map. It compares that area to the rest of the map to determine whether the steepest area represents a cone. Values greater than 1.4 are considered suspects (Fig. 14.9A,B).

6. **Index of height decentration (IHD)**

IHD describes the decentration of the values in the vertical direction. From recent data, IHD was observed to be one of the most suitable indices to differentiate between healthy and early KC cases.[20–22]

7. **Index of vertical asymmetry (IVA)**

IVA describes the comparison between superior and inferior vertical areas. IVA is an important index that can be significantly different in KC suspects when compared with normal eyes.[20,21]

8. **Surface asymmetry index (SAI)**

SAI indicates an average value of the power differences between the points spatially located at 180 degrees apart in 128 equidistant meridians.

9. **Surface regularity index (SRI)**

SRI is a local descriptor of regularity in a central area 4.5 mm in diameter. It utilizes the central 10 rings of Placido disk. SRI quantifies power gradient differences between successive pairs of rings in 256 equidistant semimeridians.

Final Considerations

Corneal topography derived from Placido capture systems remains an excellent tool for screening for KC. Constant improvement from different technologies adds valuable information in this very special field.

Scheimpflug technology generates maps of the anterior surface of the cornea with the same topometric indices already described in this chapter plus information on the posterior surface, pachymetric maps, and information from the three-dimensional (3D) reconstruction of the anterior segment of the eye.

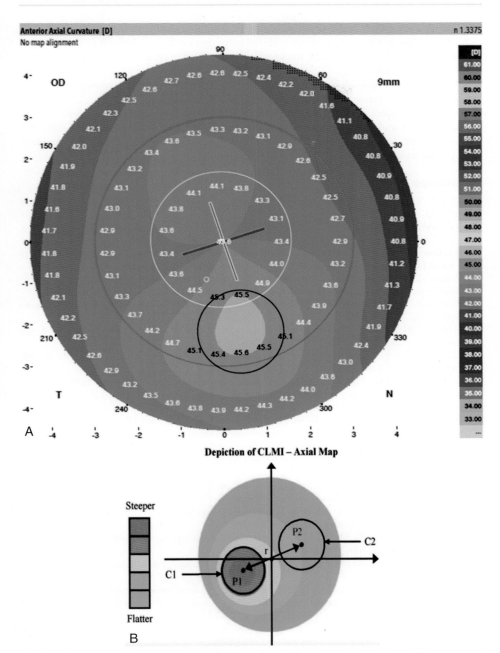

Fig. 14.9 (A) Anterior axial curvature with the *black circle* surrounding the spot size of 2 mm. This is compared with the opposite region generating a cone location and magnitude index *(CLMI)* of 1.9. (B) Demonstration of the detection of the CLMI.

To bring even greater sensitivity to screening for KC, optical coherence tomography (OCT) technology allows reconstruction of the epithelial maps that can have significant variation in corneas with KC.[22-25] Thinner epithelial thickness is observed in the apex of the cone with a thicker region outside this apex.

Combining these technologies through artificial intelligence allows the association of different indices in order to increase sensitivity and specificity in KC screening.

Despite the undeniable contribution of technology that allows total corneal (front surface, pachymetry data, and back surface) analysis in the diagnosis of KC, data consistently show that the anterior surface of the cornea remains essential to the diagnosis and is, perhaps, the most sensitive parameter in detecting earlier and subtle changes that are suggestive of KC.[20,22]

References

1. Maguire LJ, Bourne WM. Corneal topography of early keratoconus. *Am J Ophthalmol.* 1989;108(2): 107–112.
2. Rabinowitz YS, McDonnell PJ. Computerized corneal topography in keratoconus. *Refract Corneal Surg.* 1989;5:400–408.
3. Randleman JB, Crosby MB. Corneal ectatic disorders. In: Trattler WB, Majmudar PA, Luchs JI, Swartz TS, eds. *Cornea Handbook.* Thorofare, NJ: SLACK Incorporated; 2010:109–122.
4. Wilson SE, Lin DT, Klyce SD. Corneal topography of keratoconus. *Cornea.* 1991;10:2–8.
5. Randleman JB, Khandelwal SS, Hafezi F. Corneal cross-linking. *Surv Ophthalmol.* 2015;60:509–523.
6. Piñero DP, Nieto JC. Lopez-Miguel A. Characterization of corneal structure in keratoconus. *J Cataract Refract Surg.* 2012;38(12):2167–2183.
7. Henriquez MA, Hadid M Jr, Izquierdo L. A systematic review of subclinical keratoconus and forme fruste keratoconus. *J Refract Surg.* 2020;36(4):270–279.
8. Maeda N, Klyce SD, Tano Y. Detection and classification of mild irregular astigmatism in patients with good visual acuity. *Surv Ophthalmol.* 1998;43(1):53–58.
9. Klyce SD, Wilson SE. Methods of analysis of corneal topography. *Refract Corneal Surg.* 1989;5:368–371.
10. Koh S. Irregular astigmatism and higher-order aberrations in eyes with dry eye disease. *Invest Ophthalmol Vis Sci.* 2018;59(14):DES36–DES40.
11. Piñero DP, Soto-Negro R, Ruiz-Fortes P, Pérez-Cambrodí RJ, Fukumitsu H. Analysis of intrasession repeatability of ocular aberrometric measurements and validation of keratometry provided by a new integrated system in mild to moderate keratoconus. *Cornea.* 2019;38(9):1097–1104.
12. Wilson SE, Klyce SD, Husseini ZM. Standardized color-coded maps for corneal topography. *Ophthalmology.* 1993;100(11):1723–1727.
13. Cavas-Martínez F, De la Cruz Sánchez E, Nieto Martínez J, Fernández Cañavate FJ, Fernández-Pacheco DG. Corneal topography in keratoconus: state of the art. *Eye Vis (Lond).* 2016;3:5.
14. Henriquez MA, Hadid M, Izquierdo Jr L. A systematic review of subclinical keratoconus and forme fruste keratoconus. *J Refract Surg.* 2020;36(4):270–279.
15. Maguire LJ, Klyce SD, McDonald MB, Kaufman HE. Corneal topography of pellucid marginal degeneration. *Ophthalmology.* 1987;94:519–524.
16. Rabinowitz YS. Videokeratographic indices to aid in screening for keratoconus. *J Refract Surg.* 1995;11:371–379.
17. Rabinowitz YS, Rasheed K. KISA% index: a quantitative videokeratography algorithm embodying minimal topographic criteria for diagnosing keratoconus [published correction appears in *J Cataract Refract Surg.* 2000;26(4):480]. *J Cataract Refract Surg.* 1999;25(10):1327–1335.
18. Maeda N, Klyce SD, Smolek MK, Thompson HW. Automated keratoconus screening with corneal topography analysis. *Invest Ophthalmol Vis Sci.* 1994;35(6):2749–2757.
19. Mahmoud AM, Roberts CJ, Lembach RG, et al. CLMI: the cone location and magnitude index. *Cornea.* 2008;27(4):480–487.
20. Shajari M, Jaffary I, Herrmann K, et al. Early tomographic changes in the eyes of patients with keratoconus. *J Refract Surg.* 2018;34(4):254–259.

21. Bae GH, Kim JR, Kim CH, Lim DH, Chung ES, Chung TY. Corneal topographic and tomographic analysis of fellow eyes in unilateral keratoconus patients using Pentacam. *Am J Ophthalmol.* 2014;157(1):103–109.
22. Hwang ES, Perez-Straziota CE, Kim SW, Santhiago MR, Randleman JB. Distinguishing highly asymmetric keratoconus eyes using combined Scheimpflug and spectral-domain OCT analysis. *Ophthalmology.* 2018;125(12):1862–1871.
23. Li Y, Tan O, Brass R, et al. Corneal epithelial thickness mapping by Fourier-domain optical coherence tomography in normal and keratoconic eyes. *Ophthalmology.* 2012;119:2425–2433.
24. Li Y, Shekhar R, Huang D. Corneal pachymetry mapping with high-speed optical coherence tomography. *Ophthalmology.* 2006;113:792–799.e2
25. Shetty R, Rao H, Khamar P, et al. Keratoconus screening indices and their diagnostic ability to distinguish normal from ectatic corneas. *Am J Ophthalmol.* 2017;181:140–148.

CHAPTER 15

Scheimpflug Imaging for Keratoconus and Ectatic Disease

Michael W. Belin

KEY CONCEPTS

- Scheimpflug imaging provides a complete anterior segment analysis that is not possible with older Placido-based systems.
- Imaging of the posterior cornea allows identification of subclinical keratoconus prior to vision loss.
- The addition of a Placido disk to a Scheimpflug device offers no clinical advantage.
- The Belin/Ambrósio Enhanced Ectasia Display (BAD) is the most commonly used refractive screening tool.
- The Belin ABCD classification/staging eliminates the limitations of the older Amsler-Krumeich classification.
- The Belin ABCD Progression Display monitors ectatic patients over time and displays when significant progression occurs prior to permanent vision loss.

Background

There has been a dramatic increase in the need to recognize the earliest forms of keratoconus and other ectatic disorders and to eliminate the false-positives seen with some older technologies. As in other areas of medicine, imaging has played a large part in this change. The new information offered by anterior segment tomography not only allows for earlier identification of disease, but has altered our perception of what constitutes keratoconus. Tomographic imaging (Scheimpflug, ocular coherence tomography [OCT]) offers significant advantages over traditional Placido-based curvature analysis (topography) and ultrasonic pachymetry. Elevation-based tomographic imaging allows for the measurement of both the anterior and posterior corneal surfaces. The accurate measurement of both the anterior and posterior corneal surfaces and the anterior lens allows for the creation of a three-dimensional reconstruction of the anterior segment, which affords significantly more diagnostic information than was previously available.[1-5] Posterior measurements and/or changes in pachymetric distribution are often the first indicators of ectatic disease, despite completely normal anterior curvature. Examination of the posterior corneal surface can often reveal pathology that would otherwise be missed if one were relying on anterior analysis alone[2,4,6-8] (Fig. 15.1). The remainder of this chapter will deal solely with Scheimpflug tomography. For purposes of ectatic disease diagnosis and refractive screening, Scheimpflug imaging has certain advantages over OCT in that it allows for a much greater area of coverage (up to limbal to limbal coverage) typically not possible with current/older OCT technology (newer and imaging OCT systems have improved coverage). Scheimpflug imaging also covers significantly more of the cornea than was possible with Placido-based devices, the coverage of

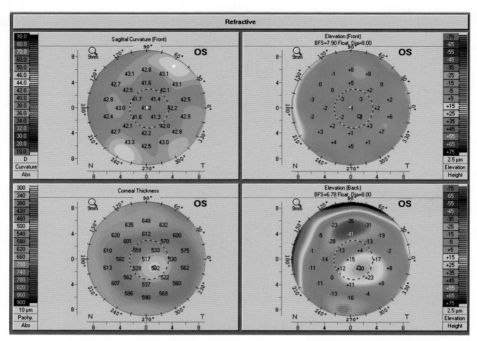

Fig. 15.1 Four-map composite display. The *upper left* map shows a normal anterior sagittal curvature with minimal astigmatism. This is also seen on the front elevation *(upper left)*. The posterior elevation *(bottom right)*, however, shows a positive island of elevation indicating early ectatic change. This is a map of subclinical keratoconus.

which is limited to, at best, 40% of the cornea. This added coverage is critical in the correct diagnosis of peripheral diseases such as pellucid marginal degeneration (PMD)[5] (Fig. 15.2). Although multiple Scheimpflug devices exist, this chapter will deal solely with the OCULUS Pentacam (OCULUS GmbH, Wetzlar, Germany), as this is the most commonly used Scheimpflug device. Other devices have combined Scheimpflug imaging with older Placido imaging. Other than offering some familiarity with older technology, the addition of a Placido disk makes little, if any, clinical sense. There has been a long-standing misconception that Placido-based curvature is in some way inherently superior to elevation-based curvature or that elevation-based curvature is derived and not a direct measurement. Both Placido systems and elevation systems derive curvature. Placido systems measure slope and derive curvature and Scheimpflug systems measure elevation (points in space) and derive curvature. Other than the greater area of coverage afforded by Scheimpflug imaging and the lower susceptibility to tear abnormalities, the curvature maps are virtually identical (Fig. 15.3). The importance of corneal coverage is not just limited to PMD. In addition to being able to measure and locate the true thinnest point, a full corneal thickness map allows the generation of pachymetric progression graphs that reflect the rate of change in corneal thickness. A single thickness reading is very limited in determining what is normal. Two corneas can have the same central corneal thickness but share dramatically different pachymetric progressions. Abnormal corneas (i.e., corneas showing ectatic change or tendency) have a more rapid thinning from the corneal periphery to the thinnest point.[4,9] This more rapid rate of pachymetric progression, when seen in a preoperative cornea, is highly suggestive of ectatic change or an eye at greater risk of postoperative ectatic change (Fig. 15.4).

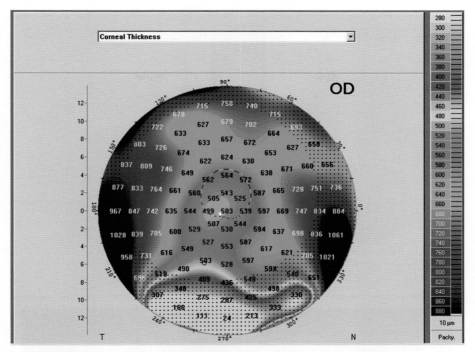

Fig. 15.2 Corneal thickness map showing an inferior band of thinning. This is pathognomonic for pellucid marginal degeneration. To display a full corneal thickness map the 9-mm restriction needs to be removed.

The biggest advantage of Scheimpflug imaging, however, is the measurement of the posterior corneal surface. Although the posterior surface contributes minimally to the overall refractive power of the eye (due to the minimal difference between the index of refraction of the cornea and aqueous) and was, in the past, considered less important, posterior surface changes are now recognized to serve as the earliest indicator of ectatic change and typically predate any changes on the anterior corneal surface[4,6,10,11] (Fig. 15.5).

Elevation Maps

That the standard anterior and posterior corneal tomographic maps are referred to as elevation maps is somewhat of a misnomer. True elevation would require displaying the data against a planar (flat) surface. Maps generated against a flat surface are not clinically useful (intuitive), as the surface changes cannot be visually appreciated. The reason is that the raw elevation data from normal eyes and markedly ectatic corneas look remarkably similar (Fig. 15.6). To make the maps clinically useful and to allow for a rapid visual inspection, the raw data are compared with some nonplanar reference surface. The purpose of the reference surface is to magnify or amplify the surface differences that would otherwise not be appreciated by the naked eye. The so-called "elevation" maps depict how the corneal surface differs from a defined reference shape. Although the appearance of the map will vary greatly depending on the reference surface used, all maps are generated using the same raw elevation data. Recognizing that the reference surface will alter the appearance of a map, but not its accuracy, is important.[12,13]

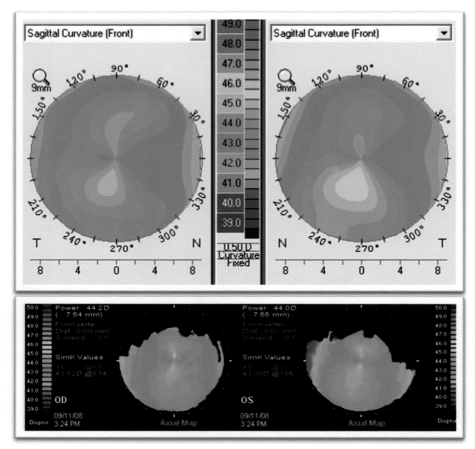

Fig. 15.3 Anterior curvature maps generated from a Scheimpflug device *(upper)* compared to a standard Placido device *(lower)*. Although the astigmatic patterns are almost identical, the Scheimpflug device has significantly more coverage and no loss of data secondary to poor tear film.

The choice of the reference surface will often depend on the clinical situation, the population being evaluated, and the specific pathology. For most applications, the best-fit-sphere (BFS) is the most qualitatively intuitive (easiest to read and understand) surface and the most commonly used. A BFS allows for the visualization of astigmatism, as the flat meridian rises above the BFS while the steep meridian drops below the BFS. The normal astigmatic pattern generated against a BFS is easily recognizable (Fig. 15.7). When screening for ectatic disease, one is trying to identify an abnormal conical protrusion. A focal protrusion will appear as an elevated area against the BFS (positive island of elevation) (Fig. 15.8). As the cornea is normally aspherical, steeper in the center, and flatter toward the periphery, normal corneas will have some central positive elevation. The goal of screening is to allow for a rapid visual inspection to separate normal from abnormal. This task, however, is made more difficult by the fact that the normal cornea is aspherical and displays, to a smaller degree, a positive elevation ("positive island of elevation"), similar to what is seen with ectatic disease. The BFS and the resultant elevation map will vary depending on how much of the

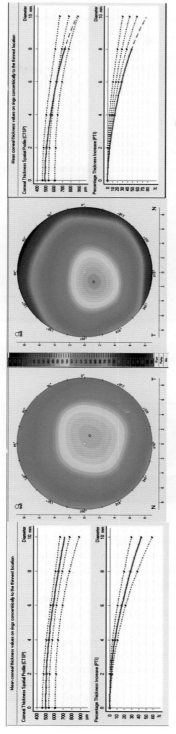

Fig. 15.4 Pachymetric progression graphs showing a thin but normal eye *(left)* compared with an eye with the same minimal thickness but a more rapid (abnormal) rate of change *(right)*. The map of the right is highly suggestive of ectatic disease.

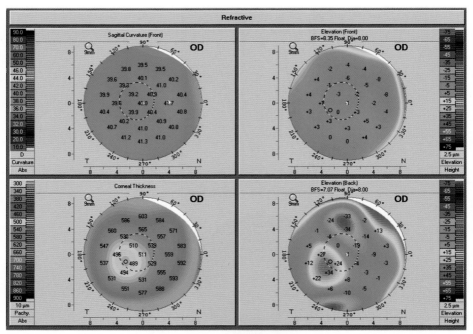

Fig. 15.5 Four-map composite display. The *bottom right* map shows a prominent posterior positive island and the corneal thickness map *(bottom left)* shows the thinnest point displacement corresponding to the posterior ectasia. *Both top* maps (anterior curvature and elevation) are normal. This is an example of subclinical keratoconus.

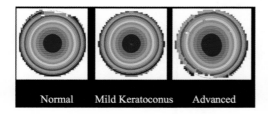

Fig. 15.6 Raw elevation maps (i.e., a planar reference surface) showing that the raw elevation data for normal, mild keratoconus, and advanced keratoconus lack sufficient surface change for visual differentiation.

cornea is utilized to construct the reference surface. If the entire cornea is used to construct the BFS, then the normal asphericity of the cornea will be clearly demonstrated. As the area (optical zone) to compute the BFS is decreased, the BFS steepens as less of the flatter periphery is incorporated into the BFS. Taking the BFS from the central 8.0-mm optical zone steepens the BFS enough to mask effectively the normal corneal asphericity (Fig. 15.9). Masking the normal asphericity makes screening for ectatic disease easier and allows for rapid visual inspection. The BFS taken from the central 8.0-mm optical zone has become somewhat standardized.

It should be understood that although the reference surface does not affect "accuracy," it does affect quantitative data. Published normal values are all reference surface specific.[14,15] Normal elevation values will not only vary based on which reference surface is used, but also on where or at what part of the cornea the values are measured. Normal elevation values have been reported at the apex, maximal values within the central 4.0-mm zone and at the thinnest point.[14–16] The thinnest

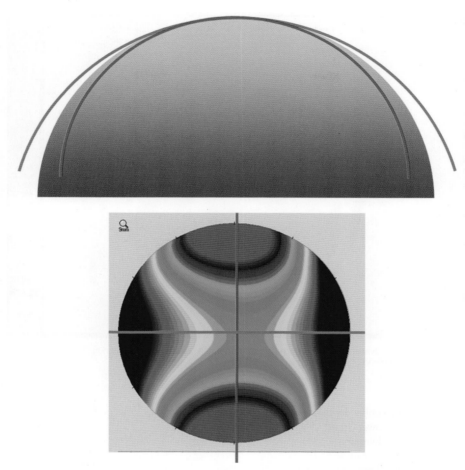

Fig. 15.7 Anterior elevation maps of regular with-the-rule astigmatism. The steep meridian *(red)* drops below the best-fit-sphere whereas the flat meridian *(blue)* rises above the best-fit-sphere.

point has some advantages as in the keratoconic cornea; it usually corresponds to the center of the cone and is reasonably reproducible.

The original basic display offered by the OCULUS Pentacam was the four-map display, where four individual maps are shown on one composite map or display. The four maps are user selected and may include any of the following:

- Corneal thickness
- Tangential curvature (front)
- Tangential curvature (back)
- Axial/sagittal curvature (front)
- Axial/sagittal curvature (back)
- Elevation (front)
- Elevation (back)
- True net power
- Keratometric power deviation

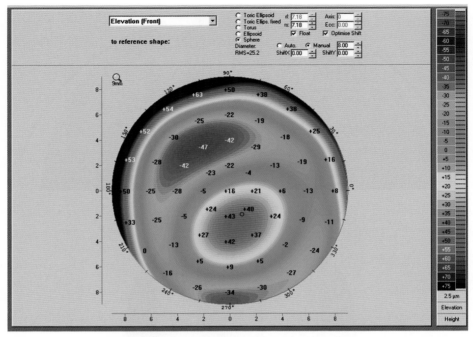

Fig. 15.8 Anterior elevation map of a cornea with moderately advanced keratoconus. The map shows a prominent positive island of elevation against the standard best-fit-sphere.

- Anterior chamber depth (internal)
- Refractive power (front)
- Relative pachymetry
- Equivalent K-reading 65 power
- Total corneal refractive power
- Cornea density average
- Cornea density maximum

The most commonly chosen four maps for the composite display for both keratoconus and refractive evaluation include corneal thickness, anterior curvature, and anterior and posterior elevation.

Enhanced Reference Surface and BAD Display

Although the BFS is the most intuitive reference surface, any of the standard reference surfaces (e.g., BFS, best-fit toric ellipsoid [BFTE], best-fit ellipse [BFE]) are susceptible to influence by the pathologic portion of an abnormal, ectatic cornea. In keratoconus, the incorporation of the ectatic region into the reference surface causes the reference surface to steepen and results in the lower height difference between the ectatic region and the reference surface. The ectatic region could be highlighted (i.e., greater elevation difference) if the reference surface more closely reflected the more normal peripheral cornea and was not influenced by the ectatic region. This was the concept for the "*enhanced reference surface*" (ERS). The ERS is generated by incorporating the same 8.0-mm diameter used in the standard BFS but excludes a small zone surrounding the thinnest portion of the cornea (Fig. 15.10). This exclusion zone varies between 3.0 and 4.0 mm

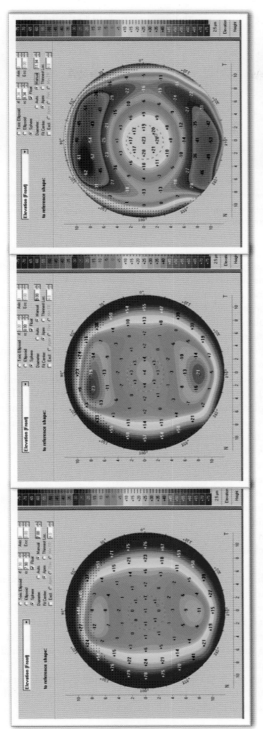

Diameter = 7.0 mm   Diameter = 9.0 mm   Diameter = 11.94 mm

Fig. 15.9 Three anterior elevation maps from the same normal cornea showing the variation in elevation appearance with changes in size of the optical zone used for the best-fit-sphere. When the full corneal diameter is used to generate the best-fit-sphere, the normal asphericity of the cornea is revealed.

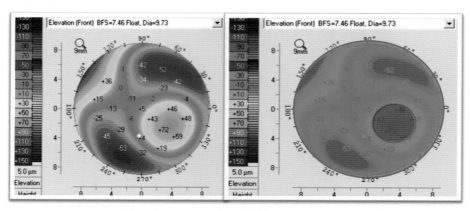

Fig. 15.10 The enhanced reference surface is generated by removing a small optical zone (shown in *red*) centered on the thinnest point from the best-fit-sphere computation.

and is based on a proprietary algorithm used in the Belin/Ambrósio Enhanced Ectasia Display (BAD). Excluding a small zone surrounding the thinnest point in the keratoconic cornea flattens the overall reference. The degree of flattening of the ERS compared with the standard BFS will vary greatly based on the presence or absence of a significant cone. Normal eyes undergo very little change from BFS to ERS, resulting in little, if any, elevation change, but in ectatic eyes eliminating the zone surrounding the ectatic region (thinnest portion of the cornea) flattens the reference surface and allows the ectatic region to be more prominent (greater height off the reference surface) and thus easier to differentiate by visual inspection (Fig. 15.11).

A comprehensive refractive screening display incorporating both the ERS and pachymetric progression graphs (BAD III) is currently offered on the Pentacam. The BAD III display combines nine different tomographic parameters in a unified screening tool. Currently, the display uses the following parameters in a regression analysis to assist the refractive surgeon in identifying patients potentially at risk for ectatic change:

- Anterior elevation at the thinnest point
- Posterior elevation at the thinnest point
- Change in anterior elevation
- Change in posterior elevation
- Corneal thickness at thinnest point
- Location of thinnest point
- Pachymetric progression
- Ambrósio relational thickness
- K_{max}

The BAD III displays each parameter and individually reports them as a standard deviation, then reports a final overall reading (final "D") that is based on a regression analysis to maximize the separation of normal corneas from those with ectatic change. Each individual parameter will be highlighted in yellow when it is ≥ 1.6 but <2.6 standard deviations and turns red if ≥ 2.6 standard deviations. The final overall reading (final "D") turns yellow at 1.6 and red at 3.0 standard deviations. Fig. 15.12 depicts a case of moderately advanced keratoconus with a final "D" reading of 8.16 with every individual parameter in the "red" zone.

It should be recognized that the BAD is a refractive screening display designed to separate normal eyes from abnormal, and although it is very helpful in diagnosing ectatic disease, it will also be abnormal in other pathologic conditions (e.g., corneal edema).

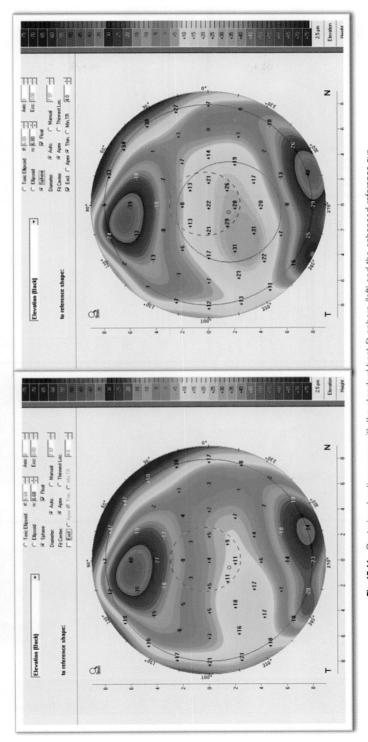

Fig. 15.11 Posterior elevation maps with the standard best-fit-sphere *(left)* and the enhanced reference surface *(right)*. The posterior positive island of elevation is much more prominent and easily visualized with the enhanced reference surface.

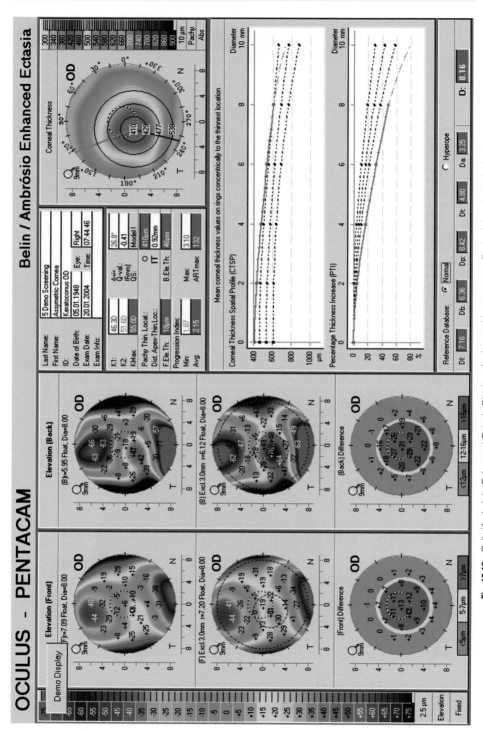

Fig. 15.12 Belin/Ambrósio Enhanced Ectasia Display of advanced keratoconus. Each of the nine individual parameters are outside the 2.6 standard deviation (*red*), with a final overall reading of 8.16 (final "D").

TABLE 15.1 ■ The Belin ABCD Classification[a]

ABCD Criteria	A	B	C	D
	ARC (3-mm Zone)	PRC (3-mm Zone)	Thinnest Pach (µm)	BDVA
Stage 0	>7.25 mm (<46.5D)	>5.90 mm	>490	≥20/20 (≥1.0)
Stage I	>7.05 mm (<48.0D)	>5.70 mm	>450	<20/20 (<1.0)
Stage II	>6.35 mm (<53.0D)	>5.15 mm	>400	<20/40 (<0.5)
Stage III	>6.15 mm (<55.0D)	>4.95 mm	>300	<20/100 (<0.2)
Stage IV	<6.15 mm (>55.0D)	<4.95 mm	≤300	<20/400 (<0.05)

[a]Generated using four parameters (anterior and posterior radius of curvature taken from a 3.0-mm optical zone centered on the thinnest point ["A" and "B" parameters], minimal corneal thickness ["C"], and best spectacle distance visual acuity ["D"]) and five stages (0–IV).
ARC, Anterior radius of curvature; BDVA, best distance visual acuity; PRC, posterior radius of curvature.

ABCD Classification

The additional information afforded by tomographic analysis provided physicians with a wealth of new information, but it also exposed the inadequacies of the older classification systems (e.g., Amsler-Krumeich [AK]) and of relying on maximum keratometry (K_{max}) as the sole predictor for both ectatic progression and cross-linking (CXL) efficacy.[17–21] The Belin ABCD classification and staging system was introduced on the OCULUS Pentacam partly in response to the shortcomings of the AK system and, in part, in response to the needs outlined in the Global Consensus on Keratoconus and Ectatic Disease published in 2015.[22] The ABCD classification utilizes four parameters: "**A**" represents the **A**nterior radius of curvature taken from a 3.0-mm optical zone centered on the thinnest point, "**B**" (for **B**ack) is the posterior radius of curvature from a 3.0-mm zone centered on the thinnest point, "**C**" is minimal corneal thickness, and "**D**" is best spectacle **D**istance visual acuity (Table 15.1). The Belin ABCD classification and staging is currently part of the Topometric/Keratoconus display. The four ABCD parameters are displayed three ways: (1) graphically, (2) with the actual radius of curvature and pachymetry values, and (3) in a five-step staging ranging from zero to five (Fig. 15.13).[23,24]

Belin ABCD Progression Display

The ABCD parameters were initially designed not just as a new classification and staging system, but to be used to determine ectatic progression. Prior progression parameters were all based on the anterior corneal surface, meaning that visual loss had to be present and further loss required to determine progressive disease. The Belin ABCD Progression Display allows up to eight examinations over time to be displayed. Each ABCD parameter is individually displayed and one-sided confidence intervals (both 80% and 95%) for change are displayed for both a normal and keratoconic population. The normal-based gates (shown in green) are suggested for young patients with early disease, whereas the keratoconic gates (shown in red) are meant for the more established cases (Fig. 15.14); the most recent iteration of the progression display incorporates confidence intervals for corneas after cross-linking. The post CXL gates only appear on exams at least 1 year post-op.

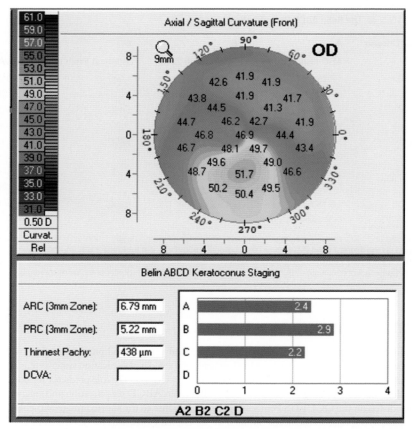

Fig. 15.13 Belin ABCD classification. The actual numerical values are shown on the left table, a graphical analysis on the right, and the staging on the bottom. Distance Corrected Visual acuity (DCVA) is operator entered (not generated by the Pentacam), as was not entered in this example. *ARC,* Anterior radius of curvature; *PRC,* posterior radius of curvature.

The clinical application of the Belin ABCD Progression Display can be seen in Fig. 15.15, where highly significant change (progression) can be seen on the posterior corneal surface ("B" parameter) in spite of a stable anterior surface ("A" parameter) and a stable K_{max} (circled in blue). The ABCD Progression Display should allow the clinician to monitor disease and to diagnose progressive disease much sooner than was possible with earlier systems that were limited to the anterior corneal surface, with the hope that earlier intervention can prevent vision loss, rather than just stabilize it after it has already occurred.[25,26]

Summary

Scheimpflug imaging provides a comprehensive anterior segment analysis that includes posterior corneal data and full corneal thickness analysis in addition to anterior surface imaging. This added information improves the ability of the corneal surgeon to screen patients for occult ectatic disease, analyze patients with keratoconus, and identify patients potentially at higher risk for post-LASIK ectasia. Rotating Scheimpflug cross-sectional analysis meets the criterion for a successful

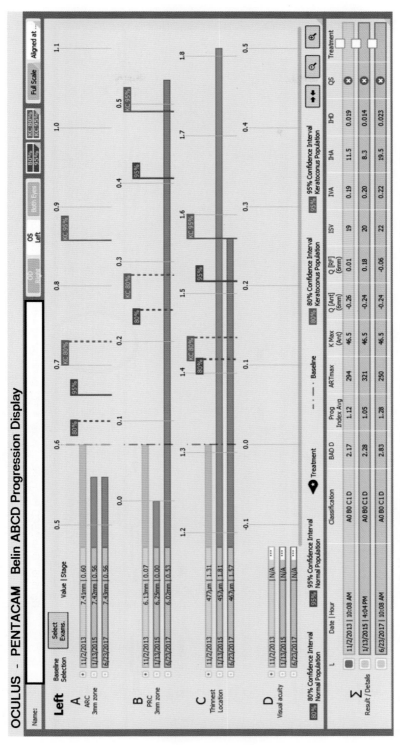

Fig. 15.14 Belin ABCD Progression Display. Individual examinations are graphically displayed (up to eight examinations) and shown against both 80% and 95% confidence intervals for change. The *green gates* are generated from a normal population and the *red gates* from patients with known keratoconus (K_{max}, Maximum keratometry.

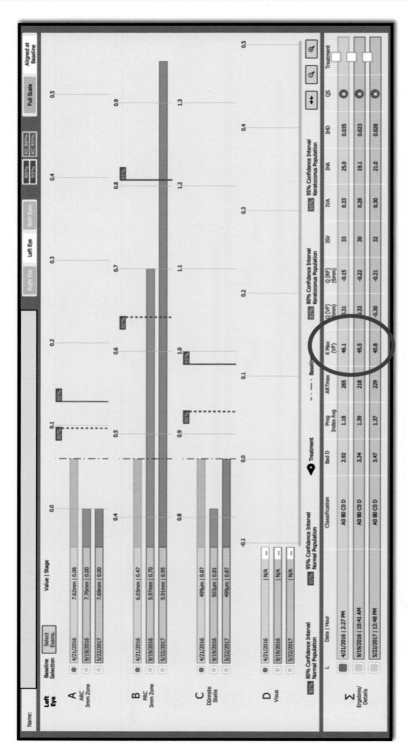

Fig. 15.15 Belin ABCD Progression Display. A 17-year-old patient with very early keratoconus (final "D" at initial examination of 2.92) followed for 13 months. Despite a stable anterior surface and stable K_{max}, the posterior cornea ("B" parameter) shows very significant progression (beyond the 95% gate). K_{max}, Maximum keratometry.

screening tool in that it not only provides the necessary data, but it does so in a manner that does not interrupt patient flow or require skills beyond those of most ophthalmic technicians.

Dr. Belin serves as consultant to OCULUS GmbH. He receives no royalties for any of the software mentioned in this chapter.

References

1. Kim SW, Sun HJ, Chang JH, Kim EK. Anterior segment measurements using Pentacam and Orbscan II 1 to 5 years after refractive surgery. *J Refract Surg.* 2009;25(12):1091–1097.
2. Yazici AT, Bozkurt E, Alagoz C, et al. Central corneal thickness, anterior chamber depth, and pupil diameter measurements using Visante OCT, Orbscan, and Pentacam. *J Refract Surg.* 2010;26:127–133.
3. Belin MW, Khachikian SS. Corneal diagnosis and evaluation with the OCULUS Pentacam. *Highlights of Ophthalmology.* 2007;35(2):5–7.
4. Ambrósio Jr R, Caiado AL, Guerra FP, et al. Novel pachymetric parameters based on corneal tomography for diagnosing keratoconus. *J Refract Surg.* 2011;27(10):753–758.
5. Walker RN, Khachikian SS, Belin MW. Scheimpflug imaging of pellucid marginal degeneration. *Cornea.* 2008;27(8):963–966.
6. Ambrósio Jr R, Dawson DG, Salomão M, Guerra FP, Caiado AL, Belin MW. Corneal ectasia after LASIK despite low risk: evidence of enhanced sensitivity based on tomographic and biomechanical findings in the unoperated, stable, fellow eye. *J Refract Surg.* 2010;26(11):906–911.
7. Belin MW, Asota IM, Ambrósio Jr R, Khachikian SS. What's in a name: keratoconus, pellucid marginal degeneration and related thinning disorders. *Am J Ophthalmol.* 2011;152(2):157–162.
8. Walker RN, Khachikian SS, Belin MW. Scheimpflug imaging of pellucid marginal degeneration. *Cornea.* 2008;27(8):963–966.
9. Belin MW, Khachikian SS. New devices and clinical implications for measuring corneal thickness. *Clin Exp Ophthalmol.* 2006;34:729–731.
10. Khachikian SS, Belin MW. Posterior elevation in keratoconus. *Ophthalmology.* 2009;116:816.
11. de Sanctus U, Loiacono C, Richiardi L, Turco D, Mutani B, Grignolo FM. Sensitivity and specificity of posterior corneal elevation measured by Pentacam in discriminating keratoconus/subclinical keratoconus. *Ophthalmology.* 2008;115:1534–1539.
12. Belin MW, Litoff D, Strods SJ, Winn SS, Smith RS. The PAR technology corneal topography system. *Refract Corneal Surg.* 1992;8:88–96.
13. Belin MW, Khachikian SS. An introduction to understanding elevation-based topography: how elevation data are displayed—a review. *Clin Exp Ophthalmol.* 2009;37:14–29.
14. Kim JT, Cortese M, Belin MW, Khachikian SS, Ambrósio Jr R. Tomographic normal values for corneal elevation and pachymetry in a hyperopic population. *J Clinic Experiment Ophthalmol.* 2011;2:130–135.
15. Feng MT, Belin MW, Ambrósio Jr R, et al. International values for corneal elevation in normal subjects by rotating Scheimpflug camera. *J Cataract Refract Surg.* 2011;37(10):1817–1821.
16. Hashemi H, Mehravaran S. Day to day clinically relevant corneal elevation, thickness and curvature parameters using the Orbscan II scanning slit topographer and Pentacam Scheimpflug imaging device. *Middle East Afr J Ophthalmol.* 2010;17(1):44–55.
17. Amsler M. [Classic keratocene and crude keratocene; unitary arguments]. *Ophthalmologica.* 1946;111:96–101.
18. Rabinowitz YS, Rasheed K. KISA% index: a quantitative videokeratography algorithm embodying minimal topographic criteria for diagnosing keratoconus. *J Cataract Refract Surg.* 1999;25:1327–1335.
19. Alió JL, Shabayek MH. Corneal higher order aberrations: a method to grade keratoconus. *J Refract Surg.* 2006;22:539–545.
20. McMahon TT, Szczotka-Flynn L, Barr JT, et al; CLEK Study Group. A new method for grading the severity of keratoconus: the keratoconus severity score (KSS). *Cornea.* 2006;25:794–800.
21. Li X, Yang H, Rabinowitz YS. Keratoconus: classification scheme based on videokeratography and clinical signs. *J Cataract Refract Surg.* 2009;35:1597–1603.
22. Gomes JA, Tan D, Rapuano CJ, et al. Global consensus on keratoconus and ectatic disease. *Cornea.* 2015;34:359–369.
23. Belin MW, Duncan JK, Ambrósio Jr R, Gomes JAP. A new tomographic method of staging/classifying keratoconus: the ABCD grading system. *Int J Kerat Ect Cor Dis.* 2015;4(3):85–93.

24. Belin MW, Duncan JK. Keratoconus: the ABCD grading system. *Klin Monbl Augenheilkd.* 2016;233(6):701–707.
25. Belin MW, Meyer JJ, Duncan JK, Gelman R, Borgstrom M, Ambrósio R. Jr. Assessing progression of keratoconus and crosslinking efficacy: the Belin ABCD progression display. *Int J Kerat Ect Cor Dis.* 2017;6(1):1–10.
26. Sedaghat MR, Momeni-Moghaddam H., Belin MW, et al. Changes in ABCD keratoconus grade after intracorneal ring implantation. *Cornea.* 2018;37:1431–1437.

CHAPTER 16

Dual Scheimpflug Tomography and Placido Topography

Carlos G. Arce

KEY CONCEPTS

- Placido-based corneal topography and Scheimpflug anterior segment optical tomography are long-established valuable technologies widely used in clinical practice and refractive surgery screening protocols.
- With the combination and integration of Placido topography and dual Scheimpflug tomography, the Galilei and the CGA color scales (by Carlos G. Arce, 2003) have facilitated the interpretation of data on maps independent of the parameter studied and without forcing the verification of numeric values.
- This chapter demonstrates the use of the Galilei system to detail the four primary signs that identify keratoconus: ectasia, steepening, asymmetry, and thinning. They are not synonyms. There are not keratoconus without ectasia however, it may be steepening, asymmetry or thinning, isolated or in combination, without ectasia.

Introduction

Keratoconus (KC) is a chronic time-dependent deformation of the cornea caused by the biomechanical failure of the corneal tissue induced or promoted by a congenital predisposition, and may be triggered by iatrogenic, surgical, traumatic, inflammatory, environmental, or unknown factors.

Our current understanding of keratectasia has been molded by the available technology. New signs in incipient cases have been discovered since the corneal profiles of Mandell[1] and the computer-assisted topography of the anterior corneal surface by Klyce.[2] We recognize Placido-based corneal topography (by Antonio Placido, 1880)[3] as a long-established valuable technology widely used in clinical practice and refractive surgery screening protocols, although it may be inadequate for early diagnosis. Modern equipment, such as slit-scan and rotational Scheimpflug tomography, have increased our knowledge of concepts such as elevation topography, wavefront, and optical pachymetry. Furthermore, despite their lesser ability to detect surface curvature differences,[4] anterior segment imaging systems based in Scheimpflug photography have introduced diagnostic strategies not possible with the assessment of the anterior corneal surface alone.

With the combination and integration of Placido topography and dual Scheimpflug tomography, the Galilei (Ziemer Ophthalmic Systems AG, Port, Switzerland) and the CGA color scales (Carlos G. Arce, 2003)[5–8] have facilitated the interpretation of data on maps independent of the parameter studied and without forcing the verification of numeric values. The CGA scales are, basically, comprehensive absolute scales with the yellow step(s) fixed in accepted normal limit values codifying the meaning of all colors. The suggested settings for all maps are summarized in

TABLE 16.1 ■ Values Used to Code Galilei Color Scales

MAP		Anterior Axial [a] or TCP [a]	Anterior Instantaneous regular [a]	Anterior Instantaneous modified [a]	Posterior Axial or Posterior Instantaneous [b]	Pachymetry [c]	BFS [d], BFA [d] or BFTA [d] Elevation	Differential Maps	Wavefront (WF)
Suggested Scale	Style	*Default*	*Default*	*German*	*Default*	*German*	*ANSI*	*American*	*American*
	Steps	CGA 1.0 D	CGA 1.50 D	CGA 1.0 D	CGA 0.25 D	CGA 20 μm	CGA 5 μm	1 D [a], 0.25 D [b], 10 μm [c], 5 μm [d]	0.50 μm or 0.50 D
TREND		Steeper	Steeper	Steeper	Steeper	Thinner	Elevated	Different	Aberrated
COLOR MEANING	GRAY	-----	-----	59.00 D to 62.00 D	-----	260 μm to 200 μm	-----	-----	-----
	RED	50.00 D to 61.00 D	51.50 D to 68.00 D	50.00 D to 58.00 D	−7.50 D to −10.25 D	440 μm to 280 μm	> 30 μm to 80 μm		
	ORANGE	48.00 D to 49.00 D	48.50 D to 50.00 D	48.00 D to 49.00 D	−7.00 D to −7.25 D	480 μm to 460 μm	20 μm to 30 μm	Positive Change	Positive HOA
	YELLOW	47.00 D	47.00 D	47.00 D	−6.75 D	500 μm	10 μm to 15 μm		
	GREEN	46.00 D to 41.00 D	45.50 D to 38.00 D	46.00 D to 39.00 D	−6.50 D to −5.25 D	520 μm to 660 μm	±5 μm	Zero (No change)	Zero (Focused)
	NAVY BLUE	40.00 D to 36.00 D	36.50 D to 30.50 D	38.00 D to 36.00 D	−5.00 D to −4.00 D	680 μm to 720 μm	≤10 μm to 90 μm	Negative Change	Negative HOA
	LIGHT BLUE	-----	-----	35.00 D to 32.00 D	-----	740 μm to 800 μm	-----	-----	-----
TREND		Flatter	Flatter	Flatter	Flatter	Thicker	Depressed	Different	Aberrated

ANSI, American National Standards Institute; *BFA*, best fit aspheric; *BFS*, best-fit-sphere; *BFTA*, best fit toric aspheric; *HOA*, high-order aberration; *TCP*, total corneal power.
Modified from Arce CG. Galilei map interpretation guide.[7]

Table 16.1. New Galilei reports and combinations of maps using posterior curvature, best fit toric aspheric (BFTA) elevation, total corneal power, and wavefront maps go beyond the traditional and insufficient four-map presentation with anterior curvature, anterior and posterior best-fit-sphere (BFS), and pachymetry (Fig. 16.1A).[8,9] Special windows, such as the refractive (see Fig. 16.1B) and asymmetry (see Fig. 16.1C) displays,[8,9] the cone location and magnitude index X (CLMI.X; Fig. 16.2),[10] the percentage tissue altered (PTA; see Fig. 16.2),[11] and the thickness progression (Fig. 16.3)[12] report, have been developed, improving our diagnostic capability with suspicious or borderline cases prior to refractive surgery.

The characteristics of the three types of primary keratectasia—KC, pellucid marginal degeneration (PMD), and keratoglobus—have been described elsewhere using the Galilei.[12-14] More recently, we identified the differences between secondary acquired keratectasia after the cornea, predisposed or not, was weakened by incisions, scars, or tissue ablation.[12,13] We also reported the detection of at least six types of corneas with KC signs that may appear before ectasia. They have been usually confused with corneas with KC despite seem to be in a pre-KC stage because do not have ectasia.[13] In this chapter, we will demonstrate the use of the Galilei system to detail the four primary signs of KC: ectasia, steepening, asymmetry, and thinning.

Tomographic Characteristics of Ectasia

KC progresses slowly from an apparent normal but predisposed susceptible eye. Ectasia is an abnormal forward protrusion of either of the two surfaces of the cornea and is the most recognized topo-tomographic sign of the biomechanical failure in KC. Nevertheless, ectasia, steepening, and KC are not synonymous.[12]

Using the Galilei system, ectasia is typically identified as a central or paracentral well-delimited zone with the steepest anterior keratometry reading (K_{max}) greater than 48 diopters (D) and/or posterior K_{max} steeper than −7.0 D, and with the anterior most-elevated best-fit-sphere point (BFS_{max}) higher than 12 μm and/or a posterior BFS_{max} of 17 μm. In the anterior tangential

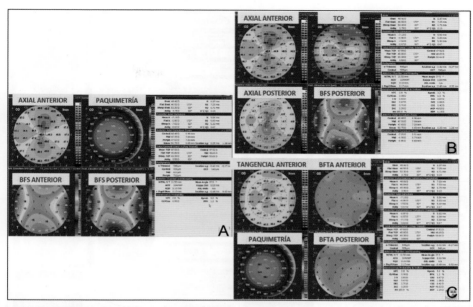

Fig. 16.1 (A) Galilei G4 old quad map of a right cornea that 6 years before was diagnosed with KC because of high K_{max} despite normal pachymetry, normal best-fit-sphere *(BFS)* maps, and with-the-rule (WTR) symmetric astigmatism. (B) The refractive report of the same cornea displays a posterior axial map, also with high K_{max} and WTR parallel astigmatism. Total corneal power (TCP) maps shows a very symmetric toric multifocal cornea. (C) The asymmetry report has an anterior tangential map of a uniform steeper toric cornea *(yellow and orange steps)*. Both central zones of BFS maps are normal green without any evidence of an ectatic lump. The central thinnest point is normal with normal thickness progression. This is a cornea with pre-KC type 1 in the sister of the patient described in Fig. 16.10. *BFTA,* Best fit toric aspheric; *KC,* keratoconus.

curvature maps, the zone of ectasia is observed as an orange-to-red central area surrounded by a yellow-green ring of variable width with normal values (Brazilian flag sign) usually located between 6- and 9-mm diameter (Fig. 16.4).[12,13] In the BFS maps, the protrusion is characteristically shown by a circular or semi-circular pattern with concentric color steps, from the normal green to the more elevated yellow, that we call 'fried-egg" pattern.

ECTASIA AND STEEPENING OF K_{MAX}

A recent controversial multicenter study did not consider the steepening of surfaces as mandatory for KC diagnosis.[15,16] However, although steepening is a classic indicator of KC progression, a keratometry value (K) alone is not the best way to discover early KC, because of its low sensitivity. In suspected cases, a simulated keratometry (SimK) greater than 45.43 D and a posterior mean K steeper than −6.41 D had 46.51% and 67.44% sensitivity and 96.19% and 73.33% specificity, respectively. In cases with established KC, a SimK greater than 45.43 D and a posterior mean K steeper than −6.62 D had 59.3% and 67.4% sensitivity, and 96.2% and 91.14% specificity, respectively.[17]

Although we believe K_{max} is a better parameter than the average K, we conclude that a single steep K value is insufficient for the diagnosis of KC, when ectasia is not demonstrated as shown by symmetric steeper toric, not hyperprolate, corneas (Figs. 16.1 and 16.5), or by asymmetric corneas with a normal range of K_{max} (see Fig. 16.5). In these cases, the biomechanical failure and forces molding the cornea were not sufficient to cause central asymmetry and/or focal bulging. We, therefore, classified them at pre-KC stages.[12,13]

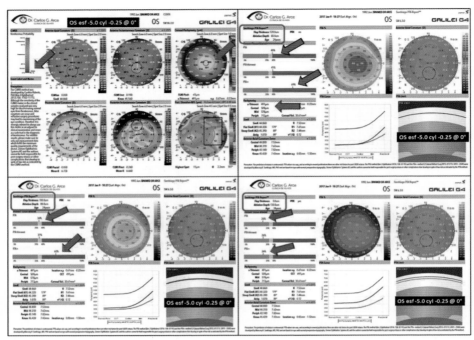

Fig. 16.2 Percentage tissue altered (PTA) report in a cornea with Rx sphere −5.0 cylinder −0.25 at 0 degrees, normal anterior and posterior curvature, 491 μm central thinnest point, and zero cone location and magnitude index X (CLMI.X) *(red arrows, top left)*. Regular PTA for LASIK with a 120 μm flap is 41% but PTA+ is 69% because cornea is thin *(top right)*. PTA fell to 36% with femtosecond flap of 100 μm but the PTA+ remained high at 60% *(bottom left)*. For PTA for photorefractive keratectomy, however (considering 50 μm of epithelium), the three PTAs were 26% *(bottom right)*.

ECTASIA, INCREASED ASPHERICITY, AND TOTAL CORNEAL SPHERICAL ABERRATION

The asphericity (Q factor) and the e^2 (squared eccentricity) of surfaces are particularly useful for identifying corneas with ectasia. Basically, both indices represent the relationship between the central and the peripheral curvature. If the center is flatter than the periphery, the surface is aspherical oblate. If the center is steeper, it is aspherical prolate. Q factor and e^2 also represent conical sections. If center and periphery have the same curvature, the surface is truly spherical ($e^2 = -Q = 0$) or is spherical on average with prolate and oblate hemimeridians that compensate one another. An $e^2 = \pm 1.0$ indicates a parabolic shape. If $0 < e^2 < 1.0$, or $0 > e^2 > -1.0$, the surface is elliptical prolate or oblate, respectively, and if $e^2 > 1.0$ or $e^2 < -1.0$, it has a hyperbolic prolate or oblate profile, respectively (Fig. 16.6).[14]

Currently, a corneal surface would be considered abnormal and hyperprolate if it has $e^2 \geq 0.8$, especially if associated with a negative total corneal spherical aberration in microns. When either or both faces reach $e^2 = 1.0$, such a cornea has KC until otherwise proven. However, there are asymmetric and misshapen corneas with sinusoid profiles (such as initial PMD or advanced KC, depressed superiorly and protruding inferiorly) that may have $e^2 < 1.0$.[14]

In the Galilei system, the e^2 and Q factor are calculated from the central 8-mm diameter aligned by default with the first Purkinje image but can be measured centered to the pupil. They

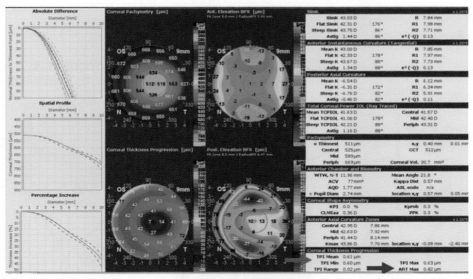

Fig. 16.3 Prototype of the thickness progression profile of a cornea with normal curvature and anterior best-fit-sphere (BFS; *top right*) and best fit toric aspheric (BFTA) elevation maps. The posterior BFS *(bottom right)* has an asymmetric peninsula pattern with 14 µm BFS_max. Pachymetry map is normal *(top center)*. The new map of thickness progression begins with blue steps at the center *(flat slope)* and ends with green at the periphery *(center bottom)*. Graphics of thickness progression *(left)* are in µm and percentage. Average thickness progression index (TPI) minimum TPI, maximum TPI, TPI range *(red arrow)*, and the Ambrosio's relational thickness (ART) maximum index *(blue arrow)* are shown among the numerical indexes.

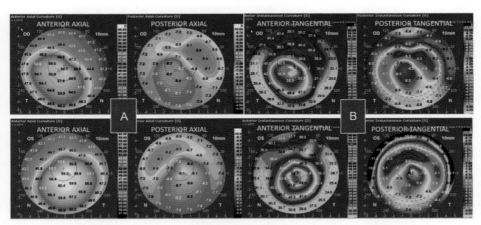

Fig. 16.4 (A) Conventional anterior and posterior axial maps with conventional scale CGA-Default with 1 D steps: *(left)* and CGA-Default with 0.25 D steps: *(right)* from a 19-year-old female patient with Down syndrome. Ectasia seems to reach the edge of the map. (B) Tangential maps of same corneas with 10-mm diameter, modified scale CGA – 1 D: German *(left)* and CGA – 0.25 D: German *(right)* show the actual size of the ectasia (orange-red-gray) delimited by a normal yellow-green curvature ring (Brazilian flag sign). Whereas the anterior surface has a flat *(navy blue)* or extremely flat *(light blue)* periphery, the periphery at the posterior surface is very steep *(red to gray)* explaining its progressive thickening.

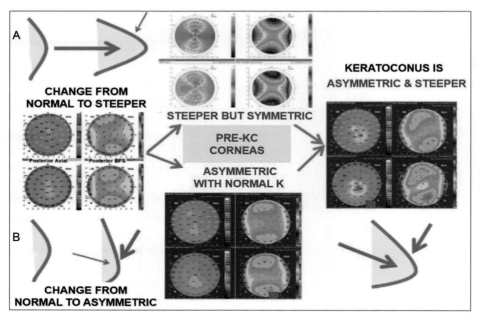

Fig. 16.5 Depending on the tissue fragility and/or the main deformation vectors over the external or internal face, normal corneas may achieve a pre-K stage without ectasia, being (A) pre-keratoconus (KC) grade 1 with toric symmetric steepening or (B) pre-KC type 3 with toric asymmetric curvature within normal range. If the tissue damage persists for long enough, the deformation would become KC after completing its four main components: steepening, asymmetry, ectasia, and thinning.

are not necessarily interchangeable with other devices as these values depend on the alignment of data and the size of the measured area, especially in asymmetric corneas.[18] Although the posterior surface is usually more prolate than the anterior, when analyzed separately, the anterior Q factor had slightly better specificity and sensitivity for corneas diagnosed with confirmed KC (Fig. 16.7).[17] An increased e^2 for both surfaces correlated directly with the loss of visual quality in eyes with KC,[19] directly with the steepening of the anterior surface, inversely with the steepening of the posterior surface (Fig. 16.8, top), and inversely with the spherical aberration (see Fig.16.8, middle).[20,21]

The total corneal spherical aberration depicts the wavefront profile of light rays focusing after crossing the cornea. Spherical aberration may be expressed in microns or in diopters, and zero spherical aberration means that the circle of least confusion is so small that all light rays focus on a common point. Positive spherical aberration in microns (negative in diopters) occurs when the cornea has greater power at the periphery, whereas negative spherical aberration in microns (positive in diopters) occurs when there is more power at the center.

When the anterior corneal surface is spherical, the total corneal spherical aberration (measured from 6-mm diameter centralized to the pupil) is between 0.25 and 0.30 μm. In oblate anterior surfaces, such as after radial keratotomy (RK) or myopic LASIK, it tends to be more positive in microns, while it is close to zero when the anterior surface is prolate and ideally aspheric ($e^2 = -Q \approx 0.60$). However, most corneas with a hyperprolated anterior surface and $e^2 = -Q \geq 0.80$ already have a negative total corneal spherical aberration in microns.[14,20–23] Some corneas with KC and a sinusoid shape, however, may have spherical aberration close to zero or even positive in microns.[12,14]

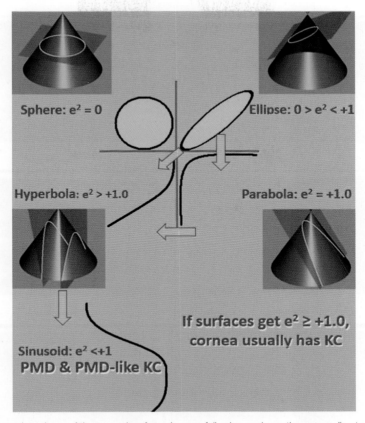

Fig. 16.6 The prolate shape of the corneal surface changes following conic sections according to keratoconus *(KC)* progression. Posterior e^2 usually is larger than anterior e^2. A spherical shape $(e^2 = 0)$ steepens to initially assume a prolate toric ellipsoid aspheric shape $(0 > e^2 < +1)$ and later a parabolic $(e^2 = +1)$ or an asymmetric hyperbolic $(e^2 > +1)$ shape. In more advanced cases, $e^2 < +1$ may be reached owing to the sinusoid shape. No normal cornea has $e^2 \geq +1$; however, there are corneas with KC or pellucid marginal degeneration *(PMD)* with $e^2 < +1$. (Modified from Arce and Trattler, 2010.)[14]

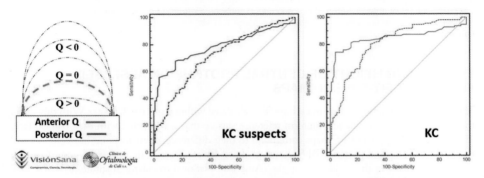

Fig. 16.7 Receiver operating characteristic (ROC) curves of specificity and sensibility of anterior and posterior Q factor assessed by the Galilei G2 to distinguish eyes suspect for keratoconus *(KC)* and with KC. (Modified from Núñez and Blanco-Marín, 2013.)[17]

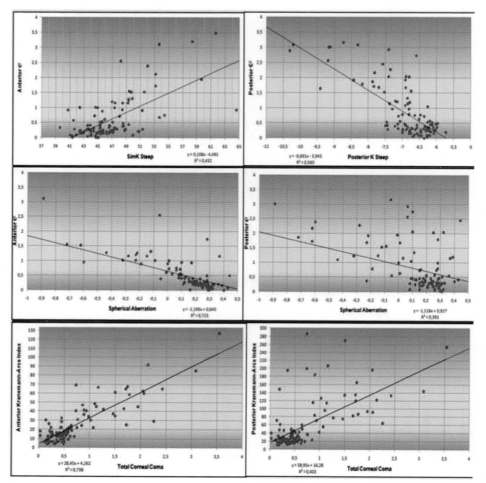

Fig. 16.8 *Top:* Direct and inverse relationship between steepening (K_{steep}) and prolaticity (e^2) of anterior *(left)* and posterior *(right)* surfaces. *Middle:* Inverse relationship between the total corneal spherical aberration (in μm) and the prolaticity (e^2) of anterior *(left)* and posterior *(right)* surfaces. *Bottom:* Direct relationship between the total corneal coma and the Kraneman-Arce index of anterior (A-KAI, *left*) and posterior (P-KAI, *right*) surfaces. (Modified from Arce, 2010.)[20,21]

ECTASIA AND HEIGHT OF CENTRAL PROTRUSION ASSESSED FROM BEST-FIT-SPHERE MAPS

The BFS is the curvature average of each surface calculated within a specific diameter. With this value, the system generates a spherical uniform reference surface that is compared with each corneal face. The values that appear in BFS maps correspond to their difference, point-to-point in microns. Currently, the anterior and posterior BFS shown in most devices is set from a central 8-mm diameter, as it was originally in the Galilei. Using the (American National Standards Institute), ANSI-CGA 5-μm scale, Galilei BFS maps of normal with-the-rule (WTR) corneas have a green horizontal band (±5 μm) with few or nonyellow steps within the 4-mm diameter central region (gray circle on maps). The BFS$_{max}$ is marked by a small dark dot (Fig. 16.9A). We use 10 to 12 μm (first yellow) as the cutoff

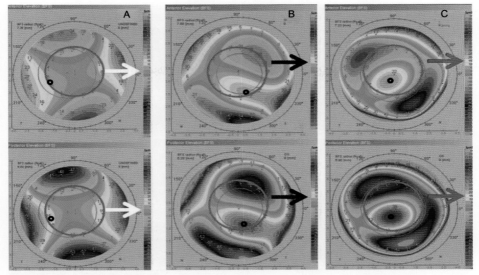

Fig. 16.9 Typical best-fit-sphere *(BFS)* maps with ANSI-CGA 5-μm scale. Green is coded for ±5 μm *(white arrows)*. First yellow (10 μm, *black arrows*) and second yellow (15 μm, *red arrows*) are limit values for anterior and posterior surface, respectively. (A) Normal anterior *(top)* and posterior *(bottom)* BFS maps with a green central band. BFS$_{max}$ is indicated by a dark spot within the 4-mm diameter central zone. (B) BFS maps from a keratoconus (KC) cornea showing a peninsula pattern with elevated BFS$_{max}$, dislocated inferiorly. (C) BFS maps from a cornea with advanced KC showing peninsula and fried-egg patterns with elevated dislocated BFS$_{max}$.

value for the front surface and 15 to 17 μm (second yellow) for the posterior.[7,14,22,23] When the cornea has a lump-like zone of ectasia, the Galilei maps typically have concentric yellow circles or semicircles forming patterns called yellow tongue (see Fig. 16.9B), fried egg, peninsula (see Fig. 16.9C), or island (Fig. 16.10A, and 16.10B).[7,12–14]

Galilei BFS values were studied using 106 normal healthy eyes, 59 eyes with forme fruste KC (FFKC), and 113 eyes with KC. The best and earliest indicator of ectasia seems to be the central posterior BFS$_{max}$[12–14,17] with a sensitivity of 73.3% and 91.2%, and a specificity of 85.7% and 85.7%, to distinguish normal corneas from those with FFKC and KC, respectively (Fig. 16.11).[17] From the functional point of view, increased anterior or posterior BFS$_{max}$ has shown good correlation with the loss of visual acuity in corneas with KC.[19] However, it is important to note that BFS values only measure the height of ectasia and do not assess its asymmetry.

Tomographic Characteristics of Asymmetry

TOPOGRAPHIC PATTERNS IN KERATOCONUS

KC phenotypes[24] have been associated with the different topographic patterns described in curvature maps.[25,26] Symmetric WTR small central bow ties (baby bow tie by Peter Stewart, 2009; Fig. 16.12A) or classic vertical orthogonal bow ties (see Fig. 16.12B) develop inferior K$_{max}$ shifting to asymmetric snowman (see Fig. 16.12C) or oblique skewed nonorthogonal duck patterns (see Fig. 16.12D). In advanced asymmetric cases, the vertical profile may become sinusoid with oblate superior depression, prolate inferior protrusion, against-the-rule (ATR) astigmatism, and incomplete (see Fig. 16.12E) or complete (see Fig. 16.12F) croissant, crab-claw or kissing bird patterns (pellucid-like KC).[12–14] There are suspects with horizontal asymmetry resembling the letter D (see Fig. 16.13C),[27] and advanced cases with an inferior oval (see Fig. 16.12G) or central round to oval zone of ectasia (see Fig. 16.12H).[28]

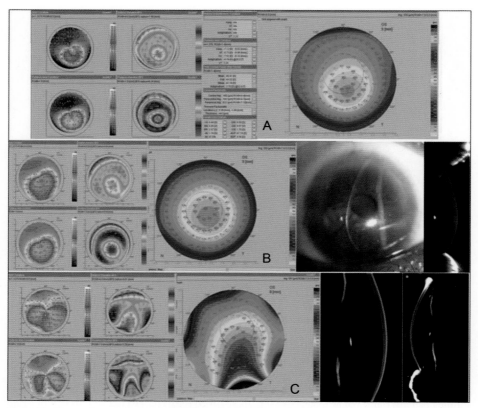

Fig. 16.10 Steepening usually goes further than what the color scale represent changing the croissant pattern (A) of anterior *(top)* or posterior *(bottom)* curvature maps to a round or a hart-like pattern (B and C). The vertical band of the anterior and posterior BFS maps may be converted to an island or peninsula pattern, always with the more elevated point (BFS$_{max}$) dislocated inferiorly. In advanced PMD, anterior K$_{max}$ of instantaneous maps *(apex)* and BFS$_{max}$ use to be located at same level or above the thinnest point *(center)* which is already below 500 μm.

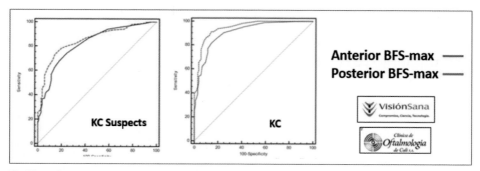

Fig. 16.11 Receiver operating characteristic (ROC) curves of anterior and posterior BFS$_{max}$ measured by the Galilei G2 to distinguish keratoconus *(KC)* suspects and corneas with KC. *BFS*, Best-fit-sphere. (Modified from Núñez and Blanco-Marín, 2013.)[17]

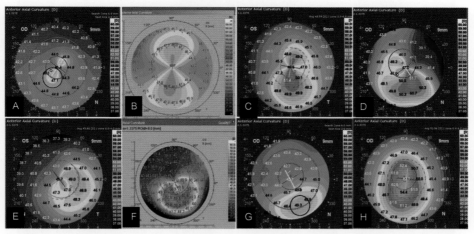

Fig. 16.12 Corneal patterns of anterior axial maps in KC. (A) Baby bow tie. (B) Orthogonal classic bow tie with inferior steepening. (C) Orthogonal asymmetric snowman bow tie in cornea with with-the-rule (WTR)/WTR, parallel anterior/posterior astigmatism. (D) Skewed duck bow tie in cornea with oblique/WTR, 45-degrees crossed anterior/posterior astigmatism. (E) Incomplete pellucid marginal degeneration (PMD)-like pattern in cornea with oblique/WTR 45-degree crossed anterior/posterior astigmatism. (F) PMD-like sinusoid pattern in cornea with against-the-rule (ATR)/WTR 90-degree crossed anterior/posterior astigmatism. (G) Inferior oval pattern. (H) Central oval with K_{max} dislocated inferiorly.

Vertical asymmetry of corneal surfaces has been a longstanding accepted indicator of and risk factor for KC, as well as postoperative ectasia.[29,30] With the Galilei, asymmetry is recognized either by the color coding of anterior or posterior curvature and elevation or by pachymetry maps and is quantified by several indices. It should be noted that both numerical indices and asymmetric patterns can vary among devices depending on the reference used as map center, either the pupil, first Purkinje, or apex.[31]

ASYMMETRIC INDICES FROM THE ANTERIOR SURFACE

Curvature indices from the anterior surface were initially created in Placido topographers[29,30,32,33] and later adapted to the Galilei.[34] The most important are the keratoconus prediction index (KPI; normal KPI range <20%),[7,34–36] KC probability (K_{prob}; normal K_{prob} <25%),[7,34–36] cone location and magnitude index (CLMI; normal CLMI <1.5 D),[34–36] percentage probability of keratoconus (PPK; normal PPK <5%),[34–36] and inferior-superior (I-S; normal I-S <1.5 D).[29,30]

The KPI is a percentage calculated as KPI = 4.62 [0.30 + 0.01 (−41.23 − 0.15 DSI + 1.18 OSI + 1.49 SAI − 0.56 SimKs + 1.08 SimKf − 3.74 IAI + 0.10 AA)] − 60.25, where DSI is the differential sector index, OSI is the opposite sector index, CSI is the center/surround index, SAI is the surface asymmetry index, SimKf is the simulated keratometry flat, SimKs is the simulated keratometry steep, IAI is the irregular astigmatism index, and AA is the analyzed area.[8] The IAI and the surface regularity index (SRI, r =− 0.695) correlated well ($P < 0.001$) with the loss of contrast sensitivity in corneas with KC.[19]

The CLMI is a variant of Rabinowitz's I-S index[25,26,29,30] not limited to the vertical meridian alone. The CLMI assesses the difference in curvature of the 2-mm circular area around the K_{max} with the opposite zone of same size located at 180 degrees and at the same distance from the center of the map.[8,34] Two independent studies demonstrated that KPI and CLMI were statistically similar in detecting KC.[17,35,36] Despite their good sensitivity and specificity, they should not be used to progress KC because of the

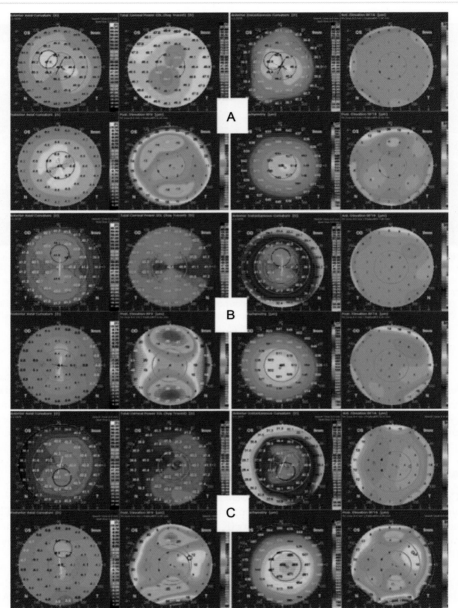

Fig. 16.13   Prekeratoconus type 5 may occur in thin corneas without ectasia. (A) A screening for myopic LASIK in an asymptomatic male myope aged 45 years, in whom we found a symmetric against-the-rule (ATR)/oblique 45-degree crossed total corneal astigmatism *(top and bottom left)* with a central thickness of 508 μm and normal thickness progression *(bottom center-right)*. All other maps and numeric indexes were within normal range. (B) Keratoconus screening of an 11-year-old female high myope patient, demonstrating a central thinnest point of 494 μm with normal thickness progression *(bottom center-right)*. Although within the normal curvature range, instantaneous mapping shows a peripheral flattening in almost 360 degrees *(top center-right)*. All other maps and numeric indexes are within normal range. (C) Asymptomatic male myope aged 30 years who came for screening before refractive surgery. Axial *(top left)* and instantaneous *(top center-right)* anterior maps have normal range curvature but with a D-like pattern that is also present on the TCP map *(top center-left)*. Instantaneous map shows a peripheral flattening in 360 degrees *(top center-right)*. Posterior axial, posterior BFS, and both BFTA maps are normal. Thinnest point is central and measures 465 μm and >200 μm superior-nasal difference is present only between 8 and 1 o'clock, indicating a faster thickness progression at this quadrant.

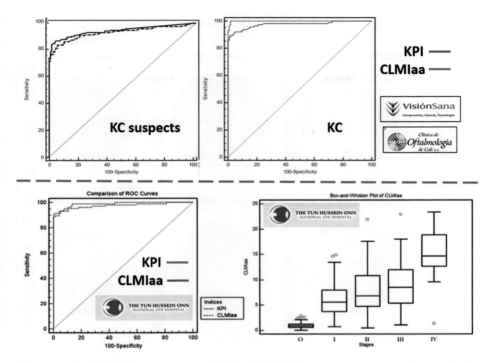

Fig. 16.14 Receiver operating characteristic (ROC) curve with specificity and sensitivity of KPI and CLMIaa assessed with the Galilei G2 to distinguish suspects for keratoconus *(KC)* and eyes with KC. Despite their good specificity and sensitivity in detecting early KC, they cannot be used to stage the disease because of overlapping of values. (Modified from Núñez and Blanco-Marín, 2012.)[35]

overlapping of values in different KC stages (Fig. 16.14).[36] Other studies have also shown the ability of CLMI, KPI, and other Galilei parameters to distinguish KC from normal corneas.[37–39]

CLMI.X

The Galilei is the only device with the CLMI.X display (Figs. 16.2, 16.15, and 16.16),[10,40] which combines curvature, pachymetry, and elevation data. This index represents the PPK, applying the regular CLMI concept of asymmetry within the 6-mm central zone not only to the anterior axial (CLMIaa), but also to the anterior instantaneous (CLMI Inst), the posterior axial (CLMI-Paxial), and the posterior instantaneous (CLMI-Pinst) maps. It also considers the SimK from the anterior axial map, the K_{max} from the anterior instantaneous map, and the mean K from the posterior axial and the posterior instantaneous maps. From the pachymetry, the CLMI.X uses the thinnest thickness value (μm) and its location to derive a new index called FLMI_Pach (flat location and magnitude index adapted to the pachymetry map), which is the difference in μm between a small zone around the thinnest point and the opposite zone of same size in the same meridian with a minimum distance of 2 mm between them.[10] Finally, the CLMI.X also considers the posterior BFS_{max} within the 4.4 mm of central zone and its location in cartesian coordinates.

Comparison of CLMIaa (only from the anterior axial map) and the CLMI.X (Fig. 16.17)[10] indicated that the CLMI.X has almost 100% sensitivity and specificity for the diagnosis of KC and a cutoff value of 25% for suspects and 80% for KC (Table 16.2). Although a false negative is extremely uncommon, we observed false positive cases when Placido or Scheimpflug data did not

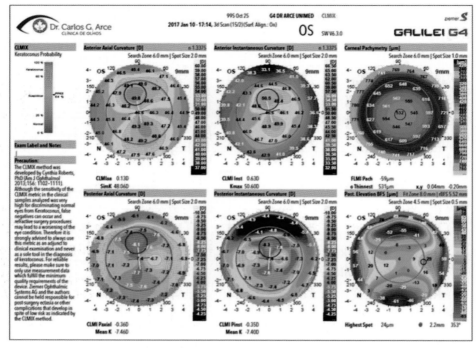

Fig. 16.15   Cone location and magnitude index X (CLMI.X) is 54% in a symmetric cornea with pre-keratoconus type 1, normal e^2, 50.60-D tangential K_{max}, posterior curvature with steeper zones, 531 µm thinnest point, and 24 µm of posterior best-fit-sphere (BFS)$_{max}$.

achieve good quality, if the upper lid covered part of the cornea, and in eyes with corneal transplant or RK despite them not having KC.[12,13]

ASYMMETRY ASSESSED BY BFTA ELEVATION MAPS AND COMA

The BFTA maps reflect the asymmetry, irregularity, or roughness of the cornea by comparing it with an ideal toric aspheric surface generated from the BFS value used as the central value zero. Different from the BFS maps, which serve to assess the height of KC, the BFTA maps show how tilted is it when the curvature slope is not the same in 360 degrees.[12,13]

In the Galilei, uniform, smooth, symmetrical, toric, and aspheric surfaces produce green BFTA maps with elevation values within ±5 µm (see Fig. 16.13, column on right). When curvature of one half of the cornea changes from the center to the periphery at a different rate from the other half, asymmetry is shown by two opposite zones on BFTA maps: one yellow (more elevated) and the other light blue (more depressed). A central narrow green band (symmetrical meridian) divides both halves (Fig. 16.18).[12-14]

The asymmetry found in BFTA maps has been quantified by the anterior (A-KAI) and posterior (P-KAI) Kranemann-Arce Index.[12-14,21,22] A-KAI and P-KAI (also called AAI or asymmetric aspheric index)[41,42] represent the difference in elevation between the most elevated positive point and the most depressed negative point within a central zone of 6-mm[41,42] or 6.5-mm[14,20,21] diameter of BFTA maps (Fig. 16.19). The P-KAI is always higher than the A-KAI in deformed corneas. A-KAI has been reported to be 10.72 ± 5.72 µm (mean ± standard deviation, Table 16.3) with a maximum normal limit between 15 and 19 µm. Normal

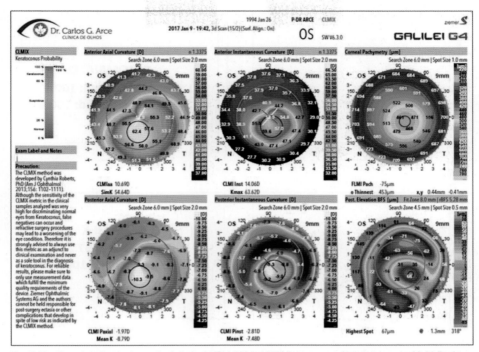

Fig. 16.16 Cone location and magnitude index X (CLMI.X) is 100% in a cornea with keratoconus, 63.62 D of tangential K_{max}, very steep posterior curvature, 453 μm thinnest point, and 67 μm of posterior best-fit-sphere (BFS)$_{max}$.

P-KAI was 22.49 ± 9.29 μm and would not be higher than 30 μm.[14,20,21] In KC grade 1, the A-KAI was 18.90 ± 7.95 μm and the P-KAI was 41.23 ± 34.97 μm. In KC grade 3, the A-KAI was 51.86 ± 23.96 μm and the P-KAI was 132.36 ± 66.22 μm.[14,20,21] In corneas with KC, a high KAI correlated well with loss of visual function.[19] Another study found that a P-KAI (or AAI) more than 21.5 μm combined with a corneal volume (from the central 8-mm diameter) less than 30.8 mm³ detected FFKC with 93.5% sensitivity and 97.2% specificity, and KC with 100% sensitivity and 99.5% specificity.[41,42]

Surface deformation causes high-order aberrations such as coma, trefoil, tetrafoil, or spherical aberration. Coma is the most important index of corneal wavefront asymmetry and is directly proportional to the asymmetry of surfaces (see Fig. 16.8, bottom).[20,21] In KC, the yellow and the light blue opposite zones of BFTA (in microns) and vertical negative coma (in diopters) maps have a similar orientation (axis) and position, with the yellow at the bottom indicating that the ectasia is steeper and more positive elevated inferiorly (see Figs. 16.18 and 16.20). The normal total corneal coma for the central 6-mm zone aligned to the pupil was 0.38 ± 0.15 D. In KC grade 1, it was 0.57 ± 0.66 D and in KC grade 3 was 1.86 ± 1.88 D.[20,21]

Central Thinning and Corneal Volume

THIN CORNEAS AND THINNEST POINT

With the Galilei, an isolated thinnest point is not a good parameter for detecting early KC,[17] as very stable uniform thin corneas with a central thinnest point of 500 μm or slightly less are not necessarily pathologic (see Fig. 16.13). The diagnosis of KC is clearer when there is a thinnest

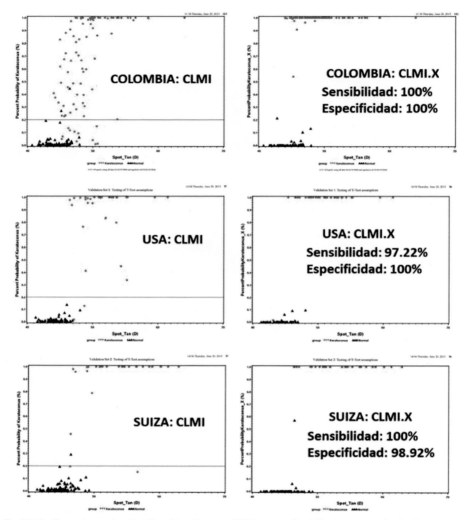

Fig. 16.17 Percentage of probability of keratoconus (PPK) versus Spot Tan (average value in diopters of a 2-mm diameter zone around tangential K_{max}) obtained with traditional cone location and magnitude index (CLMI) algorithm *(left)* and the CLMI.X *(right)* in three independent populations from Colombia *(top)*, USA *(middle)*, and Switzerland *(bottom)*. (Modified from Mahmoud et al., 2013.)[10]

point of 500 μm or less located 1 mm or more from the pupil center (Fig. 16.21)[5,14,43] Interestingly, the meridian of thinnest point dislocation, usually inferotemporal, tends to coincide with the coma axis and the meridian of asymmetry found in BFTA maps.[12]

Thin corneas, however, might have KC earlier and faster if subjected to the similar loading forces that may damage and mold thicker corneas. In fact, whereas FFKC seems to be more common in corneas with less than 30.8 mm³ of volume,[41,42] a thin cornea may indicate there is not enough tissue to maintain homeostasis. The PTA[11] is probably the strongest recognized risk factor of postoperative ectasia after LASIK or photorefractive keratectomy (PRK) developed for normal corneas. PTA plus (PTA+) uses a new algorithm considering a higher additional risk when the thinnest point is 500 μm or less (see Fig. 16.2).[11]

TABLE 16.2 ■ Sensitivity and Specificity of BFS$_{max}$, CLMI, and KPI From Galilei G2 in Recognizing Suspect Corneas and Corneas With Keratoconus[40]

Index	Type of Cornea	Sensitivity	Specificity	Cut-off Value
Anterior BFS-max	KC Suspect	68.0 %	81.9 %	> 6 µm
	With KC	73.3 %	85.7 %	> 17 µm
Posterior BFS-max	KC Suspect	81.4 %	85.7 %	> 7 µm
	With KC	91.2 %	85.7 %	> 17 µm
CLMI	KC Suspect	83.7 %	94.3 %	> 1.35 D
	With KC	100 %	98.1 %	> 1.76 D
KPI	KC Suspect	84.3%	98.1 %	> 13.1 %
	With KC	100 %	98.1 %	> 13.1 %

BFS$_{max}$, Most-elevated best-fit-sphere point; *CLMI*, cone location and magnitude index; *KC*, keratoconus; *KPI*, keratoconus prediction index.

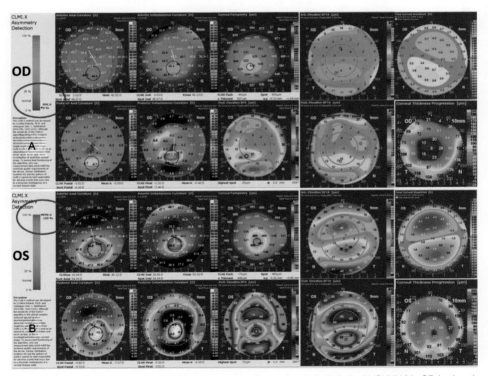

Fig. 16.18 Forme fruste keratoconus with zero cone location and magnitude index X (CLMI.X) in OD *(red oval in A)* whereas the OS has 100% CLMI.X *(red oval in B)*. Some asymmetry in anterior and posterior surface *(top left and center-left)*, steepening of K$_{max}$ in posterior instantaneous map *(bottom center-left)*, increased posterior BFS)$_{max}$ *(bottom center)*, dislocated thinnest point *(top center)*, and 0.60 D of total corneal coma *(top right)*. Recently we also found peripheral flattening of anterior surface *(top center-left)* and increased thickness progression *(bottom right)*. Left eye recently had selective Galilei-guided corneal cross-linking. Anterior best fit toric aspheric (BFTA) maps (in microns) perfectly correlate with total corneal coma maps (in diopters).

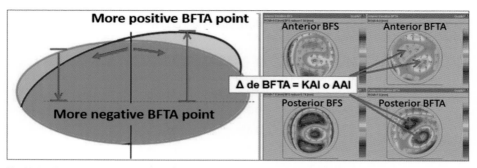

Fig. 16.19 The Kranemann-Arce index is the difference in μm between the point of maximum positive best fit toric aspheric *(BFTA)* elevation and the point of minimum negative BFTA elevation. *AAI,* Asymmetric aspheric index; *BFS,* best-fit-sphere; *KAI,* Kraneman-Arce index. (Modified from Arce, 2010.)[20,21]

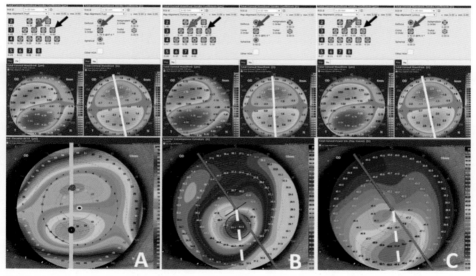

Fig. 16.20 Total corneal wave-front report from a 6-mm zone of a cornea with keratoconus aligned to the pupil *(top left)*, to first Purkinje *(top center)*, and to the center of horizontal limbus diameter (WTW, *top right*). The axis of coma *(white line)* in diopters is close with the asymmetry (A, *yellow line*) shown on the anterior best fit toric aspheric (BFTA) map (in μm) using the most positive *(blue dot)* and the more negative *(red dot)*. Both principal axes of anterior tangential (B) and TCP (C) maps are similar *(red lines)* but different than the axis of the total corneal coma (white solid lines) which seems closer to the skewed axes in the inferior half of both maps (white dot lines). Axes and values of total corneal coma *(green arrows)* are not the same in the three alignments: 1.78 D at 97.6 degrees (pupil), 1.86 D at 92.9 degrees (first Purkinje), and 1.92 D at 96.9 degrees (WTW). Trefoil values *(blue arrows)*, vertical coma *(red arrows)*, and spherical aberration also changed according to the alignment of data.

THINNED CORNEAS AND THICKNESS PROGRESSION PROFILE

The difference in pachymetry between the thinnest point and the periphery has been used to study thickness progression for some time. The absolute thickness difference (pachymetry index) was settled in the Galilei as 200 μm at 9-mm diameter.[14,22,23] From the clinical and biomechanical

TABLE 16.3 ■ Galilei G1 Indexes Found From 39 Normal Corneas of 24 Patients (Aged 32.7 ± 12.1 Years), 39 Corneas With Keratoconus Grade 1 of 22 Patients (Aged 32.1 ± 13.0 Years) and 28 Corneas With Keratoconus Grade 3 of 18 Patients (Aged 34.0 ± 10.7 Years) With no Other Ocular Pathologies

Index	Normal	KC Grade I	KC Grade III
SimK avg (D)	43.42 ±1.51	45.18 ±2.17	49.09 ±4.57
Flatter SimK (D)	42.87 ±1.50	43.84 ±2.15	45.60 ±9.39
Steeper SimK (D)	43.96 ±1.60	46.49 ±2.38	51.22 ±5.04
Cylinder SimK (D)	1.08 ±0.73	2.65 ±1.31	4.12 ±2.31
Anterior ϵ^2	0.20 ±0.16	0.42 ±0.28	1.42 ±0.88
Posterior Kavg (D)	-6.21 ±0.23	-6.56 ±0.38	-7.60 ±1.07
Flatter Kpost (D)	-6.04 ±0.23	-6.28 ±0.36	-7.18 ±1.02
Steeper Kpost (D)	-6.36 ±0.25	-6.85 ±0.42	-8.05 ±1.22
Cylinder post (D)	-0.29 ±0.19	-0.58 ±0.15	-0.66 ±0.74
Posterior ϵ^2	0.25 ±0.16	0.77 ±0.61	1.95 ±0.85
TCP mean (D)	43.04 ±1.46	44.70 ±2.21	48.20 ±4.36
Flatter TCP (D)	42.64 ±1.52	43.46 ±2.20	46.29 ±4.53
Steeper TCP (D)	42.53 ±6.85	45.82 ±2.49	50.25 ±4.67
Cylinder TCP (D)	0.96 ±0.68	2.28 ±1.61	4.05 ±2.25
Defocus (D)	-0.24 ±0.11	-0.21 ±0.21	0.22 ±0.80
Astigmatism (D)	0.77 ±0.49	1.91 ±1.04	2.63 ±1.57
Coma (D)	0.38 ±0.15	0.57 ±0.66	1.86 ±1.88
Trefoil (D)	0.20 ±0.13	0.26 ±0.20	1.04 ±1.24
Spherical Aberration (D)	-0.18 ±0.08	-0.11 ±0.14	0.31 ±0.61
5th order HOAs (D)	0.08 ±0.08	0.11 ±0.09	0.67 ±1.16
RMS (D)	1.01 ±0.40	2.74 ±1.27	3.83 ±2.04
Maximum anterior BFS (μm)	5.79 ±2.45	12.49 ±5.75	22.64 ±10.91
Maximum posterior BFS (μm)	11.85 ±3.59	22.90 ±6.34	51.61 ±24.56
Anterior Kranemman-Arce Index (μm)	10.72 ±5.72	18.90 ±7.95	51.86 ±23.96
Posterior Kranemann-Arce Index (μm)	22.49 ±9.29	41.23 ±34.97	132.36 ±66.22
I-S Rabinovitch Index (D)	0.78 ±0.46	1.53 ±1.73	6.54 ±4.47
KPI (%)	3.23 ±6.48	10.58 ±16.13	77.94 ±30.19
KProb Index (%)	4.85 ±12.46	16.20 ±26.39	81.90 ±26.44

BFS, Best-fit-sphere; *HOA,* high-order aberration; *I-S,* inferior-superior; *KPI,* keratoconus prediction index; *RMS,* root mean square; *SimK,* simulated keratometry; *TCP,* total corneal power.
Modified from Arce, 2010.[20,21]

point of view, the progression of corneal thickness from the center to the periphery is more important than the simple measurement of the thinnest point. As the peripheral pachymetry is less affected than the center, thickness progression ratio is faster beyond the central thinned zone with ectasia, as it is well shown in thickness progression graphics[44] and in the new thickness progression maps of Galilei.[12,13]

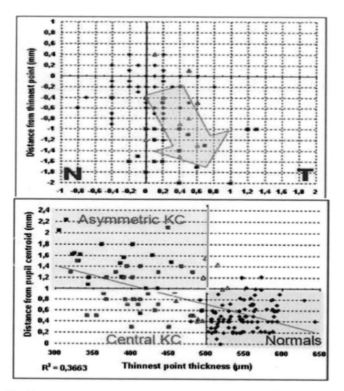

Fig. 16.21 The thinnest point is central in normal corneas *(blue dots)* but in corneas with keratoconus (KC; *red dots)* tends to be temporally-inferior dislocated farther *(top)*. Most normal corneas have a central thinnest point of more than 500 µm. All corneas with an asymmetric thinnest point of 500 µm or less located 1 mm or more from the pupil center had KC *(bottom)*. (Modified from Arce and Trattler, 2010.)[14]

The Galilei thickness progression maps depict, point-to-point, the slope of thickening and seem to be able to separate corneas with normal thickness progression (Figs. 16.3 and 16.22A–D) from corneas with increased progression (see Fig. 16.22E, F). Corneas uniformly thin (see Fig. 16.22D) end in a green-yellow periphery whereas those thinned at the center end in orange-red color steps (see Fig. 16.22E). Further, the graphic of percentage increase typically ends at the vertical edge when there is a normal progression but ends at the corner or the horizontal edge when there is a faster abnormal thickness progression.[12,13]

In summary, the technology embraced by the Galilei system provides expanded information by combining and integrating data from Placido topography and dual Scheimpflug tomography. With new features and color scales it facilitates the interpretation of maps and KC signs. Recent applications developed with the incorporation of optical biometry with reflectometry-interferometry have converted the Galilei Lens Professional into a complete platform for all specialists dedicated to the anterior segment of the eye.

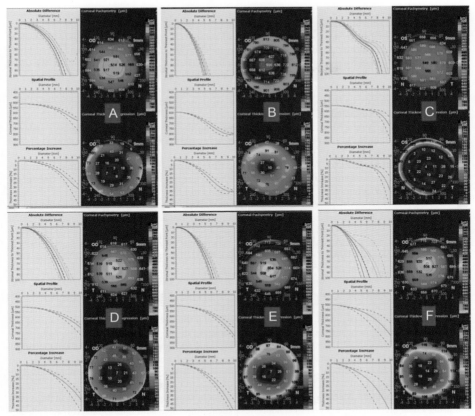

Fig. 16.22 Thickness progression profile and graphics of (A) cornea with normal curvature, pachymetry, and thickness progression; (B) thick normal cornea with normal thickness progression; (C) cornea with normal curvature and pachymetry without ectasia but with flat thickness progression at center and steep progression at the periphery; (D) cornea with normal curvature, 506 μm central thinnest point, and normal thickness progression, meaning that it is a uniformly thin cornea; (E) cornea with normal curvature, 504 μm central thinnest point, and steeper peripheral thickness progression, meaning that it is a thinned cornea at the center; (F) cornea with keratoconus, 503 μm central thinnest point, and steeper peripheral thickness progression, meaning that it is a thinned cornea at center.

References

1. Mandell RB. Profile methods of measuring corneal curvature. *J Amer Optom Assoc.* 1961;32:627–631.
2. Klyce SD. Computer-assisted corneal topography: high resolution graphical presentation and analysis of keratoscopy. *Invest Ophthalmol Vis Sci.* 1984;25:1426–1435.
3. Plácido A. Novo instrumento de exploração da córnea. *Periódico d'oftalmologia prática (Lisbon).* 1880;5:27–30.
4. Studer H. Accurate anterior segment topography. Online training—Galilei—Introduction to the system—GALILEI G4 and G6 key features-2. https://e-learning.ziemergroup.com/index.php?p=2. Port, Switzerland: Ziemer Ophthalmic Systems AG.
5. Schor P, Arce CG. Aspectos básicos do Orbscan. In: Alves MR, Chamon W, Nosé W, eds. *Cirurgia Refrativa. Brazilian Council of Ophthamology.* Rio de Janeiro, Brazil: Cultura Médica; 2003:21–49, chap 3B.

6. Arce CG. Galilei™ color scales and report formats: new features in software release 5.0. Galilei Technical Bulletin No. 4. Port, Switzerland: Ziemer Ophthalmic Systems AG; 2010.

7. Arce CG. Galilei™ map interpretation guide: Software version 5.2. Port, Switzerland: Ziemer Ophthalmic Systems AG; 2011. https://adaptltda.com.br/galilei/assets/files/GALILEI_Map_Interpretation_Guide.pdf.

8. Ziemer Ophthalmic Systems AG. Galilei G4 operator manual. Doc. No. CM3941-0081-03; 2016. https://www.e-learning.ziemergroup.com/uploads/1466413051.pdf.

9. Arce CG, Forseto A, de Abreu GP. *New map settings to facilitate preoperative and postoperative laser refractive surgery evaluation and keratoconus diagnosis.* Oral paper presented at: ESCRS-Winter Congress, February; 20-22, 2015; Istanbul, Turkey.

10. Mahmoud AM, Nunez MX, Blanco C, et al. Expanding the cone location and magnitude index to include corneal thickness and posterior surface information for the detection of keratoconus. *Am J Ophthalmol.* 2013;156:1102–1111.

11. Santhiago MR, Smadja D, Gomes BF, et al. Association between the percent tissue altered and post-laser in situ keratomileusis ectasia in eyes with normal preoperative topography. *Am J Ophthalmol.* 2014;158(1):87–95.e1.

12. Arce CG. Diagnóstico del queratocono con tomografía de duplo Scheimpflug y topografía de Placido. In: Albertazzi R, ed. *Queratocono.* Buenos Aires, Argentina: Argentinian Council of Ophthalmology; 2020. In press.

13. Keratoconus. Up to date Arce CGA. Galilei™ for keratoconus diagnosis. In: Almodin E, Nassaralla B, eds. *Brazilian Society of Ophthalmology.* Panama: Jaypee Highlights Medical Publishers; 2020: chap 1.6.3. In press.

14. Arce CG, Trattler W. Keratoconus and keratoectasia. In: Boyd S, Gutiérrez AM, McCulley JP, eds. *Atlas and Text of Corneal Pathology and Surgery.* Panama: Jaypee Highlights Medical Publishers; 2010:161–225, chap 13.

15. Gomes JA, Tan D, Rapuano CJ, et al. Group of panelists for the global Delphi panel of keratoconus and ectatic diseases. Global consensus on keratoconus and ectatic diseases. *Cornea.* 2015;34:359–369.

16. Randelman JB, Dupps WJ, Santhiago MR, et al. Screening for keratoconus and related ectatic corneal disorders. *Cornea.* 2015;34(8):e20–e22. https://www.ncbi.nlm.nih.gov/pmc/articles/PMC6392063/.

17. Núñez XM, Blanco-Marín C. Tomographic detection of keratoconus suspects. Paper presented at: ASCRS Meeting, April 19–23, 2013, San Francisco, CA.

18. Torquetti L, Arce CG, Merayo-Lloves J, et al. Evaluation of anterior and posterior surfaces of the cornea using a dual Scheimpflug analyzer in keratoconus patients implanted with intrastromal corneal ring segments. *Int J Ophthalmol.* 2016;9:1283–1288.

19. Bayraktar Bilen N, Hepsen IF, Arce CG. Correlation between visual function and refractive, topographic, pachymetric and aberrometric data in eyes with keratoconus. *Int J Ophthalmol.* 2016;9:1127–1133.

20. Arce CG. Corneal shape and HOAs may be used to distinguish corneas with keratoconus. *Poster presented at: ASCRS Meeting,* April 9–14 2010; Boston, MA.

21. Arce CG. *Corneal shape and HOAs may be used to distinguish corneas with keratoconus. Poster presented at: ESCRS Congress,* September 4–8, 2010; Paris, France.

22. Arce CG. Galilei™: Topografía de Plácido y tomografía del segmento anterior con doble Scheimpflug. In: Castillo A, ed. *Métodos Diagnósticos en Segmento Anterior (Monografías SECOIR), Sección 2, Evaluación Preoperatoria.* Madrid, Spain: Spanish Society of Implant-Refractive Ocular Surgery; 2011:211–236, chap 18.

23. Galilei Arce CG. Topografia de Plácido e tomografia do segmento anterior com duplo Scheimpflug. In: Ambrósio R Jr, Chalita MR, Vieira Netto M, Schor P, Chamon W, Fontes BM, eds. *Wavefront & Topografia, Tomografia e Biomecânica da Córnea.* 7th ed. Rio de Janeiro, Brazil: Cultura Médica; 2013:165–202, chap 14.

24. Fernández-Vega L. *New keratoconus classification guides customization of intracorneal ring segment implantation.* Ocular Surgery News Europe July 08, 2016. Classification of keratoconus. Presented at: European Meeting of Young Ophthalmologists. Oviedo, Spain. June 24. https://www.healio.com/news/ophthalmology/20160711/new-keratoconus-classification-guides-customization-of-intracorneal-ring-segment-implantation.

25. Rabinowitz YS, McDonnell PJ. Computer-assisted corneal topography in keratoconus. *Refract Corneal Surg.* 1989;5(6):400–408.

26. Rabinowitz YS, Yang H, Brickman Y, et al. Videokeratography database of normal human corneas. *Br J Ophthalmol.* 1996;80:610–616. https://www.ijkecd.com/doi/IJKECD/pdf/10.5005/jp-journals-10025-1114.

27. Abad JC, Rubinfeld RS, Del Valle M, Belin MW, Kurstin JM. A novel topographic pattern in some keratoconus suspects. *Opthalmology.* 2007;114(5):1020–1026.

28. Perry HD, Buxton JN, Fine BS. Round and oval cones in keratoconus. *Ophthalmology.* 1980;87(9):905–909.

29. Rabinowitz YS. Videokeratographic indices to aid in screening for keratoconus. *J Refract Surg.* 1995;11:371–379.

30. Rabinowitz YS, Rasheed K. KISA% index: a quantitative videokeratography algorithm embodying minimal topographic criteria for diagnosing keratoconus. *J Cataract Refract Surg.* 1999;25:1327–1335.

31. Arce CG, Campos M, Schor P. Overlooked features of corneal topographers. *J Cataract Refract Surg.* 2008;34:719–720.

32. Maeda N, Klyce SD, Smolek MK, Thompson HW. Automated keratoconus screening with corneal topography analysis. *Invest Ophthalmol Vis Sci.* 1994;35(6):2749–2757.

33. Mahmoud AM, Roberts C, Lembach R, Herderick EE, McMahon TTClek Study Group. Simulation of machine-specific topographic indices for use across platforms. *Optom Vis Sci.* 2006;83:682–693.

34. Roberts CJ. KPI analysis with the GALILEI™. Galilei Technical Bulletin No. 4. Port, Switzerland: Ziemer Ophthalmic Systems AG; 2010.

35. Núñez MX, Blanco C. Comparison between CLMI and KPI. Paper presented at: AAO Meeting, November, 10–13, 2012; Chicago, IL.

36. Ramani V. Wrap-up on keratoconus detection using the GALILEI dual Scheimpflug analyzer. Online training—Galilei—Applications—Keratoconus Screening and Detection III-2. Port, Switzerland: Ziemer Ophthalmic Systems AG. https://e-learning.ziemergroup.com/index.php?p=3.

37. Reddy JC, Rapuano CJ, Cater JR, Suri K, Nagra PK, Hammersmith KM. Comparative evaluation of dual Scheimpflug imaging parameters in keratoconus, early keratoconus, and normal eyes. *J Cataract Refract Surg.* 2014;40(4):582–592.

38. Feizi S, Yaseri M, Kheiri B. Predictive ability of Galilei to distinguish subclinical keratoconus and keratoconus from normal corneas. *J Ophthalmic Vis Res.* 2016;11(1):8–16. doi:10.4103/2008-322X.180707.

39. Shetty R, Rao H, Khamar P, et al. Keratoconus screening indices and their diagnostic ability to distinguish normal from ectatic corneas. *Am J Ophthalmol.* 2017;181:140–148.

40. Lewis JR, Frueh BE, Tappeiner C, Mahmoud AM, Roberts CJ. Keratoconus screening based on broader applications of CLMI algorithm. Paper presented at ARVO annual meeting, April 2011. *Invest Ophthalmol Vis Sci.* 2011;52(14):5167. https://iovs.arvojournals.org/article.aspx?articleid=2357710.

41. Smadja D, Santhiago MR, Mello GR, Krueger RR, Colin J, Touboul D. Influence of the reference surface shape for discriminating between normal corneas, subclinical keratoconus, and keratoconus. *J Refract Surg.* 2013;29:274–281.

42. Smadja D, Touboul D, Cohen A, et al. Detection of subclinical keratoconus using an automated decision tree classification. *Am J Ophthalmol.* 2013;156:237–246.

43. Arce CG, Francesconi CM. Topografia da córnea por varredura de fenda de luz — Orbscan I, II e IIZ. In: Ruiz-Alves M, Campos M, Ambrosio R Jr, Chamon W, Diniz CHR, eds. *Cirurgia Refrativa. Serie Oftalmológica Brasileira. Brazilian Council of Ophthamology.* 3rd ed. Rio de Janeiro, Brazil: Cultura Médica; 2013:71–86, sect B, chap 7C.

44. Ambrósio R, Alonso RS, Luz A. Coca Velarde LG. Corneal-thickness spatial profile and corneal-volume distribution: tomographic indices to detect keratoconus. *J Cataract Refract Surg.* 2006;32:1851–1859.

CHAPTER 17

Ocular Wavefront Analysis

Fernando Faria-Correia ▪ Jorge Haddad ▪ Renato Ambrósio Jr.

KEY CONCEPTS

- Wavefront sensing has renewed interest in understanding and correcting ocular irregularities and improving human visual acuity. The different systems used to analyze wavefront aberrations of the eye are classically divided into ingoing and outgoing systems.
- Each imaging device reconstructs Zernike terms differently, using smoothing functions from the acquired data. From the wavefront aberration data, mathematical calculations enable simulation of the appearance of the retinal image.
- The integration of total and corneal wavefront data improves diagnostic accuracy of keratoconus.
- The application of wavefront analysis in cases of corneal ectasia is unquestionably valuable for diagnosis, staging, and treatment planning.

Introduction

Along with corneal imaging, major advances in image enhancement within the field of astronomy were adopted by ophthalmology for enhancing optical analysis of the eye.[1] These concepts have been used to characterize refractive errors of the human eye using polynomial terms beyond sphere and cylinder, so that "irregular astigmatism" can be quantified and detailed. The difference between classical refraction, based on the sphere and cylinder, and wavefront aberrometry is analogous to the difference between keratometry and corneal topography. An understanding of the ocular wavefront has enabled a new era in customized refractive ablation techniques to improve optical results.[2,3] This chapter is focused on the clinical applications of ocular wavefront analysis for the evaluation of keratoconus (KC).

Understanding Wavefront Aberrations

In a "perfect" optical system, rays emanating from an object point are refracted to converge to the unique image point expected from Gaussian ray-tracing theory. If we consider divergent wavefront rays spreading out from the object to be changed by the optical system into convergent wavefront rays (such as the rays exiting the eye), in a "perfect" optical medium, the wavefronts will be perpendicular to the rays for any phase analyzed (Fig. 17.1A). However, if there are aberrations, the refracted rays no longer perfectly converge to the unique image point, and the wavefronts are no longer parallel to the rays (see Fig. 17.1B). The wavefront aberration is the distance, usually measured in micrometers (μm) between an actual wavefront and an ideal "perfect" plano wavefront measured at the pupil. This distance is a difference in the optical path, which is referenced to the center of the exit pupil of the system, where the wavefront aberration should be zero.[4]

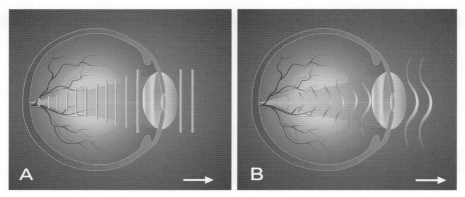

Fig. 17.1 Perfect optical system with a plano wavefront (A) and wavefront aberrations in a representation of a relatively normal eye (B).

Use of Zernike polynomial terms is recognized as the best method for the diagnostic characterization of wavefront aberrations (Fig. 17.2). The terms were developed by Frits Zernike (1888–1966).[1,4] The Zernike polynomials are used in geometry to describe mathematically best-fit curves. These equations function as building blocks to better describe the details of the wavefront shape. Therefore, more terms included in the equation, the better the fit. In optical terms, this means that the more Zernike terms that are calculated, the more completely the aberrations will be characterized. The degree of aberration is calculated with the root mean square (RMS) of difference between the real and ideal wavefront for every term. These terms can be combined or presented as an isolated RMS term. It is critical to understand that the larger the pupil diameter, the greater the amount of aberrations, which will increase the RMS (Fig. 17.3).[4]

Other mathematical methods use wavefront data for planning custom ablations, which have a potential benefit because of the limitations of Zernike's terms for describing very irregular shapes.[5] However, Zernike's polynomials excel in extracting clinically useful information for describing the wavefront aberrations of vision optics.[6–8] The lower order aberrations (LOAs) include the components zero (piston), one (tilt), and two (defocus and astigmatism) of the Zernike polynomials pyramid (see Fig. 17.2). The second order terms are the ones that can be corrected by glasses. The higher order aberrations (HOAs) are considered from the third order onward and represent irregular astigmatism. The third (coma and trefoil) and fourth (spherical aberrations) orders are the most important high order coefficients and have higher impact on the quality of vision in patients with corneal irregularities, including KC and other types of ectasia.

From the wavefront aberration data, we can calculate the point-spread function, as well as the modulation transfer function for the contrast, as a function of the spatial frequency. Mathematical calculations for determining image formation allow for simulating the appearance of the retinal image, which can be used, for example, for a Snellen letter of any chosen size (Fig. 17.4).[4,9]

Types of Wavefront Systems

Currently, there are several commercially available systems that analyze wavefront aberrations of the eye. These are classically divided into ingoing and outgoing systems.[4] *Ingoing* optical systems study the optical aberrations of a light beam projected onto the retina, such as the Tscherning aberrometer, which projects a grid, and the sequential retinal ray tracing of individual point scanning.[10] The scanning of individual points allows measurement in corneas with more pronounced optical distortions and is very useful in cases of KC. In the analysis of *outgoing* optics, the wavefront is

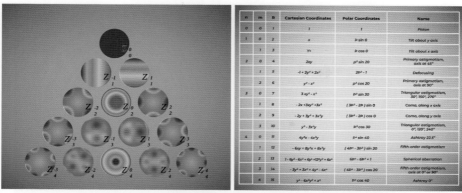

n	m	R	Cartesian Coordinates	Polar Coordinates	Name
0	0	1	1	1	Piston
1	0	2	x	$\rho \sin \theta$	Tilt about y axis
1	1	3	y	$\rho \cos \theta$	Tilt about x axis
2	0	4	2xy	$\rho^2 \sin 2\theta$	Primary astigmatism, axis at 45°
2	1	5	$-1+2y^2+2x^2$	$2\rho^2-1$	Defocusing
2	2	6	y^2-x^2	$\rho^2 \cos 2\theta$	Primary astigmatism, axis at 90°
3	0	7	$3xy^2-x^3$	$\rho^3 \sin 3\theta$	Triangular astigmatism, 30°, 150°, 270°
3	1	8	$-2x+3xy^2+3x^3$	$(3\rho^3-2\rho)\sin\theta$	Coma, along x axis
3	2	9	$-2y+3y^3+3x^2y$	$(3\rho^3-2\rho)\cos\theta$	Coma, along y axis
3	3	10	y^3-3x^2y	$\rho^3 \cos 3\theta$	Triangular astigmatism, 0°, 120° 240°
4	0	11	$4y^3x-4x^3y$	$\rho^4 \sin 4\theta$	Ashtray 22.5°
4	1	12	$-6xy+8y^3x+8x^3y$	$(4\rho^4-3\rho^2)\sin 2\theta$	Fifth-order astigmatism
4	2	13	$1-6y^2-6x^2+6y^4+12x^2y^2+6x^4$	$6\rho^4-6\rho^2+1$	Spherical aberration
4	3	14	$-3y^2+3x^2+4y^4-4x^4$	$(4\rho^4-3\rho^2)\cos 2\theta$	Fifth-order astigmatism, axis at 0° or 90°
4	4	15	$y^4-6x^2y^2+x^4$	$\rho^4 \cos 4\theta$	Ashtray 0°

Fig. 17.2 Zernike polynomial pyramid and equations.

assessed exiting the eye. A light beam is projected and reflected from the retina, exiting the eye, and is analyzed by a sensor such as the Hartmann-Shack, which is the most popular system available in commercial instruments.[11] One drawback of wavefront analysis for evaluating KC patients is that it is necessary to have a high dynamic range wavefront sensor to enable the optical analysis in more advanced cases. This measurement can be achieved by using a shorter focal length lenslet array in a Hartmann-Shack system. Dynamic skiascopy, which utilizes the scanning infrared slit refractometer, is another option.[12,13] Recently, pyramidal sensor wavefront analysis became available in the market (Osiris-T, Costruzione Strumenti Oftalmici, CSO, Florence, Italy). This system combines a corneal topographer with a total ocular aberrometer. This sensor design allows the aberrometer to measure aberrations with a resolution of 45,000 points (at the maximum pupil diameter), with a broad dynamic range.[14]

Corneal Wavefront Measurements

Polynomial mathematical calculations may also be used to describe front and back corneal elevation data from tomography systems, as well as front surface data from topography systems. The integration of wavefront data from the whole eye and from the cornea enables the characterization of the impact of distinct ocular elements in the overall optical property of the eye.[15] Using corneal aberrations to describe the optical quality of the cornea is highly relevant. The detection of KC based on Zernike coefficients from the corneal front surface was pioneered by Schwiegerling.[16] However, there are some discrepancies in the performance of such parameters to discriminate KC

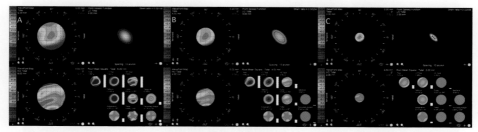

Fig. 17.3 Impact of the scanned pupil area (A) 6 mm, (B) 4 mm, and (C) 2 mm for calculating wavefront aberrations. The original scan was 7.44 mm, which enables calculation of the PSF Point Spread Function, root mean square, and all maps up to 2 mm.

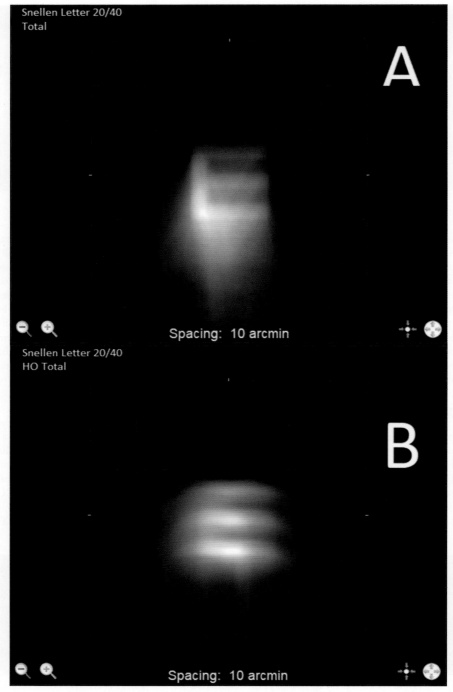

Fig. 17.4 Impact of total (A) and only the higher order aberrations (B) on the convolving simulated image of a Snellen E with 20/40 size.

from normal corneas. For example, Gobbe showed that the best detector to differentiate between suspected KC and normal corneas was vertical coma with a specificity of 71.9% and sensitivity of 89.3%.[17] Buhren and coworkers have successfully utilized first surface HOAs for diagnosing subclinical KC, with an area under the receiver operating characteristic curve (AUC) of 0.98.[18] However, it is important to note that each instrument will reconstruct Zernike terms differently, using smoothing functions from the acquired data.

Total Wavefront for Diagnosing Keratoconus

Maeda and coworkers reported corneal and ocular wavefront aberrations of normal and keratoconic eyes.[19] Thirty-five keratoconic eyes and 38 normal controls had HOAs in total refraction measured with the KR-9000 Analyzer (Topcon Corporation, Tokyo, Japan), which is a Hartmann-Shack sensor combined with a Placido disk–based topography. Significantly more total ocular HOAs were found in the KC eyes, such as coma, which was found to be 2.32 times more frequent than spherical-like aberrations in keratoconic eyes. In this study, wavefront sensing enabled not only evaluation of the quality of vision but also differentiation of KC eyes from normal eyes by analysis of the characteristics of the HOAs. In another prospective case-control study involving 55 eyes of 30 patients with KC and 100 eyes of 50 refractive surgery candidates, Miháltz and coworkers evaluated total wavefront aberrations with a Hartmann-Shack sensor.[20] The results revealed a statistically higher level of aberration in KC eyes compared with normal controls. The authors also described the changes in the axis of line of sight (LoS) among keratoconic patients. A significant displacement of the LoS was observed in these eyes, which relates to the position of the cone on topography and the vertical coma measured by aberrometry. Saad and Gatinel also investigated the application of anterior corneal and ocular aberrations in detecting mildly ectatic corneas.[21] The authors used the NIDEK Corneal Navigator System automated corneal classification software (NIDEK, Gamagori, Japan) to classify the patients. Corneal and ocular tilt, vertical coma, and trefoil were significantly different in the forme fruste keratoconus (FFKC) group when compared with the normal control group. The discriminating functions between the FFKC and the normal group, and between the KC and the normal group, reached an AUC of 0.98 and 0.96, respectively.

Ray-Tracing Aberrometry for Ectasia Diagnosis

We also performed a study to describe and compare the ocular and anterior corneal wavefront data derived from normal, KC, and FFKC eyes. The iTrace (Tracey Technologies, Houston, TX) was used for the wavefront analysis. The aberrometer uses the ray-tracing principle, which sequentially projects 256 near-infrared laser beams into the eye in a specific scanning pattern.[22,23] Topographies were captured using the Placido-based corneal topographer (EyeSys Vision LLC, Houston, TX) mounted on the same device. Demographic data for each group are presented in Table 17.1. The data from the Pentacam HR (OCULUS Optikgeräte GmbH, Wetzlar, Germany) were also used to classify these patients. The normal (N) group comprised 84 eyes randomly selected from 84 vision correction candidates. These patients presented unremarkable Scheimpflug tomography in both eyes (Ambrósio Relational Thickness Maximum [ART Max] greater than 400 microns; BAD [Belin Ambrósio Display] D value less than 1.60), based on previous reports. The Amsler-Krumeich KC (TKC) grading score, which is derived from the front corneal surface indices, was also null in these eyes. Fig. 17.5 illustrates a cornea with unremarkable topographic and tomographic findings on the Pentacam examination. The KC group included 70 eyes randomly selected from 70 patients who had bilateral KC. All eyes of this group presented a positive score on the TKC grading system. The FFKC group enrolled 31 topographically normal eyes of patients with clinical KC in the fellow eye (Figs. 17.6 and 17.7).[24–26]

TABLE 17.1 ■ Demographic Characteristics of Each Group

	N	KC	FFKC
Eyes (n)	84	70	31
Age (mean ± SD)	28.869 ± 6.655 [10; 40]	28.329 ± 6.814 [17; 41]	31.806 ± 7.968 [17; 45]
Sphere (D) [range]	−3.138 ± 3.683 [−11; 8.25]	−1.898 ± 3.482 [−13.25; 2.62]	−1.064 ± 2.632 [−10.12; 2.5]
Cylinder (D) [range]	−1.560 ± 1.399 [−5.75; 0]	−3.969 ± 2.181 [−9.12; −0.12]	−1.417 ± 1.288 [−4.12; −0.25]

FFKC, Forme fruste keratoconus; *KC*, keratoconus; *N*, normal.

The wavefront data were decomposed for only one pupil size (5.0 mm). Only the individual Zernike terms were selected for analysis, using the available data automatically extracted from each scan into an Excel spreadsheet (Microsoft Corporation, Redmond, Washington DC) by the software. Tables 17.2 and 17.3 display the cutoff values, the AUC, and the standard error 95% confidence intervals of the individual corneal and ocular Zernike coefficients that were statistically different between the N versus KC groups and N versus FFKC groups, respectively. The overall performance of using individual Zernike terms to identify KC and FFKC eyes was comparable to previous studies. Nevertheless, the differences in the AUC and cutoff values of the Zernike terms are justified by the methodology implemented in the studies, such as distinct scanning technology and patient selection criteria. Similar to previous reports, individual Zernike coefficients derived from the corneal topography demonstrated better performance than those derived from the total wavefront.[18,21]

To improve the detection of mild forms of ectasia, linear discriminant functions were created based on the N and FFKC groups' topography and ocular wavefront data. The function Ocular Coefficients (CO) included only ocular wavefront Zernike coefficients, the Corneal Coefficients (CC) was derived only from the anterior corneal Zernike terms, and the Corneal and Ocular Coefficients (CCO) enrolled the corneal and ocular Zernike coefficients. Regarding these functions, statistically significant differences were found between the three study groups ($P < 0.0001$ for all comparisons). The Corneal and Ocular Coefficients (CCO) obtained the best discriminant ability to separate the N and the FFKC groups (Table 17.4). Fig. 17.8 demonstrates graphically the receiver operating characteristic curves of all the discriminant functions. In the pairwise comparisons of the discriminant functions, there was a statistically significant difference between the Corneal and Ocular Coefficients (CCO) and the other two function models (Table 17.5). All three discriminant functions achieved an AUC higher than 0.9 for the differentiation between the N and KC groups (Table 17.6).

Impact of Wavefront Analysis in Refraction of Keratoconus

In a previous study, we described that ray-tracing wavefront analysis was also relevant in facilitating refraction in these patients.[27] In a retrospective chart review of 46 patients (89 eyes) with KC, we described a best-corrected distance visual acuity (BCVA) improvement in cases with some degree of contact lens intolerance. Fifty-two eyes (58.4%) of 28 patients showed improvement in BCVA with wavefront-based refraction (average improvement was 0,13 logMAR or 1,3 lines on Snellen chart).

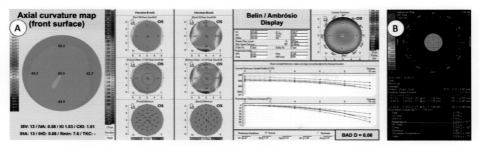

Figure 17.5   Representative case from a normal group with unremarkable topometric and tomographic examination (A) and related higher order aberrations map (B).

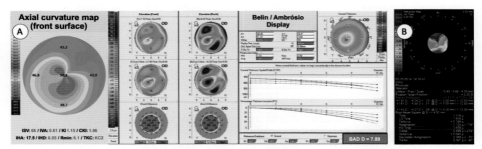

Fig. 17.6   Topometric and tomographic evaluation of keratoconus. The contralateral eye (Fig. 17.7) has no clinical or topometric signs of ectasia (A). Higher order aberrations map (B).

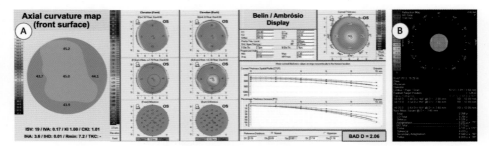

Fig. 17.7   Topometric and tomographic (A) and higher order aberrations (B) map evaluation of a forme fruste keratoconus (FFKC). The FFKC eye reveals relatively normal corneal topography and tomographic changes, which are indicative of susceptibility to corneal ectasia. The Amsler-Krumeich keratoconus (TKC) grading displayed a null score.

TABLE 17.2 ■ Data Summary From ROC Curves of the Individual Corneal and Ocular Zernike Coefficients That Were Statistically Different Between the N and KC Groups

Variable	Area Under the ROC Curve	Standard Error	95% Confidence Interval	Significance Level (P Value)
Corneal Zernike Coefficients				
ZC_1^{-1}	0.981	0.0107	0.945–0.996	0.0001
ZC_1^{1}	0.749	0.0388	0.673–0.816	0.0001
ZC_2^{-2}	0.879	0.0277	0.816–0.926	0.0001
ZC_2^{0}	0.661	0.0434	0.580–0.735	0.0002
ZC_2^{2}	0.660	0.0444	0.579–0.734	0.0003
ZC_3^{-3}	0.774	0.0385	0.700–0.838	0.0001
ZC_3^{-1}	0.984	0.00983	0.949–0.997	0.0001
ZC_3^{1}	0.759	0.0382	0.683–0.824	0.0001
ZC_3^{3}	0.699	0.0417	0.620–0.770	0.0001
ZC_4^{-4}	0.609	0.0452	0.527–0.686	0.0164
ZC_4^{-2}	0.837	0.0338	0.768–0.891	0.0001
ZC_4^{0}	0.708	0.0412	0.630–0.779	0.0001
ZC_4^{2}	0.743	0.0394	0.666–0.810	0.0001
ZC_4^{4}	0.661	0.0444	0.580–0.736	0.0003
ZC_5^{-3}	0.709	0.0415	0.630–0.780	0.0001
ZC_5^{-1}	0.887	0.0283	0.826–0.933	0.0001
ZC_5^{1}	0.653	0.0451	0.571–0.729	0.0007
ZC_5^{3}	0.671	0.0442	0.590–0.744	0.0001
ZC_5^{5}	0.645	0.0448	0.562–0.721	0.0012
ZC_6^{-6}	0.629	0.0476	0.543–0.710	0.0067
ZC_6^{-2}	0.670	0.0445	0.587–0.746	0.0001
ZC_6^{2}	0.710	0.0429	0.630–0.782	0.0001
ZC_6^{4}	0.645	0.0451	0.562–0.722	0.0013
Ocular Zernike Coefficients				
ZO_1^{-1}	0.896	0.0257	0.836–0.939	0.0001
ZO_1^{1}	0.637	0.0443	0.556–0.713	0.002
ZO_2^{-2}	0.837	0.032	0.769–0.892	0.0001
ZO_2^{2}	0.711	0.0422	0.632–0.781	0.0001
ZO_3^{-3}	0.651	0.0447	0.570–0.725	0.0008
ZO_3^{-1}	0.912	0.0236	0.855–0.951	0.0001
ZO_3^{1}	0.672	0.043	0.592–0.746	0.0001
ZO_3^{3}	0.778	0.0369	0.704–0.841	0.0001
ZO_4^{-4}	0.616	0.045	0.535–0.693	0.0097
ZO_4^{-2}	0.738	0.0408	0.661–0.806	0.0001
ZO_4^{2}	0.809	0.0344	0.738–0.868	0.0001
ZO_4^{4}	0.700	0.0429	0.621–0.771	0.0001
ZO_5^{3}	0.680	0.0437	0.600–0.753	0.0001
ZO_6^{2}	0.616	0.0457	0.534–0.693	0.0113

KC, Keratoconus; N, normal; ROC, receiver operating characteristic.

TABLE 17.3 ▪ Data Summary From ROC Curves of the Individual Corneal and Ocular Zernike Coefficients That Were Statistically Different Between the N and FFKC Groups

Variable	Area Under the ROC Curve	Standard Error	95% Confidence Interval	Significance Level (P Value)
Corneal Zernike Coefficients				
ZC_1^{-1}	0.75	0.0468	0.661–0.826	0.0001
ZC_3^{-1}	0.735	0.0482	0.645–0.813	0.0001
ZC_3^{3}	0.711	0.0503	0.619–0.792	0.0001
Ocular Zernike Coefficients				
ZO_4^{2}	0.695	0.0516	0.602–0.777	0.0002

FFKC, Forme fruste keratoconus; *N*, normal; *ROC*, receiver operating characteristic.

TABLE 17.4 ▪ Data Summary From ROC Curves of the Discriminant Functions for Differentiating the N and FFKC Groups

Variable	Area Under the ROC Curve	Standard Error	95% Confidence Interval	Significance Level (P Value)
CO	0.889	0.0298	0.817–0.940	0.0001
CC	0.915	0.0255	0.848–0.959	0.0001
CCO	0.980	0.0115	0.935–0.997	0.0001

FFKC, Forme fruste keratoconus; *N*, normal; *ROC*, receiver operating characteristic.

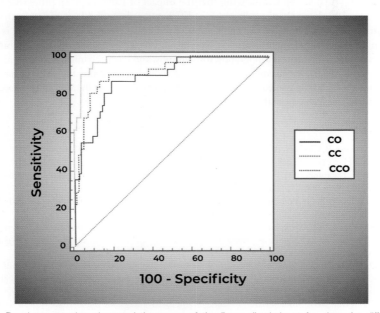

Fig. 17.8 Receiver operating characteristic curves of the linear discriminant functions for differentiation between the N and KC groups.

TABLE 17.5 ■ Pairwise Comparisons of the AUC for Discriminant Functions

	CO	CC	CCO
CO		0.490	0.001
CC			0.006
CCO			0.345 ± 0.284 [−0.506 − 0.752]

AUC, Area under the receiver operating characteristic curve.

TABLE 17.6 ■ Data Summary From ROC Curves of the Discriminant Functions for Differentiating the N and KC Groups

Variable	Area Under the ROC Curve	Standard Error	95% Confidence Interval	Significance Level (P Value)
CO	0.926	0.0215	0.873–0.962	0.0001
CC	0.947	0.0181	0.899–0.977	0.0001
CCO	0.970	0.0135	0.930–0.991	0.0001

KC, Keratoconus; *N,* normal; *ROC,* receiver operating characteristic.

Conclusion

Wavefront sensing has renewed interest in understanding and correcting HOAs of the eye to improve human visual acuity. Considering that the impact of KC on optical properties occurs as the result of corneal shape changes, diagnosis of KC based only on total wavefront analysis of the eye is relatively limited. However, the application of total wavefront in cases of ectasia is unquestionably valuable, to complement diagnosis, staging, and treatment planning. The combination of wavefront analysis with corneal topography, tomography, and biomechanical data may also enable a higher level of diagnostic accuracy. The clinician should understand the differences between these technologies, and the clinical guidelines for interpretation of the data should be used accordingly, specific to the instrumentation used.

References

1. Liang J, Grimm B, Goelz S, Bille JF. Objective measurement of wave aberrations of the human eye with the use of a Hartmann-Shack wave-front sensor. *J Opt Soc Am A Opt Image Sci Vis.* 1994;11:1949–1957.
2. Mrochen M, Kaemmerer M, Seiler T. Wavefront-guided laser in situ keratomileusis: early results in three eyes. *J Refract Surg.* 2000;16:116–121.
3. Netto MV, Dupps W Jr, Wilson SE. Wavefront-guided ablation: evidence for efficacy compared to traditional ablation. *Am J Ophthalmol.* 2006;141:360–368.
4. Ambrósio R Jr, Chalita MR, Netto MV, Schor P, Chamon W, Fontes BM. *Wavefront, Topografia, Tomografia e Biomecânica da Córnea e Segmento Anterior—Atualização Propedêutica em Cirurgia Refrativa.* 2nd ed. Rio de Janeiro, Brazil: Cultura Médica; 2013.
5. Koch DD, Wang L, Chernyak DA. Wavefront reconstruction methods. *J Refract Surg.* 2009;25:9–10.
6. Smolek MK, Klyce SD. Goodness-of-prediction of Zernike polynomial fitting to corneal surfaces. *J Cataract Refract Surg.* 2005;31:2350–2355.
7. Klyce SD, Karon MD, Smolek MK. Advantages and disadvantages of the Zernike expansion for representing wave aberration of the normal and aberrated eye. *J Refract Surg.* 2004;20:S537–S541.

8. Smolek MK, Klyce SD. Zernike polynomial fitting fails to represent all visually significant corneal aberrations. *Invest Ophthalmol Vis Sci.* 2003;44:4676–4681.

9. Applegate RA, Marsack JD, Ramos R, Sarver EJ. Interaction between aberrations to improve or reduce visual performance. *J Cataract Refract Surg.* 2003;29(8):1487–1495.

10. Mrochen M, Kaemmerer M, Mierdel P, Krinke HE, Seiler T. Principles of Tscherning aberrometry. *J Refract Surg.* 2000;16:S570–S571.

11. Thibos LN. Principles of Hartmann-Shack aberrometry. *J Refract Surg.* 2000;16:S563–S565.

12. McAlinden C, Moore JE. Higher order aberrations using the NIDEK OPD-Scan and AMO WaveScan. *J Refract Surg.* 2010;26:1–4.

13. Cervino A, Hosking SL. Montes-Mico R. Comparison of higher order aberrations measured by NIDEK OPD-Scan dynamic skiascopy and Zeiss WASCA Hartmann-Shack aberrometers. *J Refract Surg.* 2008;24:790–796.

14. Singh N, Jaskulski M, Ramasubramanian V, et al. Validation of a clinical aberrometer using pyramidal wavefront sensing. *Optom Vis Sci.* 2019;96(10):733–744.

15. Naseri A, McLeod SD, Lietman T. Evaluating the human optical system: corneal topography and wavefront analysis. *Ophthalmol Clin North Am.* 2001;14:269–273; vii.

16. Schwiegerling J, Greivenkamp JE. Keratoconus detection based on videokeratoscopic height data. *Optom Vis Sci.* 1996;73:721–728.

17. Gobbe M, Guillon M. Corneal wavefront aberration measurements to detect keratoconus patients. *Cont Lens Anterior Eye.* 2005;28:57–66.

18. Buhren J, Kuhne C, Kohnen T. Defining subclinical keratoconus using corneal first-surface higher-order aberrations. *Am J Ophthalmol.* 2007;143:381–389.

19. Maeda N, Fujikado T, Kuroda T, et al. Wavefront aberrations measured with Hartmann-Shack sensor in patients with keratoconus. *Ophthalmology.* 2002;109:1996–2003.

20. Miháltz K, Kránitz K, Kovács I, Takács A, Németh J, Nagy ZZ. Shifting of the line of sight in keratoconus measured by a Hartmann-Shack sensor. *Ophthalmology.* 2010;117:41–48.

21. Saad A, Gatinel D. Evaluation of total and corneal wavefront high order aberrations for the detection of forme fruste keratoconus. *Invest Ophthalmol Vis Sci.* 2012;53:2978–2992.

22. Molebny VV, Panagopoulou SI, Molebny SV, Wakil YS. Pallikaris IG. Principles of ray tracing aberrometry. *J Refract Surg.* 2000;16:S572–S575.

23. Faria-Correia F, Lopes B, Monteiro T, Franqueira N, Ambrósio R Jr. Scheimpflug lens densitometry and ocular wavefront aberrations in patients with mild nuclear cataract. *J Cataract Refract Surg.* 2016;42(3):405–411.

24. Ambrósio R Jr, Ramos I, Faria-Correia F, Luz A, Valbon BF. Scheimpflug imaging for laser refractive surgery. *Curr Opin Ophthalmol.* 2013;24(4):310–320.

25. Ambrósio R Jr, Ramos I, Lopes B, et al. Ectasia susceptibility before laser vision correction. *J Cataract Refract Surg.* 2015;41(6):1335–1336.

26. Ambrósio Jr R, Lopes B, Faria-Correia F, et al. Integration of Scheimpflug-based corneal tomography and biomechanical assessments for enhancing ectasia detection. *J Refract Surg.* 2017;33(7):434–443.

27. Ambrósio R Jr, Caldas DL, da Silva RS, Pimentel LN, Valbon BF. Impact of the wavefront analysis in refraction of keratoconus patients. *Rev Bras Oftalmol.* 2010;69(5):294–300.

CHAPTER 18

Epithelial Thickness Mapping for Keratoconus Screening by VHF Digital Ultrasound or Anterior Segment OCT

Dan Z. Reinstein ■ Timothy J. Archer ■ Ryan S. Vida

KEY CONCEPTS

- Epithelial thickness maps provide a higher sensitivity and specificity in the detection of keratoconus than topography and tomography alone.
- Epithelial thickness maps may help *identify* keratoconus in patients who have an otherwise *normal* topography/tomography.
- Epithelial thickness maps can be used to help *rule out* keratoconus in some patients with *equivocal* topography/tomography.
- Epithelial thickness maps are also essential for evaluating complex corneas in the assessment and therapeutic planning of refractive surgery.
- Epithelial thickness maps are becoming the gold standard in corneal laser refractive surgery for detecting or excluding keratoconus.

Introduction

Keratoconus is a progressive corneal disorder that manifests as corneal thinning and the formation of a cone-shaped protrusion. Because laser refractive surgery may lead to accelerated postoperative ectasia in patients with keratoconus,[1,2] the accurate detection of early keratoconus is a major safety concern. The reported prevalence of keratoconus in the Caucasian population is approximately 1/2000.[3] The incidence of undiagnosed keratoconus presenting to refractive surgery clinics tends to be much higher than this, as patients with keratoconus develop astigmatism that is more difficult to correct by contact lenses or glasses, leading them to consider refractive surgery.[4] The challenge for keratoconus screening is to have high sensitivity, combined with high specificity to minimize the number of atypical normal patients who are denied surgery.

Significant efforts have been made to develop methods for screening of early keratoconus over the last 30 years. In 1984 Klyce[5] introduced color-coded maps derived from computerized front surface Placido topography, which have made the diagnosis of keratoconus easier, as patterns including inferior steepening, asymmetric bow tie, and skew bow tie typical of keratoconus can be seen early in the progression of the disease.[6,7] Placido-based instruments producing maps of anterior surface topography and curvature became available by the early 1990s and their use in keratoconus screening was demonstrated.[7–16] Characterization of corneal thickness and topography of both corneal surfaces using scanning-slit tomography was introduced commercially in the mid-1990s by the Orbscan scanning-slit system (Bausch & Lomb, Rochester, NY)[17–19] and later by the

Pentacam rotating Scheimpflug-based system (OCULUS Optikgeräte, Wetzlar, Germany)[20,21] and other tomography scanners. Wavefront assessment[22] and biomechanical parameter evaluation with the Ocular Response Analyzer (Reichert, Depew, NY)[23] and Corvis ST (OCULUS Optikgeräte, Wetzlar, Germany)[24–26] have also been employed as means to detecting early keratoconus.

Topographic and tomographic evaluation has evolved from qualitative observation[7] to quantitative measurements, and many parameters have been described to aid the differentiation of normal from keratoconus eyes.[7–16] Several statistical and machine-based or computerized learning models have been employed for keratoconus detection, and automated systems for screening based on front and back surface topography and whole corneal tomography and pachymetric profile have been developed.[20,27–34]

Although these approaches have improved the effectiveness of keratoconus screening, there are still equivocal cases where a confident diagnosis cannot be made, and undiagnosed keratoconus probably remains the leading cause of corneal ectasia after LASIK.[35–47] The addition of quantitative parameters that are independent of those now obtained by topographic and tomographic analysis could potentially improve screening.

The corneal epithelial and stromal thickness profiles may represent such an independent parameter and will be the focus of this chapter. As will be described later, the corneal epithelium has the ability to alter its thickness profile to reestablish a smooth, symmetrical optical outer corneal surface and either partially or totally mask the presence of an irregular stromal surface from front surface topography.[48,49] Therefore the epithelial thickness profile would be expected to follow a distinctive pattern in keratoconus to partially compensate for the cone.

History of the Measurement of Epithelial Thickness

The first real measurement of the epithelium in vivo was made in 1979 by Holden and Payor using optical pachymetry.[50] In 1993[51] we started measuring epithelial thickness using very-high-frequency (VHF) digital ultrasound and published a 3-mm diameter map in 1994.[52–55] By 2000 this method had been improved to generate a 10-mm map.[48,56–72] VHF digital ultrasound was further developed and is now commercially available as the Artemis Insight 100 VHF digital ultrasound arc-scanner (ArcScan Inc, Golden, CO), which has been previously described in detail.[52,56,59]

During the 1990s, optical pachymetry was used for a number of studies measuring epithelial thickness.[73–75] Epithelial thickness was studied using histology from 1992,[76–79] Moller-Pedersen et al.[80–82] started using confocal microscopy in 1997, and optical coherence tomography (OCT) was first used for measuring the epithelium in 2001.[83–86] Epithelial thickness maps in an 8-mm diameter using OCT were published by Haque et al. in 2008,[87] followed Li et al. in 2012,[88] and are now commercially available using the RTVue/Avanti OCT (Optovue, Fremont, CA). Since then, other OCT devices have been developed that include epithelial thickness mapping, such as the MS-39 OCT (CSO, Florence, Italy) and Cirrus HD-OCT (Carl Zeiss Meditec, Jena, Germany).

EPITHELIAL THICKNESS PROFILE IN NORMAL EYES

Before looking at more complicated situations, it is useful to consider the epithelial thickness profile in a population of 110 normal eyes.[59] We have demonstrated using VHF digital ultrasound that the epithelium is not a layer of homogeneous thickness as had previously been thought but follows a very distinct pattern. On average, the epithelium was 5.7 μm thicker inferiorly than superiorly and 1.2 μm thicker nasally than temporally, with a mean central thickness of 53.4 μm (Fig. 18.1). The average central epithelial thickness was 53.4 μm and the standard deviation was only 4.6 μm.[59] This indicated that there was little variation in central epithelial thickness in the population. The thinnest epithelial point within the central 5 mm of the cornea was displaced on average 0.33 mm (±1.08 mm) temporally and 0.90 mm (±0.96 mm) superiorly with reference to

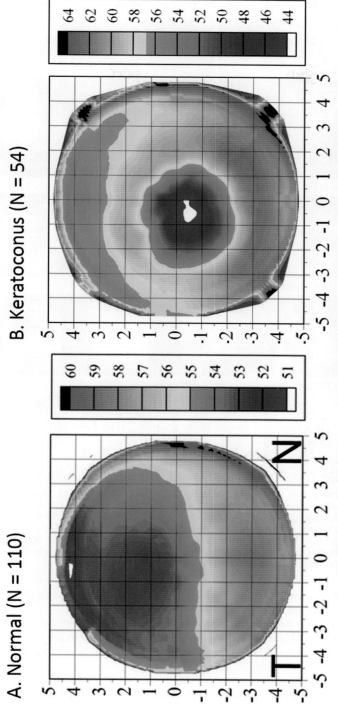

Fig. 18.1 Mean epithelial thickness profile for a population of 110 normal eyes (A) and a population of 54 keratoconic eyes (B). The epithelial thickness profiles for all eyes in each population were averaged using mirrored left eye symmetry. The color scale represents epithelial thickness in microns. A Cartesian 1-mm grid is superimposed with the origin at the corneal vertex. (Reprinted with permission from SLACK Incorporated: Reinstein DZ, Gobbe M, Archer TJ, Silverman RH, Coleman DJ. Epithelial, stromal, and total corneal thickness in keratoconus: three-dimensional display with Artemis very-high frequency digital ultrasound. *J Refract Surg.* 2010;26(4):259–271.)

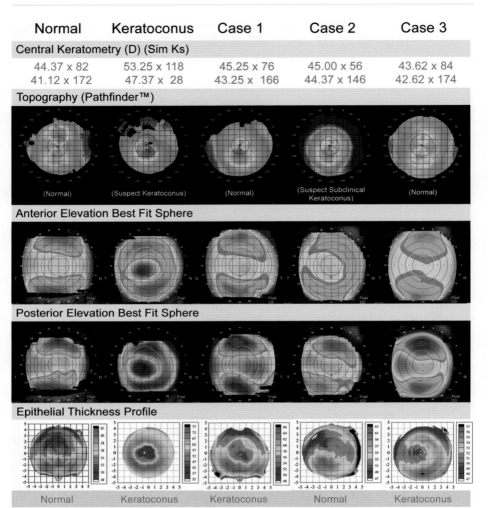

Normal	Keratoconus	Case 1	Case 2	Case 3
Central Keratometry (D) (Sim Ks)				
44.37 x 82	53.25 x 118	45.25 x 76	45.00 x 56	43.62 x 84
41.12 x 172	47.37 x 28	43.25 x 166	44.37 x 146	42.62 x 174

Fig. 18.2 Central keratometry, Atlas corneal topography and PathFinder corneal analysis, Orbscan anterior and posterior elevation best-fit-sphere, and Artemis epithelial thickness profile for one normal eye, one keratoconic eye, and three example eyes where the diagnosis of keratoconus might be misleading from topography. The final diagnosis based on the epithelial thickness profile is shown at the bottom of each example. (Reprinted with permission from SLACK Incorporated: Reinstein DZ, Gobbe M, Archer TJ, Silverman RH, Coleman DJ. Epithelial, stromal, and total corneal thickness in keratoconus: three-dimensional display with Artemis very-high frequency digital ultrasound. *J Refract Surg.* 2010;26(4):259–271.)

the corneal vertex. Studies using OCT have confirmed this superior-inferior and nasal-temporal asymmetric profile for epithelial thickness in normal eyes.[88]

Fig. 18.2, column 1 shows the keratometry, Atlas 995 (Carl Zeiss Meditec, Jena, Germany) corneal topography map and PathFinder corneal analysis, Orbscan II (software version 3.00) anterior elevation best-fit-sphere (BFS), Orbscan II posterior elevation BFS, and Artemis epithelial thickness profile of a normal eye.

This normal non-uniformity seems to provide evidence that the epithelial thickness is regulated by eyelid mechanics and blinking, as we suggested in 1994.[51] The eyelid might effectively be chafing the surface epithelium during blinking, and the posterior surface of the semirigid tarsus provides a template for the outer shape of the epithelial surface. During blinking, which occurs on average between 300 and 1500 times per hour,[89] the vertical traverse of the upper lid is much greater than that of the lower lid. Doane[90] studied the dynamics of eyelid anatomy during blinking and found that during a blink the descent of the upper eyelid reaches its maximum speed at about the time it crosses the visual axis. As a consequence, it is likely that the eyelid applies more force on the superior cornea than inferior cornea. Similarly, the friction on the cornea during lid closure is likely to be greater temporally than nasally as the outer canthus is higher than the inner canthus (mean intercanthal angle = 3 degrees), and the temporal portion of the lid is higher than the nasal lid (mean upper lid angle = 2.7 degrees).[91] Therefore, it seems that the nature of the eyelid completely explains the nonuniform epithelial thickness profile of a normal eye.

Further evidence for this theory is provided by the epithelial thickness changes observed in orthokeratology.[63] In orthokeratology, a shaped contact lens is placed on the cornea overnight that sits tightly on the cornea centrally but leaves a gap in the midperiphery. Therefore the natural template provided by the posterior surface of the semirigid tarsus of the eyelid is replaced by an artificial contact lens template designed to fit tightly to the center of the cornea and loosely paracentrally. We found significant epithelial thickness changes with central thinning and mid-peripheral thickening showing that the epithelium had remodeled according to the template provided by the contact lens, that is, the epithelium is chafed and squashed by the lens centrally whereas the epithelium is free to thicken paracentrally where the lens is not so tightly fitted.

EPITHELIAL THICKNESS PROFILE IN KERATOCONIC EYES

It is well known that the epithelial thickness changes in keratoconus as extreme steepening leads to epithelial breakdown, as is often seen clinically. Epithelial thinning over the cone has been demonstrated using histopathologic analysis of keratoconic corneas by Scroggs and Proia[92] and later using custom software and a Humphrey-Zeiss OCT system (Humphrey Systems, Dublin, CA) by Haque et al.[93]

We have characterized the in vivo epithelial thickness profile in a population of 54 eyes with keratoconus.[64] The average epithelial thickness profile in keratoconus revealed significantly greater irregularity compared with a normal population. The epithelium was thinnest at the apex of the cone and this thin epithelial zone was surrounded by an annulus of thickened epithelium (see Fig. 18.1). Whereas all eyes exhibited the same epithelial doughnut pattern, characterized by a localized central zone of thinning surrounded by an annulus of thick epithelium, the thickness values of the thinnest point and the thickest point as well as the difference in thickness between the thinnest and thickest epithelium varied greatly between eyes. There was a statistically significant correlation between the thinnest epithelium and the steepest keratometry (D), indicating that as the cornea became steeper, the epithelial thickness minimum became thinner. In addition, there was a statistically significant correlation between the thickness of the thinnest epithelium and the difference in thickness between the thinnest and thickest epithelium. This indicated that as the epithelium thinned, there was an increase in the irregularity of the epithelial thickness profile, that is, there was an increase in the severity of the keratoconus. The location of the thinnest epithelium within the central 5 mm of the cornea was displaced on average 0.48 mm (±0.66 mm) temporally and 0.32 mm (±0.67 mm) inferiorly with reference to the corneal vertex. The mean epithelial thickness for all eyes was 45.7 ± 5.9 μm (range: 33.1–56.3 μm) at the corneal vertex, 38.2 ± 5.8 μm (range: 29.6–52.4 μm) at the thinnest point, and 66.8 ± 7.2 μm (range: 54.1–94.4 μm) at the thickest point.[64]

Fig. 18.2, column 2 shows the keratometry, Atlas 995 corneal topography map and PathFinder corneal analysis, Orbscan II anterior elevation BFS, Orbscan II posterior elevation BFS, and Artemis epithelial thickness profile of a keratoconic eye. As expected, the front surface topography shows inferotemporal steepening with steep average keratometry and high astigmatism; the anterior and posterior elevation BFS maps demonstrate that the apex of the cone is located inferotemporally; the epithelial thickness profile shows epithelial thinning at the apex of the cone surrounded by an annulus of thicker epithelium. The steepest cornea coincides with the apex of the anterior and posterior elevation BFS as well as with the location of the thinnest epithelium.

Recently, the MS-39 OCT device has been introduced, which combines Placido topography with OCT scanning. This enables the MS-39 to simultaneously capture front surface topography and pachymetry data, producing epithelial thickness, corneal thickness, front surface topography, and back surface elevation maps that are all registered to the same measurement location (Fig. 18.3). This greatly helps to assess coincidence between these maps.

The epithelial thickness profile for keratoconus as described here has been confirmed by studies using OCT.[88,94–96] The study by Sandali et al.[96] elegantly described the different stages of advanced keratoconus, demonstrating that as keratoconus moves into its latter stages, a very different epithelial thickness profile becomes apparent. In advanced keratoconus, there is stromal loss often in the location of the cone, for example, because of hydrops. This means that rather than the cone being elevated relative to the rest of the stroma, this region is now a depression. Therefore, the epithelium changes from being thinnest over the cone to being thickest in this region, as it is compensating for a depression instead of an elevation (see next section). Stromal loss in such advanced keratoconus can be significant, so the epithelium can be as thick as 200 μm in some cases. Examples of this epithelial thickening were also reported by Rocha et al.[94] who concluded that focal central epithelial thinning was suggestive but not pathognomonic for keratoconus (i.e., the presence of an epithelial doughnut pattern did not prove beyond any doubt that an eye has keratoconus). However, as described by Sandali et al., these cases only appear in very advanced keratoconus, which means that they are of no interest with respect to keratoconus screening. Eyes with early keratoconus will never present with epithelial thickening in the location of the cone, as by definition if there has been stromal loss, the keratoconus must be more advanced and the cornea will be obviously abnormal.

Understanding the Predictable Behavior of the Corneal Epithelium

Epithelial thickness changes in keratoconus provide another example of the very predictable mechanism of the corneal epithelium to compensate for irregularities on the stromal surface. Epithelial thickness changes have also been described after myopic excimer laser ablation,[60,70,74,97] hyperopic excimer laser ablation,[66] radial keratotomy,[69] intracorneal ring segments,[57] irregularly irregular astigmatism after corneal refractive surgery,[48,55,72,98–100] and in ectasia.[67]

In all these cases, the epithelial thickness changes are clearly a compensatory response to the change to the stromal surface and can all be explained by the theory of eyelid template regulation of epithelial thickness.[49] Compensatory epithelial thickness changes can be summarized by the following rules:

1. The epithelium thickens in areas where tissue has been removed or the curvature has been flattened (e.g., central thickening after myopic ablation[60,70,74] or radial keratotomy[69] and peripheral thickening after hyperopic ablation[66]).
2. The epithelium thins over regions that are relatively elevated or the curvature has been steepened (e.g., central thinning in keratoconus,[64,88,94–96] ectasia,[67] and after hyperopic ablation[66]).
3. The magnitude of epithelial changes correlates to the magnitude of the change in curvature (e.g., more epithelial thickening after higher myopic ablation,[60,74,97] after higher hyperopic ablation,[66] and in more advanced keratoconus[64,88,94–96]).
4. The amount of epithelial remodeling is defined by the rate of change of curvature of an irregularity[49,101]; there will be more epithelial remodeling for a more localized irregularity.[48,72,98–100] The epithelium effectively acts as a low pass filter, smoothing local changes

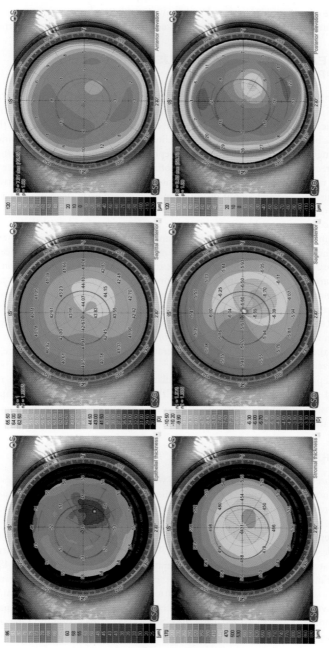

Fig. 18.3 MS-39 (CSO, Florence, Italy) six-map display showing a patient with mild keratoconus demonstrating correspondence between epithelial thinning, pachymetric thinning, curvature, and elevation maps.

(high curvature gradient) almost completely, but only partially smoothing global changes (low curvature gradient). For example, there is almost twice as much epithelial thickening after a hyperopic ablation[66] compared with a myopic ablation,[60,74,97] and there is almost total epithelial compensation for small, very localized stromal loss such as after a corneal ulcer.[66]

DIAGNOSING EARLY KERATOCONUS USING EPITHELIAL THICKNESS PROFILES

Mapping of the epithelial thickness reveals a very distinct thickness profile in keratoconus compared with that of normal corneas, owing to the compensatory mechanism of the epithelium for stromal irregularities. The epithelial thickness profile changes with the progression of the disease. As the keratoconus becomes more severe, the epithelium at the apex of the cone becomes thinner, and the surrounding annulus of epithelium in the epithelial doughnut pattern becomes thicker. Therefore the degree of epithelial abnormality in both directions (thinner and thicker than normal) can be used to confirm or exclude a diagnosis of keratoconus in eyes suggestive but not conclusive of a diagnosis of keratoconus on topography at a very early stage in the expression of the disease.[61]

In early keratoconus, we would expect to see the pattern of localized epithelial thinning surrounded by an annulus of thick epithelium coincident with a suspected cone on posterior elevation BFS. The coincidence of epithelial thinning together with an eccentric posterior elevation BFS apex may reveal whether to ascribe significance to an eccentric posterior elevation BFS apex occurring *concurrently with* a normal front surface topography. In other words, in the presence of normal or questionable front surface topography, thinning of the epithelium coincident with the location of the posterior elevation BFS apex would represent total masking or compensation for a subsurface stromal cone that *does* represent keratoconus (see Fig. 18.2). Conversely, finding thicker epithelium over an area of topographic steepening or an eccentric posterior elevation BFS apex would imply that the steepening is *not* due to a keratoconic subsurface stromal cone, but more likely due to localized epithelial thickening.

Evaluation of epithelial thickness profile irregularities provides a very sensitive method of examining stromal surface topography—by proxy. Therefore epithelial thickness mapping provides increased sensitivity and specificity to a diagnosis of keratoconus and, in many cases, before there is any detectable corneal front surface topographic change.

Case Examples

Fig. 18.2 shows three further selected examples in which epithelial thickness profiles helped to interpret and diagnose anterior and posterior elevation BFS abnormalities. In each case, the epithelial thickness profile appears to be able to differentiate cases in which the diagnosis of keratoconus is uncertain, from normal.[61]

Case 1 (OS) represents a 25-year-old male, with a manifest refraction of −1.00 −0.50 × 150 and a best spectacle-corrected visual acuity of 20/16. Atlas corneal topography demonstrated inferior steepening that would traditionally indicate keratoconus. The keratometry was 45.25/43.25 D × 76, and PathFinder corneal analysis classified the topography as normal. Orbscan II posterior elevation BFS showed that the posterior elevation BFS apex was decentered inferotemporally. Corneal pachymetry minimum by handheld ultrasound was 479 μm. Contrast sensitivity was slightly below the normal range measured using the CSV-1000 (Vector Vision Inc, Greenville, OH). There was −0.30 μm (OSA notation) of vertical coma on WASCA aberrometry. Corneal hysteresis was 7.5 mmHg and corneal resistance factor was 7.1 mmHg, which are low, but these could be affected by the low corneal thickness. The combination of inferior steepening, an eccentric posterior elevation BFS apex, and thin cornea raised the suspicion of keratoconus although there was no suggestion of keratoconus by refraction, keratometry, or PathFinder corneal analysis. Artemis epithelial thickness profile showed a pattern typical of keratoconus with an epithelial doughnut shape characterized by a localized zone of epithelial thinning displaced inferotemporally over the eccentric posterior elevation BFS apex, surrounded by an annulus of thick epithelium. The coincidence of an area of epithelial thinning with the apex of the posterior elevation BFS, as well as the increased irregularity of the epithelium, confirmed the diagnosis of early keratoconus.

Case 2 (OD) represents a 31-year-old female, with a manifest refraction of −2.25 −0.50 × 88 and a best spectacle-corrected visual acuity of 20/16. Atlas corneal topography demonstrated a very similar pattern to case 1 of inferior steepening, therefore suggesting that the eye could also be keratoconic. The keratometry was 44.12/44.75 D × 148, and PathFinder corneal analysis classified the topography as suspect subclinical keratoconus. Orbscan II posterior elevation BFS showed that the apex was slightly decentered nasally. Corneal pachymetry minimum by handheld ultrasound was 538 μm. Contrast sensitivity was in the normal range. There was 0.32 μm (OSA notation) of vertical coma on WASCA aberrometry. Corneal hysteresis was 10.1 mmHg and corneal resistance factor was 9.8 mmHg, which are well within normal range. The combination of inferior steepening, against-the-rule astigmatism, and high degree of vertical coma raised the suspicion of keratoconus, which was also noted by PathFinder corneal analysis. Artemis epithelial thickness profile showed a typical normal pattern with thicker epithelium inferiorly and thinner epithelium superiorly. Thicker epithelium inferiorly over the suspected cone (inferior steepening on topography) was inconsistent with an underlying stromal surface cone, and therefore the diagnosis of keratoconus was excluded. This patient would have been rejected for surgery given a documented PathFinder corneal analysis warning of suspect subclinical keratoconus, but given the epithelial thickness profile, this patient was deemed a suitable candidate for LASIK.

The anterior corneal topography in case 3 (OD) bears no features related to keratoconus. The patient is a 35-year-old female with a manifest refraction of −4.25 −0.50 × 4 and a best spectacle-corrected visual acuity of 20/16. The refraction had been stable for at least 10 years, and the contrast sensitivity was within normal limits. The keratometry was 43.62/42.62 D × 74 and PathFinder analysis classified the topography as normal. Orbscan II posterior elevation BFS showed that the apex was slightly decentered inferotemporally, but the anterior elevation BFS apex was well centered. Corneal pachymetry minimum by handheld ultrasound was 484 μm. Pentacam (OCULUS, Wetzlar, Germany) keratoconus screening indices were normal. WASCA ocular higher-order aberrations were low (RMS = 0.19 μm), as was the level of vertical coma (coma = 0.066 μm). Corneal hysteresis was 8.9 mmHg and corneal resistance factor was 8.8 mmHg, both within normal limits. In this case, only the slightly eccentric posterior elevation BFS apex and the low-normal corneal thickness were suspicious for keratoconus, whereas all other screening methods gave no indication of keratoconus. However, the epithelial thickness profile showed an epithelial doughnut pattern characterized by localized epithelial thinning surrounded by an annulus of thick epithelium, coincident with the eccentric posterior elevation BFS apex. Epithelial thinning with surrounding annular thickening over the eccentric posterior elevation BFS apex indicated the presence of probable subsurface keratoconus. In this case, it seems that the epithelium had fully compensated for the stromal surface irregularity so that the anterior surface topography of the cornea appeared perfectly regular. Given the regularity of the front surface topography and the normality of nearly all other screening parameters, it is feasible that this patient could have been deemed suitable for corneal refractive surgery and subsequently developed ectasia. As we were able to also consider the epithelial thickness profile, this patient was rejected for corneal refractive surgery. This kind of case may explain some reported cases of ectasia "without a cause."[102]

Fig. 18.4 shows an example of early keratoconus in which the front surface topography and Pentacam tomography appear normal; however, the epithelial thickness profile demonstrates focal thinning that is identified as keratoconus by this automated algorithm.

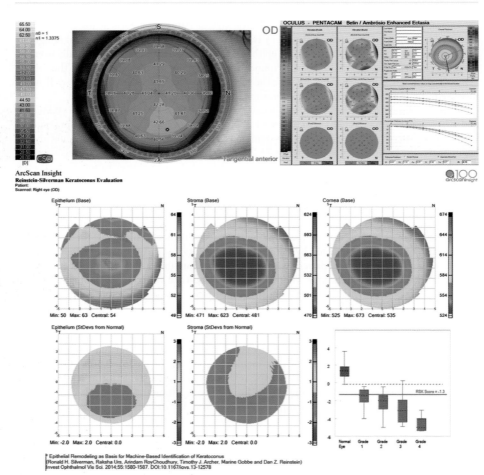

Fig. 18.4 MS-39 *(top left)* shows a relatively normal corneal curvature with a slight superior to inferior difference in keratometry. The corresponding Pentacam Belin/Ambrósio Display *(top right)* shows a normal front and back surface elevation. The ArcScan Insight 100 shows an area of epithelial thinning with surrounding thickening. This is further highlighted in the *bottom left* map, which shows the thickness standard deviations from the normal population. The epithelial map confirms that despite the topography and tomography findings, the patient has keratoconus.

Automated Algorithm for Classification by Epithelium

Based on this qualitative diagnostic method, we set out to derive an automated classifier to detect keratoconus using epithelial thickness data, together with Silverman et al. at Columbia University.[103] We used stepwise linear discriminant analysis (LDA) and neural network (NN) analysis to develop multivariate models based on combinations of 161 features comparing a population of 130 normal and 74 keratoconic eyes. This process resulted in a six-variable model that provided an area under the receiver operating curve of 100%, indicative of complete separation of keratoconic from normal corneas. Test-set performance averaged over 10 trials gave a specificity of 99.5% ± 1.5% and sensitivity of 98.9% ± 1.9%. Maps of the average epithelium and LDA function values were also found to be well correlated with keratoconus severity grade (Figs. 18.5 and 18.6). Other

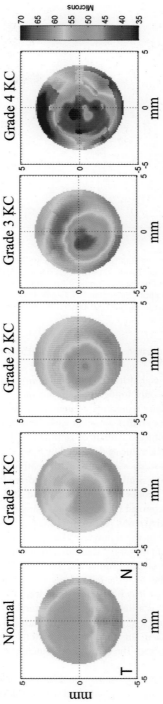

Fig. 18.5 Epithelial thickness maps averaged over all normal corneas and for each keratoconus grade. The departure from the normal epithelial distribution is evident even in grade 1 keratoconus, but becomes more obvious with severity. (Reprinted with permission from IOVS: Silverman RH, Urs R, Roychoudhury A, Archer TJ, Gobbe M, Reinstein DZ. Epithelial remodeling as basis for machine-based identification of keratoconus. *Invest Ophthalmol Vis Sci.* 2014;55(3):1580–1587.) *KC,* Keratoconus.

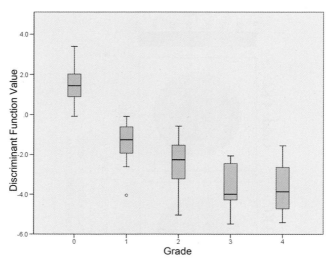

Fig. 18.6 Box and whisker plot of discriminant function value versus keratoconus severity grade. Grade 0 represents normal subjects. Grades 1 to 4 are based on Krumeich classification. Boxes represent ±1 quartile about median value *(horizontal line)*, and whiskers represent full range of values for each group. *Circles* indicate outliers. (Reprinted with permission from Silverman RH, Urs R, Roychoudhury A, Archer TJ, Gobbe M, Reinstein DZ. Epithelial remodeling as basis for machine-based identification of keratoconus. *Invest Ophthalmol Vis Sci.* 2014;55(3):1580–1587.)

groups have also been working on automated classification algorithms based on epithelial thickness data obtained by OCT.[88,104]

Following this study, we applied the algorithm to a population of 10 patients with unilateral keratoconus (clinically and algorithmically topographically normal in the fellow eyes), on the basis that the fellow eye in such patients represents a latent form of keratoconus, and, as such, has been considered a gold standard for studies aimed at early keratoconus detection. These eyes were also analyzed using the Belin-Ambrósio Enhanced Ectasia Display (BAD-D parameter and ART_{max})[20,27,105] and the Orbscan SCORE value as described by Saad and Gatinel.[31–33]

The most interesting finding of this study was that more than 50% of the fellow eyes were classified as normal by all methods. This was similar to the result reported by Bae et al.,[29] who found no difference in the BAD-D or ART_{max} values between normal and topographically normal fellow eyes of keratoconus patients. This is in contrast to other studies using unilateral keratoconus populations in which a much higher sensitivity was reported. However, these studies often included patients with a suspicious topography in the fellow eye (i.e., some studies use a more rigorous definition of unilateral keratoconus than others).[30] Therefore, the main conclusion from the study was to put into question the validity of using unilateral keratoconus patients for keratoconus screening studies. The fact that a number of these fellow eyes showed absolutely no indication of keratoconus by any method implies that it is likely that these were truly normal eyes. However, it is generally agreed that keratoconus as a disease must be bilateral.[106] Therefore it appears that these cases are patients who do not have keratoconus but have induced an ectasia in one eye, for example, by eye rubbing or trauma. This means that using "unilateral keratoconus" populations to study keratoconus screening may be flawed. The significant influence of eye rubbing is becoming increasingly apparent.[107]

The alternative is somewhat more alarming, as this would mean that there are eyes with keratoconus that are literally undetectable by any existing method. This would, however, explain any case of "ectasia without a cause."[102,108] Detection of keratoconus in such cases may require development of new in vivo measurements of corneal biomechanics, although this appears to be outside the scope of current methods such as the Ocular Response Analyzer[24,25,109] and Corvis[24,25] owing to the wide scatter in the data acquired. Another factor, as has been described using Brillouin micros-copy,[110] may be that the biomechanical tensile strength of the cornea may not be different from normal in early keratoconus when measuring the whole cornea globally, but there may only be a difference in the region localized of the cone (or in the location of a future cone). Another poten-tial and final solution would be whether a genotype or other molecular marker for keratoconus could be found.[111–113]

Finally, another interpretation of this result is that keratoconus may not necessarily be a disease of abnormal stromal substance. The localization of the reduced corneal biomechanics found in ker-atoconus suggests that this may be caused by a local defect in Bowman's layer owing to eye rubbing or other trauma. A break in Bowman's layer would reduce the tension locally and the asymmetric stress concentration would then cause the stroma to bulge in this location. Evidence for changes in Bowman's layer in keratoconus has been reported using ultrahigh resolution OCT. Abou Shousha et al.[114] showed that Bowman's layer was thinner inferiorly in keratoconus and described a Bow-man's ectasia index (BEI) to use for keratoconus screening. Yadav et al.[115] also described differences in the thickness of Bowman's layer in keratoconus, as well as a difference in light scatter.

Factors Influencing the Epithelium

Although the epithelium is the most sensitive method for detecting very early keratoconus, it is important to recognize some other factors that may affect the epithelial pattern. Epithelial changes associated with anterior basement membrane dystrophy (ABMD) may cause focal areas of a thickening that can be identified on clinical slit-lamp examination. These clinical findings will often have corresponding changes in the epithelial thickness map (Fig. 18.7). If there is paracen-tral thickening, the epithelial thickness profile can resemble a keratoconus pattern, as can be seen in Fig. 18.8. In addition to ABMD, dry eye can also affect the epithelium. Kanellopoulos and Asi-mellis[116] found the central epithelial thickness in dry eye patients to be 59.5 ± 4.2 μm compared with 53.0 ± 2.7 μm in the control group. Fig. 18.9 shows an extreme example of this in a patient who had an episode of Bell's palsy resulting in an incomplete blink. The right eye epithelium thickened by 14 μm centrally during the episode and subsequently returned to normal to match the left eye once blinking function recovered.

Conclusion

Keratoconus detection is ever evolving. We have demonstrated that the epithelial thickness pro-file was significantly different between normal eyes and keratoconic eyes. Whereas the epithe-lium in normal eyes was relatively homogeneous in thickness with a pattern of slightly thicker epithelium inferiorly than superiorly, the epithelium in keratoconic eyes was irregular, showing a doughnut-shaped pattern and a marked difference in thickness between the thin epithelium at the center of the doughnut and the surrounding annulus of thick epithelium. We have shown that the epithelial thickness profile progresses with the evolution of keratoconus. More advanced keratoconus produces greater irregularity in the epithelial thickness profile. We have found that the distinctive epithelial doughnut pattern associated with keratoconus can be used to confirm or exclude the presence of an underlying stromal surface cone in cases with normal or suspect front surface topography, as well as be a "qualifier" for the finding of an eccentric posterior elevation BFS apex.

Knowledge of the differences in epithelial thickness profile between the normal population and the keratoconic population allowed us to identify several features of the epithelial thickness profile that might help to discriminate between normal eyes and keratoconus suspect eyes.

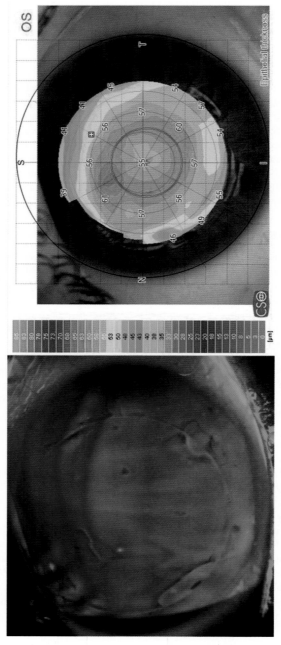

Fig. 18.7 Slit-lamp photograph under heavy fluorescein staining showing focal anterior basement membrane dystrophy *(left)* and the associated thickening seen on the MS-39 epithelial map *(right)*.

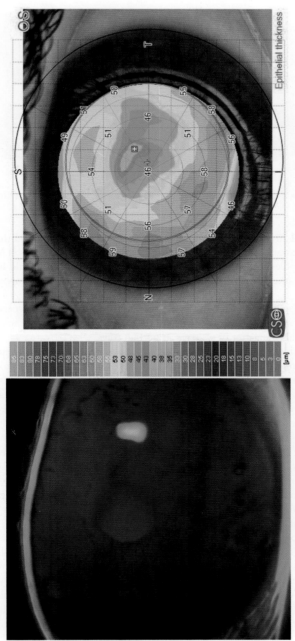

Fig. 18.8 Slit-lamp photography under heavy fluorescein staining showing diffuse anterior basement membrane dystrophy (*left*) and the associated thickening seen on the MS-39 epithelial map (*right*). The epithelial pattern mimics that seen in keratoconus with an area of central thinning, surrounding by thickening.

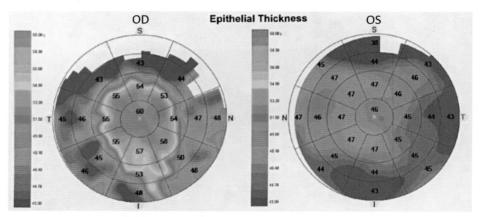

Fig. 18.9 Cirrus HD-OCT epithelial thickness map showing thickening in the right eye owing to decreased blinking ability during a Bell's palsy episode. The left eye epithelial thickness is normal. *OD*, right eye; *OS*, left eye.

Randleman et al., in their paper assessing risk factors for ectasia, reported that ectasia might still occur after uncomplicated surgery in appropriately screened candidates.[36] Mapping of epithelial thickness profiles might provide an explanation for these cases; it could be that a stromal surface cone was masked by epithelial compensation and the front surface topography appeared normal.

Mapping of the epithelial thickness profile may increase sensitivity and specificity of screening for keratoconus compared with current conventional corneal topographic screening alone and may be useful in clinical practice in two very important ways.

First, epithelial thickness mapping can exclude the appropriate patients by detecting keratoconus earlier or confirming keratoconus in cases where topographic changes may be clinically judged as being "within normal limits." Epithelial information allows an earlier diagnosis of keratoconus, as epithelial changes will occur before changes on the front surface of the cornea become apparent. Epithelial thinning coincident with an eccentric posterior elevation BFS apex, in particular if surrounded by an annulus of thicker epithelium, is consistent with keratoconus. Excluding early keratoconic patients from laser refractive surgery will reduce and potentially eliminate the risk of iatrogenic ectasia of this etiology and therefore increase the safety of laser refractive surgery. From our data, 136 eyes out of 1532 consecutive myopic eyes screened for refractive surgery demonstrated abnormal topography suspect of keratoconus. All 136 eyes were screened with Artemis VHF digital ultrasound arc-scanning and individual epithelial thickness profiles were mapped. Out of 136 eyes with suspect keratoconus, only 22 eyes (16%) were confirmed as keratoconus.[62]

Second, epithelial thickness profiles may be useful in excluding a diagnosis of keratoconus despite suspect topography. Epithelial thickening over an area of topographic steepening implies that the steepening is not due to an underlying ectatic surface. In such cases, excluding keratoconus using epithelial thickness profiles appears to allow patients who otherwise would have been denied treatment because of suspect topography to be deemed suitable for surgery. From our data, out of the 136 eyes with suspect keratoconus screened with Artemis VHF digital ultrasound arc-scanning, 114 eyes (84%) showed normal epithelial thickness profile and were diagnosed as non-keratoconic and deemed suitable for corneal refractive surgery. One-year post-LASIK follow-up data[62] and preliminary 2-year follow-up data[117] on these demonstrated equal stability and refractive outcomes as matched control eyes.

In summary, it is important to obtain a full clinical picture for the patient including demographic, diagnostic, and clinical examination data. With advancements in keratoconus screening to include topography to tomography, and now epithelium, we are seeing a shift in standard of care, and we are able to better serve our patients. In the future, advancements in algorithms keratoconus by this automated and deep machine learning may prove to be yet another tool to aid in the early detection of keratoconus.

References

1. Ambrósio R Jr, Wilson SE. Complications of laser in situ keratomileusis: etiology, prevention, and treatment. *J Refract Surg*. 2001;17:350–379.
2. Seiler T, Koufala K, Richter G. Iatrogenic keractectasia after laser in situ keratomileusis. *J Refract Surg*. 1998;14:312–317.
3. Krachmer JH, Feder RF, Belin MW. Keratoconus and related non-inflammatory corneal thinning disorders. *Surv Ophthalmol*. 1984;28:293–322.
4. Wilson SE, Klyce SD. Screening for corneal topographic abnormalities before refractive surgery. *Ophthalmology*. 1994;101:147–152.
5. Klyce SD. Computer-assisted corneal topography. High-resolution graphic presentation and analysis of keratoscopy. *Invest Ophthalmol Vis Sci*. 1984;25:1426–1435.
6. Rabinowitz YS, Yang H, Brickman Y, et al. Videokeratography database of normal human corneas. *Br J Ophthalmol*. 1996;80:610–616.
7. Rabinowitz YS, McDonnell PJ. Computer-assisted corneal topography in keratoconus. *Refract Corneal Surg*. 1989;5:400–408.
8. Rabinowitz YS. Videokeratographic indices to aid in screening for keratoconus. *J Refract Surg*. 1995;11:371–379.
9. Rabinowitz YS. Tangential vs. sagittal videokeratographs in the "early" detection of keratoconus. *Am J Ophthalmol*. 1996;122:887–889.
10. Rabinowitz YS, Rasheed K. KISA% index: a quantitative videokeratography algorithm embodying minimal topographic criteria for diagnosing keratoconus. *J Cataract Refract Surg*. 1999;25:1327–1335.
11. Smolek MK, Klyce SD. Current keratoconus detection methods compared with a neural network approach. *Invest Ophthalmol Vis Sci*. 1997;38:2290–2299.
12. Maeda N, Klyce SD. Smolek MK. Comparison of methods for detecting keratoconus using videokeratography. *Arch Ophthalmol*. 1995;113:870–874.
13. Nesburn AB, Bahri S, Salz J, et al. Keratoconus detected by videokeratography in candidates for photorefractive keratectomy. *J Refract Surg*. 1995;11:194–201.
14. Chastang PJ, Borderie VM, Carvajal-Gonzalez S, Rostène W, Laroche L. Automated keratoconus detection using the EyeSys videokeratoscope. *J Cataract Refract Surg*. 2000;26:675–683.
15. Maeda N, Klyce SD, Smolek MK, Thompson HW. Automated keratoconus screening with corneal topography analysis. *Invest Ophthalmol Vis Sci*. 1994;35:2749–2757.
16. Kalin NS, Maeda N, Klyce SD, Hargrave S, Wilson SE. Automated topographic screening for keratoconus in refractive surgery candidates. *CLAO J*. 1996;22:164–167.
17. Auffarth GU, Wang L, Volcker HE. Keratoconus evaluation using the Orbscan topography system. *J Cataract Refract Surg*. 2000;26:222–228.
18. Rao SN, Raviv T, Majmudar PA, Epstein RJ. Role of Orbscan II in screening keratoconus suspects before refractive corneal surgery. *Ophthalmology*. 2002;109:1642–1646.
19. Tomidokoro A, Oshika T, Amano S, Higaki S, Maeda N, Miyata K. Changes in anterior and posterior corneal curvatures in keratoconus. *Ophthalmology*. 2000;107:1328–1332.
20. Ambrósio R Jr, Alonso RS, Luz A. Coca Velarde LG. Corneal-thickness spatial profile and corneal-volume distribution: tomographic indices to detect keratoconus. *J Cataract Refract Surg*. 2006;32:1851–1859.
21. de Sanctis U, Loiacono C, Richiardi L, Turco D, Mutani B, Grignolo FM. Sensitivity and specificity of posterior corneal elevation measured by Pentacam in discriminating keratoconus/subclinical keratoconus. *Ophthalmology*. 2008;115:1534–1539.
22. Saad A, Gatinel D. Evaluation of total and corneal wavefront high order aberrations for the detection of forme fruste keratoconus. *Invest Ophthalmol Vis Sci*. 2012;53:2978–2992.
23. Luce DA. Determining in vivo biomechanical properties of the cornea with an Ocular Response Analyzer. *J Cataract Refract Surg*. 2005;31:156–162.
24. Vellara HR, Patel DV. Biomechanical properties of the keratoconic cornea: a review. *Clin Exp Optom*. 2015;98:31–38.

25. Piñero DP, Alcón N. Corneal biomechanics: a review. *Clin Exp Optom.* 2015;98(2):107–116.
26. Vinciguerra R, Ambrósio R Jr, Elsheikh A, et al. Detection of keratoconus with a new biomechanical index. *J Refract Surg.* 2016;32:803–810.
27. Ambrósio R Jr, AL Caiado, Guerra FP, et al. Novel pachymetric parameters based on corneal tomography for diagnosing keratoconus. *J Refract Surg.* 2011;27:753–758.
28. Fontes BM, Ambrósio R Jr, Salomao M, Velarde GC. Nose W. Biomechanical and tomographic analysis of unilateral keratoconus. *J Refract Surg.* 2010;26:677–681.
29. Bae GH, Kim JR, Kim CH, Lim DH, Chung ES, Chung TY. Corneal topographic and tomographic analysis of fellow eyes in unilateral keratoconus patients using Pentacam. *Am J Ophthalmol.* 2014;157:103–109. e101.
30. Muftuoglu O, Ayar O, Ozulken K, Ozyol E, Akinci A. Posterior corneal elevation and back difference corneal elevation in diagnosing forme fruste keratoconus in the fellow eyes of unilateral keratoconus patients. *J Cataract Refract Surg.* 2013;39:1348–1357.
31. Chan C, Ang M, Saad A, et al. Validation of an objective scoring system for forme fruste keratoconus detection and post-LASIK ectasia risk assessment in Asian eyes. *Cornea.* 2015;34:996–1004.
32. Saad A, Gatinel D. Validation of a new scoring system for the detection of early forme of keratoconus. *Int J Kerat Ect Cor Dis.* 2012;1:100–108.
33. Saad A, Gatinel D. Topographic and tomographic properties of forme fruste keratoconus corneas. *Invest Ophthalmol Vis Sci.* 2010;51:5546–5555.
34. Mahmoud AM, Nunez MX, Blanco C, et al. Expanding the cone location and magnitude index to include corneal thickness and posterior surface information for the detection of keratoconus. *Am J Ophthalmol.* 2013;156:1102–1111.
35. Randleman JB, Trattler WB., Stulting R.D. Validation of the ectasia risk score system for preoperative laser in situ keratomileusis screening. *Am J Ophthalmol.* 2008;145:813–818.
36. Randleman JB, Woodward M, Lynn MJ, Stulting RD. Risk assessment for ectasia after corneal refractive surgery. *Ophthalmology.* 2008;115:37–50.
37. Seiler T, Quurke AW. Iatrogenic keratectasia after LASIK in a case of forme fruste keratoconus. *J Cataract Refract Surg.* 1998;24:1007–1009.
38. Speicher L, Gottinger W. Progressive corneal ectasia after laser in situ keratomileusis (LASIK). *Klin Monatsbl Augenheilkd.* 1998;213:247–251.
39. Geggel HS, Talley AR. Delayed onset keratectasia following laser in situ keratomileusis. *J Cataract Refract Surg.* 1999;25:582–586.
40. Amoils SP, Deist MB, Gous P, Amoils PM. Iatrogenic keratectasia after laser in situ keratomileusis for less than -4.0 to -7.0 diopters of myopia. *J Cataract Refract Surg.* 2000;26:967–977.
41. McLeod SD, Kisla TA, Caro NC, McMahon TT. Iatrogenic keratoconus: corneal ectasia following laser in situ keratomileusis for myopia. *Arch Ophthalmol.* 2000;118:282–284.
42. Holland SP, Srivannaboon S, Reinstein DZ. Avoiding serious corneal complications of laser assisted in situ keratomileusis and photorefractive keratectomy. *Ophthalmology.* 2000;107:640–652.
43. Schmitt-Bernard CF, Lesage C, Arnaud B. Keratectasia induced by laser in situ keratomileusis in keratoconus. *J Refract Surg.* 2000;16:368–370.
44. Rao SN, Epstein RJ. Early onset ectasia following laser in situ keratomileusus: case report and literature review. *J Refract Surg.* 2002;18:177–184.
45. Malecaze F, Coullet J, Calvas P, Fournie P, Arne JL, Brodaty C. Corneal ectasia after photorefractive keratectomy for low myopia. *Ophthalmology.* 2006;113:742–746.
46. Randleman JB, Russell B, Ward MA, Thompson KP., Stulting R.D. Risk factors and prognosis for corneal ectasia after LASIK. *Ophthalmology.* 2003;110:267–275.
47. Leccisotti A. Corneal ectasia after photorefractive keratectomy. *Graefes Arch Clin Exp Ophthalmol.* 2007;245:869–875.
48. Reinstein DZ, Archer T. Combined Artemis very high-frequency digital ultrasound-assisted transepithelial phototherapeutic keratectomy and wavefront-guided treatment following multiple corneal refractive procedures. *J Cataract Refract Surg.* 2006;32:1870–1876.
49. Reinstein DZ, Archer TJ, Gobbe M. Rate of change of curvature of the corneal stromal surface drives epithelial compensatory changes and remodeling. *J Refract Surg.* 2014;30:800–802.
50. Holden BA, Payor S. Changes in thickness in the corneal layers. *Am J Optom.* 1979;56:821.

51. Reinstein DZ, Silverman RH, Coleman DJ. High-frequency ultrasound measurement of the thickness of the corneal epithelium. *Refract Corneal Surg.* 1993;9:385–387.
52. Reinstein DZ, Silverman RH, Trokel SL, Coleman DJ. Corneal pachymetric topography. *Ophthalmology.* 1994;101:432–438.
53. Cusumano A, Coleman DJ, Silverman RH, et al. Three-dimensional ultrasound imaging. Clinical applications. *Ophthalmology.* 1998;105:300–306.
54. Silverman RH, Reinstein DZ, Raevsky T, Coleman DJ. Improved system for sonographic imaging and biometry of the cornea. *J Ultrasound Med.* 1997;16:117–124.
55. Reinstein DZ, Silverman RH, Sutton HF, Coleman DJ. Very high-frequency ultrasound corneal analysis identifies anatomic correlates of optical complications of lamellar refractive surgery: anatomic diagnosis in lamellar surgery. *Ophthalmology.* 1999;106:474–482.
56. Reinstein DZ, Silverman RH, Raevsky T, et al. Arc-scanning very high-frequency digital ultrasound for 3D pachymetric mapping of the corneal epithelium and stroma in laser in situ keratomileusis. *J Refract Surg.* 2000;16:414–430.
57. Reinstein DZ, Srivannaboon S, Holland SP. Epithelial and stromal changes induced by Intacs examined by three-dimensional very high-frequency digital ultrasound. *J Refract Surg.* 2001;17:310–318.
58. Reinstein DZ, Rothman RC, Couch DG, Archer TJ. Artemis very high-frequency digital ultrasound-guided repositioning of a free cap after laser in situ keratomileusis. *J Cataract Refract Surg.* 2006;32:1877–1882.
59. Reinstein DZ, Archer TJ, Gobbe M, Silverman RH, Coleman DJ. Epithelial thickness in the normal cornea: three-dimensional display with Artemis very high-frequency digital ultrasound. *J Refract Surg.* 2008;24:571–581.
60. Reinstein DZ, Srivannaboon S, Gobbe M, et al. Epithelial thickness profile changes induced by myopic LASIK as measured by Artemis very high-frequency digital ultrasound. *J Refract Surg.* 2009;25:444–450.
61. Reinstein DZ, Archer TJ, Gobbe M. Corneal epithelial thickness profile in the diagnosis of keratoconus. *J Refract Surg.* 2009;25:604–610.
62. Reinstein DZ, Archer TJ, Gobbe M. Stability of LASIK in corneas with topographic suspect keratoconus, with keratoconus excluded by epithelial thickness mapping. *J Refract Surg.* 2009;25:569–577.
63. Reinstein DZ, Gobbe M, Archer TJ, Couch D, Bloom B. Epithelial, stromal, and corneal pachymetry changes during orthokeratology. *Optom Vis Sci.* 2009;86:E1006–E1014.
64. Reinstein DZ, Archer TJ, Gobbe M, Silverman RH, Coleman DJ. Epithelial, stromal and corneal thickness in the keratoconic cornea: three-dimensional display with Artemis very high-frequency digital ultrasound. *J Refract Surg.* 2010;26:259–271.
65. Reinstein DZ, Archer TJ, Gobbe M, Silverman RH, Coleman DJ. Repeatability of layered corneal pachymetry with the Artemis very high-frequency digital ultrasound arc-scanner. *J Refract Surg.* 2010;26:646–659.
66. Reinstein DZ, Archer TJ, Gobbe M, Silverman RH, Coleman DJ. Epithelial thickness after hyperopic LASIK: three-dimensional display with Artemis very high-frequency digital ultrasound. *J Refract Surg.* 2010;26:555–564.
67. Reinstein DZ, Gobbe M, Archer TJ, Couch D. Epithelial thickness profile as a method to evaluate the effectiveness of collagen cross-linking treatment after corneal ectasia. *J Refract Surg.* 2011;27:356–363.
68. Reinstein DZ, Archer TJ, Gobbe M. Very high-frequency digital ultrasound evaluation of topography-wavefront-guided repair after radial keratotomy. *J Cataract Refract Surg.* 2011;37:599–602.
69. Reinstein DZ, Archer TJ, Gobbe M. Epithelial thickness up to 26 years after radial keratotomy: three-dimensional display with Artemis very high-frequency digital ultrasound. *J Refract Surg.* 2011;27:618–624.
70. Reinstein DZ, Archer TJ, Gobbe M. Change in epithelial thickness profile 24 hours and longitudinally for 1 year after myopic LASIK: three-dimensional display with Artemis very high-frequency digital ultrasound. *J Refract Surg.* 2012;28:195–201.
71. Reinstein DZ, Archer TJ, Gobbe M. Stability of epithelial thickness during 5 minutes immersion in 33 degrees C 0.9% saline using very high-frequency digital ultrasound. *J Refract Surg.* 2012;28:606–607.
72. Reinstein DZ, Archer TJ, Gobbe M. Improved effectiveness of trans-epithelial phototherapeutic keratectomy versus topography-guided ablation degraded by epithelial compensation on irregular stromal surfaces [plus video]. *J Refract Surg.* 2013;29:526–533.

73. Gauthier CA, Holden BA, Epstein D, Tengroth B, Fagerholm P, Hamberg-Nystrom H. Factors affecting epithelial hyperplasia after photorefractive keratectomy. *J Cataract Refract Surg.* 1997;23:1042–1050.

74. Gauthier CA, Holden BA, Epstein D, Tengroth B, Fagerholm P., Hamberg-Nystrom H. Role of epithelial hyperplasia in regression following photorefractive keratectomy. *Br J Ophthalmol.* 1996;80:545–548.

75. Gauthier CA, Epstein D, Holden BA, et al. Epithelial alterations following photorefractive keratectomy for myopia. *J Refract Surg.* 1995;11:113–118.

76. Shieh E, Moreira H, D'Arcy J, Clapham TN, McDonnell PJ. Quantitative analysis of wound healing after cylindrical and spherical excimer laser ablations. *Ophthalmology.* 1992;99:1050–1055.

77. Beuerman RW, McDonald MB, Shofner RS, et al. Quantitative histological studies of primate corneas after excimer laser photorefractive keratectomy. *Arch Ophthalmol.* 1994;112:1103–1110.

78. Lohmann CP, Patmore A, Reischl U, Marshall J. The importance of the corneal epithelium in excimer-laser photorefractive keratectomy. *Ger J Ophthalmol.* 1996;5:368–372.

79. Lohmann CP, Reischl U, Marshall J. Regression and epithelial hyperplasia after myopic photorefractive keratectomy in a human cornea. *J Cataract Refract Surg.* 1999;25:712–715.

80. Li HF, Petroll WM, Moller-Pedersen T, Maurer JK, Cavanagh HD, Jester JV. Epithelial and corneal thickness measurements by in vivo confocal microscopy through focusing (CMTF). *Curr Eye Res.* 1997;16:214–221.

81. Moller-Pedersen T, Li HF, Petroll WM, Cavanagh HD, Jester JV. Confocal microscopic characterization of wound repair after photorefractive keratectomy. *Invest Ophthalmol Vis Sci.* 1998;39:487–501.

82. Moller-Pedersen T, Vogel M, Li HF, Petroll WM, Cavanagh HD, Jester JV. Quantification of stromal thinning, epithelial thickness, and corneal haze after photorefractive keratectomy using in vivo confocal microscopy. *Ophthalmology.* 1997;104:360–368.

83. Feng Y, Varikooty J, Simpson TL. Diurnal variation of corneal and corneal epithelial thickness measured using optical coherence tomography. *Cornea.* 2001;20:480–483.

84. Wirbelauer C, Pham DT. Monitoring corneal structures with slitlamp-adapted optical coherence tomography in laser in situ keratomileusis. *J Cataract Refract Surg.* 2004;30:1851–1860.

85. Haque S, Fonn D, Simpson T, Jones L. Corneal and epithelial thickness changes after 4 weeks of overnight corneal refractive therapy lens wear, measured with optical coherence tomography. *Eye Contact Lens.* 2004;30:189–193; discussion 205–186.

86. Sin S, Simpson TL. The repeatability of corneal and corneal epithelial thickness measurements using optical coherence tomography. *Optom Vis Sci.* 2006;83:360–365.

87. Haque S, Jones L, Simpson T. Thickness mapping of the cornea and epithelium using optical coherence tomography. *Optom Vis Sci.* 2008;85:E963–E976.

88. Li Y, Tan O, Brass R, Weiss JL, Huang D. Corneal epithelial thickness mapping by Fourier-domain optical coherence tomography in normal and keratoconic eyes. *Ophthalmology.* 2012;119:2425–2433.

89. Bentivoglio AR, Bressman SB, Cassetta E, Carretta D, Tonali P, Albanese A. Analysis of blink rate patterns in normal subjects. *Mov Disord.* 1997;12:1028–1034.

90. Doane MG. Interactions of eyelids and tears in corneal wetting and the dynamics of the normal human eyeblink. *Am J Ophthalmol.* 1980;89:507–516.

91. Young G, Hunt C, Covey M. Clinical evaluation of factors influencing toric soft contact lens fit. *Optom Vis Sci.* 2002;79:11–19.

92. Scroggs MW., Proia A.D. Histopathological variation in keratoconus. *Cornea.* 1992;11:553–559.

93. Haque S, Simpson T, Jones L. Corneal and epithelial thickness in keratoconus: a comparison of ultrasonic pachymetry, Orbscan II, and optical coherence tomography. *J Refract Surg.* 2006;22:486–493.

94. Rocha KM, Perez-Straziota CE, Stulting RD, Randleman JB. SD-OCT analysis of regional epithelial thickness profiles in keratoconus, postoperative corneal ectasia, and normal eyes. *J Refract Surg.* 2013;29:173–179.

95. Kanellopoulos AJ, Aslanides IM, Asimellis G. Correlation between epithelial thickness in normal corneas, untreated ectatic corneas, and ectatic corneas previously treated with CXL; is overall epithelial thickness a very early ectasia prognostic factor?. *Clin Ophthalmol.* 2012;6:789–800.

96. Sandali O, El Sanharawi M, Temstet C, et al. Fourier-domain optical coherence tomography imaging in keratoconus: a corneal structural classification. *Ophthalmology.* 2013;120:2403–2412.

97. Kanellopoulos AJ, Asimellis G. Longitudinal postoperative Lasik epithelial thickness profile changes in correlation with degree of myopia correction. *J Refract Surg.* 2014;30:166–171.

98. Reinstein DZ, Archer TJ, Gobbe M. Refractive and topographic errors in topography-guided ablation produced by epithelial compensation predicted by three-dimensional Artemis very high-frequency digital ultrasound stromal and epithelial thickness mapping. *J Refract Surg.* 2012;28:657–663.

99. Reinstein DZ, Gobbe M, Archer TJ, Youssefi G, Sutton HF. Stromal surface topography-guided custom ablation as a repair tool for corneal irregular astigmatism. *J Refract Surg.* 2015;31:54–59.

100. Reinstein DZ, Archer TJ, Dickeson ZI, Gobbe M. Trans-epithelial phototherapeutic keratectomy protocol for treating irregular astigmatism based on population epithelial thickness measurements by Artemis very high-frequency digital ultrasound. *J Refract Surg.* 2014;30:380–387.

101. Vinciguerra P, Roberts CJ, Albe E, et al. Corneal curvature gradient map: a new corneal topography map to predict the corneal healing process. *J Refract Surg.* 2014;30:202–207.

102. Klein SR, Epstein RJ, Randleman JB., Stulting R.D. Corneal ectasia after laser in situ keratomileusis in patients without apparent preoperative risk factors. *Cornea.* 2006;25:388–403.

103. Silverman RH, Urs R, Roychoudhury A, Archer TJ, Gobbe M, Reinstein DZ. Epithelial remodeling as basis for machine-based identification of keratoconus. *Invest Ophthalmol Vis Sci.* 2014;55:1580–1587.

104. Temstet C, Sandali O, Bouheraoua N, et al. Corneal epithelial thickness mapping using Fourier-domain optical coherence tomography for detection of forme fruste keratoconus. *J Cataract Refract Surg.* 2015;41:812–820.

105. Ambrósio R Jr, F Faria-Correia, Ramos I, et al. Enhanced screening for ectasia susceptibility among refractive candidates: the role of corneal tomography and biomechanics. *Curr Ophthalmol Rep.* 2013;1:28–38.

106. Gomes JA, Tan D, Rapuano CJ, et al. Global consensus on keratoconus and ectatic diseases. *Cornea.* 2015;34:359–369.

107. Najmi H, Mobarki Y, Mania K, et al. The correlation between keratoconus and eye rubbing: a review. *Int J Ophthalmol.* 2019;12:1775–1781.

108. Ambrósio R Jr, Dawson DG, Salomao M, Guerra FP, Caiado AL, Belin MW. Corneal ectasia after LASIK despite low preoperative risk: tomographic and biomechanical findings in the unoperated, stable, fellow eye. *J Refract Surg.* 2010;26:906–911.

109. Dupps WJ Jr, Kohnen T, Mamalis N, et al. Standardized graphs and terms for refractive surgery results. *J Cataract Refract Surg.* 2011;37:1–3.

110. Scarcelli G, Besner S, Pineda R, Yun SH. Biomechanical characterization of keratoconus corneas ex vivo with Brillouin microscopy. *Invest Ophthalmol Vis Sci.* 2014;55:4490–4495.

111. Abu-Amero KK, Al-Muammar AM, Kondkar AA. Genetics of keratoconus: where do we stand?. *J Ophthalmol.* 2014;2014:641708.

112. Burdon KP, Vincent AL. Insights into keratoconus from a genetic perspective. *Clin Exp Optom.* 2013;96:146–154.

113. Rabinowitz YS, Dong L, Wistow G. Gene expression profile studies of human keratoconus cornea for NEIBank: a novel cornea-expressed gene and the absence of transcripts for aquaporin 5. *Invest Ophthalmol Vis Sci.* 2005;46:1239–1246.

114. Abou Shousha M, Perez VL, Fraga Santini Canto AP, et al. The use of Bowman's layer vertical topographic thickness map in the diagnosis of keratoconus. *Ophthalmology.* 2014;121:988–993.

115. Yadav R, Kottaiyan R, Ahmad K, Yoon G. Epithelium and Bowman's layer thickness and light scatter in keratoconic cornea evaluated using ultrahigh resolution optical coherence tomography. *J Biomed Opt.* 2012;17:116010.

116. Kanellopoulos AJ, Asimellis G. In vivo 3-dimensional corneal epithelial thickness mapping as an indicator of dry eye: preliminary clinical assessment. *Am J Ophthalmol.* 2014;157:63–68. e62.

117. Reinstein DZ, Archer TJ, Gobbe M. Stability of LASIK in Corneas With Topographic Suspect Keratoconus Confirmed Non-Keratoconic by Epithelial Thickness Mapping: 2-Years Follow-Up. *San Francisco*: AAO; 2009.

CHAPTER 19

Confocal Microscopy

Manuel Ramirez

KEY CONCEPTS

- Superficial corneal epithelium cells show an elongated shape in keratoconus patients.
- Stromal corneal nerves are thicker in keratoconus patients.
- After cross-linking treatment, stromal keratocytes become activated.
- Vogt striae can be seen as vertical and dark linear images.

Introduction

By using confocal microscopy systems, the study of in vivo tissues is possible, noninvasively and in real time, and with high-quality images.[1–4]

In 1955 Minsky developed the first confocal microscope,[5] a technique based on conjugation of the microscope objective lens and light in a small tissue portion to acquire high-quality images.[3,6] The cornea provides an excellent tissue for study by confocal microscopy because of its easy access and transparency.[7,8]

The purpose of this chapter is to describe corneal confocal microscopic findings in keratoconus (KC) and corneal tissue changes after cross-linking treatment.

Corneal Epithelium and Subepithelial Nerve Plexus

In normal conditions, confocal microscopic images of superficial corneal epithelium cells show regular and symmetric shapes. In contrast, superficial epithelium cells in KC patients show regular elongated shapes (Fig. 19.1A, B). Basal epithelial cells are similar in both patients with normal eyes and KC patients (Fig. 19.2). Bowman's layer cannot be seen by confocal microscopy, but the subepithelial nerve plexus, which rests above it, can be observed, and those nerves do not show morphological differences between KC and normal eyes (Fig. 19.3).[9]

Corneal Stroma

With confocal microscopy, evaluating the stromal corneal nerves is possible. Stromal corneal nerves are more visible at slit lamp examination in KC patients compared with normal corneas,[10] and several studies have shown this finding.[11] With corneal confocal microscopy, it has been possible to verify these differences in corneal nerves, as these nerves appear as linear hyperreflective structures in corneal confocal microscopy, can be measured and compared between KC and normal eyes and are thicker in KC patients. By using confocal microscopy, corneal stromal nerve thickness has been measured. The mean stromal nerve thickness in KC patients is 7.2 ± 1.9 (range 3.5–12.0) microns, compared with 5.7 ± 1.7 (range 3.3–10.4) microns in normal eyes (Fig. 19.4A,B).[12]

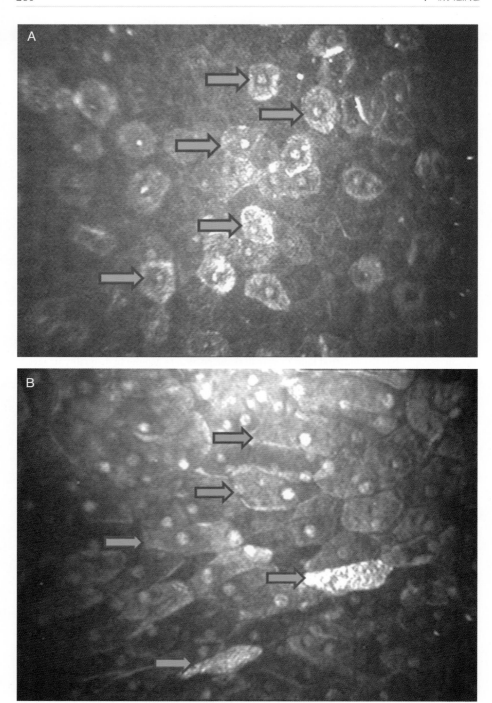

Fig. 19.1 Confocal microscopy images at the superficial epithelial cell layer showing regular and symmetric shape in a normal eye (A) and elongated shapes in a keratoconus patient (B) *(arrows)* (340 × 255 μm).

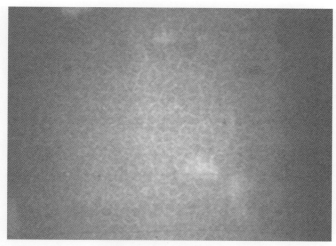

Fig. 19.2 Confocal microscopy image from keratoconus patient, showing basal epithelial cells (340 × 255 μm).

Stromal keratocytes do not show morphological differences between KC and normal eyes by confocal microscopy; normally, only the nuclei of the keratocytes can be seen (Fig. 19.5). However, it is possible to evaluate the healing process in the corneal stroma and the changes in keratocytes after cross-linking treatment during the healing process. The keratocytes become activated under these conditions, and the cytoplasmic cells can be seen with brightened nuclei by confocal microscopy.

Standard epi-off cross-linking technique shows more changes by confocal microscopy in the corneal stroma after treatment, when compared with transepithelial techniques, demonstrating activated keratocytes from the first corneal stromal image to a depth more than 300 microns (324.9 ± 66.0 mirc μm) at 1 month after cross-linking treatment (Fig. 19.5A,B). These changes could explain in part the concept that cross-linking treatment provides a real effect in stabilizing KC progression.[13]

Descemet Membrane

The Descemet membrane is not observed by confocal microscopy in normal conditions, but Vogt striae seen in KC patients can be seen, and it is possible to find them in the deep cornea anterior to the endothelium, visible as vertical and dark linear images with a mean thickness of 7.5 ± 4.3 (range 4.8–18.0) microns (Fig. 19.6).[9]

Corneal Endothelium

With confocal microscopy, corneal endothelial cells do not show morphological differences between KC and normal eyes. However, obtaining a flat image is not possible because of the corneal ectasia, so a single image will show both the corneal endothelium and a small portion of the anterior chamber (Fig. 19.7).[9]

Chapter Acknowledgment

Erika A. Guillen, MD.

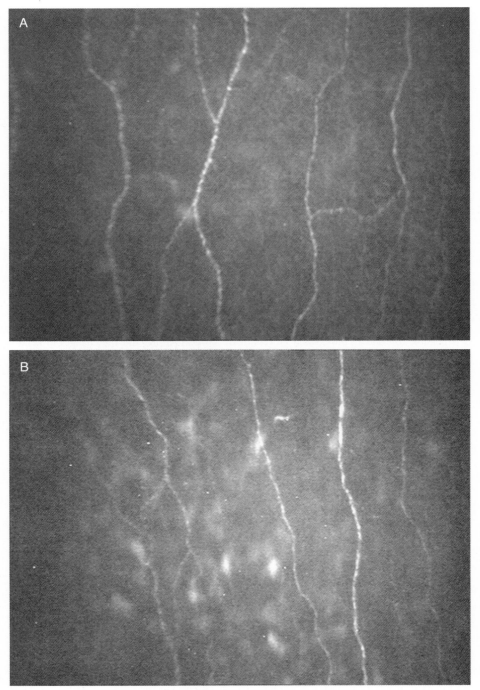

Fig. 19.3 Confocal microscopy image of the subepithelial nerve plexus; no morphological differences between keratoconus (A) and normal eyes (B) are observed (340 × 255 µm).

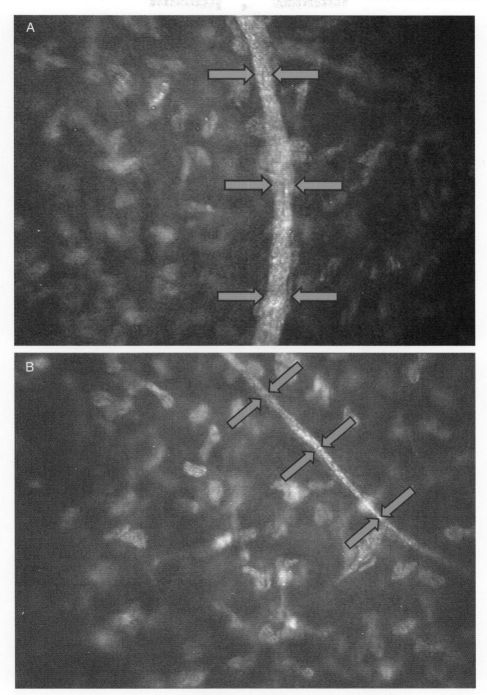

Fig. 19.4 Confocal microscopy images showing that stromal corneal nerves are thicker in keratoconus patients (A) than in those with normal eyes (B) *(arrows)* (340 × 255 μm).

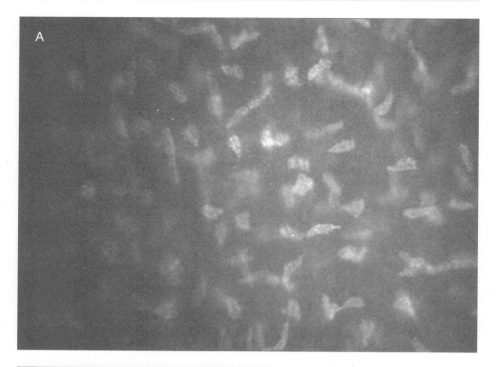

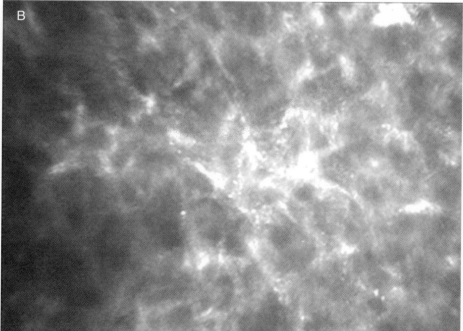

Fig. 19.5 Confocal microscopy images of a keratoconus patient at the corneal stromal level, showing normal keratocytes image before cross-linking treatment (A) and activated keratocytes after cross-linking treatment (B) (340 × 255 µm).

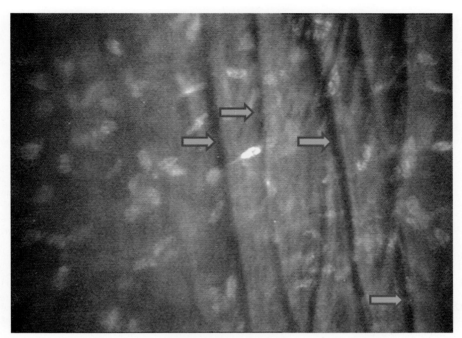

Fig. 19.6 Confocal microscopy image at the Descemet membrane level, showing Vogt striae as vertical and dark linear images (indicated by *arrows*) (340 × 255 μm).

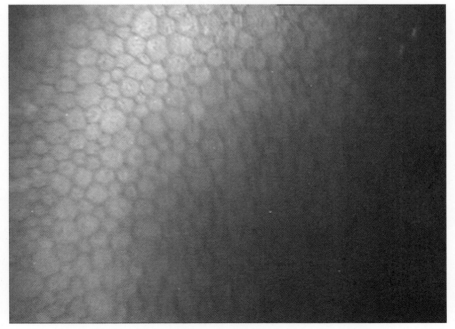

Fig. 19.7 Confocal microscopy image showing, in the same image, the corneal endothelium and a small portion of the anterior chamber (340 × 255 μm).

References

1. Jester JV, Andrews PM, Petroll WM, Lemp MA, Cavanagh HD. In vivo, real-time confocal imaging. *J Electron Microsc Tech.* 1991;18:50–60.
2. Andrews PM, Petroll WM, Cavanagh HD, Jester JV. Tandem scanning confocal microscopy (TSCM) of normal and ischemic living kidneys. *Am J Anat.* 1991;191:95–102.
3. Petroll WM, Jester JV, Cavanagh HD. In vivo confocal imaging: general principles and applications. *Scanning.* 1994;16:131–149.
4. Rigby PJ, Goldie RG. Confocal microscopy in biomedical research. *Croat Med J.* 1999;40:346–352.
5. Minsky M. Memoir on inventing the confocal scanning microscope. *Scanning Journal.* 1988;10:128–138.
6. Boyde A, Petran M, Hadravsky M. Tandem scanning reflected light microscopy of internal features in whole bone and tooth samples. *J Microsc.* 1983;132:1–7.
7. Erie JC, Patel SV, McLaren JW, Maguire LJ, Ramirez M, Bourne W. Keratocyte density in vivo after photorefractive keratectomy in humans. *Am J Ophthalmol.* 2000;129:703.
8. Sanchez-Huerta V, Ramirez Fernandez M, Castro Muñoz-Ledo F, Kuri Harchuc W, Naranjo Tackman R. Cambios en el estroma corneal in vivo secundarios a quemadura por álcali. *Revista Mexicana de Oftalmologia.* 2001;75:145–150.
9. Gaecia AM, Ramirez M. *Hallazgos mediante microscopia confocal en epitelio y capa de Descemet en pacientes con queratocono.* Cornea. Mexico City: Universidad Nacional Autonoma de Mexico; 2019.
10. Krachmer JH, Feder RS, Belin MW. Keratoconus and related noninflammatory corneal thinning disorders. *Surv Ophthalmol.* 1984;28:293–322.
11. Simo Mannion L, Tromans C, O'Donnell C. An evaluation of corneal nerve morphology and function in moderate keratoconus. *Cont Lens Anterior Eye.* 2005;28:185–192.
12. Ramírez Fernández M, Hernández Quintela E, Naranjo Tackman R. Comparison of stromal corneal nerves between normal and keratoconus patients using confocal microscopy. *Arch Soc Esp Oftalmol.* 2014;89:308–312.
13. Ramírez M, Hernández -Quintela E, Naranjo-Tackman R. Early confocal microscopy findings after cross-linking treatment. *Arch Soc Esp Oftalmol.* 2013;88:179–183.

CHAPTER 20

Other Diagnostic Imaging Tools for Keratoconus

Jose Luis Reyes Luis ■ Roberto Pineda

KEY CONCEPTS

Diagnosis, refractive screening, and collagen cross-linking changes in keratoconus with:
- Ocular Response Analyzer (ORA) and Corvis ST
- Brillouin microscopy
- Ex vivo assessment of corneal biomechanics.

Background

Since 1854, when John Nottingham published the first detailed description of keratoconus (KC),[1] corneal diagnostic devices have been evolving. In 1880 Placido developed the first keratoscope based on corneal reflections of a series of concentric rings.[1] In 1980 Klyce refined this technology and introduced computerized videokeratoscopy, allowing for better evaluation of the anterior corneal curvature and improving KC detection.[1] In the 1990s, with the proliferation of refractive surgery, the need for better screening for KC increased. This became yet more relevant in 1998 when the first case of iatrogenic ectasia was reported in a patient with forme fruste keratoconus (FFKC).[2] Reports of postrefractive surgery ectasia steadily increased. Fortunately, advances in KC diagnostic imaging methods also continued.

Currently, the anterior and posterior corneal surfaces of the cornea can be evaluated with corneal tomography, and pachymetric distribution patterns can be assessed with anterior segment optical coherence tomography (AS-OCT).[1] In addition, confocal microscopy and wavefront analysis have resulted in a greater capacity to evaluate corneal characteristics such as structural alterations and corneal aberrations.[3] However, current options for evaluating corneal biomechanics—properties of the cornea that have been demonstrated to play an important role in KC—are limited.[3]

Biomechanics

In the field of biomechanics the micro and macro effects of forces acting on living organisms are studied.[4] Our understanding of the biomechanical features of human tissues has contributed to improving understanding of diseases and has enhanced the prediction of tissue alterations.[4] To comprehend the biomechanical response of living tissues, two concepts are fundamental: Young's modulus and viscoelasticity (Box 20.1).[4]

In Vivo Assessment of Corneal Biomechanics

OCULAR RESPONSE ANALYZER

In 2005 Reichert Technologies launched the first device for in vivo evaluation of corneal biomechanics.[5,6] The device, named Ocular Response Analyzer (ORA; Reichert Ophthalmic Instruments, Depew, NY), works by emitting an air-pulse in the central 3 mm of the cornea capable of producing an inward deformation of the tissue.[4] When the first applanation moment is detected (also called first state of applanation), the air-pulse signal is terminated. However, the inertia of the air pulse continues to raise the air pressure, and the cornea reaches a concavity configuration peak. Subsequently, the air pressure diminishes allowing the cornea to gradually return to its original configuration. During the outgoing phase, a second moment of applanation (or second state of applanation) is also detected (Fig. 20.1).[5] An infrared emitter detects the two states of applanation and measures the emitted air pressure at those moments (see P1 and P2) (see Fig. 20.1).[4,7] From these measurements, the ORA software obtains several important corneal biomechanical parameters (Box 20.2).

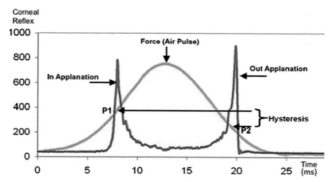

Fig. 20.1   Ocular Response Analyzer (ORA) (Reichert Ophthalmic Instruments, Depew, NY) diagram showing the applanation and air pulse from one measurement. The corneal hysteresis (CH) is derived from the difference between *P1* and *P2* applanation pressures. (Image reproduced from Esporcatte LPG, Salomão MQ, Lopes BT, et al. Biomechanical diagnostics of the cornea. *Eye Vis (Lond).* 2020;7:9. [http://creativecommons.org/licenses/by/4.0/.])

ORA in Keratoconus (Table 20.1)

Studies have shown a significant decrease in both corneal hysteresis (CH) and corneal resistance factor (CRF).[8,9] However, ORA has poor sensitivity and specificity for detecting mild KC (Fig. 20.2).[10,11]

ORA in Refractive Surgery

After refractive surgery, a decrease in CH and CRF has been reported.[12,13] This effect is more pronounced after LASIK surgery than with photorefractive keratectomy (PRK).[14]

ORA in Cross-Linking

No changes in CH and CRF have been detected after collagen cross-linking (CXL) for KC.[15–18]

ORA Limitations

According to some studies, there is an unclear relationship between corneal mechanical properties, such as Young's modulus, and CH and CRF, as well as an overlap between elasticity and viscosity. These circumstances make data difficult to interpret.[3,6] Moreover, the new ORA software provides

TABLE 20.1 ■ **Biomechanical Parameters of ORA in Normal and Keratoconus**[11]

Parameter	Normal	Keratoconus	Sensitivity	Specificity
CH (mmHg)	>8.50	≤8.50	52%	95.4%
CRF (mmHg)	>8.60	≤8.60	77.6%	86%
HLA	>92.629	≤92.629	88.8%	88.9%

CH, Corneal hysteresis; *CRF,* corneal resistance factor; *HLA,* hysteresis loop area; *mmHg,* millimeters of mercury; *ORA,* Ocular Response Analyzer.

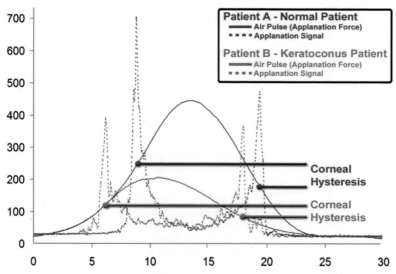

Fig. 20.2 Ocular Response Analyzer in a normal patient *(blue)* and a keratoconus patient *(red)*. A decrease in corneal hysteresis is seen in keratoconus. (Image courtesy Reichert.)

42 new variables; however, more studies are needed to determine their clinical significance.[3] Also, air-puff pressure is not constant, making measurements difficult to compare between eyes.[4]

CORVIS ST

In 2009 Oculus introduced the Corvis ST noncontact tonometer (OCULUS Optikgeräte GmbH, Wetzlar, Germany) for biomechanical evaluation of the cornea. This device combines dynamic applanation with an ultra-high-speed Scheimpflug camera (4330 frames/second) that records an 8-mm wide horizontal section of the cornea (Fig. 20.3).[3,4,7] The air emitted by the noncontact tonometer does not vary from one measurement to another and the corneal response, recorded by the Scheimpflug camera, is analyzed to obtain the corneal biomechanical variables (Box 20.3).[4]

Corvis ST in Keratoconus (Table 20.2)

Studies have found higher deformation amplitude (DA) values in KC patients; however, this parameter cannot differentiate between healthy and KC corneas (due to its low sensitivity and specificity).[19,20]

Both the Corvis biomechanical index (CBI) with a 0.5 cutoff and the tomographical/biomechanical index (TBI) with a 0.79 cutoff demonstrated high sensitivity and specificity for KC detection (100% sensitivity with 94.1% specificity and 100% of sensitivity with 100% specificity, respectively).[5,21,22]

In Fig. 20.4, the Ambrósio, Roberts, Vinciguerra (ARV) Corvis ST display of a patient with a very asymmetric ectasia (normal tomography in the right eye [VAE-NT], and ectasia in the left eye [VAE-E]) is shown. The display shows abnormalities in the tomographic assessment, the CBI index, the TBI index, and the Belin/Ambrósio deviation index (BAD-D, Box 20.4).

Corvis ST in Suspected Keratoconus/Forme Fruste Keratoconus

The original Corvis ST software did not detect suspected keratoconus/forme fruste keratoconus (SC/FFKC). New software includes two new indices that can be used for the diagnosis of SC/FFKC: the CBI index (63% sensitivity and 80.3% specificity) and the TBI index (84% sensitivity and 86% specificity).[23] Fig. 20.5 presents the ARV Corvis ST display of a patient with a very asymmetric ectasia. The normal tomography (VAE-NT) contrasts with three abnormal indices on the ARV display (CBI, TBI, and BAD-D). Patients with very asymmetric ectasias have high risk of developing postrefractive ectasias.

Corvis ST in Refractive Surgery

It is important to emphasize that current studies may be not powered enough to detect the biomechanical changes produced by refractive surgery. However, several authors have reported an increase in the first and second applanation lengths, as well as in the DA, after LASIK surgery.[24] Similarly, Small Incision Lenticule Extraction (SMILE) surgery was capable of inducing a rise in those parameters, although its effect was transitory.[25] However, an increase in DA combined with a decrease in stiffness at first applanation and at highest concavity after PRK and PRK with CXL has been documented (with changes significantly larger in the first group).[26]

Corvis ST in Cross-Linking

Several studies have reported the biomechanical effects of CXL. Those effects consist of a decrease in strain and an increase in stiffness that were proved in a parametric study to persist for up to 4 years after treatment.[27] Moreover, the development of the stress-strain index (SSI) currently allows objective estimation of the stiffening changes after CXL.[5,28]

Corvis ST Limitations

Unfortunately, the relationship between the mechanical response parameters (measured by both the Corvis ST and the ORA), and Young's modulus and other corneal properties (measured in

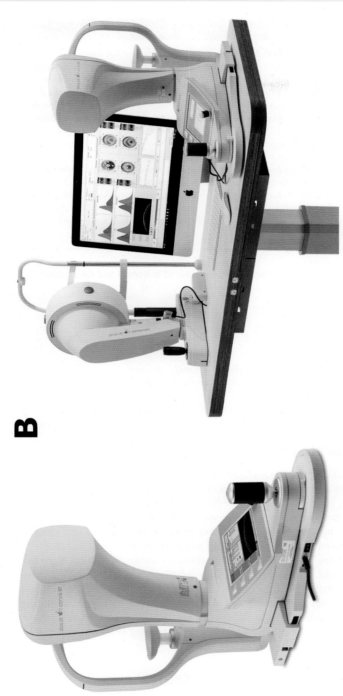

Fig. 20.3 (A) Corvis ST and (B) Pentacam (OCULUS Optikgeräte GmbH, Wetzlar, Germany). (Images courtesy OCULUS.)

BOX 20.3 ■ Corvis ST Biomechanical Parameters

- ***Deformation Amplitude (DA).*** Maximum inward movement of the corneal apex.[7]
- ***First Applanation.*** Event that occurs during the first flattening of the cornea during the air puff (in milliseconds). The length of the applanation at this moment is measured in millimeters.[5]
- ***Second Applanation.*** Event that occurs during the second flattening of the cornea during the air puff (in milliseconds). The length of the applanation at this moment is measured in millimeters.[5]
- ***Corneal Velocities (CVel).*** Maximum velocities in ingoing and outgoing phases. Expressed in meters per second.[5]
- ***Highest Concavity.*** The length distance between the two peaks (in millimeters) during the air puff (in milliseconds).[5]
- ***Ambrósio Relational Thickness Over the Horizontal Meridian (ARTh).*** Index that represents the characterization of the thickness data on the horizontal Scheimpflug image.[5]
- ***Corvis Biomechanical Index (CBI).*** Index based on combining ARTh with 16 dynamic corneal response (DCR) parameters.[21]
- ***Tomographical/Biomechanical Index (TBI).*** Index that combines tomographic and biomechanical data.[5,22]

TABLE 20.2 ■ Biomechanical Parameters of Corvis ST in Normal and Keratoconus.[5,20,21]

Parameter	Normal	Keratoconus	Sensitivity	Specificity
DA (mm)	<1.18	≥1.18	81.7%	83.3%
CBI	<0.5	≥0.5	100%	94.1%
TBI	<0.79	≥0.79	100%	100%

CBI, Corvis biomechanical index; *DA,* deformation amplitude; *TBI,* tomographical/biomechanical index.

---

experimental studies) has not been clearly defined.[4] Moreover, Corvis ST and ORA cannot evaluate the spatial differences in those parameters across the cornea (in depth and width).[3]

BRILLOUIN SPECTROSCOPY

In 1980 Brillouin spectroscopy was introduced to ophthalmology.[29] It was initially used to determine the ex vivo biomechanical properties of the lens and cornea, and required an integration time that varied from 10 minutes to 1 hour.[30,31] Technological advances have reduced the acquisition and integration times needed to calculate spatially resolved measurements and included imaging.

Brillouin spectroscopy uses the quantum principle of Brillouin scattering to measure the relationship between a narrow-banded light and ***phonons*** in matter (Box 20.5).[3,29] This principle occurs when pressure waves, generated by intrinsic thermodynamic fluctuations within a material, scatter incident light.[3] Therefore when a laser light is applied to a biological tissue, it undergoes a frequency shift, called the Brillouin frequency shift.[29] This shift is proportional to the velocity of the interacting phonons and is fundamental for calculating the bulk elastic and the Brillouin modulus.[29,32] An empirical relationship between the Brillouin modulus and conventional Young's modulus has been described; however, a clear understanding of their correlation has not yet been thoroughly elaborated.[30,33,34]

BRILLOUIN OPTICAL SCATTERING SYSTEM

Brillouin Optical Scattering System (BOSS; Intelon Optics, Boston, MA) is the first device capable of measuring the Brillouin frequency shift in vivo.[3] This equipment is in the process of being commercialized and consists of a light source, a human scanning interface, and a double

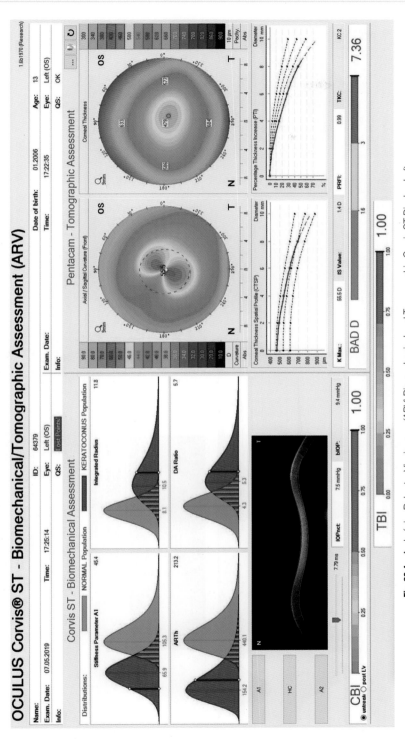

Fig. 20.4 Ambrósio, Roberts, Vinciguerra (ARV) Biomechanical and Tomographic Corvis ST Display. Left eye of a patient with very asymmetric ectasia (VAE-E). Abnormal reported indices are represented in *red*. (Image reproduced from Esporcatte LPG, Salomão MQ, Lopes BT, et al. Biomechanical diagnostics of the cornea. *Eye Vis (Lond)*. 2020;7:9. [http://creativecommons.org/licenses/by/4.0/.])

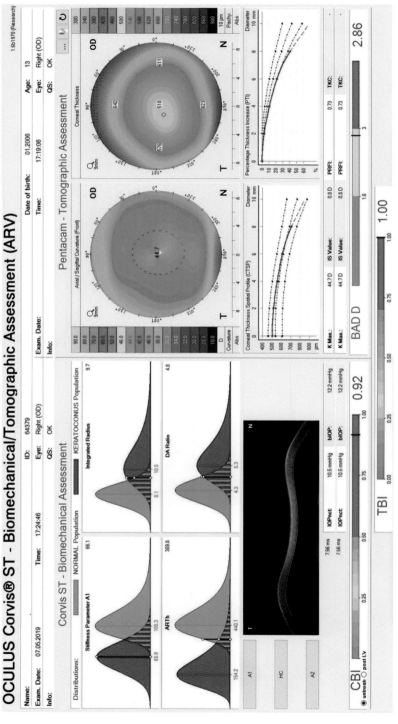

Fig. 20.5 Ambrósio, Roberts, Vinciguerra *(ARV)* Biomechanical and Tomographic Corvis ST Display. Right eye of a patient with VAE-E and normal tomography (VAE-NT). Abnormal reported indices are represented in *yellow* and *red*. (Image reproduced from Esporcatte LPG, Salomão MQ, Lopes BT, et al. Biomechanical diagnostics of the cornea. *Eye Vis (Lond)*. 2020;7:9. [http://creativecommons.org/licenses/by/4.0/.])

BOX 20.4 ■ The Ambrósio, Roberts, Vinciguerra (ARV) Corvis ST Display

The combined indices *CBI, TBI,* and *BAD-D* performed better than any individual biomechanical parameter.[22]

BOX 20.5 ■ Phonon Definition

Wavelets produced by molecular vibrations. These wavelets occur in every tissue at room temperature and are capable of traveling inside matter. Velocity of phonons is determined, among other methods, by the Young's modulus.[29]

---

virtually imaged phased array (VIPA) spectrometer.[30,34-36] The laser light that it employs has an output spectrum in the near-infrared wavelength (~780 nm) and is polarized by a polarization-maintaining fiber. This polarization-maintaining fiber also directs the backscattered light to a single-mode fiber. The collected light is then delivered to the VIPA, which achieves a free-spectral range of ~16 GHz, a resolution ~0.3 GHz and an extinction efficiency of –65 dB. Then an electron multiplying charge-coupled device (EM-CCD) records ~6000 Brillouin photons per second and with this information, at an integration time of 0.2 seconds, BOSS obtains the Brillouin frequency shift (Fig. 20.6).[29,34-36]

In corneal pathology, Brillouin microscopy is capable of mapping Young's modulus, creating the expectation for identifying specific corneal weak areas with great precision.[3] Moreover, unlike air-puffed devices, it elucidates intrinsic viscoelastic properties of the cornea without applying pressure and without being dependent on structural information.[5] Unlike other methods and owing to its high spatial resolution images, BOSS applications may extend beyond anterior and posterior segment structures.[3]

Normal Corneas

Evidence demonstrates a low Young's modulus in the epithelial region, a high Young's modulus in the anterior stroma (that decreases with depth), and a low Young's modulus in the endothelium.[30]

A significant correlation between age and Brillouin frequency (average increase rate of 4 MHz per decade) has been described.[29]

Keratoconus Corneas

Some studies have revealed a regional variation in the Brillouin shift of the cone region and the periphery (with lower values toward the apex of the cone).[29,34,37] In addition, Brillouin frequency shift has correlated with geometric KC indices at the point of maximum posterior elevation.[29] This asymmetric distribution may be useful for the diagnosis of early onset and progression of KC; however, more studies are needed to determine suitable criteria for making the diagnosis (Fig. 20.7).[29,34,37]

Cross-Linking

Studies have shown an increase in Brillouin frequency shift after CXL on bovine corneal samples. This would indicate that, after the procedure, the corneal tissue stiffens, with a greater effect in the anterior stroma.[30]

Limitations of Brillouin Spectroscopy

Clinically relevant Young's modulus values have been identified in a surface-parallel plane; nevertheless, measurements with the actual Brillouin devices are assessed using a surface-perpendicular direction.[29]

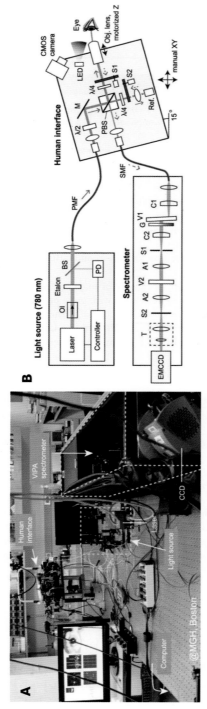

Fig. 20.6 (A) The Brillouin ocular analyzer system. (B) Schematic representation of the Brillouin imaging system with the light source, the human interface, and the double virtually imaged phased array (VIPA) spectrometer and the electron multiplying charge-coupled device (EM-CCD) camera. A1/2, Achromatic lens; BS, beam-sampler; C1/C2, cylindrical lens; M, mirror; Obj; L, objective lens; OI, optical isolator; PBS, polarizing beam-splitter; PD, photodiode; PMF, polarization maintaining; Ref, reference materials; S1/S2, optical shutters; SMF, single mode fiber; V1/V2, VIPAs; λ/4, quarter waveplate; λ/2, half waveplate; λ/4, quarter waveplate. (Imaged reproduced from Shao P, Eltony AM, Seiler TG, et al. Spatially-resolved Brillouin spectroscopy reveals biomechanical abnormalities in mild to advanced keratoconus in vivo. *Sci Rep.* 2019;9(1):7467. [http://creativecommons.org/licenses/by/4.0/.])

This Page Is Left Intentionally Blank

Before performing Brillouin spectroscopy, a tomographic characterization of the cornea is essential for detecting the thinnest point and the point of maximum posterior elevation of the cornea. This will allow correlation of the geometric KC indices with the Brillouin frequency shift.[29]

Additional disadvantages include the high price and long acquisition time (~15 minutes), which has greatly improved but remains impractical for routine clinical use.[29]

Today, the Brillouin frequency shift has been measured in normal and KC corneas, providing the opportunity to detect age-related and pathologic changes. Studies have demonstrated the potential for diagnosis of early forms of KC, screening for laser vision correction procedures, and follow-up after corneal CXL. Nevertheless, the utility of this technology in diagnosing early KC remains controversial, as some current limitations to Brillouin microscopy need to be addressed and better correlation with Young's modulus achieved. In addition, better techniques of measurement, such as impulsive stimulated Brillouin scattering, are being developed.[38] This may open possibilities for better diagnosis and for evaluation of other ocular structures such as the crystalline lens. Undoubtedly, this is a thriving field of study with potential for continued advancement.

Ex Vivo Devices

This technology is used in experimental models only, some of which are in development for potential in vivo use. This category includes:

- Elastography. A class of medical imaging modalities in which the aim is to describe the elastic properties of soft tissue for diagnostic purposes. Cornea elastography depends primarily on imaging such as optical coherence tomography, ultrasound, and, more recently, magnetic resonance.[3]
    - Ultrasound elastography. This imaging modality includes the ultrasound elasticity microscope, corneal transient elastography (CTE), and ocular pulse elastography. CTE is the method most used and employs echographic pulses, applied to different parts of the cornea, to create three-dimensional (3D) images of the different layers of the cornea (with a resolution of 150 μm).[3,39]
    - OCT elastography. The inclusion of OCT provides a significant improvement in tissue displacement measurements (from micrometers to depths of 1 mm).[3,40]
    - Magnetic resonance elastography. This technique has only been applied to evaluate ex vivo bovine corneas.[3, 41]
- Interferometry. Interferometry employs the basic principle of interferometry that coherent light scattered from an irregular surface will generate a pattern of constructive and destructive interference, and includes the interferometry-electronic speckle pattern interferometer (ESPI), the electronic speckle pattern shearing interferometer (ESPSI), and quantitative ultrasound spectroscopy.[3]

Conclusions

Corneal biomechanics is the area of science in which the relationship between the microstructure, macrostructure, and optical function of the cornea is analyzed. It provides a new way to conceptualize the cornea, as did topography and tomography, with the ultimate goal of enhancing the ability of the ophthalmologist to diagnose pathology in the anterior segment, determine treatment options, and document and measure its evolution.

Air-puff devices have contributed to a better understanding of the complexity of this anatomical structure, although some limitations in distinguishing the early forms of KC have been encountered.[4] However, Brillouin spectroscopy has been proven, with its spatially resolved method, to locate weak areas in the cornea and promises improvements in the diagnosis of KC.[3] Other prototypes of new technologies directly quantify Young's modulus and may herald a new era in imaging tools for corneal biomechanics.[3] Finally, with artificial intelligence (AI), the integration and combination of biomechanical and tomographic data are possible, providing an opportunity to better understand the interconnection between structure and optical function.

References

1. Imbornoni LM, McGhee CNJ, Belin MW. Evolution of keratoconus: from diagnosis to therapeutics. *Klin Monbl Augenheilkd.* 2018;235(6):680–688.
2. Seiler T, Quurke AW. Iatrogenic keratectasia after LASIK in a case of forme fruste keratoconus. *J Cataract Refract Surg.* 1998;24(7):1007–1009.
3. Yuan A, Pineda R. Developments in imaging of corneal biomechanics. *Int Ophthalmol Clin.* 2019;59(4):1–17.
4. De Stefano VS, Dupps WJ Jr. Biomechanical diagnostics of the cornea. *Int Ophthalmol Clin.* 2017;57(3):75–86.
5. Esporcatte LPG, Salomão MQ, Lopes BT, et al. Biomechanical diagnostics of the cornea. *Eye Vis (Lond).* 2020;7:9.
6. Roy A, Shetty R, Kummelil M. Keratoconus: a biomechanical perspective on loss of corneal stiffness. *Indian J Ophthalmol.* 2013;61(8):392.
7. Gokul A, Vellara HR, Patel DV. Advanced anterior segment imaging in keratoconus: a review. *Clin Exp Ophthalmol.* 2018;46(2):122–132.
8. Piñero DP, Alcón N. In vivo characterization of corneal biomechanics. *J Cataract Refract Surg.* 2014;40(6):870–887.
9. Shah S, Laiquzzaman M, Bhojwani R, Mantry S, Cunliffe I. Assessment of the biomechanical properties of the cornea with the Ocular Response Analyzer in normal and keratoconic eyes. *Invest Ophthalmol Vis Sci.* 2007;48(7):3026.
10. Luce DA. Determining in vivo biomechanical properties of the cornea with an Ocular Response Analyzer. *J Cataract Refract Surg.* 2005;31(1):156–162.
11. Hallahan KM, Roy AS, Ambrósio R, Salomao M, Dupps WJ Jr. Discriminant value of custom Ocular Response Analyzer waveform derivatives in keratoconus. *Ophthalmology.* 2014;121(2):459–468.
12. Ortiz D, Piñero D, Shabayek MH, Arnalich-Montiel F, Alió JL. Corneal biomechanical properties in normal, post-laser in situ keratomileusis, and keratoconic eyes. *J Cataract Refract Surg.* 2007;33(8):1371–1375.
13. Chen MC, Lee N, Bourla N, Hamilton RD. Corneal biomechanical measurements before and after laser in situ keratomileusis. *J Cataract Refract Surg.* 2008;34(11):1886–1891.
14. Kamiya K, Shimizu K, Ohmoto F. Comparison of the changes in corneal biomechanical properties after photorefractive keratectomy and laser in situ keratomileusis. *Cornea.* 2009;28(7):765–769.
15. Terai N, Raiskup F, Haustein M, Pillunat LE, Spoerl E. Identification of biomechanical properties of the cornea: the Ocular Response Analyzer. *Curr Eye Res.* 2012;37(7):553–562.
16. Hallahan KM, Rocha K, Sinha RA, Randleman JB, Stulting RD, Dupps WJ Jr. Effects of corneal cross-linking on Ocular Response Analyzer waveform-derived variables in keratoconus and postrefractive surgery ectasia. *Eye Contact Lens.* 2014;40(6):339–344.
17. Sedaghat M, Naderi M, Zarei-Ghanavati M. Biomechanical parameters of the cornea after collagen crosslinking measured by waveform analysis. *J Cataract Refract Surg.* 2010;36(10):1728–1731.
18. Goldich Y, Marcovich AL, Barkana Y, et al. Clinical and corneal biomechanical changes after collagen cross-linking with riboflavin and UV irradiation in patients with progressive keratoconus. *Cornea.* 2012;31(6):609–614.
19. Ali NQ, Patel DV, Mcghee CNJ. Biomechanical responses of healthy and keratoconic corneas measured using a noncontact Scheimpflug-based tonometer. *Invest Ophthalmol Vis Sci.* 2014;55(6):3651.
20. Tian L, Huang YF, Wang LQ, et al. Corneal biomechanical assessment using corneal visualization Scheimpflug technology in keratoconic and normal eyes. *J Ophthalmol.* 2014;2014:1–8.
21. Vinciguerra R, Ambrósio R, Elsheikh A, et al. Detection of keratoconus with a new biomechanical index. *J Refract Surg.* 2016;32(12):803–810.
22. Sedaghat MR, Momeni-Moghaddam H, Ambrósio R, et al. Diagnostic ability of corneal shape and biomechanical parameters for detecting frank keratoconus. *Cornea.* 2018;37(8):1025–1034.
23. Wang YM, Chan TC, Yu M, Jhanji V. Comparison of corneal dynamic and tomographic analysis in normal, forme fruste keratoconic, and keratoconic eyes. *J Refract Surg.* 2017;33(9):632–638.

24. Frings A, Linke S, Bauer E, Druchkiv V, Katz T, Steinberg J. Effects of laser in situ keratomileusis (LASIK) on corneal biomechanical measurements with the Corvis ST tonometer. *Clin Ophthalmol.* 2015;9:305–311.

25. Mastropasqua L, Calienno R, Lanzini M, et al. Evaluation of corneal biomechanical properties modification after small incision lenticule extraction using Scheimpflug-based noncontact tonometer. *Biomed Res Int.* 2014;2014:1–8.

26. Lee H, Roberts CJ, Ambrósio R, Elsheikh A, Kang DSY, Kim TI. Effect of accelerated corneal crosslinking combined with transepithelial photorefractive keratectomy on dynamic corneal response parameters and biomechanically corrected intraocular pressure measured with a dynamic Scheimpflug analyzer in healthy myopic patients. *J Cataract Refract Surg.* 2017;43(7):937–945.

27. Hashemi H, Ambrósio R, Vinciguerra R, et al. Two-year changes in corneal stiffness parameters after accelerated corneal cross-linking. *J Biomech.* 2019;93:209–212.

28. Eliasy A, Chen KJ, Vinciguerra R, et al. Determination of corneal biomechanical behavior in-vivo for healthy eyes using Corvis ST tonometry: stress-strain index. *Front Bioeng Biotechnol.* 2019;7:105.

29. Seiler TG, Shao P, Eltony A, Seiler T, Yun SH. Brillouin spectroscopy of normal and keratoconus corneas. *Am J Ophthalmol.* 2019;202:118.

30. Scarcelli G, Yun SH. In vivo Brillouin optical microscopy of the human eye. *Optics Express.* 2012;20(8):9197.

31. Vaughan JM, Randall JT. Brillouin scattering, density and elastic properties of the lens and cornea of the eye. *Nature.* 1980;284(5755):489–491.

32. Scarcelli G, Kim P, Yun SH. In vivo measurement of age-related stiffening in the crystalline lens by Brillouin optical microscopy. *Biophysical J.* 2011;101(6):1539–1545.

33. Lepert G, Gouveia RM, Connon CJ, Paterson C. Assessing corneal biomechanics with Brillouin spectromicroscopy. *Faraday Discuss.* 2016;187:415–428.

34. Scarcelli G, Besner S, Pineda R, Yun SH. Biomechanical characterization of keratoconus corneas ex vivo with Brillouin microscopy. *Invest Ophthalmol Vis Sci.* 2014;55(7):4490.

35. Scarcelli G, Pineda R, Yun SH. Brillouin optical microscopy for corneal biomechanics. *Invest Ophthalmol Vis Sci.* 2012;53(1):185.

36. Shao P, Eltony AM, Seiler TG, et al. Spatially-resolved Brillouin spectroscopy reveals biomechanical abnormalities in mild to advanced keratoconus in vivo. *Sci Rep.* 2019;9(1):7467.

37. Scarcelli G, Besner S, Pineda R, Kalout P, Yun SH. In vivo biomechanical mapping of normal and keratoconus corneas. *JAMA Ophthalmol.* 2015;133(4):480.

38. Ballmann CW, Meng Z, Yakovlev VV. Nonlinear Brillouin spectroscopy: what makes it a better tool for biological viscoelastic measurements. *Biomedical Optics Express.* 2019;10(4):1750.

39. Tanter M, Touboul D, Gennisson JL, Bercoff J, Fink M. High-resolution quantitative imaging of cornea elasticity using supersonic shear imaging. *IEEE Trans Med Imaging.* 2009;28(12):1881–1893.

40. Schmitt JM. OCT elastography: imaging microscopic deformation and strain of tissue. *Optics Express.* 1998;3(6):199.

41. Pavlatos E, Chen H, Clayson K, Pan X, Liu J. Imaging corneal biomechanical responses to ocular pulse using high-frequency ultrasound. *IEEE Trans Med Imaging.* 2018;37(2):663–670.

Non-Surgical Management

CHAPTER 21

Keratoconus: Diagnosis and Management With Spectacles and Contact Lenses

Melissa Barnett ■ Karen Lee ■ Mark Mannis

KEY CONCEPTS

- Retinoscopy can play an important role in keratoconus screening, because of its portability, affordability, sensitivity, and easy accessibility.
- With progression in keratoconus, contact lenses are recommended for vision restoration and delayed surgical intervention.
- Corneal gas permeable contact lenses play a large role in keratoconus management and continue to be the initial lens of choice among practitioners when fitting the irregular cornea.
- Hybrid lenses are a good lens option for those who are intolerant of corneal gas permeable contact lenses.
- Scleral lenses are large diameter gas permeable contact lenses that vault the cornea and land on the scleral conjunctiva.
- SLs offer visual improvement and neutralize irregularities of the corneal surface. Compared to corneal lenses, SLs have improved centration and stability.

Introduction

Early detection and management of keratoconus (KC) is critical and may impact quality of life. Glasses and contact lenses (CLs) may be utilized to aid function early in the course of the disease. However, CLs do not slow or stop the advancement of KC. Spectacle correction may be used in mild cases of KC, or used at home in addition to CLs. Vision may be limited, since glasses do not correct irregular astigmatism. Soft contact lenses (SCLs) are an option in early cases. In moderate to advanced cases, rigid corneal gas permeable (GP), piggyback, hybrid, and scleral lenses (SL) improve vision by correcting irregular astigmatism induced by an irregular cornea. In this chapter we will review various types of spectacles and CLs in the optical management of KC.

RETINOSCOPY

The retinoscope, a common tool utilized by optometrists and ophthalmologists for objective refraction, has been available since the early 1900s and may play an important role in KC screening, as it is portable, affordable, sensitive, and easily accessible. During retinoscopy, a streak of light is directed into the patient's eye and reflects off the retina, producing a light reflex that can be neutralized by correcting the patient's refractive error. High myopia, irregular astigmatism, and a scissoring reflex are commonly observed during retinoscopy in a KC patient.[1,2] The scissoring reflex is more prominently noted in those with advanced disease and is a strong indicator of KC. When compared with the Belin and Ambrósio Enhanced Ectasia display on the Pentacam (OCULUS GmbH, Wetzlar, Germany), the retinoscope had a 98% sensitivity and 78% specificity in KC diagnosis.[2]

Pinhole visual acuity may help to demonstrate an approximate improvement in vision; however, the amount of improvement in pinhole acuity may not be a true gauge of best-corrected acuity. In patients with KC, spectacle or CL acuity may not match the pinhole acuity because of posterior corneal irregularities and/or corneal scarring.

REFRACTION

A baseline refraction is beneficial in determining best-corrected visual acuity (BCVA). In patients with KC and irregular astigmatism, BCVA may be reduced and may not be improved with manifest refraction. Reduced vision with manifest refraction and spectacle correction may be a strong motivator for the use of GP CLs. Conversely, if vision is relatively good with manifest refraction, the patient may not be as motivated to wear GP CLs. Improvement of visual acuity with CLs compared with manifest refraction and documentation of visual improvement may be important for legal and insurance purposes. Even if vision is poor, glasses to wear at home after CL removal may be beneficial.

A manifest refraction can aid the type of CL selected and in deciding whether CLs or glasses should be recommended. If refractive error is relatively symmetrical, glasses are tolerable, visual acuity meets driving standards, and glasses are comfortable to wear, spectacle correction may be an acceptable option. However, glasses may not optimally correct visual acuity, reduce glare and halos, nor correct higher-order aberrations. In these instances, CLs are a better option. If a prescription for glasses is given, one should consider postponing the refraction until after the CL fitting is finalized, to minimize spectacle blur.

A study of 90 eyes in 61 patients with KC compared corrected distance visual acuity with autorefraction and manifest refraction.[3] Superior vision was achieved with manifest refraction compared with autorefraction. Additionally, the difference between the autorefraction and manifest refraction increases as the cornea steepens. This study concluded that autorefraction is not reliable in patients with KC. However, evaluation of the mires when performing autorefraction may be diagnostic of KC. Irregular mires may be indicative of high and/or irregular astigmatism.

SOFT CONTACT LENSES

As KC progresses and spectacles no longer provide adequate visual acuity, patients and practitioners turn to CLs for vision restoration and delayed surgical intervention.[4,5] Viable options are abundant and include commercially available SCLs, custom SCLs, specialty KC SCLs, corneal GP lenses, hybrid lenses, piggyback lens systems, and scleral lenses (SLs). Ideally, the CL should feel comfortable, not compromise ocular health, and provide functional vision. It is important to note that the ability of CLs to treat or prevent KC progression is a common misconception, especially among patients, and has been disproven.[6]

Early or mild KC patients may do well in commercially available SCLs as toric and extended range parameters are readily manufactured (Table 21.1). If decreased acuity or lens decentration is noted with commercially available SCLs, numerous laboratories also offer custom SCLs with greater power ranges and parameter availability. These made-to-order lenses may provide improved vision, a better fit, and greater comfort as they are tailored specifically for the patient (Table 21.2). These SCLs are limited when fitting the more advanced KC patient, as they tend to contour to and assume the irregular keratoconic cornea.

TABLE 21.1 ■ Commercially Available Soft Contact Lenses With Extended Ranges for Those With High Myopia and Astigmatism

Contact Lens Name and Manufacturer	Sphere Power Range	Cylinder Power Range	Axis	Replacement Schedule
Biofinity XR (CooperVision)	−12.50 D to −20.00 D +8.50 D to +15.00 D (0.50-D steps)	N/A	N/A	1 month
Biofinity Toric XR (CooperVision)	±10.00 D (0.50-D steps after ±6.00)	−0.75 to −5.75 (0.50-D steps)	5–180 degrees (5-degree steps)	1 month
Proclear Toric XR (CooperVision)	±10.00 D (0.50-D steps after −6.50 D and +6.00 D)	−0.75 to −5.75 (0.50-D steps)	5–180 degrees (5-degree steps)	1 month

TABLE 21.2 ■ Example of Custom Soft Contact Lens Parameter Availabilities. Numerous Designs Are Available and Are Manufacturer Dependent

Diameter	Base Curve	Sphere Power Range	Cylinder Power Range	Axis	Replacement Schedule
10.0 mm–16.0 mm	6.9–9.5 mm (0.1-mm steps)	+/-30.00 D (0.10-D steps)	−0.25 to −8.00 (0.1-D steps)	0–360 degrees (1-degree steps)	Practitioner discretion

SPECIALTY SOFT CONTACT LENSES FOR KERATOCONUS

Masking front surface corneal irregularity requires a neutralizing tear lens under a smooth refractive plane and may be achieved with a GP lens.[7] Specialty SCLs designed specifically for the KC patient exhibit characteristics similar to a GP lens and mask low amounts of corneal irregularity as they are lathed in higher modulus (stiffer) materials or are designed with greater lens center thicknesses. Many KC SCLs are available in silicone hydrogel materials or even utilize fenestrations to prevent corneal hypoxia. Diagnostic fitting and following the manufacturer fit guide are recommended as numerous designs are available and vary greatly in fitting philosophy (Table 21.3). If a patient is adamantly against wearing GP lenses or is intolerant of them, overlay spectacles may be prescribed in addition to SCL wear for possible further vision rehabilitation.

CORNEAL GAS PERMEABLE CONTACT LENSES

Corneal GP lenses play a large role in KC management and continue to be the initial lens of choice among practitioners when fitting the irregular cornea.[10] Fitting goals for a corneal GP lens are that they vault minimally over the corneal apex to prevent epithelial disruption, and provide midperipheral bearing and moderate peripheral clearance. In early KC, an ideal fit is easier to obtain. In moderate to advanced KC, it is more difficult to obtain an optimal fit because of corneal irregularities.

KC patients with paracentral "nipple" cones often do well with smaller diameter corneal GP lenses, whereas patients with larger "oval" cones or decentered cones fare better with medium or large diameter corneal GP lenses (Table 21.4). A poor-fitting GP lens may be uncomfortable and compromise ocular health. A known risk factor for corneal scarring is a flat-fitting GP lens with

TABLE 21.3 ■ **Specialty Soft Contact Lenses for Keratoconus**

Manufacturer	Contact Lens Name
ABB Optical Group	Concise K
	KeraSoft IC and KeraSoft Thin
Acculens	Soft K
Advanced Vision Technologies	Soft K and Soft K Definitive
	NaturaSOFT IC and ICR
Bausch+Lomb	NovaKone and NovaKone Toric
Art Optical	KeraSoft Thin
Continental	Continental Kone
GP Specialists	YamaKone IC
Gelflex USA	Keratoconus Lens
Marietta	Soflex
Metro Optics	Revitaleyes and Revitaleyes Definitive
	KeraSoft Thin
Ocu-Ease, Optech	Ocu-Flex K
TruForm Optics	KeraSoft IC and KeraSoft Thin
United Contact Lens	UCL K-Lens
Visionary Optics	HydroKone and HydroKone Toric
X-Cel Contacts	Flexlens ARC and Flexlens Tri-Curve

Adapted from Bennett ES, Barr JT, Szczotka-Flynn L. Keratoconus. In: Bennett ES, Henry VA, eds. *Clinical Manual of Contact Lenses*. 5th ed. Wolters Kluwer; 2020:590–591[8] and Thompson TT. *Tyler's Quarterly Soft Contact Lens Parameter Guide: TQ*. Vol. 38. Avisha Vision, LLC; 2021:18–18.[9]

TABLE 21.4 ■ **Corneal Gas Permeable Lens (GPs) Types, Diameters, and Keratoconic Considerations**

Corneal GP Type	Diameter Range	Keratoconus Indication
Small diameter corneal GP	8.5–9.5 mm	Central/paracentral "nipple" cone
Medium diameter corneal GP	9.3–10.9 mm	Larger cone
		Decentered cone
Large diameter or intralimbal GP	11.0–12.2 mm	Oval cone
		Decentered cone

associated corneal staining.[11] Patients in flat-fitting GP lenses also experienced more lens discomfort and a greater propensity for corneal transplantation.[12] It is imperative that a harsh apical bearing relationship be avoided when fitting the KC patient, regardless of the GP lens diameter utilized. Two common fitting philosophies strive for either very light apical bearing (three-point touch) or mild apical clearance first definite apical clearance lens (FDACL) fluorescein pattern.[13] Adequate peripheral edge lift and movement on blink is also necessary to facilitate tear exchange and debris removal. Lens design software available in some corneal topographers may simplify the fitting process by relaying information directly to GP lens laboratories. Advanced lathing technologies can also be used to fabricate asymmetric peripheral curves, creating a more uniform edge during GP lens wear. Numerous corneal GP lens designs of various diameters are available from every GP lens laboratory.

In general, corneal GP lenses for KC comprise a small diameter, steep base curve radius, and spherical or aspheric peripheral curves. A type of conventional lens design is the Collaborative Longitudinal Evaluation of Keratoconus (CLEK) design. More recent designs include Rose K2, ComfortKone, TruKone, Dyna Z Cone, V Cone, C Cone, and E Cone. Intralimbal designs include Dyna Intra-Limbal, Rose K2 IC, and the G.B.L. For detailed information on each lens design, we advise referencing the fitting guide from the specific manufacturer.

PIGGYBACK CONTACT LENS SYSTEM

Poor corneal GP lens centration, lens discomfort, and ejection with blink are often noted in the advanced KC patient. Although these patients are often better suited for a hybrid or SL, refitting into these advanced designs can be cost prohibitive. A piggyback system comprising an SCL under a corneal GP lens may be a viable solution that maintains ocular health while simultaneously improving both lens fit and vision (Fig. 21.1). A plus-powered SCL will not only act as a bandage, but will also provide a centralized convex surface to aide GP lens centration. Approximately 20.9% of the SCL power is contributed toward the total refractive error correction.[14] One can minimize GP lens power modifications by selecting a low-powered, well-fitting silicone hydrogel lens of high Dk (Contact lens oxygen permeability). Both the SCL and corneal GP lens should exhibit good independent lens movement to allow adequate tear exchange and facilitate debris removal. Selecting a lens with a lower modulus or steeper base curve may decrease any noted edge fluting (Fig. 21.2). The piggyback system may be cumbersome, as it requires the proper care and handling of two different sets of CLs. Prescribing a daily disposable SCL will simplify the process but may increase patient cost.

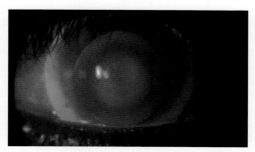

Fig. 21.1 A piggyback lens system highlighted with high molecular weight sodium fluorescein. (Image credit Karen Lee, OD.)

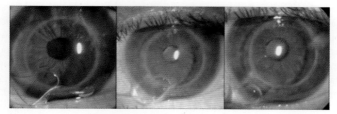

Fig. 21.2 Lens edge fluting in three different soft contact lenses. *left*, Edge fluting noted with a lens of modulus 1.4 MPa; *middle*, decreased fluting noted, with an 8.8-mm base curvature radius (BCR) lens and modulus of 0.72 MPa; and *right*, least edge fluting when an 8.4-mm BCR lens with 0.72 MPa modulus is used. (Image courtesy Karen Lee, OD.)

HYBRID CONTACT LENSES

Hybrid lenses are a good lens option for those who are intolerant of corneal GP lenses and dislike SLs. The only KC hybrid lens currently on the market in the United States is UltraHealth (SynergEyes, Carlsbad, CA). This lens design consists of a corneal GP lens bonded with a soft peripheral silicone hydrogel skirt. The central GP lens provides crisp optics and offers ultraviolet protection, whereas the soft skirt enhances lens comfort, stability, and centration. An ideal fitting hybrid lens should vault over corneal irregularities and move freely, ensuring adequate tear exchange. UltraHealth lenses can also be ordered empirically from patient data. This may increase likelihood of success and decrease necessary after time. Outside of the US, EyeBridTM hybrid lenses are used for keratoconus and irregular corneas. An extensive range of EyeBridTM parameters are available, including spherical, bitoric, back surface toric, front surface toric, and for presbyopia with astigmatism. multifocal

SCLERAL LENSES

SLs are large-diameter GP CLs that vault the cornea and land on the scleral conjunctiva.[15] SLs made of blown glass shells were first described in the late 1800s.[16–18] Optical correction of corneal irregularity in patients with KC was described by Fick and Kalt.[16,17] In the early 1900s, SLs were manufactured from polymethyl methacrylate (PMMA) material and impression molds were used to shape these lenses. Shortcomings of conventional SLs were reproducibility, hypoxia, and design limitations. Interest in SLs has continued to expand since Don Ezekiel's description in 1983 of rigid gas permeable (RGP) SLs in the management of KC, high ametropia, corneal scarring, and ocular surface disease. Modern SLs have highly oxygen-permeable materials, are very reproducible with repeatable computer-assisted lathes, and are highly customized with sophisticated designs. The main indications of SLs are visual rehabilitation in irregular corneas, therapeutic treatment of ocular surface disease, and correction of refractive error in normal or healthy eyes.[15] Fluid in the SL post-lens fluid reservoir corrects corneal irregularities and provides continuous corneal lubrication and ocular protection.

SLs offer visual improvement and neutralize irregularities of the corneal surface. Compared to corneal lenses, SLs have improved centration and stability. As SLs do not touch the cornea, there is improved comfort due to less lens awareness. A recent study compared the comfort and visual performance of corneal RGP CLs and SLs in participants with corneal ectasia successfully wearing habitual corneal RGP lenses. Significantly improved comfort was reported for SLs compared with RGP lenses.[19] SLs are less likely to reshape the cornea mechanically and cause corneal warpage than corneal GP lenses. The use of SLs in the management of corneal ectasias, both primary and secondary, has been described extensively. Primary corneal ectasia includes KC, keratoglobus, and pellucid marginal degeneration. Secondary corneal ectasia may occur after refractive surgery, corneal transplantation, or after traumatic scarring.

According to the published literature, KC is the single most common indication for SL fitting.[20–23] Use of SLs may delay or even avoid surgical intervention. A retrospective study investigated the success and failure rates of SL correction in severe KC.[4] Patients with KC with maximal keratometry values ≥70 diopters (D, determined by Scheimpflug tomography sagittal curvature map) examined in a KC clinic between January 1, 2010 and December 31, 2014 were included in the study. SLs were prescribed in 51 of 75 eyes. In patients with severe KC that would otherwise have undergone corneal transplant surgery, 40 of 51 eyes were successfully treated with long-term SL wear. Thus the indication for keratoplasty was more than halved in the KC population. A different study evaluated the association of SL use on the risk for keratoplasty for people with KC.[24] Electronic health records were viewed between August 1, 2012, and December 31, 2018. Patients with keratoconus or corneal ectasia without a history of keratoplasty were included. Using a multivariable Cox regression model, associations between SCL use and keratoplasty were tested and adjusted for sociodemographic factors, maximum keratometry, and current CL wear. Out of 2806 eyes, 36.2% wore contact lenses (7.2% soft, 33.9% GP, and 22.7% scleral). Of all eyes, 3.2% underwent keratoplasty. Contact lens wear significantly lowered the risk of undergoing keratoplasty. Keratoplasty was not associated with sex, insurance, or maximum keratometry measurements.

SPECIAL CONSIDERATIONS FOR SCLERAL LENSES IN KERATOCONUS

There are multiple considerations when selecting a SL for KC. Corneal and scleral topography and/or tomography are beneficial to determine the type of KC and areas of elevation. Corneal diameter, the presence of ocular surface disease, palpebral aperture, and disease severity are all considerations for initial lens selection. In a patient with mild KC, a smaller diameter SL may be used. In a patient with advanced KC or keratoglobus, a larger diameter SL may be preferred. For those with progressive KC, a SL may be fitted with additional sagittal depth to allow room for progression.

In cases of extreme ectasia, a specialized design such as BostonSight Scleral or EyePrintPRO may be preferable. A retrospective study evaluated indications and outcomes of patients fitted with an EyePrintPRO therapeutic SL. There was improvement in quality of vision and the comfort of lenses, and a reduction in dry eye, eye redness, and pain symptoms.[25]

SLs have been utilized to minimize visual distortion after corneal collagen cross-linking for KC. A prospective cohort study evaluated subjective and objective SL tolerance in 18 unilateral eyes in habitual SL wearers who underwent corneal cross-linking.[26] There was no significant change between preprocedure distance visual acuity and acuity with SLs 1 year after cross-linking. Median wearing time of 16 hours per day and subjective tolerance were stable. This study demonstrated the benefits of SLs in the management of primary corneal ectasia and that lenses may be used in combination with other modalities.

SLs have been utilized to improve vision and reduce higher-order aberrations after intracorneal ring segment (ICRS) implantation for KC. Twenty-seven eyes of 27 patients with KC had SLs fitted after ICRS implantation.[27] There was improvement in visual acuity, decreased high-order aberrations, and improvement of spatial frequencies of contrast sensitivity. Quality of vision and lens wear time were improved. No adverse effects were reported nor changes in corneal parameters, visual quality, comfort scores, or wearing time. Thus, those with KC after ICRS implantation may successfully wear SLs.

SCLERAL LENS SOLUTIONS

Proper handwashing is critical prior to handling SLs. Washing hands with soap and water decreases the risk of contamination. To avoid risk of contamination, hands must be completely dried using a clean towel.

SLs require two solutions, one for lens application and one for disinfection. SLs should be filled with preservative-free solution since there is longer contact time to the cornea compared with corneal GP lenses. Preservative-free saline is used for lens application. Since the solution does not contain preservatives, it must be discarded after a single use to avoid an infiltrative event or microbial keratitis. It is important to overfill the SL with preservative-free saline, until the solution is convex above the lens.

SLs are worn during the day, removed prior to sleeping, and require overnight storage in a disinfecting solution that kills pathogens associated with eye infections. The two types of disinfection systems are multipurpose and hydrogen peroxide disinfection care systems. Multipurpose disinfecting solutions clean and disinfect with a single product. A digital rub is utilized with multipurpose solutions. Hydrogen peroxide disinfecting solutions are effective for SLs, particularly for those sensitive to chemicals and preservatives in multipurpose solutions. Hydrogen peroxide systems require a disinfection process in which the hydrogen peroxide neutralizes into saline. This process occurs over a period of 4 to 6 hours. A surfactant cleaner may be added to either care system to improve the cleaning process for SLs.

Surface treatments may be applied to the SL to improve the lens wearing experience. Plasma treatment is used to enhance wettability on the SL surface. A finished lens is bombarded with high-energy radio waves in an oxygen-rich environment. The GP lens surface undergoes radiofrequency ionized oxygen that makes hydrophobic surfaces more hydrophilic, thus improving surface wettability. Exotic oxygen radicals strike the surface of the lens and dislodge hydrocarbons such as oils. Molecules on the lens surface are rearranged as carbon migrates away from the surface and oxygen and nitrogen migrate toward the surface. The lens surface becomes ionized, increasing its ability to attract liquids, which increases surface wettability and resists protein and bacterial deposits.

Plasma treatment is the first step in Tangible Hydra-PEG treatment. Tangible Hydra-PEG is a novel surface treatment comprising a 90% water polyethylene glycol (PEG)-based polymer mixture that is permanently bonded to the surface of the CL, made from the lubricant PEG. Tangible Hydra-PEG shields the lens surface from the tear film and ocular surface, minimizes friction and deposition, and improves lens wettability, tear film breakup time, and deposit resistance, ultimately enhancing CL comfort. A study compared lens comfort and dry eye symptoms of SL wearers with dry eye, fitted with Tangible Hydra-PEG treated and untreated SLs. PEG-treated SL wear led to significantly improved lens comfort; reduced dry eye symptoms; reduced corneal sodium fluorescein staining and temporal conjunctival lissamine green staining; reduced lid wiper epitheliopathy, reduction of conjunctival papillae, lower frequency of foggy vision, and increased tear breakup time and increased comfortable lens wearing time compared with untreated lens wear.[28]

SCLERAL LENS APPLICATION

Difficulty with SL application and removal is the main reason for discontinuing lens wear.[28] Reported dropout rates range from 25% to 49%.[30,31] Patient education materials are available from the Scleral Lens Education Society (SLS) and other resources at no charge. The SLS YouTube page has a video titled *Scleral Contact Lens Insertion, Removal, Troubleshooting and Lens Care* that reviews SL care and handling in detail (Fig. 21.3).

Patients may initially find it easier to apply and remove the lens with a rubber plunger. SL plungers should be cleaned nightly with 70% isopropyl rubbing alcohol and replaced every 3 to 4 months as the surface erodes. The SL should be rinsed thoroughly with preservative-free saline (Fig. 21.4). The patient should overfill the SL with preservative-free saline, position the head parallel to the table, raise the SL towards the eye and gently close the eye around the plunger once the SL is in contact with the conjunctiva. The eye is then gently closed around the plunger, and once the SL is in contact with the eye, the plunger is pulled away, separating it from the SL. With increased experience, patients may forgo the application plunger and opt to use the tripod method when applying their SL (Fig. 21.5).

One should check for the presence of application bubbles or poor surface wetting immediately after lens application. If an application bubble or fluctuating vision occurs, the lens should be

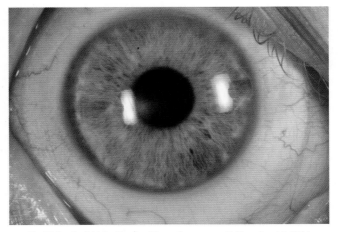

Fig. 21.3   An ideally fit scleral lens. (Image credit Tom Arnold, OD.)

A

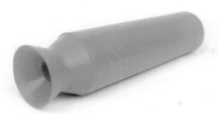

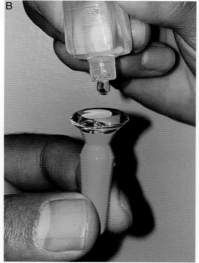

Fig. 21.4   (A and B) DMV Scleral Cup for scleral lens application.

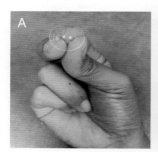
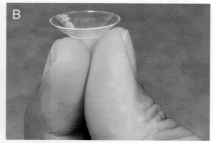

Fig. 21.5   (A and B) Tripod (Inserter) method.

removed, cleaned, and reapplied, as longstanding bubbles may cause ocular discomfort and corneal epithelium desiccation, and alter the overrefraction over the lens.

Scleral Lens Removal

After washing the hands and drying with a lint-free towel, the patient moistens the removal plunger with a few drops of saline and opens the eye as wide as possible before gently placing the removal plunger on the lens periphery (Figs. 21.6 and 21.7). The plunger and lens are gently

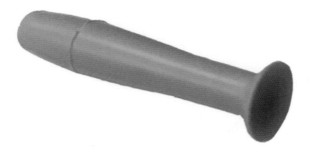

Fig. 21.6 DMV Ultra removal plunger.

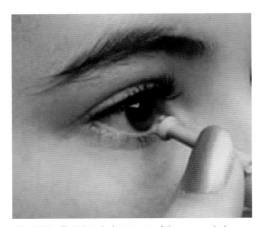

Fig. 21.7 Peripheral placement of the removal plunger.

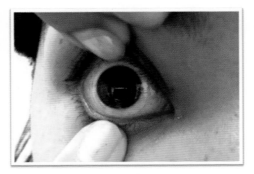

Fig. 21.8 Patient removing scleral lens with finger method.

pulled away from the eye. Central placement of the removal plunger is discouraged as increased SL suction may be experienced. Patients may also break SL suction by gently indenting the bulbar conjunctiva adjacent to the lens edge and allowing air bubbles into the lens reservoir.

SLs can be removed without the aid of a plunger, using just fingers. The lids are controlled by placing the pointer finger of the nondominant hand on the middle of the upper eyelid and the pointer finger of the dominant hand on the middle of the lower eyelid margin (Fig. 21.8). The patient then pulls the lids apart and gently presses the lower eyelid margin in toward the globe and up and under the lens edge (Fig. 21.9).

Additional application and removal challenges may be experienced by those with poor uncorrected visual acuity or poor finger dexterity owing to arthritic joints or tremors. Alternative

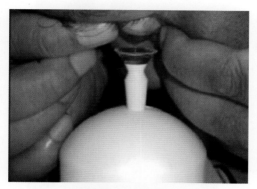

Fig. 21.9 Patient applying scleral lens with the use of the plunger stand.

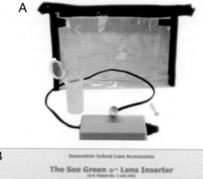

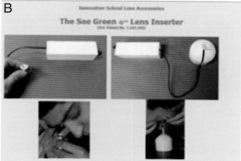

Fig. 21.10 (A and B) See-Green Lens Inserter system.

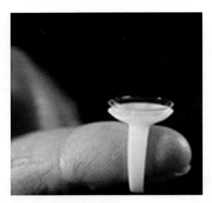

Fig. 21.11   EZi scleral lens applicator on finger with scleral lens.

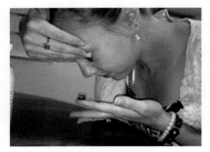

Fig. 21.12   Patient applying scleral lens with #8 O ring.

application devices such as a plunger stand, See-Green Lens inserter system (Fig. 21.10), Ezi ring applicator (Fig. 21.11), or a standard #8 O ring (Fig. 21.12) should be considered. These devices may further aid those who are unsuccessful with the traditional methods of applying and removing a SL.

It is critical to diagnose and manage keratoconus early in the disease process prior to loss of vision. If possible, corneal collagen cross-linking should be performed prior to the progression of KC. Whereas glasses and SCLs may be adequate in mild cases of KC, in more advanced cases, rigid corneal GP, piggyback, hybrid, and scleral lenses provide a greater improvement in visual acuity and comfort.

References

1. Krachmer JH, Feder RS, Belin MW. Keratoconus and related noninflammatory corneal thinning disorders. *Surv Ophthalmol.* 1984;28(4):293–322.
2. Al-Mahrouqi H, Oraba SB, Al-Habsi S, et al. Retinoscopy as a screening tool for keratoconus. *Cornea.* 2019;38(4):442–445.
3. Soeters N, Muijzer MB, Molenaar J. Godefrooij DA, Wisse RPL. Autorefraction versus manifest refraction in patients with keratoconus. *J Refract Surg.* 2018;34(1):30–34.
4. Koppen C, Kreps EO, Anthonissen L, Van Hoey M, Dhubhghaill SN, Vermeulen L. Scleral lenses reduce the need for corneal transplants in severe keratoconus. *Am J Ophthalmol.* 2018;185:43–47.
5. Rathi VM, Mandathara PS, Dumpati S. Contact lens in keratoconus. In: *Indian J Ophthalmol.* 2013 61(8):410.
6. Edrington TB, Szczotka LB, Barr JT, et al. Rigid contact lens fitting relationships in keratoconus. Collaborative Longitudinal Evaluation of Keratoconus (CLEK) Study Group. *Optom Vis Sci.* 1999;76(10):692–699.

7. Jupiter DG, Katz HR. Management of irregular astigmatism with rigid gas permeable contact lenses. *CLAO J.* 2000;26(1):14–17.
8. Bennett ES, Barr JT, Szczotka-Flynn L, *Keratoconus. In: Bennett ES, Henry VA, eds. Clinical Manual of Contact Lenses.* 5th ed. Wolters Kluwer; 2020:590–591.
9. Thompson TT. Tyler's quarterly soft contact lens parameter guide: TQ. Vol 38. *Avisha Vision, LLC;* 2021:18–18.
10. Shorter E, Harthan J, Nau CB, et al. Scleral lenses in the management of corneal irregularity and ocular surface disease. *Eye Contact Lens.* 2018;44(6):372–378.
11. Barr JT, Zadnik K, Wilson BS, et al. Factors associated with corneal scarring in the collaborative longitudinal evaluation of keratoconus (CLEK) study. *Cornea.* 2000;19(4):501–507.
12. Zadnik K, Barr JT, Steger-May K, Edrington TB, McMahon TT, et al. Gordon M. Comparison of flat and steep rigid contact lens fitting methods in keratoconus. *Optom Vis Sci.* 2005;82(12):1014–1021.
13. Edrington TB, Barr JT, Zadnik K, et al. Standardized rigid contact lens fitting protocol for keratoconus. *Optom Vis Sci.* 1996;73(6):369–375.
14. Michaud L, Brazeau D, Corbeil ME, Forcier P, Bernard PJ. Contribution of soft lenses of various powers to the optics of a piggy-back system on regular corneas. *Cont Lens Anterior Eye.* 2013;36(6):318–323.
15. Schornack M. Medical indications for scleral lens use. In: Barnett M, Johns LK, eds.. *Contemporary Scleral Lenses: Theory and Application.* Vol. 4 1st ed. Bentham Science; 2017: 135–141.
16. Efron N, Pearson RM. Centenary celebration of Fick's eine Contactbrille. *Arch Ophthalmol.* 1988;106(10):1370–1377.
17. Pearson RM. Kalt, keratoconus, and the contact lens. *Optom Vis Sci.* 1989;66(9):643–646.
18. Pearson RM, Efron N. Hundredth anniversary of August Muller's inaugural dissertation on contact lenses. *Surv Ophthalmol.* 1989;34(2):133–141.
19. Levit A, Benwell M, Evans BJW. Randomised controlled trial of corneal vs. scleral rigid gas permeable contact lenses for keratoconus and other ectatic corneal disorders. *Cont Lens Anterior Eye.* 2020;43(6):543–552.
20. Tan DT, Pullum KW, Buckley RJ. Medical applications of scleral contact lenses. *Cornea.* 1995;14(2):121–129.
21. Rosenthal P, Croteau A. Fluid-ventilated, gas-permeable scleral contact lens is an effective option for managing severe ocular surface disease and many corneal disorders that would otherwise require penetrating keratoplasty. *Eye Contact Lens.* 2005;31(3):130–134.
22. Pullum KW, Whiting MA, Buckley RJ. Scleral contact lenses: the expanding role. *Cornea.* 2005;24(3):269–277.
23. Visser ES, Visser R, van Lier HJ, Otten HM. Modern scleral lenses part I: clinical features. *Eye Contact Lens.* 2007;33(1):13–20.
24. Ling, J, Shahzad M, Stein J, et al. Impact of Scleral Contact Lens Use on the Rate of Corneal Transplantation for Keratoconus. *Cornea* 2021 Jan:40(1):39-42. doi: 10.1097.
25. Nguyen MTB, Thakrar V, Chan CC. EyePrintPRO therapeutic scleral contact lens: indications and outcomes. *Can J Ophthalmol.* 2018;53(1):66–70.
26. Visser ES, Soeters N, Tahzib NG. Scleral lens tolerance after corneal cross-linking for keratoconus. *Optom Vis Sci.* 2015;92(3):318–323.
27. Montalt JC, Porcar E, España-Gregori E, Peris-Martínez C. Visual quality with corneo-scleral contact lenses after intracorneal ring segment (ICRS) implantation for keratoconus management. *Cont Lens Anterior Eye.* 2019;42(1):111–116.
28. Mickles C, Harthan J, Barnett M. A surface treatment solution for scleral lens wearers with dry eye. Free Paper GSLS. 2019.
29. Fadel D, Toabe M. Scleral lens issues and complications related to handling, care and compliance. *J Contact lens Res Sci.* 2018;2(2):1–13.
30. Barnett M, Lien V, Li JY, Durbin-Johnson B, Mannis MJ. Use of scleral lenses and minischeral lenses after penetrating keratoplasty. *Eye Contact Lens.* 2016;42(3):185–189.
31. Asena L, Altınörs DD. Clinical outcomes of scleral Misa lenses for visual rehabilitation in patients with pellucid marginal degeneration. *Cont Lens Anterior Eye.* 2016;39(6):420–424.

Surgical Management

CHAPTER 22

Surgical Planning in Keratoconus

Luis Izquierdo Jr. ▪ Or Ben-Shaul ▪ Isabel Gomez

KEY CONCEPTS

- Before performing any refractive intervention in keratoconus, it is important to recognize the progressive nature of the disease and to treat appropriately.
- The only surgical treatment that has been shown to halt the progression of keratoconus is corneal collagen cross-linking.
- Surface laser ablation in patients with keratoconus is safe in nonprogressive early stages.
- Intrastromal corneal ring segment implantation is an option in patients with best corrected visual acuity equal to or worse than 20/40, achieving a significant effect in visual acuity improvement, correction of high cylinder, and reduction of corneal aberrations.
- The use of phakic intraocular lenses may be a useful tool for the correction of high ametropia in patients with keratoconus and can be combined with corneal regularization techniques to improve the result.
- In advanced keratoconus and intolerance to scleral lenses, keratoplasty is the treatment option. Depending on the depth of the corneal scar, deep anterior lamellar keratoplasty or penetrating keratoplasty can be performed.

Background

Surgical procedures play a fundamental role in the treatment of keratoconus. The final result in visual rehabilitation depends on an appropriate indication as well as surgical performance. Eye rubbing has proven to be a trigger factor for the disease,[1-5] and warning the patient to stop eye rubbing is a nonsurgical measure that should always be present as a mainstay of treatment. However, in cases of progression despite cessation of eye rubbing or in patients who are not adherent to changes in lifestyle, corneal cross-linking (CXL) has proven to be the only procedure that halts the progression of ectasia.[6,7]

The patient with keratoconus is a daily challenge in clinical practice, because of high ametropia and anisometropia, which makes correction difficult with conventional optical aids. Despite progress in their fitting, the use of contact lenses requires a learning curve and daily insertion and removal routines that often lead the patient to request a "more definitive" therapeutic option. Surface ablation for higher order aberrations and refractive error, intracorneal ring segments (ICRSs), phakic intraocular lenses (pIOLs), and keratoplasty, in advanced stages, are the procedures that are currently employed. This chapter will deal with the planning and the decision-making necessary when considering surgical intervention in keratoconus. After presenting the surgical solutions that are currently available, we will offer a flowchart that can assist the reader in choosing the proper strategy based on the patient's needs and condition.

ASSESSING SEVERITY AND PROGRESSION

The management of a keratoconus patient varies according to disease severity. Therefore the first step is to determine the disease stage. Although the Amsler-Krumeich classification system is widely accepted, it does not combine tomographic indicators or biomechanical parameters. Newer classification systems combine other parameters. The ABCD grading system[8] incorporates anterior and posterior curvature, the thinnest pachymetric values, and distance visual acuity. It consists of five stages (0 to 4). In Table 22.1 both classification systems are shown.

Many studies show that a criterion for ectasia progression is a change of at least 1 diopter (D) in the maximum and/or steeper and/or mean keratometry or corneal apex power. Another sign of progression is a 0.5-D change in manifest spherical equivalent (SE) and thinning of more than 2% or 30 μm in central corneal thickness from the baseline, in a 1-year period.[9] The Global Consensus on Keratoconus and Ectatic Diseases[10] defines ectasia progression by a consistent change in at least two of the following parameters: (1) steepening of the anterior corneal surface, (2) steepening of the posterior corneal surface, and (3) thinning and/or an

TABLE 22.1 ■ **Keratoconus Severity Classification According to Amsler-Krumeich and Belin ABCD Grading System**

Stage	Amsler-Krumeich Classification System	ABCD Grading System
0		ARC >7.25 mm (<46.5 D) PRC >5.9 mm Thinnest pachymetry >490 μm BCDVA ≥20/20 Scarring –
1	Eccentric steepening Myopia, induced astigmatism, or both <5.00 D Mean central k readings <48 D	ARC >7.05 mm (<48.0 D) PRC >5.7 mm Thinnest pachymetry >450 μm BCDVA <20/20 Scarring –, +, ++
2	Myopia, induced astigmatism, or both from 5.00 to 8.00 D Mean central k readings <53 D Absence of scarring Corneal thickness >400 μm	ARC >6.35 mm (<53.0 D) PRC >5.15 mm Thinnest pachymetry >400 μm BCDVA ≥20/40 Scarring –, +, ++
3	Myopia, induced astigmatism, or both from 8.00 to 10.00 D Mean central k readings >53 D Absence of scarring Corneal thickness 300–400 μm	ARC >6.15 mm (<55.0 D) PRC >4.95 mm Thinnest pachymetry >300 μm BCDVA ≥20/100 Scarring –, +,++
4	Refraction not measurable Mean central k readings >55 D Central corneal scarring Corneal thickness <200 μm	ARC <6.15 mm (>55.0 D) PRC <4.95 mm Thinnest pachymetry 450 μm BCDVA ≤20/400 Scarring –, +, ++

ARC, Anterior radius of curvature; *BCDVA,* best corrected distance visual acuity; *K,* keratometry; *PRC,* posterior radius of curvature.

increase in the rate of corneal thickness change. In the majority of the criteria used, progression of keratoconus usually leads to a deterioration in best spectacle-corrected visual acuity (BSCVA).

Surgical Procedures

To provide an evidence-based review of the different procedures that can be performed in keratoconus, the level of evidence of each of the currently used treatments was classified according to the Oxford Centre for Evidence-Based Medicine (OCEBM)[11] levels of evidence, shown in Table 22.2.

CROSS-LINKING

Whereas nonsurgical refractive solutions for keratoconus do not affect the disease progression,[12] CXL does appear to halt the ectatic process.[13] CXL increases the stiffness and rigidity of the anterior cornea by creating photochemical cross-linking and covalent binding between collagen fibers.[13–16] Although it is an effective treatment for halting the progression of keratoconus, the improvement in visual acuity after CXL is usually not enough to improve patient quality of life or dependency on contact lenses.[17–20]

The evidence available to evaluate the effectiveness of CXL in halting the progression of keratoconus has been reviewed in meta-analyses (Level 1a). In a study published by Li et al. in 2015, the authors found a significant reduction in K_{max} and K_{min} in the analysis of subgroups with homogeneity.[6] In 2017 Kobashi and Rong published another meta-analysis of randomized controlled trials (RCTs, Level 1a). They found a statistically significant difference in the improvement of BSCVA in the CXL group and no difference in the minimum pachymetry and cylindrical refraction between the control group and the CXL group.[7] The evidence for recommending CXL in patients with progressive keratoconus (Level 1a) is demonstrated by the decrease in K_{min} and K_{max}, without evidence of a significant change in thinnest pachymetry and refractive cylinder, as well as evidence of improvement in BSCVA when compared with the control group.

TABLE 22.2 ■ Level of Evidence According to OCEBM

Level	Description
1a	SR (with homogeneity) of RCTs
1b	Individual RCT (with narrow confidence interval)
1c	All or none
2a	SR (with homogeneity) of cohort studies
2b	Individual cohort study (including low-quality RCT, e.g., <80% follow up)
2c	"Outcomes" research; ecological studies
3a	SR (with homogeneity) of case-control studies
3b	Individual case-control study
4	Case series (and poor-quality cohort and case-control studies)
5	Expert opinion without explicit critical appraisal, or based on physiology, bench research or "first principles"

OCEBM, Oxford Centre for Evidence-Based Medicine; *RCT,* randomized controlled trial; *SR,* systematic review.

In 2017 McAnena et al. published a meta-analysis of CXL in children under 18 years of age in which they included case-control studies (Level 3a). They found improvement in uncorrected distance visual acuity (UCDVA) in the standard CXL group at 6 months and 1 year but with no difference at 2 years. K_{max} did not show differences at 6 months and 1 year but did show a statistically significant reduction at 2 years in the standard CXL group.[21] Henriquez et al. conducted a prospective cohort study (Level 2b) of CXL epi-off versus epi-on in children under 18 years of age. Their recently published results at 5 years found a significant flattening in the K_{mean} in the epi-off group and a progression rate of 9.37% in the epi-on group compared with 0% in the epi-off group.[22]

A randomized controlled trial (Level 1b) was published by Eissa and Yassin in which they compared accelerated CXL and conventional CXL in patients with keratoconus aged 9 to 16 years. They found an improvement in both groups in the UCDVA and the BSCVA, as well as flattening of the K_{max}, with no cases of progression in either of the groups at 36 months of follow up.[23]

Our group performs CXL in all patients with documented progression and those with a high risk of progression, defined as suspicious keratoconus by tomography and young age. We can do this alone or in combination with the fitting of a contact lens or a surgical procedure (like wavefront or corneal-guided photorefractive keratectomy [PRK], ICRS, pIOL) according to our goal.

PHOTOREFRACTIVE KERATECTOMY

In PRK, the excimer laser is used to ablate tissue and change the profile of the central anterior part of the cornea. Although several studies have demonstrated that PRK in keratoconus patients may be considered a risk factor for progression of ectasia,[24,25] other studies have shown improvement in visual acuity, slowing of disease progression, and a decrease in high order aberrations.[26-28]

Evidence for performing PRK in patients with suspected or diagnosed keratoconus as the only treatment is scarce; A study published by Guedj et al. retrospectively described a series of cases (Level 4) of patients who underwent PRK between 2004 and 2006, demonstrating stability and no progression of ectasia in the 62 eyes studied. The average age was 34.6 ± 15.1 years, mean SE 3.96 ± 3.05 D, and average thinnest point 522.14 ± 34.65 μm.[29] Chelala et al. published a prospective cohort with a 5-year follow up of 78% (Level 4) in which they performed PRK in patients with grades 1 and 2 keratoconus according to the Amsler-Krumeich classification. The inclusion criteria were stable keratoconus, maximum ablation of 50 μm with a minimum residual stromal bed of 450 μm, and BCDVA better than or equal to 20/30. In this study, they reported that 2 eyes out of 119 treated (1.7%) presented with disease progression at 5 years of follow up.[30]

This chapter's authors recommend only performing PRK without CXL in patients with no associated risks for progression, older than 35 years, with mild keratoconus, without evidence of progression over at least 2 years of follow-up assessed with corneal topography and tomography, and with BSCVA equal or better than 20/30.

PRK AND CXL

The adjunctive use of CXL has been proposed to perform surface ablation safely on ectatic corneas while improving corneal stiffness and halting keratoconus progression. The objective of surface ablation in patients with keratoconus is to reduce corneal irregularity and/or, partially, refractive error with a maximum ablation of 50 μm in the center and minimal residual stromal bed between 350 and 400 μm. Between 2007 and 2012, different authors published case reports and case series of topography-guided surface ablation and CXL in patients with keratoconus both sequentially and simultaneously, demonstrating stability and refractive improvement up to 36 months of follow up.[31-35] Non–topography-guided PRK has also been performed with success.[36]

Kanellopoulos compared the effect of performing CXL and PRK in the same procedure versus performing PRK 6 months after CXL. He found that simultaneous treatment allows a single procedure, improving the patient's visual rehabilitation time.[37]

Gore et al. published a prospective case series (Level 4). They simultaneously performed CXL plus transepithelial PRK wavefront-guided only high order aberrations with average ablation at the apex of the cone of 35 ± 15 μm; This group was compared with a historical cohort of patients who underwent CXL alone. Both groups had 2 years of follow up, with three cases in each group that presented one keratometry parameter indicative of progression. Only one case in the CXL group presented two keratometry parameters indicative of progression. They found that the mean gain in BSCVA was just over one line, from 0.28 ± 0.21 preoperatively to 0.15 ± 0.14 ($P = 0.01$) at 2 years. Clinically significant visual gains (≥2 lines of BSCVA) were more common after transepithelial PRK-CXL (30%) than after CXL alone (6%).[38]

Besides the increased risk for ectasia mentioned earlier, when treating a patient with CXL-PRK combination, we also expose them to possible (but rare) CXL complications: postoperative infection/ulcer, corneal haze, endothelial damage, peripheral sterile infiltrates, herpes reactivation, and treatment failure.[39] We prefer to perform corneal wavefront or ocular wavefront transepithelial PRK (after at least 6 months of CXL) or simultaneous with CXL focusing on correcting higher order aberration. We target improvement in BSCVA, so later we can correct the ametropia with spectacles or a pIOL. Fig. 22.1 shows a case of trans-PRK wavefront-guided treatment, 6 months after CXL.

Intracorneal Ring Segments (ICRS)

ICRS are miniature polymethylmethacrylate (PMMA) ring segments used to make the cornea's surface more regular and make a correction in the patient refractive error. Because of the flattening effect of ICRS, this technique was first developed for myopia[40] but is now a widely used treatment for keratoconus.[41]

Corneal clarity and a minimal pachymetry of 400 μm in the insertion site are mandatory for ICRS and, therefore, it is commonly used in mild to moderate keratoconus. One or two ring segments are implanted into the stroma in a safe and reversible process. This procedure may improve best and uncorrected visual acuity (UCVA), contact lens tolerance, and high order corneal aberrations,[42–45] and it can also delay the need for keratoplasty.[43] There are two optional techniques for stromal tunnel creation: manual and femtosecond laser (FSL)–assisted. Using mechanical dissection is associated with higher rate of complications such as epithelial defects, depth asymmetry, and corneal perforation.[46–48]

Creating the tunnel with an FSL is also possible, predetermining the segment depth and orientation with high precision. This technique is considered by many to be more precise and more predictable than the mechanical technique.[49]

PATIENT SELECTION

Choosing the right patient for ICRS implantation is important. Criteria are not fixed, but most authors suggest the following guidelines (Table 22.3): corneal thickness at the thinnest point greater than 400 μm, K_{max} lower than 60 D, refractive error in SE lower than 6 D, BSCVA equal or worse than 20/40, and absence of cornea scarring. In cases of higher keratometry values, thin cornea, and corneal scarring, ICRS is contraindicated. Other contraindications include pregnancy, uncontrolled autoimmune disease, or excessive eye rubbing.

INTRACORNEAL RING CALCULATION

Several companies supply ICRS, and each offers a nomogram that determines the recommended ring segment or segments according to the patient's refraction, pachymetry, and topography. The surgeon can then customize the nomogram based on their surgical experience. A few parameters influence the ICRS mechanism of action that we need to understand to choose the right segment or segments for a specific patient.[50] The Barraquer thickness law states that a flattening effect is

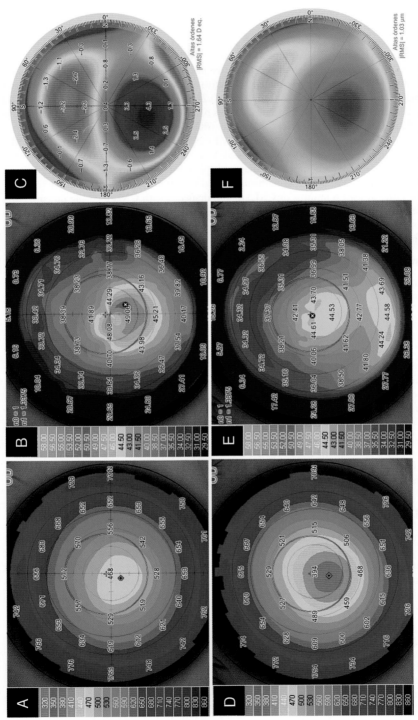

Fig. 22.1 Trans-PRK wavefront-guided treatment in keratoconus post-CXL. Patient with −0.75 −3.00 × 55 degrees. (A) Pachymetry pretreatment. (B) Tangential map pretreatment. (C) Wavefront map pretreatment with total corneal HOAs at 6 mm 1.64, coma 1.51. (D) Pachymetry 6 months post-treatment. (E) Tangential map 6 months post-treatment. (F) Wavefront map 6 months post-treatment with total corneal HOAs at 6 mm 1.03, coma 0.93. UCDVA at 6 months was 20/25, refraction 0.00 −0.50 × 80. BSCVA 20/20. *CXL*, Corneal cross-linking; *HOAs*, higher order aberrations; *PRK*, photorefractive keratectomy; *UCDVA*, uncorrected distance visual acuity.

TABLE 22.3 ■ Guidelines for ICRS Implantation

ICRS	Recommended	Relative Contraindication	Contraindicated
Corneal thickness	>400 μm	350–400 μm	<350 μm
K_{max}	<60 D	60–65 D	>65 D
Refractive error (SE)	<6 D	>6 D	
Corneal transparency	Clear	Paracentral scars	Central scars or opacities

D, Diopters; *ICRS,* intracorneal ring segment; K_{max}, maximum keratometry; *SE,* spherical equivalent.

achieved when adding material to the periphery of the cornea or subtracting material from the center. Therefore ICRSs have a flattening effect that is directly proportional to the thickness of the segment and inversely proportional to the corneal diameter where it is implanted.

The ring has a flattening effect at its parallel axis and between ring segments (Fig. 22.2) and a steepening effect at the perpendicular axis—the shorter the arc, the lower the flattening effect. Another important factor is the distance from the center or the diameter, a smaller diameter will produce a higher flatening effect.

In some cases, implanting one segment is enough, and in others, two may be needed. Alió et al. demonstrated that the topographic pattern could help in making that decision. For example, in symmetrical cones, implantation of two segments offers better results, whereas in inferior steepening, one implant may be enough.[51] Recently Izquierdo et al. showed a great flattening effect (average of 6 D), with the use of long arc rings with no differences when comparing two different techniques (tunnel vs. pocket) for two different rings (340 degrees and complete circular of 360 degrees) with an average of one to two lines of BSCVA improvement.[52]

Izquierdo et al. published a systematic review of 18 trials, including clinical trials, cohort studies, and case-control studies (Level 2b) with high heterogeneity. UCDVA improved by 0.23 ± 0.28 logMAR, and corrected distance visual acuity improved by 0.06 ± 0.21 logMAR. Sphere improved by 2.81 ± 1.54 D, cylinder improved by 1.49 ± 0.83 D, and mean keratometry improved by 3.41 ± 2.13 D within 12 months of follow up. ICRS implantation combined with CXL improved UCVA, refraction, and keratometry to a greater degree than ICRS implantation alone.[53]

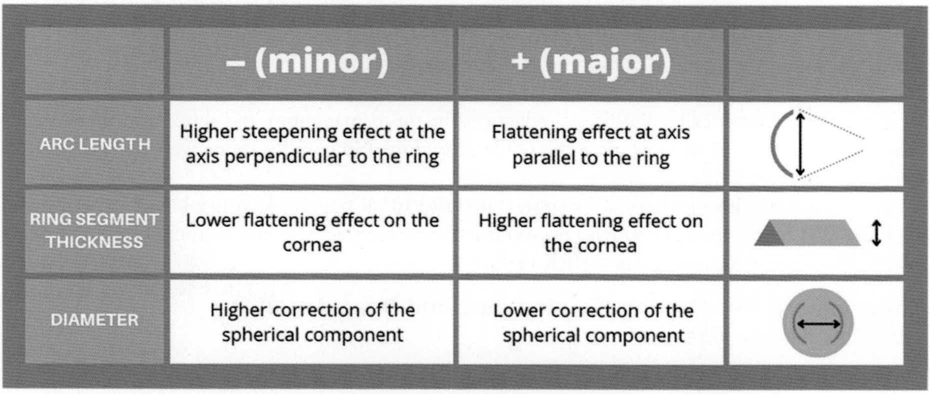

	– (minor)	+ (major)	
ARC LENGTH	Higher steepening effect at the axis perpendicular to the ring	Flattening effect at axis parallel to the ring	
RING SEGMENT THICKNESS	Lower flattening effect on the cornea	Higher flattening effect on the cornea	
DIAMETER	Higher correction of the spherical component	Lower correction of the spherical component	

Fig. 22.2 Factors affecting ICRS corneal correction. *ICRS,* Intracorneal ring segment.

Many studies have demonstrated the benefit of combining CXL with ICRS. Hashemi et al. published a systematic review and meta-analysis of clinical studies (Level 2a) where they evaluated the appropriate sequence of combining ICRS with CXL. In this study, they compared three groups: CXL first, ICRS first, and simultaneous CXL + ICRS, and found that at 12 months of follow up there were no statistically significant differences in UCVA, BSCVA, and refractive cylinder. However, when comparing spherical refractive error, flat keratometry, and steep keratometry, the group with simultaneous CXL + ICRS was superior to the others.[54]

We implant ICRS for patients with more advanced disease than those for which we use PRK. On average, we expect two to three lines of BSCVA improvement using ICRS. Commonly, for asymmetric cones, we use a single ICRS (arc of 160 degrees or less). We use the longer arc (240 degrees or more) for central cones with higher spherical components with significant spherical component correction. Fig. 22.3 shows a case of keratoconus at diagnosis and 1 month after ICRS implantation.

Phakic Intraocular Lens

The implantation of pIOLs in patients with keratoconus is presented as a safe option to correct elevated refractive errors without putting the cornea at risk in patients with stable keratoconus. The baseline endothelial count and the depth of the anterior chamber are two parameters that must be considered in all patients considered for a pIOL, regardless of its indication. In a recent study, Galvis et al. found that 7.5% of myopic patients have loss of 25% or more of endothelial cells over 5 years. They concluded that to guarantee long-term safety and minimize the loss of endothelial cells, a minimum anterior chamber depth of 3.0 mm and a minimum endothelial count of 3000 cells is necessary for patients under 25 years of age.[55]

Emerah et al. published a series of cases of patients with stable keratoconus in whom a collamer toric phakic lens was implanted with good refractive results and with no change in high order aberrations.[56] A retrospective case series found that in patients with grades I and II keratoconus (according to Amsler-Krumeich), good refractive results and predictability were achieved for both the iris-claw phakic lens and the posterior chamber collameric phakic lens, with no statistically significant difference in the postoperative results.[57] In 2012 Güell et al. published a series of cases in which they performed CXL followed by implantation of an iris-claw toric phakic lens. With a follow up of 36.9 ± 15.0 months, 94% of the eyes achieved UCVA of 20/40 or better, and no eyes lost CDVA lines.[58]

In 2011 Izquierdo et al. published a comparative prospective case series (Level 4) of anterior foldable iris-claw pIOL implants. The inclusion criteria were progressive keratoconus (Amsler-Krumeich classification grades I and II) with no corneal opacities, corneal thickness greater than 450 μm, endothelial cell count greater than 2500 cells/mm^2, anterior chamber depth greater than 3.2 mm, SE refraction greater than 4.50 D, and no other treatment for keratoconus other than a contact lens. Each patient underwent CXL in the keratoconus eye, with implantation of the Artiflex pIOL 6 months later. In 12 months of follow up, they found all eyes achieved UCDVA of 0.3 logMAR or better. Final spherical and cylindrical errors ranged from 0 to –1.50 D and 0 to –1.75 D, respectively. Statistically significant reductions in mean maximum and minimum keratometry values were present 12 months after the CXL procedure. No complications were associated with the procedure.[59]

We use phakic lens (spherical or spherical-toric) in all contact lens intolerant patients who have BSCVA better than 20/40 who need refractive correction. This can be implanted in patients post-CXL, after wavefront-guided PRK or ICRS.

Keratoplasty: Penetrating Keratoplasty and Deep Anterior Lamellar Keratoplasty

Keratoconus is one of the leading indications for corneal transplants,[60–62] and penetrating keratoplasty (PKP) was considered, until recently, the treatment of choice for advanced forms of

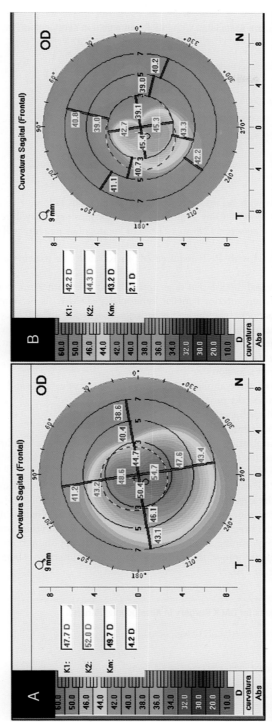

Fig. 22.3 Intracorneal ring segment (ICRS) implantation in keratoconus. (A) Sagittal map pre-ICRS with steeper keratometry (K2) 52.0 D and "corneal astigmatism" 4.2. (B) Sagittal map 6 months after steeper keratometry (ICRS) implantation with K2 44.3 D and Cyl 4.1.

TABLE 22.4 ■ Risk Factors Associated With PKP Requirement in Keratoconus Patients

- Corneal scarring
- Contact lens corrected visual acuity <20/40
- Keratometry >55 D
- Corneal astigmatism >10 D
- Early age of keratoconus development
- Poor contact lens tolerance

D, Diopters; *PKP,* penetrant keratoplasty.

keratoconus. In patients with keratoconus who have contact lens failure or apical scarring, PKP is a well-accepted treatment.[60,63] Only a minority of keratoconus patients will require PKP; long-term follow ups estimate between 12% and 21.6% of keratoconus patients will ever require such procedure.[64–66]

Risk factors associated with PKP requirement in Keratoconus patients are listed in Table 22.4.[62,66,67]

When treating a corneal disease that does not include the endothelium, as in keratoconus, it is understandable that deep anterior lamellar keratoplasty (DALK) is becoming more popular. Indications for DALK surgery in keratoconus patients are listed in Table 22.5.

Although PKP in keratoconus patients is considered a relatively low-risk surgery, and results are good in terms of rejection and graft clarity, DALK still offers certain advantages[60,62–64,67–70]:

- Better long-term graft survival
- Lower rates of graft rejection
- Minimal steroid-related complications—lower incidence of cataract and glaucoma
- Avoidance of an open sky procedure
- Lower risk of endothelial cell loss
- Lower-quality donor cornea can be used.

One advantage of implanting only the anterior part of the cornea is avoiding graft rejection. Brierly et al. showed that the rejection rate in PKP for keratoconus was 17.9%[71] but this can vary between 2.3% and 68%, according to several authors.[72,73]

When comparing PKP with DALK, another issue is visual acuity. Several studies have shown better visual acuity results after PKP.[69,74] These results could be explained by residual stroma above the recipient Descemet membrane because of incomplete dissection. When using the popular big bubble technique,[75–80] the bare Descemet membrane is revealed, and visual acuity is better.[81] In fact, electron microscopy scanning and in vivo confocal microscopy showed that when DALK is done with the big bubble technique, the quality of the achieved interface is better compared with manual, microkeratome, or FSL.[82]

TABLE 22.5 ■ Indications for DALK Surgery in Keratoconus Patients

- Anterior corneal scars/stress lines and clear cornea
- K_{max} >65 D
- Pachymetry at thinnest location <350 μm
- Very high refractive error (sphere/astigmatism >−6 D)

D, Diopters; *DALK,* deep anterior lamellar keratoplasty, K_{max}, maximum keratometry.

DALK requires surgical skill and has its limitations. For instance, previous hydrops may make DALK a challenging surgery, as may neovascularization and certain deep corneal scars.[83] The most common complication for DALK surgery is perforation of the Descemet membrane during dissection,[84] more common in young patients. This complication, in some cases, may require conversion of the surgery to PKP.

A prospective, randomized study (Level 1b) compared visual results between DALK and the big bubble technique and PKP and found no statistically significant differences in SE, maximum keratometry, and aberrometry parameters.[85] Some meta-analyses have attempted to compare PKP and DALK, but only one of them, which included two RCTs and 16 nonrandomized studies (Level 2a), could provide definitive outcome data. When analyzing only the RCTs, they found results that favor PKP over DALK in BCDVA at 6 months postoperatively. UCDVA was reported in three studies at 12 months and was better in patients in whom PKP was performed. Postoperative astigmatism did not show statistically significant differences. Concerning episodes of graft rejection, DALK had a better prognosis. The rest of the outcomes presented high heterogeneity.[73]

FEMTOSECOND LASER IN PKP AND DALK

Since the invention of the FSL, many studies have been performed to demonstrate the advantages of integrating FSL in both PKP and DALK. When performing PKP, FSL allows us to customize wound trephination patterns, improve the way the donor tissue fits the host, and facilitate better wound healing.[86] We can also form different wound configurations such as the "zig-zag," "top hat," "mushroom," and "Christmas-tree," creating more biomechanical stability.[87] Some studies show better incision integrity using this kind of configuration[88,89]; they also show earlier suture removal, less surgically induced astigmatism, and more rapid visual recovery.[86,90–93] Other studies found no significant difference in refractive and visual outcomes after FSL-assisted PK compared with conventional keratoplasty.[94]

Surgical Planning

There are many possible treatments for keratoconus, and the effectiveness of each modality varies with the patient's exact clinical condition. Presenting a simple and clear-cut indication paradigm for all cases is a challenge. Instead, we offer a few guidelines that consider the different factors in the staging of the patient's condition. The experienced clinician can match the patient's specific details to these guidelines and find the best surgical treatment to match their needs and expectations. The main factors that aid us in the surgical management of a keratoconus patient are summarized in Fig. 22.4.

DEMOGRAPHY

The patient's age, sex, geography, and genetics are factors we need to consider when deciding on a surgical plan. The older the patient is, the less chance the disease is active and progressing. When a patient is under 30 years, checking for progression before deciding to treat is important; age is also important when considering CXL, as it is less advised over 35 years of age. When treating a female patient, we should keep in mind that CXL and ICRS are not possible during pregnancy. Another issue related to progression assessment is geography. Patients from higher, drier, and colder regions are prone to more aggressive disease and may require more aggressive management.

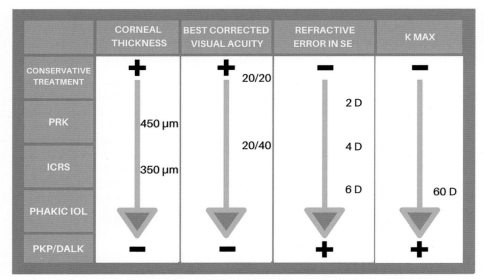

Fig. 22.4 Different factors and their effect on keratoconus surgical management. The *arrows* indicate progression of the disease: corneal thickness and BCVA decreases with progression, and maximum keratometry and the spherical equivalent (*SE*) increases with progression. *BCVA,* Best corrected visual acuity; *D,* diopters; *DALK,* deep anterior lamellar keratoplasty; *ICRS,* intracorneal ring segments; *IOL,* intraocular lens; *PKP,* penetrant keratoplasty; *PRK,* photorefractive keratectomy.

CORNEAL THICKNESS

The decrease in corneal thickness correlates with the severity of the disease. We must consider corneal thickness when considering CXL and PRK. They are not recommended when ICRS is under 400 μm, and when under 350 μm, contact lenses or corneal transplant are usually indicated.

VISUAL ACUITY AND REFRACTION

The best corrected visual acuity (BCVA) and the ability to achieve it (efficient refractive correction) are critical when deciding about the need for a surgical procedure. Good visual acuity contraindicates aggressive treatment. Guided PRK may be a good option for patients with good BCVA and with low spherical cylinder. ICRS may be an option in patients with decreased BCVA (equal to or worse than 20/40), and with a refractive error between 3 D and 6 D. Very low BCVA usually indicates scleral lenses or corneal transplant.

K_{max}

CXL is less effective and more prone to complication over 58 D,[17] and ICRSs are also not recommended in high K_{max} (>55–60 D). Correlating the clinical condition and the patient's needs with the appropriate surgical solution is important. We suggest a flowchart that will help with patient management (Fig. 22.5). After establishing keratoconus diagnosis and emphasizing the importance of stopping eye rubbing, the disease should be classified.

At stages 0 and 1 (Belin) and I (Amsler-Krumeich), consistent with corneal ectasia with low keratometry, adequate corneal thickness, and good visual acuity with correction, the recommended initial treatment is observation with close monitoring for signs that suggest progression. CXL

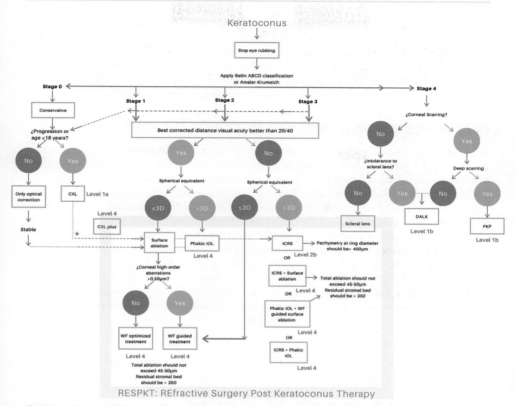

Fig. 22.5 Suggested flowchart for surgical management of keratoconus patient. *CXL,* Corneal cross-linking; *D,* diopters; *DALK,* deep anterior lamellar keratoplasty; *IOL,* intraocular lens; *ICRS,* intracorneal ring segments; *PKP,* penetrant keratoplasty; *WF,* wavefront.

is recommended only in the case of documented progression or in young patients, for example, under 18 years of age, for whom follow up may be difficult. These patients have a greater risk of progression than the older population; likewise, this progression can occur in less than a year.[95] For cases that remain stable over the years, correction with optical aids or surface ablation and/or pIOL implantation may be chosen after carefully evaluating the risk score.

In stages 2 and 3 (Belin) and II and III (Amsler-Krumeich), the disease's progressive nature should also be determined, ideally before performing any surgical procedure.

For those with BCDVA better than 20/32 or 0.63 in decimal units, indicative of low corneal irregularity, the procedure is chosen according to the SE. For lower SE, PRK would be the option of choice with the following considerations:

- The stromal ablation should not be greater than 45 to 50 μm at the cone's apex,
- The surgeon should leave a residual stromal bed thicker than 350 μm.

For those patients with higher degrees of SE, phakic lenses are an excellent option.

When high order corneal aberrations are significant (>0.50 μm) with BCVA of 20/40 or better, and if the total stromal ablation remains within the allowed value, PRK wavefront-guided ablation focusing on correcting high order aberrations would be the choice. The goal is to improve patients' symptoms and BCVA. Subsequently, we can use spectacles or a refractive procedure. If the BCVA is worse than 20/40, other corneal regularization techniques such as ICRS implantation alone or combined with a phakic lens or surface ablation may be employed.

In advanced disease—stage 4 (Belin) IV (Amsler-Krumeich) with poor visual acuity, thin cornea, and high keratometry—corneal transplantation may be required. Deep central scarring that affects visual acuity is also an indication for keratoplasty. DALK will be the treatment of choice for cases of significant corneal irregularity that do not improve with scleral lenses, or in patients with demonstrated contact lens intolerance. In cases of corneal scars and post hydrops, it is up to the surgeon to decide the best approach according to their experience and abilities.

REFRACTIVE SURGERY POST KERATOCONUS THERAPY (RESPKT)

Finally, keratoconus surgical planning should not only be considered to stop disease progression and/or correct corneal irregularity. Understanding the patient with keratoconus as an individual who needs to have the greatest visual potential in both eyes is important. Because of the frequent anisometropia in these patients, achieving this with conventional optical aids is challenging. Patients with KC can present with high anisometropia; Therefore, it can be challenging to achieve their best bilateral visual acuity with contact lenses or frames. In these cases, combined procedures may represent an option to provide these patients with the greatest visual potential bilaterally.

In conclusion, surgical planning in keratoconus is an art that is based on experience and evidence, which should start by determining the progression of the disease and, if it is progressive, halting the process. Subsequently, based on the clinical stage, choosing the best visual rehabilitation option for each patient helps to accelerate the probability of visual improvement.

We have developed an application based on artificial intelligence to help decide on the treatment of keratoconus. It can be found on the website keratoconus: www.keratoconus.app.

Acknowledgment

Vadim Igal, MD, Ophthalmology Department at Carmel Medical Center, Israel.

References

1. Rabinowitz YS. The genetics of keratoconus. *Ophthalmol Clin N Am*. 2003;16(4):607–620 vii.
2. Henriquez MA, Cerrate M, Hadid MG, Cañola-Ramirez LA, Hafezi F, Izquierdo L Jr. Comparison of eye-rubbing effect in keratoconic eyes and healthy eyes using Scheimpflug analysis and a dynamic bidirectional applanation device. *J Cataract Refract Surg*. 2019;45(8):1156–1162.
3. Moran S, Gomez L, Zuber K, Gatinel D. A case-control study of keratoconus risk factors. *Cornea*. 2020;39(6):697–701.
4. Mazharian A, Panthier C, Courtin R, et al. Incorrect sleeping position and eye rubbing in patients with unilateral or highly asymmetric keratoconus: a case-control study. *Graefes Arch Clin Exp Ophthalmol*. 2020;258(11):2431–2439.
5. Hashemi H, Heydarian S, Hooshmand E, et al. The prevalence and risk factors for keratoconus: a systematic review and meta-analysis. *Cornea*. 2020;39(2):263–270.
6. Li J, Ji P, Lin X. Efficacy of corneal collagen cross-linking for treatment of keratoconus: a meta-analysis of randomized controlled trials. *PLoS One*. 2015;10(5):e0127079.
7. Kobashi H, Rong SS. Corneal collagen cross-linking for keratoconus: systematic review. *BioMed Res Int*. 2017;2017:8145651.
8. Belin MW, Duncan JK. Keratoconus: the ABCD grading system. *Klin Monatsbl Augenheilkd*. 2016;233(6):701–707.
9. Hersh PS, Greenstein SA, Fry KL. Corneal collagen crosslinking for keratoconus and corneal ectasia: one-year results. *J Cataract Refract Surg*. 2011;37(1):149–160.
10. Gomes JAP, Tan D, Rapuano CJ, et al. Global consensus on keratoconus and ectatic diseases. *Cornea*. 2015;34(4):359–369.
11. Phillips B. Oxford Centre for Evidence-Based Medicine: Levels of Evidence (March 2009). https://www.cebm.ox.ac.uk/resources/levels-of-evidence/oxford-centre-for-evidence-based-medicine-levels-of-evidence-march-2009.

12. Wollensak G, Spoerl E, Seiler T. Riboflavin/ultraviolet-A-induced collagen crosslinking for the treatment of keratoconus. *Am J Ophthalmol.* 2003;135(5):620–627.
13. Asri D, Touboul D, Fournié P, et al. Corneal collagen crosslinking in progressive keratoconus: multicenter results from the French National Reference Center for Keratoconus. *J Cataract Refract Surg.* 2011;37(12):2137–2143.
14. Wollensak G, Spoerl E, Seiler T. Stress-strain measurements of human and porcine corneas after riboflavin-ultraviolet-A-induced cross-linking. *J Cataract Refract Surg.* 2003;29(9):1780–1785.
15. Kohlhaas M, Spoerl E, Schilde T, Unger G, Wittig C, Pillunat LE. Biomechanical evidence of the distribution of cross-links in corneas treated with riboflavin and ultraviolet A light. *J Cataract Refract Surg.* 2006;32(2):279–283.
16. Spoerl E, Wollensak G, Seiler T. Increased resistance of crosslinked cornea against enzymatic digestion. *Curr Eye Res.* 2004;29(1):35–40.
17. Koller T, Mrochen M, Seiler T. Complication and failure rates after corneal crosslinking. *J Cataract Refract Surg.* 2009;35(8):1358–1362.
18. Greenstein SA, Fry KL, Hersh PS. Corneal topography indices after corneal collagen crosslinking for keratoconus and corneal ectasia: one-year results. *J Cataract Refract Surg.* 2011;37(7):1282–1290.
19. Sakla H, Altroudi W, Muñoz G. Albarrán-Diego C. Simultaneous topography-guided partial photorefractive keratectomy and corneal collagen crosslinking for keratoconus. *J Cataract Refract Surg.* 2014;40(9):1430–1438.
20. Vinciguerra P, Albè E, Trazza S, et al. Refractive, topographic, tomographic, and aberrometric analysis of keratoconic eyes undergoing corneal cross-linking. *Ophthalmology.* 2009;116(3):369–378.
21. McAnena L, Doyle F, O'Keefe M. Cross-linking in children with keratoconus: a systematic review and meta-analysis. *Acta Ophthalmol (Copenh).* 2017;95(3):229–239.
22. Henriquez MA, Hernandez-Sahagun G, Camargo J, Izquierdo L Jr. Accelerated epi-on versus standard epi-off corneal collagen cross-linking for progressive keratoconus in pediatric patients: five years of follow-up. *Cornea.* 2020;39(12):1493–1498.
23. Eissa SA, Yassin A. Prospective, randomized contralateral eye study of accelerated and conventional corneal cross-linking in pediatric keratoconus. *Int Ophthalmol.* 2019;39(5):971–979.
24. Doyle SJ, Hynes E, Naroo S, Shah S. PRK in patients with a keratoconic topography picture. The concept of a physiological "displaced apex syndrome". *Br J Ophthalmol.* 1996;80(1):25–28.
25. Dawson DG, Randleman JB, Grossniklaus HE, et al. Corneal ectasia after excimer laser keratorefractive surgery: histopathology, ultrastructure, and pathophysiology. *Ophthalmology.* 2008;115(12):2181–2191.e1.
26. Kasparova EA. [Pathogenetic basis for treatment of primary keratoconus by a combined method of excimer laser surgery (combination of photorefraction and phototherapeutic keratectomy)]. *Vestn Oftalmol.* 2002;118(5):21–25.
27. Bahar I, Levinger S, Kremer I. Wavefront-supported photorefractive keratectomy with the Bausch & Lomb Zyoptix in patients with myopic astigmatism and suspected keratoconus. *J Refract Surg.* 2006;22(6):533–538.
28. Alpins N, Stamatelatos G. Customized photoastigmatic refractive keratectomy using combined topographic and refractive data for myopia and astigmatism in eyes with forme fruste and mild keratoconus. *J Cataract Refract Surg.* 2007;33(4):591–602.
29. Guedj M, Saad A, Audureau E, Gatinel D. Photorefractive keratectomy in patients with suspected keratoconus: five-year follow-up. *J Cataract Refract Surg.* 2013;39(1):66–73.
30. Chelala E, Rami HE, Dirani A, Fadlallah A, Fakhoury O, Warrak E. Photorefractive keratectomy in patients with mild to moderate stable keratoconus: a five-year prospective follow-up study. *Clin Ophthalmol.* 2013;7:1923–1928.
31. Kymionis GD, Kontadakis GA, Kounis GA, et al. Simultaneous topography-guided PRK followed by corneal collagen cross-linking for keratoconus. *J Refract Surg.* 2009;25(9):S807–S811.
32. Krueger RR, Kanellopoulos AJ. Stability of simultaneous topography-guided photorefractive keratectomy and riboflavin/UVA cross-linking for progressive keratoconus: case reports. *J Refract Surg.* 2010;26(10):S827–S832.
33. Tuwairqi WS, Sinjab MM. Safety and efficacy of simultaneous corneal collagen cross-linking with topography-guided PRK in managing low-grade keratoconus: 1-year follow-up. *J Refract Surg.* 2012;28(5):341–345.

34. Kanellopoulos AJ, Binder PS. Collagen cross-linking (CCL) with sequential topography-guided PRK: a temporizing alternative for keratoconus to penetrating keratoplasty. *Cornea.* 2007;26(7):891–895.
35. Stojanovic A, Zhang J, Chen X, Nitter TA, Chen S, Wang Q. Topography-guided transepithelial surface ablation followed by corneal collagen cross-linking performed in a single combined procedure for the treatment of keratoconus and pellucid marginal degeneration. *J Refract Surg.* 2010;26(2):145–152.
36. Mukherjee AN, Selimis V, Aslanides I. Transepithelial photorefractive keratectomy with crosslinking for keratoconus. *Open Ophthalmol J.* 2013;7:63–68.
37. Kanellopoulos AJ. Comparison of sequential vs same-day simultaneous collagen cross-linking and topography-guided PRK for treatment of keratoconus. *J Refract Surg.* 2009;25(9):S812–S818.
38. Gore DM, Leucci MT, Anand V, Fernandez-Vega Cueto L, Arba Mosquera S, Allan BD. Combined wavefront-guided transepithelial photorefractive keratectomy and corneal crosslinking for visual rehabilitation in moderate keratoconus. *J Cataract Refract Surg.* 2018;44(5):571–580.
39. Dhawan S, Rao K, Natrajan S. Complications of corneal collagen cross-linking. *J Ophthalmol.* 2011;2011:869015.
40. Nosé W, Neves RA, Burris TE, Schanzlin DJ, Belfort Júnior R. Intrastromal corneal ring: 12-month sighted myopic eyes. *J Refract Surg.* 1996;12(1):20–28.
41. Colin J, Cochener B, Savary G, Malet F. Correcting keratoconus with intracorneal rings. *J Cataract Refract Surg.* 2000;26(8):1117–1122.
42. Tomalla M, Cagnolati W. Modern treatment options for the therapy of keratoconus. *Cont Lens Anterior Eye.* 2007;30(1):61–66.
43. Zare MA, Hashemi H, Salari MR. Intracorneal ring segment implantation for the management of keratoconus: safety and efficacy. *J Cataract Refract Surg.* 2007;33(11):1886–1891.
44. Shabayek MH, Alió JL. Intrastromal corneal ring segment implantation by femtosecond laser for keratoconus correction. *Ophthalmology.* 2007;114(9):1643–1652.
45. Heikal MA, Abdelshafy M, Soliman TT, Hamed AM. Refractive and visual outcomes after Keraring intrastromal corneal ring segment implantation for keratoconus assisted by femtosecond laser at 6 months follow-up. *Clin Ophthalmol.* 2016;11:81–86.
46. Kanellopoulos AJ, Pe LH, Perry HD, Donnenfeld ED. Modified intracorneal ring segment implantations (INTACS) for the management of moderate to advanced keratoconus: efficacy and complications. *Cornea.* 2006;25(1):29–33.
47. Bourcier T, Borderie V, Laroche L. Late bacterial keratitis after implantation of intrastromal corneal ring segments. *J Cataract Refract Surg.* 2003;29(2):407–409.
48. Ruckhofer J, Stoiber J, Alzner E, Grabner G; Multicenter European Corneal Correction Assessment Study Group. One year results of European Multicenter Study of intrastromal corneal ring segments. Part 2: complications, visual symptoms, and patient satisfaction. *J Cataract Refract Surg.* 2001;27(2):287–296.
49. Ertan A, Bahadir M. Topography-guided vertical implantation of Intacs using a femtosecond laser for the treatment of keratoconus. *J Cataract Refract Surg.* 2007;33(1):148–151.
50. Vega-Estrada A, Alio JL. The use of intracorneal ring segments in keratoconus. *Eye Vis (Lond).* 2016;3:8.
51. Alió JL, Artola A, Hassanein A, Haroun H, Galal A. One or 2 Intacs segments for the correction of keratoconus. *J Cataract Refract Surg.* 2005;31(5):943–953.
52. Izquierdo Jr L, Rodríguez AM, Sarquis RA, Altamirano D, Henriquez MA. Intracorneal circular ring implant with femtosecond laser: pocket versus tunnel. *Eur J Ophthalmol.* 2022;32(1):176–182.
53. Izquierdo Jr L, Mannis MJ, Mejías Smith JA, Henriquez MA. Effectiveness of intrastromal corneal ring implantation in the treatment of adult patients with keratoconus: a systematic review. *J Refract Surg.* 2019;35(3):191–200.
54. Hashemi H, Alvani A, Seyedian MA, Yaseri M, Khabazkhoob M, Esfandiari H. Appropriate sequence of combined intracorneal ring implantation and corneal collagen cross-linking in keratoconus: a systematic review and meta-analysis. *Cornea.* 2018;37(12):1601–1607.
55. Galvis V, Villamil JF, Acuña MF, et al. Long-term endothelial cell loss with the iris-claw intraocular phakic lenses (Artisan®). *Graefes Arch Clin Exp Ophthalmol.* 2019;257(12):2775–2787.
56. Emerah SH, Sabry MM, Saad HA, Ghobashy WA. Visual and refractive outcomes of posterior chamber phakic IOL in stable keratoconus. *Int J Ophthalmol.* 2019;12(5):840–843.
57. Alió JL, Peña-García P, Abdulla G F, Zein G. Abu-Mustafa SK. Comparison of iris-claw and posterior chamber collagen copolymer phakic intraocular lenses in keratoconus. *J Cataract Refract Surg.* 2014;40(3):383–394.

58. Güell JL, Morral M, Malecaze F, Gris O, Elies D, Manero F. Collagen crosslinking and toric iris-claw phakic intraocular lens for myopic astigmatism in progressive mild to moderate keratoconus. *J Cataract Refract Surg.* 2012;38(3):475–484.
59. Izquierdo Jr L, Henriquez MA, McCarthy M. Artiflex phakic intraocular lens implantation after corneal collagen cross-linking in keratoconic eyes. *J Refract Surg.* 2011;27(7):482–487.
60. Kelly TL, Williams KA, Coster DJ; Australian Corneal Graft Registry. Corneal transplantation for keratoconus: a registry study. *Arch Ophthalmol.* 2011;129(6):691–697.
61. Rabinowitz YS. Keratoconus. *Surv Ophthalmol.* 1998;42(4):297–319.
62. Sray WA, Cohen EJ, Rapuano CJ. Laibson PR. Factors associated with the need for penetrating keratoplasty in keratoconus. *Cornea.* 2002;21(8):784–786.
63. Tan DTH, Por YM. Current treatment options for corneal ectasia. *Curr Opin Ophthalmol.* 2007;18(4):284–289.
64. Gordon MO, Steger-May K, Szczotka-Flynn L, et al. Baseline factors predictive of incident penetrating keratoplasty in keratoconus. *Am J Ophthalmol.* 2006;142(6):923–930.
65. Kennedy RH, Bourne WM, Dyer JA. A 48-year clinical and epidemiologic study of keratoconus. *Am J Ophthalmol.* 1986;101(3):267–273.
66. Tuft SJ, Moodaley LC, Gregory WM, Davison CR, Buckley RJ. Prognostic factors for the progression of keratoconus. *Ophthalmology.* 1994;101(3):439–447.
67. Reeves SW, Stinnett S, Adelman RA, Afshari NA. Risk factors for progression to penetrating keratoplasty in patients with keratoconus. *Am J Ophthalmol.* 2005;140(4):607–611.
68. Pramanik S, Musch DC, Sutphin JE, Farjo AA. Extended long-term outcomes of penetrating keratoplasty for keratoconus. *Ophthalmology.* 2006;113(9):1633–1638.
69. Watson SL, Ramsay A, Dart JKG, Bunce C, Craig E. Comparison of deep lamellar keratoplasty and penetrating keratoplasty in patients with keratoconus. *Ophthalmology.* 2004;111(9):1676–1682.
70. Vabres B, Bosnjakowski M, Bekri L, Weber M, Pechereau A. [Deep lamellar keratoplasty versus penetrating keratoplasty for keratoconus]. *J Fr Ophtalmol.* 2006;29(4):361–371.
71. Brierly SC, Izquierdo Jr L, Mannis MJ. Penetrating keratoplasty for keratoconus. *Cornea.* 2000;19(3):329–332.
72. Jones MNA, Armitage WJ, Ayliffe W, Larkin DF, Kaye SB; NHSBT Ocular Tissue Advisory Group and Contributing Ophthalmologists (OTAG Audit Study 5). Penetrating and deep anterior lamellar keratoplasty for keratoconus: a comparison of graft outcomes in the United kingdom. *Invest Ophthalmol Vis Sci.* 2009;50(12):5625–5629.
73. Henein C, Nanavaty MA. Systematic review comparing penetrating keratoplasty and deep anterior lamellar keratoplasty for management of keratoconus. *Cont Lens Anterior Eye.* 2017;40(1):3–14.
74. Parker JS, van Dijk K, Melles GRJ. Treatment options for advanced keratoconus: a review. *Surv Ophthalmol.* 2015;60(5):459–480.
75. Fontana L, Parente G, Tassinari G. Clinical outcomes after deep anterior lamellar keratoplasty using the big-bubble technique in patients with keratoconus. *Am J Ophthalmol.* 2007;143(1):117–124.
76. Sarnicola V, Conti L, Bellirine D. Clinical results using different DALK techniques. In: Fontana L, Tassinari G, eds. *Atlas of Lamellar Keratoplasty.* Italy: Fabiano Editore; 2007:155–162.
77. Fogla R, Padmanabhan P. Results of deep lamellar keratoplasty using the big-bubble technique in patients with keratoconus. *Am J Ophthalmol.* 2006;141(2):254–259.
78. Vajpayee RB, Tyagi J, Sharma N, Kumar N, Jhanji V, Titiyal JS. Deep anterior lamellar keratoplasty by big-bubble technique for treatment corneal stromal opacities. *Am J Ophthalmol.* 2007;143(6):954–957.
79. Anwar M, Teichmann KD. Big-bubble technique to bare Descemet's membrane in anterior lamellar keratoplasty. *J Cataract Refract Surg.* 2002;28(3):398–403.
80. Anwar M, Teichmann KD. Deep lamellar keratoplasty: surgical techniques for anterior lamellar keratoplasty with and without baring of Descemet's membrane. *Cornea.* 2002;21(4):374–383.
81. Lu Y, Grisolia AB, Ge YR, et al. Comparison of femtosecond laser-assisted descemetic and predescemetic lamellar keratoplasty for keratoconus. *Indian J Ophthalmol.* 2017;65(1):19–23.
82. Mastropasqua L, et al. Morphological analysis of lamellar keratoplasty interface. In: Fontana L, Tassinari G, eds. *Atlas of Lamellar Keratoplasty.* Italy: Fabiano Editore; 2007:165–174.
83. Sarnicola V, Toro P, Gentile S, Hannush SB. Descemetic DALK and predescemetic DALK: outcomes in 236 cases of keratoconus. *Cornea.* 2010;29(1):53–59.
84. Den S, Shimmura S, Tsubota K, Shimazaki J. Impact of the descemet membrane perforation on surgical outcomes after deep lamellar keratoplasty. *Am J Ophthalmol.* 2007;143(5):750–754.

85. Javadi MA, Feizi S, Yazdani S, Mirbabaee F. Deep anterior lamellar keratoplasty versus penetrating keratoplasty for keratoconus: a clinical trial. *Cornea*. 2010;29(4):365–371.
86. Farid M, Steinert RF, Gaster RN, Chamberlain W, Lin A. Comparison of penetrating keratoplasty performed with a femtosecond laser zig-zag incision versus conventional blade trephination. *Ophthalmology*. 2009;116(9):1638–1643.
87. Bahar I, Kaiserman I, McAllum P, Rootman D. Femtosecond laser-assisted penetrating keratoplasty: stability evaluation of different wound configurations. *Cornea*. 2008;27(2):209–211.
88. Steinert RF, Ignacio TS, Sarayba MA. "Top hat"-shaped penetrating keratoplasty using the femtosecond laser. *Am J Ophthalmol*. 2007;143(4):689–691.
89. Maier P, Böhringer D, Birnbaum F, Reinhard T. Improved wound stability of top-hat profiled femtosecond laser-assisted penetrating keratoplasty in vitro. *Cornea*. 2012;31(8):963–966.
90. Asota I, Farid M, Garg S, Steinert RF. Femtosecond laser-enabled keratoplasty. *Int Ophthalmol Clin*. 2013;53(2):103–114.
91. Farid M, Steinert RF. Femtosecond laser-assisted corneal surgery. *Curr Opin Ophthalmol*. 2010;21(4):288–292.
92. Farid M, Kim M, Steinert RF. Results of penetrating keratoplasty performed with a femtosecond laser zigzag incision initial report. *Ophthalmology*. 2007;114(12):2208–2212.
93. Shtein RM, Kelley KH, Musch DC, Sugar A, Mian SI. In vivo confocal microscopic evaluation of corneal wound healing after femtosecond laser-assisted keratoplasty. *Ophthalmic Surg Lasers Imaging*. 2012;43(3):205–213.
94. Daniel MC, Böhringer D, Maier P, Eberwein P, Birnbaum F, Reinhard T. Comparison of long-term outcomes of femtosecond laser-assisted keratoplasty with conventional keratoplasty. *Cornea*. 2016;35(3):293–298.
95. Romano V, Vinciguerra R, Arbabi EM, et al. Progression of keratoconus in patients while awaiting corneal cross-linking: a prospective clinical study. *J Refract Surg*. 2018;34(3):177–180.

CHAPTER 23

Intrastromal Corneal Ring Segments Mechanism and Techniques

Efekan Coşkunseven ■ Belma Kayhan

KEY CONCEPTS

Mechanism:

- An intrastromal corneal ring segment (ICRS) acts as a spacer, shortens arc length, and increases thickness in the cornea.
- The corrective effect is correlated in direct proportion to the thickness of the implant and in inverse proportion to its diameter (optical zone).
- New, progressive asymmetrical ICRSs have been designed for specific types of keratoconus such as asymmetric bowtie (snowman), oval (duck), or pellucid-like (lobster claw) types, because this design provides a more flattening effect on the steeper part of cornea with its thicker end and vice versa.
- ICRSs with long arc lengths, like 320 degrees or 360 degrees, act as an artificial limbus biomechanically and are effective in nipple-type and advanced keratoconus.

Techniques:

- There are two main techniques for ICRS implantation: manual (mechanical) and femtosecond laser techniques.
- Reference centers for the channel location, channel depth, and proper incision site are the main considerations in ICRS implantation.
- The limbus center, the pupil center, Purkinje reflex, or the point between the pupil center and Purkinje reflex can be considered as the center to determine the channel location.
- The depth of the incision site and the channel track should be measured accurately and 70% to 80% of the thinnest point should be taken into account for ICRS implantation.
- Migration of the segment to the incision site is responsible for most of the complications of extrusion and melting at the incision location. To avoid migration, the incision site should be far from the ring tip. Distance of the incision site to tips of the rings should be approximately 10 degrees in case of implantation of two segments. However, for single ring implantation, the incision site should be created much farther from the tip of the segment.
- In either technique, properly implanted segments should be in a symmetrical position, placed in deep stroma, and with tips far from the incision.
- The femtosecond laser technique allows more accurate stromal dissection and yields good visual and refractive results with much lower complication rates.

Mechanism

Jose I. Barraquer published his article on the thickness law, "The modification of the refraction by means of intracorneal inclusions," in 1966. He noted that the addition of material to the corneal

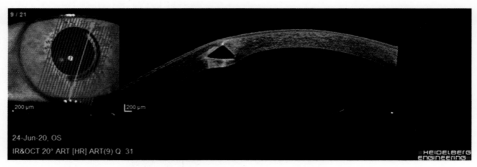

Fig. 23.1   The anterior segment optical coherence tomography image of an intrastromal corneal ring segment (ICRS). ICRS forms a spacer and thickens the cornea.

periphery flattened the central cornea. One of the considered action mechanisms for intracorneal ring segment (ICRS) implantation is related to thickness addition to obtain flattening. As the thickness of the segment increases, the anterior displacement of the cornea with the segment and sequentially central corneal flattening also increase.[1,2] Another explanation is the spacer effect. An ICRS forms a new, additional space within collagen fibers of the corneal stroma (Fig. 23.1). This spacer effect of the ICRS shortens the central arc length of the cornea (arc-shortening effect) and induces central corneal flattening.[3,4] In a normal cornea, this effect can induce a predictable, direct proportion. However, keratoconic corneas have different biomechanical properties because of the irregular distribution of collagen fibers, unlike the orthogonal alignment of collagen lamellae in the normal cornea. Hence, the effect of ICRSs in eyes with keratoconus is expected to be different from the normal corneas.

ICRSs have a flattening effect on the line that passes through both ends of the segment and a steepening effect on the line perpendicular to the segment arc. It is known that the corrective effect is correlated in direct proportion to the thickness of the implant and in inverse proportion to its diameter (optical zone) (Fig. 23.2). A shorter segment induces a greater astigmatic correction compared with long arc segments, whereas long arc segments decrease the prolate shape in advanced cases and produces flattening in nipple and oval keratoconus. Studies of rings with long arc lengths (320-degree arc segments or the full ring of 360-degree designs) demonstrate that these ring types act as an artificial limbus biomechanically. This effect separates the load on the cornea, separating the intraocular pressure into two independent loads, one inside the inner

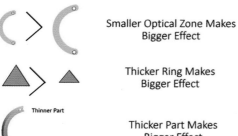

Smaller Optical Zone Makes
Bigger Effect

Thicker Ring Makes
Bigger Effect

Thicker Part Makes
Bigger Effect

Fig. 23.2   Diagrams demonstrating the effect of thickness and optical zone on flattening. As the thickness increases and the optical zone decreases, the flattening effect of the intrastromal corneal ring segment increases.

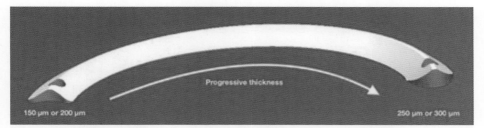

Fig. 23.3 Progressive thickness intrastromal corneal ring segment. This design provides a greater flattening effect on the steeper part of cornea with its thicker end.

diameter of the implant and the other one between the outer diameter of the implant and the limbus.[5,6]

Based on the proportional correction effect of the ICRS thickness, progressive, asymmetric ring segments have been developed.[7,8] These segments are designed as thicker at one end and thinner at the other end (Fig. 23.3). This design provides a greater flattening effect on the steeper part of cornea with its thicker end and vice versa and, therefore, allows the surgeon to remodel the corneal irregularity in specific types of keratoconus such as asymmetric bowtie (snowman), oval (duck), or pellucid-like (lobster claw) types (23.4A,B and Fig. 23.5).

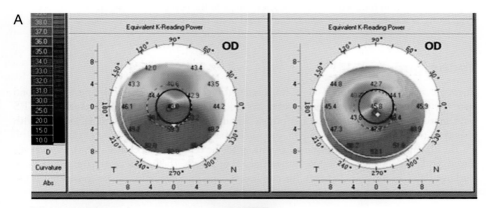

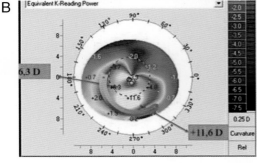

Fig. 23.4 (A) Preoperative *(left)* and postoperative *(right)* topographic maps of pellucid-like (lobster claw) type of keratoconus. (B) The topographic map of the difference. The thicker end of the progressive intrastromal corneal ring segment provides +11.6 D correction, the thinner end provides +6.3 D correction.

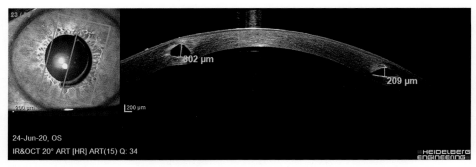

Fig. 23.5 The anterior segment optical coherence tomography image of the progressive intrastromal corneal ring segment.

The availability of various types of ICRS with different thicknesses, optical zones, and designs enables surgeons to treat several corneal irregularities together with keratoconus. ICRS implantation can be performed to regularize irregular astigmatism after penetrating or anterior lamellar keratoplasty, after radial keratotomy, and in post-LASIK/photorefractive keratectomy (PRK) ectasia.

A novel, customized ring presented by Mediphacos at the XXXIII Congress of European Society of Cataract and Refractive Surgeons in 2015 was based on the idea of a corneal endoskeleton. This segment, called Keraring Second Generation, acts like a tent skeleton or a bra wire after implantation within the cornea and gives a new shape to the cornea according to its own curvature (Fig. 23.6). It is a double arc segment. The optical zone of 5 mm is bound to a surrounding arc of 8 mm. The second arc is considered as an artificial limbus.

Techniques

There are two main techniques for ICRS implantation: manual (mechanical) and femtosecond laser techniques. Three key points should be considered to achieve successful outcomes in ICRS implantation, independent of the performed technique. These are the channel location with respect to the center, the channel depth, and the proper incision site.

The channel location is determined according to the center of the cornea. However, the preferred center may change according to the surgeon's approach. The limbus center, the pupil center, Purkinje reflex, or the point between the pupil center and Purkinje reflex can be considered as the center to determine the channel location (Fig. 23.7).

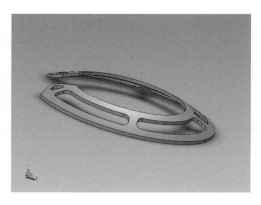

Fig. 23.6 Keraring Second Generation.

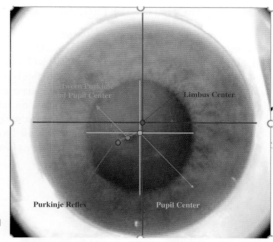

Fig. 23.7 Centers to determine the channel location.

The creation of channels at appropriate depth is another important point in implantation. The thickness of the incision site and along the channel track should be measured accurately, and 70% to 80% of the thinnest point should be taken into account for ICRS implantation (Fig. 23.8). Otherwise, inaccurate measurement of the thickness in the channel track and the incision site will lead to improper creation of the channels and consequently, to complications such as perforation or anterior or posterior dislocations of the segments.

Determination of the incision site is the third key point that should be planned before implantation. The steepest keratometric axis is the commonly preferred place for the incision site in case of implantation of two segments. The type of keratoconus may affect this decision. Temporal incision in patients with oval and central cones is reported in some studies.[9–12] Some authors propose the axis of coma aberration as the reference line for the channel location and the incision site.[13] Wherever the incision site is placed, it should be far away enough from the ends of the segments to minimize complications such as segment migration, extrusion, and corneal melting.

Properly implanted segments in either technique should be:
- in a symmetrical position,
- placed in deep stroma,
- with tips far from the incision.

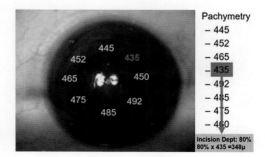

Fig. 23.8 Measuring the thickness along the channel track to determine the appropriate depth for implantation.

MANUAL (MECHANICAL) TECHNIQUE

The first ICRS implantations were performed with the manual technique. Special surgical instruments were developed for this technique (Fig. 23.9). Steps are as follows in the manual technique:

1. Firstly, the visual axis is determined. The patient is asked to look at the fixation light of the operation microscope, and the Purkinje reflex is marked (Fig. 23.10).
2. The planned optical zone and incision site are marked using a marker stained with gentian violet and centralizing the determined Purkinje reflex (Figs. 23.11A,B).
3. A calibrated micrometer diamond knife with square blade (1 mm) is set to 70% to 80% of corneal thickness at the incision site and is used to make the incision (Figs. 23.12A,B).
4. Starter intrastromal pockets are created using a Grupenmacher delaminator on each side of the incision at a uniform depth.

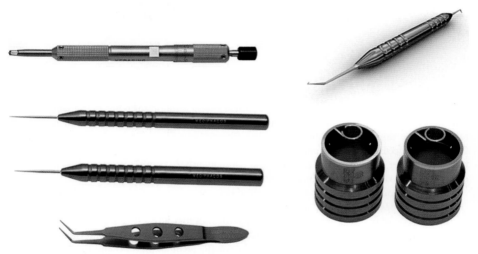

Fig. 23.9 Instruments used in manual (mechanical) technique. *(Left)* Diamond knife, Grupenmacher delaminator, Suarez spreader, Albertazzi forceps. *(Right)* Sinskey hook, blunt round stromal tunnel creator (trephines).

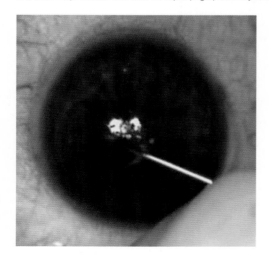

Fig. 23.10 Marking of Purkinje reflex.

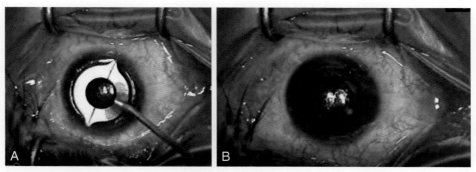

Fig. 23.11 Marking of channel tracks. (A) Marking channel tracks using an optic zone marker. (B) The image of channel track markings on the cornea.

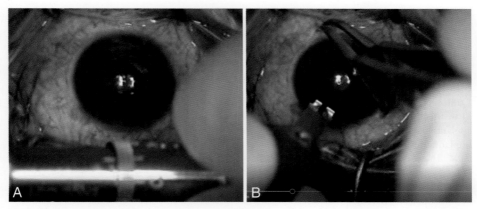

Fig. 23.12 Formation of incision using a diamond knife. (A) The diamond knife is set to the planned incision depth. (B) The incision is made by the diamond knife at the determined site.

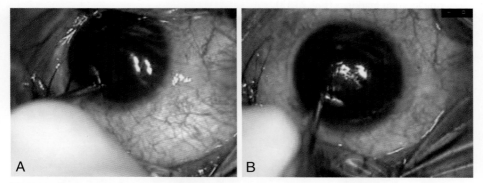

Fig. 23.13 Creation of intrastromal pockets by Suarez spreader on each side. (A) To the left and (B) to the right.

5. Intrastromal pockets are created by Suarez spreader on each side (Figs. 23.13A,B).
6. Channels are created in a clockwise and counterclockwise movement by trephines (Fig. 23.14A,B). (In the implantation of some ICRS types, a semiautomated suction ring is placed around the corneal limbus to fixate the eye during the dissection of the corneal stroma).

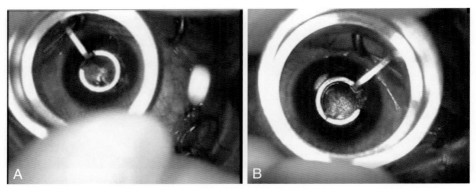

Fig. 23.14   Creation of channels by trephines. (A) To the left and (B) to the right.

7. Segments are implanted with Albertazzi forceps.
8. Segments are directed with the flat side down.
9. Each segment is inserted all the way to the end of the tunnel with the aid of a Sinskey hook.

FEMTOSECOND LASER TECHNIQUE

Femtosecond laser enables ICRSs to be implanted more easily and safely. The basic difference in this technique is in the creation of channels. A disposable single-use set of docking rings and applanation cones are used (Fig. 23.15). The steps of the femtosecond laser technique in ICRS implantation are as follows:

- The cornea is marked at 3 and 9 o'clock positions using a slit-lamp biomicroscopy to avoid cyclotorsion.
- The Purkinje reflex is chosen as the central point and is marked under the operating microscope (Fig. 23.16).
- A 5-mm marker is used to locate the exact ring channel (Fig. 23.17).
- The corneal thickness is measured during surgery using an ultrasonic pachymetry along the ring location markings (Fig. 23.18).
- The tunnel depth in the femtosecond laser is set at 80% of the thinnest corneal thickness along the tunnel location (Fig. 23.19).
- An incision site is set according to nomogram recommendations.
- A disposable suction ring is placed, and special attention is given to centralizing the disposable suction ring to mark the central point to minimize decentration (Fig. 23.20).

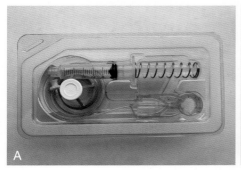
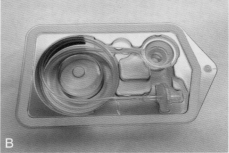

Fig. 23.15   Disposable cone sets of femtosecond lasers: (A) Intralase, (B) VisuMax.

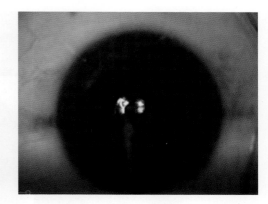

Fig. 23.16 Marking of Purkinje reflex under the operating microscope of a femtosecond laser after marking of 0-degree and 180-degree axis using a slit-lamp microscope.

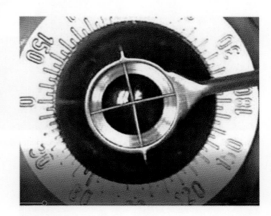

Fig. 23.17 Marking of the channel tracks.

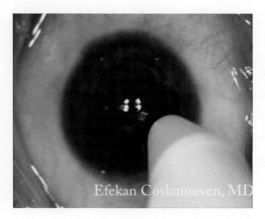

Fig. 23.18 Measurement of the corneal thickness using an ultrasonic pachymetry along the ring location markings.

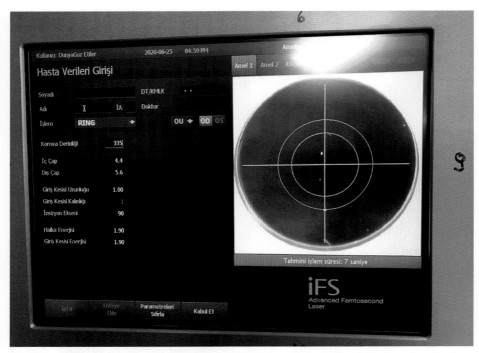

Fig. 23.19 The image of the Intralase femtosecond laser screen with the setting of the channel creation in an intrastromal corneal ring segment implantation.

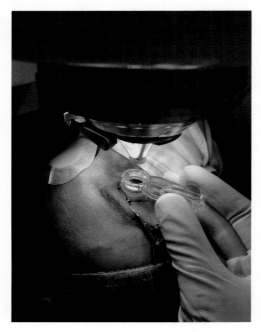

Fig. 23.20 Placement of the suction ring and applanation cone for the Intralase femtosecond laser.

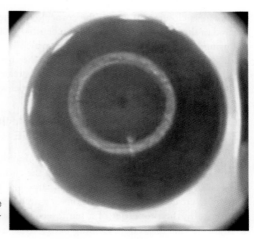

Fig. 23.21 Bubbles seen immediately after the creation of the channel and incision using femto-second laser.

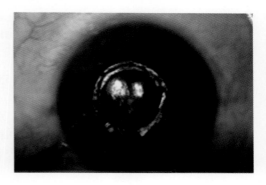

Fig. 23.22 Insertion of the intrastromal corneal ring segment through the channel.

- The cornea is flattened with a disposable applanation cone.
- After complete docking providing a precise distance from the laser head to the focal point, laser pulses are delivered to create the tunnels, including location and thickness (Fig. 23.21).
- The ICRSs are inserted immediately after channel creation before the disappearance of the bubbles, with Albertazzi forceps (Fig. 23.22).

Channel dimensions can be arranged using the femtosecond laser, and different, preferred variations of inner and outer diameter can be selected. For example, 4.4- to 5.6-mm inner and outer diameters, which are actual dimensions of Keraring SI-5 (5-mm optical zone), can be set to create channels for this type of ICRS.[14] However, some authors prefer the channel dimensions for the same segment to be 4.8- or 5.0-mm inner diameter and 6.0- or 6.6-mm outer diameter.[15,16] For Keraring SI-6 (6-mm optical zone), channels with 5.8-mm inner diameter and 6.8-, 7-, or 7.95-mm outer diameter can be formed when using the femtosecond laser technique.[17]

Currently, 90-, 120-, 160-, 210-, and 320-degree arc segments are on the market. Some types of ICRS require special attention during implantations. ICRS with arc lengths longer than 160 degrees can cause difficulties in manipulation because of their length.

POCKETMAKER ULTRAKERATOME

The PocketMaker Ultrakeratome was primarily designed by Dioptex for MyoRing implantation. This device allows the creation of almost entirely closed corneal pockets of up to 9 mm in diameter, as close as 50 μm to the corneal endothelium. In MyoRing implantation, a pocket is created in the 9-mm central cornea at a depth of 300 microns via a 4- to 5-mm wide corneal tunnel using a PocketMaker Ultrakeratome, which is a device that uses a guided vibrating diamond blade. The MyoRing is then implanted into the corneal pocket.

The femtosecond laser can also be used to create a stromal pocket for MyoRing implantation at the desired depth, diameter, and corneal tunnel width.

COMPARISON OF MANUAL (MECHANICAL) VERSUS FEMTOSECOND LASER TECHNIQUE

Mechanical dissection was the first method described for facilitating the insertion of ring segments. The use of the femtosecond laser in the corneal tunnel creation made the procedure faster and easier, especially for inexperienced surgeons. The use of the femtosecond laser allows the surgeon to create tunnels and incisions at a predetermined depth with a high degree of precision. Theoretically, the properties of a femtosecond laser-assisted procedure would generate a more accurate stromal dissection, yielding better visual and refractive results with lower complication rates.[18–20]

The Advantages of Femtosecond Laser Technique

SHORT TIME

Channel formation lasts 6 to 8 seconds, instead of 5 to 8 minutes in the mechanical technique.

LESS EPITHELIAL DEFECT

The femtosecond laser technique necessitates less handling and touch of the corneal epithelium, compared with the mechanical technique. Therefore the incidence of the epithelial defect formation is less in the femtosecond technique.

LESS DISCOMFORT

The femtosecond laser technique induces less discomfort in patients because of its shorter duration and lesser epithelial damage.

LESS RISK OF INFLAMMATION

Every intervention in the cornea will produce additional inflammation and corneal edema. The femtosecond laser technique decreases the amount of inflammation and edema compared with the mechanical technique.

ASEPTIC TECHNIQUE

Sterile single-use disposable applanation cones are used in the femtosecond technique and minimal handling reduces infection risk to minimum.

UNIFORM DISSECTION

The maximum depth for channel preparation with the femtosecond laser technique is 400 μm with the Intralase femtosecond laser. The femtosecond laser enables the creation of channels at the intended reliable and constant depth. Anterior or posterior misdirection of channels is not expected.

GOOD CENTRALIZATION

Marking the reference center under the operation microscope is necessary before operation with the Intralase femtosecond laser. Otherwise, centralization is easily mistaken in corneas with an inferior apex. However, with the VisuMax femtosecond laser, a round-shaped cone is used, and it is sufficient for the patient to look at the fixation light during the operation.

BETTER SYMMETRY

Despite the use of the stromal tunnel separator with vacuum, the tunnel shape may not be symmetrical and round during ICRS implantation, especially with the manual separator. However, tunnels of the intended depth and width can be created in 6 to 8 seconds with a femtosecond laser, and this factor increases the success of the implantation remarkably.

LOW VACUUM

The suction ring attaches to the eye with about 35 mmHg pressure lasting only a constant 8 seconds during the femtosecond laser technique.

CUSTOMIZING THE SIZE OF THE TUNNEL

Modifying channel diameters can lead to obtain different outcomes with the same ICRS.

ALLOWING ICRS IMPLANTATION IN EYES WITH A HISTORY OF PREVIOUS REFRACTIVE SURGERY

The femtosecond laser allows the surgeon to create channels in eyes previously subjected to corneal refractive surgery. Irregularities in the cornea after keratoplasty (Fig. 23.23) and radial keratotomy can be treated safely with ICRS implantation using the femtosecond laser.[21,22] In addition, previously long-diameter ICRS-implanted eyes that still have irregularities can also be treated with ICRS implantation with shorter diameters. Post-LASIK ectasia is another indication for ICRS implantation using the femtosecond laser technique.

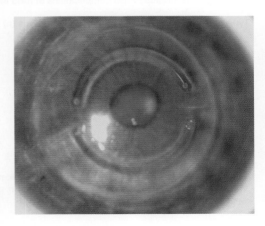

Fig. 23.23 Intrastromal corneal ring segment implantation for postkeratoplasty irregularity.

Complications Encountered During Implantation

Although the femtosecond laser provides many advantages, complications can be encountered during ICRS implantations (Table 23.1).

INCOMPLETE CHANNEL FORMATION

Insufficient laser energy levels can cause incomplete channel formation. This is minimized by regulating the energy levels and spot separation. Procedures can be completed with the use of a mechanical spreader.

Incomplete channel formation can be recognized by the difficulty in inserting the ring. The surgeon feels a blockage because bridges and blind pouches are formed by insufficient energy. To overcome this problem, the surgeon can pull the ring back slightly and advance in a different plane. If the blockage continues, the second ring can be inserted from the other side to bypass the pouches and bridges (Fig. 23.24). Irregularities of the channel wall can be seen on follow-ups (Fig. 23.25).

GALVANOMETER LAG ERROR

A technical problem encountered with the femtosecond laser is the galvanometer lag error in the memory system.

Maintenance of vacuum is important during the procedure. In the case of galvanometer lag error, surgery should be postponed. If surgery is repeated, the same cone should be used by adjusting depth to about 30 μm superficial to the previous one. If the same problem occurs during incision site formation, the incision can be completed by using a blade.

ENDOTHELIAL PERFORATION

Incorrect measurement of the thickness along channel tracks and at the incision site may lead to endothelial perforation. Bubbles are seen in the anterior chamber. When the endothelial perforation is recognized, surgery should be stopped immediately.

TABLE 23.1 ■ Intraoperative Complications of ICRS Implantation With Femtosecond Laser

Type of Complications	Eyes (n)	Percentage (%)
Incomplete tunnel formation	22	2.6
Galvo error during incision	5	0.6
Endothelial perforation	5	0.6
Incorrect entry of the channel	2	0.2
Vacuum loss	1	0.1
Total	35	4.1

ICRS, Intrastromal corneal ring segment.
From Coskunseven E, Kymionis GD, Tsiklis N, et al. Complications of intrastromal corneal ring segment implantation using a femtosecond laser for channel creation: a survey of 850 eyes with keratoconus. *Acta Ophthalmol.* 2011;89:54–57.

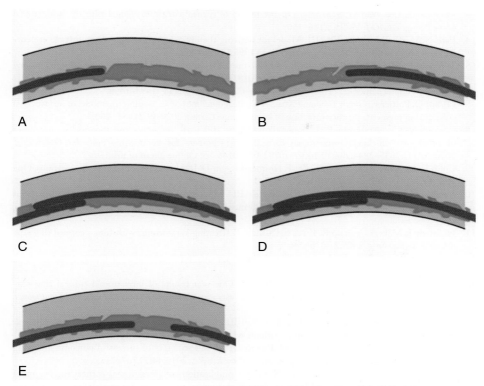

Fig. 23.24 Surgical manipulations to overcome incomplete channel. The surgeon (A) feels difficulty in inserting the ring, (B) inserts the second ring from other side, (C) inserts the first ring under the second ring, (D) advances the first ring bypassing the blockage, and (E) pulls back the second ring.

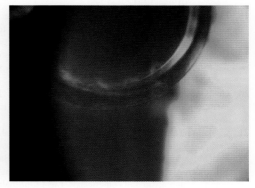

Fig. 23.25 Scars around the ring because of incomplete channel formation and bridges on the wall.

References

1. Nosé W, Neves RA, Jr, Schanzlin DJ, Belfort R. Intrastromal corneal ring one-year results of first implants in humans: a preliminary nonfunctional eye study. *Refract Corneal Surg*. 1993;9(6):452–458.
2. Burris TE, Baker PC, Ayer CT, Loomas BE, Mathis ML, Silvestrini TA. Flattening of central corneal curvature with intrastromal corneal rings of increasing thickness: an eye-bank eye study. *J Cataract Refract Surg*. 1993;19(Suppl):182–187.

3. Fleming JF, Lee Wan W, Schanzlin DJ. The theory of corneal curvature change with the intrastromal corneal ring. *CLAO J*. 1989;15:146–150.
4. Patel S, Marshall J, Fitzke FW III. Model for deriving the optical performance of the myopic eye corrected with an intracorneal ring. *J Refract Surg*. 1995;11:248–252.
5. Torquetti L, Cunha P, Luz A, et al. Clinical outcomes after implantation of 320°-arc length intrastromal corneal ring segments in keratoconus. *Cornea*. 2018;37(10):1299–1305.
6. Daxer A. Biomechanics of corneal ring implants. *Cornea*. 2015;34(11):1493–1498.
7. Prisant O, Pottier E, Guedj T, Hoang Xuan T. Clinical outcomes of an asymmetric model of intrastromal corneal ring segments for the correction of keratoconus. *Cornea*. 2020;39(2):155–160.
8. Coşkunseven E, Ambrósio R, Jr, Smorádková A, et al. Visual, refractive and topographic outcomes of progressive thickness intrastromal corneal ring segments for keratoconic eyes. *Int Ophthalmol*. 2020;40(11):2835–2844. doi:10.1007/s10792-020-01467-5. Online ahead of print.
9. Colin J, Cochener B, Savary G, Malet F, Holmes-Higgin D. Intacs inserts for treating keratoconus. One year results. *Ophthalmology*. 2001;108:1409–1414.
10. Kanellopoulos AJ, Pe LH, Perry HD, Donnenfeld ED. Modified intracorneal ring segment implantations (Intacs) for the management of moderate to advanced keratoconus. Efficacy and complications. *Cornea*. 2006;25:29–33.
11. Hellstedt T, Mäkelä Uusitalo R, Emre S, Uusitalo R. Treating keratoconus with Intacs corneal ring segments. *J Refract Surg*. 2005;21:236–246.
12. Kwitko S, Severo NS. Ferrara intracorneal ring segments for keratoconus. *J Cataract Refract Surg*. 2004;30:812–820.
13. Coskunseven E, Kymionis GD, Tsiklis NS, et al. One-year results of intrastromal corneal ring segment implantation (KeraRing) using femtosecond laser in patients with keratoconus. *Am J Ophthalmol*. 2008;145(5):775–779.
14. Wilde CL, Naylor SG, Varga Z, Morrell A, Ball JL. Keraring implantation using the Zeiss Visumax femtosecond laser in the management of patients with keratoconus. *Eye (Lond)*. 2017;31(6):916–923.
15. Sedaghat MR, Momeni-Moghaddam H, Piñero DP, et al. Predictors of successful outcome following intrastromal corneal ring segments implantation. *Curr Eye Res*. 2019;44(7):707–715.
16. Coskunseven E, Kymionis GD, Tsiklis N, et al. Complications of intrastromal corneal ring segment implantation using a femtosecond laser for channel creation: a survey of 850 eyes with keratoconus. *Acta Ophthalmol*. 2011;89:54–57.
17. Monteiro T, Alfonso JF, Freitas R, et al. Comparison of complication rates between manual and femtosecond laser-assisted techniques for intrastromal corneal ring segments implantation in keratoconus. *Curr Eye Res*. 2019;44(12):1291–1298.
18. Piñero DP, Alio JL, El Kady B, et al. Refractive and aberrometric outcomes of intracorneal ring segments for keratoconus: mechanical versus femtosecond-assisted procedures. *Ophthalmology*. 2009;116(9):1675–1687.
19. Coskunseven E, Kymionis GD, Talu H, et al. Intrastromal corneal ring segment implantation with the femtosecond laser in a post-keratoplasty patient with recurrent keratoconus. *J Cataract Refract Surg*. 2007;33(10):1808–1810.
20. Coskunseven E, Kymionis GD, Bouzoukis DI, Aslan E, Pallikaris I. Single intrastromal corneal ring segment implantation using the femtosecond laser after radial keratotomy in a keratoconic patient. *J Cataract Refract Surg*. 2009;35(1):197–199.
21. Coskunseven E, Kymionis GD, Grentzelos MA, et al. INTACS followed by KeraRing intrastromal corneal ring segment implantation for keratoconus. *J Refract Surg*. 2010;26(5):371–374.
22. Fernández-Vega-Cueto Luis, Lisa Carlos, Alfonso-Bartolozzi Belén, Madrid-Costa David, Alfonso José F Intrastromal corneal ring segment implantation in paracentral keratoconus with perpendicular topographic astigmatism and comatic axis. Eur J Ophthalmol. 2021;31(4):1540–1545. 1724-6016. doi:10.11 77/1120672120952346.32830575.

CHAPTER 24

Anatomy of Intracorneal Ring Segments for the Treatment of Keratoconus and Other Corneal Ectasias

Roberto Albertazzi

KEY CONCEPTS

- There is an inverse relationship between the diameter of the ring and its effect on the cornea.
- The width of the intrastromal corneal ring segments is related to their diameter and this is of fundamental importance to the effect of the implant.
- Intrastromal corneal ring segments with a flat profiles have more effect at their ends and in the center than segments with conical profiles.
- Conical profile segments will release less tension compared with flat profile segments because their inclination is parallel to the cornea.

Anatomy of an Intracorneal Segment

The effect that intrastromal corneal ring segments (ISCRs) produce on the cornea can be explained in part by Blavatskaia et al.'s first law which states that the smaller the diameter, the greater the effect.[1] For example, small-diameter segments, such as the Ferrara type (5 mm diameter), have a greater effect on the visual axis than large-diameter segments such as Intacs 7 mm ISCRs are available in various diameters: 5, 6, and 7 mm (Fig. 24.1A).

MATERIAL

The material used to manufacture the segments is polymethyl methacrylate (PMMA) (see Fig. 24.1B). This material is a PMMA-Perspex QC that absorbs ultraviolet (UV) radiation and is manufactured to the specifications of the US Food and Drug Administration (FDA), ISO 9001, and EN46001.[2]

APICAL DIAMETER

The apical diameter (see Fig. 24.1B) is described by the line that passes through the center of the body of the segments, thus indicating the diameter of the optical zone that the segments enclose

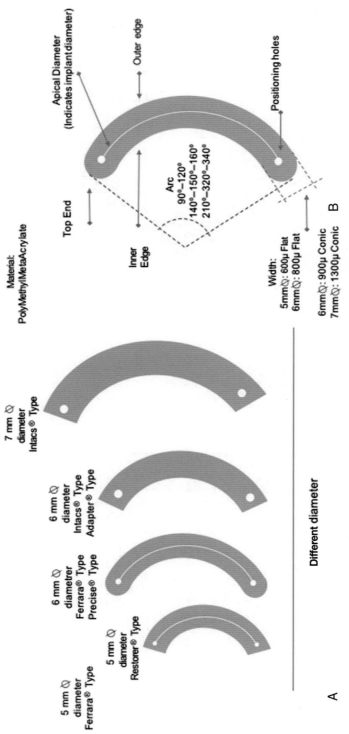

Fig. 24.1 (A) Different diameter segments (5, 6, and 7 mm). (B) Anatomy of an intracorneal ring: apical diameter.

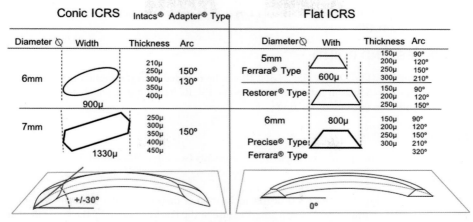

Fig. 24.2 *Top left*: conical shape (Intacs type/Adapter type) base segments indicating diameter, width, thickness, and arcs; *bottom left*: graphic of a conical design; *Top right*: Ferrara type/Precise type with flat-based segments indicating diameter, width, thickness, and arc; *bottom right*: graphic of a flat of the 0-degree angle that they present. *ICRS*, Intrastromal corneal ring segment.

(5-, 6-, or 7-mm optical zone). Although this is not the actual optical zone, this system simplifies the method of classification by segment diameter.

WIDTH

The width of the ISCRs is the measure of the side where the segment rests (Fig. 24.2), toward the corneal endothelium. The width of segments is related to their diameter and this is of fundamental importance to the effect of the implant. The width determines the profile of the segment, along with its angulation.[3]

Older, flat-bottomed 5-mm diameter segments were 600 microns in length,[4] whereas the 7-mm diameter conical segments required length up to 1330 microns to produce an effect. Fig. 24.1 demonstrates the most frequent sizes found in the market.

SIZES

Some segment manufacturers use millimeters to indicate the characteristics of their implants (Ferrara Ring)[4]; however, refractive surgeons are used to describing them in microns, for example, a 0.25-mm segment is equivalent to 250 microns.

ARC

The segment of a circle is called an arc. ISCRs are described according to their central angle, the arcs of segments found on the market range from 60 degrees to 340 degrees, but the most frequently used are 90, 120, and 150 degrees. The surgeon selects them according to the pattern of the ectasia to be treated (see Figs. 24.1 and 24.2).

INNER EDGE

The inner edge of the segment delimits the optical zone (see Fig. 24.1). The placement of the smallest segments (5 mm of the optic zone) must be precise to avoid causing glare symptoms, which occur if slightly off-center. Segments of 6-mm diameter are used in the majority of cases, with 5-mm segments used only for special cases such as severe asymmetries or high post-penetrating keratoplasty (PK) astigmatism.[6]

EXTREMES (END POINT)

Segment terminals (Figs. 24.1A and 24.3[1,2]) can be rounded as in the Ferrara type ISCRs or have a flat configuration as in Intacs segments. Some ISCRs have a notch, which allows locating the correct insertion position of the ring.

SECTION

There are two sections[8]: profiles or slopes of the segments (see Figs. 24.2 and 24.3).

Flat Segments

Flat segments (Ferrara type) have a 0-degree inclination at their base. These segments are more difficult to implant within a conical structure, because of the tension created by the structure that houses them (flat segment in conical cornea) (see Fig. 24.2). This tension translates into a decrease in the keratometric values just above the body of the segment and elevation of the tissue at its ends.

These flat segments, originally designed by Ferrara and currently marketed by several companies (Ferrara Rings, Keraring, Mediphacos, Intraseg), present a base with a flat design, which must be parallel to the corneal endothelium, without angulation.

Conical

Intacs, Intacs SK,[2] and Adapter[6] are conical section segments designed with an inclination of their base of approximately 26 to 34 degrees (see Figs. 24.2 and 24.3). These designs mimic corneal curvature making them easier to insert, and they generate very little intracorneal tension. They generate an increase in volume, which produces their effect.

Conical segments maintain a prolate corneal shape without generating astigmatism.

Thickness. Blavatskaia et al.[1] described the direct relationship between the effect of thickness and the effect of the ring: the greater the thickness of the implant, the greater the effect, and the smaller the thickness, the smaller the effect[9] (see Figs. 24.2 and 24.3).

Fig. 24.3 shows the associated complications related to the thickness of the ISCRs (minor complications are shown in *green*, major complications are shown in *red*, and contraindications are shown in violet).

Asymmetric Segments

Asymmetrical segments have different profiles on each of their ends.[10] The profile in Fig. 24.3(4) demonstrates the gradual increase in segment height from the proximal to the distal end. The segment that is 150 microns at its proximal end is 250 microns at its distal end, the segment that is 200 microns at proximal end is 300 microns at its distal end.

Profiles of ISCRs

The ISCRs modify the corneal architecture in three main areas: (1) the area where the ring is located where an increase in corneal thickness occurs, (2) at the end of the extremities of the ring (where the tension vectors are released), and (3) in the center of the cornea, where corneal flattening occurs. Fig. 24.4.

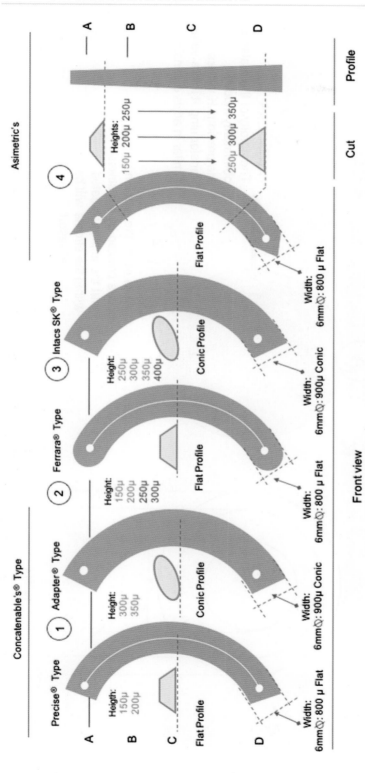

Fig. 24.3 **A:** ICRs endpoint, **B:** Height of the ICRs, **C:** ICRs profile, **D:** ICRs widht. (1) Ring segments: flat profile (Precise) and conical profile (Adapter) with flat end point that ensures safe movement within the same channel, potentially allowing multiple combinations of profiles and arcs; heights are limited to reduce possible complications. (2) Ferrara Ring, with flat profile and thicknesses. (3) Intacs SK, with conical profile and thicknesses (*B*). (4) Asymmetric segments: several companies have produced these types of flat design that vary in height from the distal to the proximal end point.

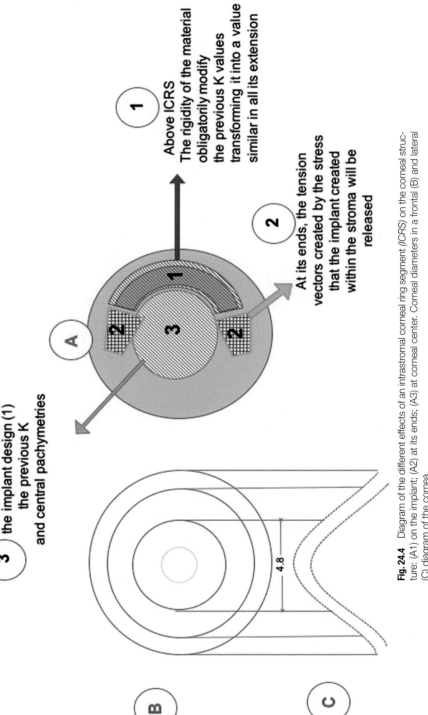

Above ICRS
The rigidity of the material obligatorily modify the previous K values transforming it into a value similar in all its extension

1

2

At its ends, the tension vectors created by the stress that the implant created within the stroma will be released

3

The tensions between: stress vectors (2) the implant design (1) the previous K and central pachymetries

A

2

3

2

1

B

4.8

C

Fig. 24.4 Diagram of the different effects of an intrastromal corneal ring segment (*ICRS*) on the corneal structure: (A1) on the implant; (A2) at its ends; (A3) at corneal center. Corneal diameters in a frontal (B) and lateral (C) diagram of the cornea.

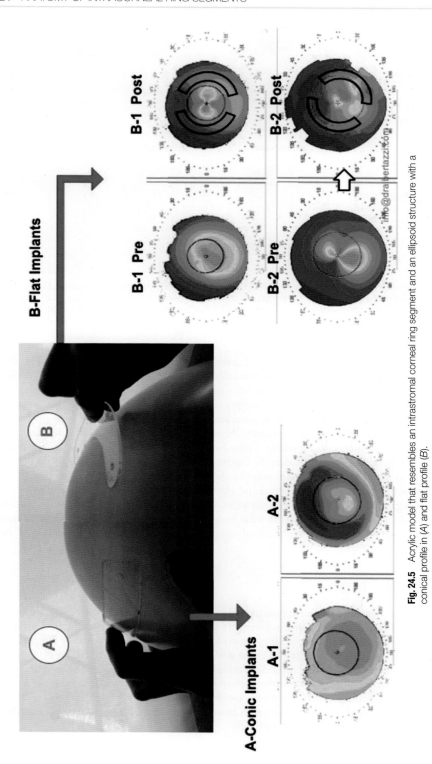

Fig. 24.5 Acrylic model that resembles an intrastromal corneal ring segment and an ellipsoid structure with a conical profile in (A) and flat profile (B).

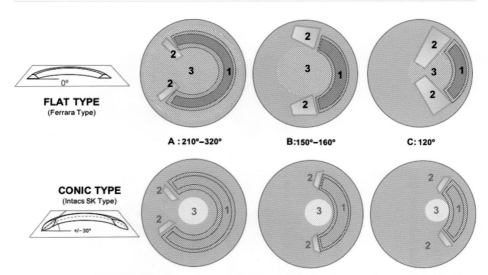

Fig. 24.6 Behavior of the different arcs (A: 210–320, B: 150–160 and C: 120 degrees) according to the intra-stromal corneal ring segment profile. (1) Increase in corneal thickness, (2) corneal effect (released tension) at the ends of the ISCRs, (3) corneal effect at the center of the cornea. Flat profiles have greater effect than conic profiles despite has same arc lenght.

To demonstrate the different behavior of these implants according to their profile, Fig. 24.5 uses a balloon and an acrylic model that resembles an ICRS. It is easy to see that the conical segment (A) will offer less resistance, as it has a similar inclination to the structure represented by the balloon, whereas it is difficult to imagine the flat segment (B) being part of the structure because significant resistance will be generated once inside. These relationships are evident during surgery when the rings are inserted. The conical ring segments do not offer resistance whereas the flat segments do, especially if they have large arcs. In Fig. 24.5, A-1 demonstrates presurgical spherical topography before the insertion of two conical segments of 150-degrees arc and 6 mm in diameter, and A-2 demonstrates the effect of the segments once implanted. The corneal structure maintains its prolate shape, but with lower keratometric values and without induced astigmatism. The same figure, shows the presurgical spherical topographic image (B-1) of a cornea in which two segments with a flat base of 150-degrees arc and 6-mm diameter were implanted, B-2 shows induced high central astigmatism as a result of the flat design of the segments.[11]

Arcs of the ISCRs

Like rings, arc segments of different profiles behave differently. This is demonstrated by the graph in Fig. 24.6, on which the flat profile segments[13] have greater effect at the ends and in the center than the conical profile segments,[11] as they release less tension. The effect will also be reduced, and this is reflected not only in the extremities but also in the corneal center (see Fig. 24.6).

Rigid segments, once implanted, modify corneal structural behavior in the following ways:

- The stroma remains rigid where the implant is located (see Fig. 24.6, area 1).
- Stress vectors are released at their ends (see Fig. 24.6, area 2).
- Flat profile segments will release much more tension (see Fig. 24.6, area 3) because their design opposes the corneal architecture.

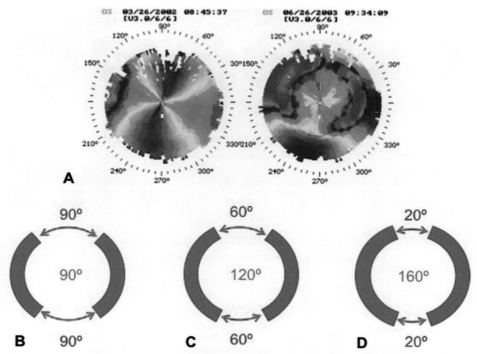

Fig. 24.7 (A) Astigmatism treated with flat segments (Ferrara type) 50 mm in diameter and 120 degrees; (B) 90-degree segments (C) 120-degree segments; (D) 160-degree segments. The greater the arc of the ISCRs, the lower the corneal space to release the tension.

- Conical profile segments will release less tension than flat profile segments, because their inclination is parallel to the corneal one (see Fig. 24.6 [*bottom*]).
- In ICRSs greater than 180-degree arc, the release of the tension vectors blocks at their ends and the entire pattern uniformly lowers the keratometric values but maintaining its topographic characteristics (see Fig. 24.6A).

Using ISCRs in Different Topographic Patterns

Most of the manufacturers have various nomograms that suggest what type of ring should be implanted, based on a variety of parameters (keratometry, topographic pattern, coma, corneal thickness, etc.). Many of these nomograms take the following into consideration:

TREATMENT OF BOW-TIE PATTERNS (BOW TIE)

When considering the surgical anatomy, symmetrical patterns are those that present symmetry within 6 mm of the optical zone:
- Symmetrical with-the-rule bow-tie pattern requires treatment with symmetrical segments
- Pellucid marginal degeneration (PMD) is treated against-the-rule, with asymmetric design segments.

The surgical procedures for the bow-tie pattern is the simplest, because they will always be symmetrical, determining the incision. Fig. 24.7 shows one of the first refractive treatments of astigmatism with intracorneal segments, performed in 2002.

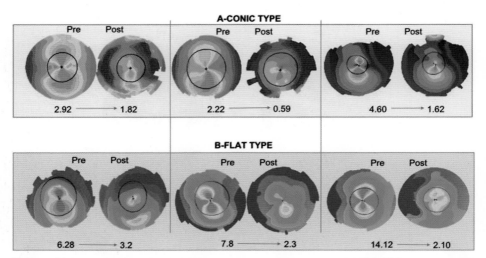

Fig. 24.8   (A) Cases treated with flat-design intrastromal corneal ring segments (ICRSs). (B) Cases treated with ICRSs of conical design.

The last of these configurations (see Fig. 24.7D) causes instability. As a result, the authors have abandoned the use of 160-degree segments and use segments of up to 140 degrees.

Fig. 24.8 A shows three cases of low astigmatism treated with 150-degree arc conical segments. Fig. 24.8B shows three cases treated with 150-degree arc flat-design segments. Both have been implanted in such a way that their ends face each other in an area of steep keratometry. The different effects on the cornea are shown by the graph in Fig. 24.9.

TREATMENT OF DUCK OR DUCK AND CROISSANT PATTERNS

Main Segment and Secondary or Accessory Segment

Asymmetric ectasias have unique characteristics[11,13–16]:

- Astigmatic values are lower
- They are frequently treated with asymmetrical segments.

The main segments will always be the inferotemporal, and they function to reduce corneal curvatures at the site of implantation. Fig. 24.10 shows the behavior of an inferotemporal main segment: 150 degrees × 150 microns, flat design, in "duck and croissant"–type ectasias. The effect will be beneficial when asymmetry is minimal, and the corneal structure still works relatively normally so that its reaction resembles a water mattress, that is, one side is pressed and a distant area rises. The accessory segments increase the corneal curvature and are shorter.

In Figs. 24.11–24.14 duck and croissant–type ectasias show a dissociation of their keratometric axis (Figs. 24.12–24.15). These patterns can be treated with different combinations of flat profile segments (Ferrara type and Precise type) and conical segments (Intacs SK type and Adapt type).[11,16] In Fig. 24.11, the first cases of these combinations are shown, in which the same arches were used for the main (inferior-temporal) and secondary (superior-temporal) segments and Fig. 24.12–24.14 show some cases where different combinations in arcs and thickness of the ISCRs are employed.

The behavior of the different profiles to treat Astigmatism or Bow Tie ectasia

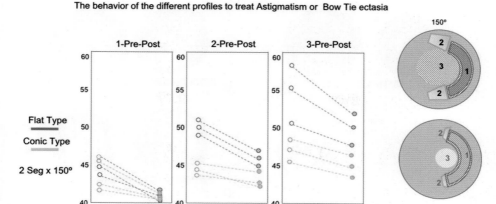

Fig. 24.9 Effect of the various intrastromal corneal ring segment designs according to the different tension release zones. (1) Effect on the implant zone; (2) effect where the tension vectors are released at their ends; (3) effect in the central cornea, showing the modification of the keratometric values within the optic zone.

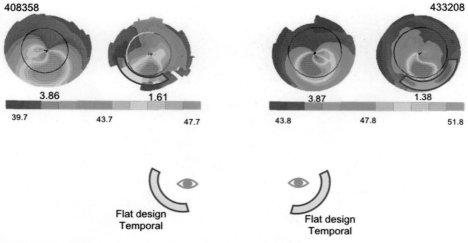

Fig. 24.10 Behavior of an inferotemporal main segment of 150 degrees × 150 microns, flat design, in duck and croissant–type ectasias.

Topographic Stages and Their Most Frequent Patterns

Fig. 24.15 shows the characteristics of 273 cases of primary ectasia according to Amsler-Krumeich classification.[20]

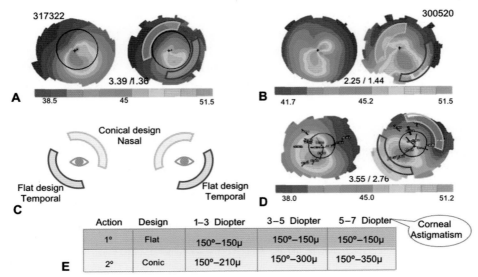

Fig. 24.11 In (A), (B), and (D) the presurgical *(left)* and postsurgical *(right)* topography and corneal astigmatism are shown; (C) is a diagram of their placement and (E) shows the guide used for their selection.

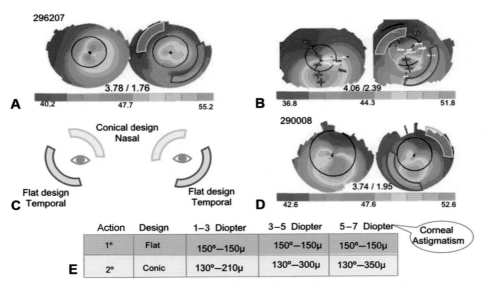

Fig. 24.12 Shorter 130-degree arc with conical profile. In (A), (B), and (D) the presurgical *(left)* and postsurgical *(right)* topographic changes are shown. (C) is a diagram of their placement and (E) is the guide used for their selection.

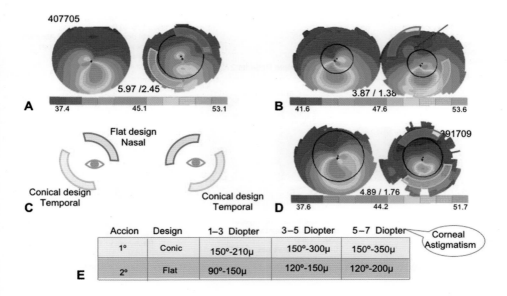

Fig. 24.13 Conical main segment and flat secondary segment. The *red arrow* in (B) shows the positive effect on the flatter quadrant (upper nasal). In (A), (B), and (D) the presurgical *(left)* and postsurgical *(right)* topography and corneal astigmatism are shown. (C) is a diagram of their placement and (E) is the guide used for the choice of placement.

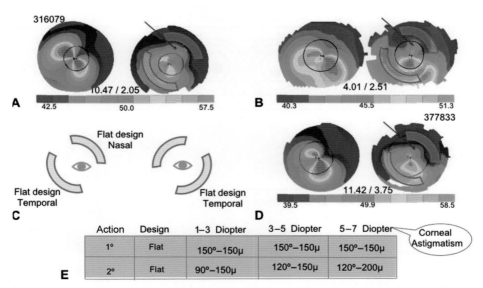

Fig. 24.14 In cases with very high astigmatism, the effect is greater when both segments are flat. The *red arrows* indicate the effect of the segments. (A), (B), and (D) show the presurgical *(left)* and postsurgical *(right)* topography and corneal astigmatism. (C) is diagram of their placement. (E) shows the guide used for the choice of placement.

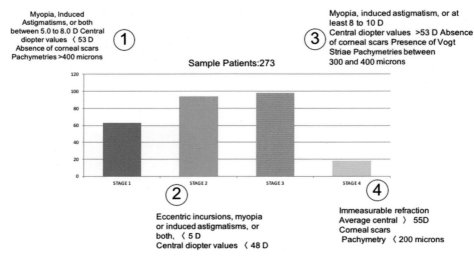

Fig. 24.15 Characteristics of a sample of 273 consecutive cases of primary ectasia.[19] These stages were proposed by Krumeich.[20]

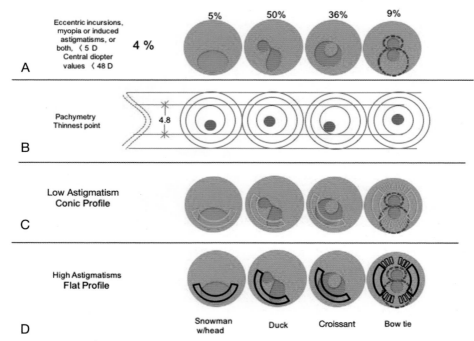

Fig. 24.16 (A) Topographic patterns. (B) Location of the minimum corneal thickness. (C) Topographic patters showing mild asymmetries treated with a single segment. In cases with less than 2.5 D of astigmatism, the implantation of conical segments between 300 and 350 microns is recommended. (D) In cases with 2.5 to 4 D of astigmatism, the use of flat profile segments not exceeding 150 microns is recommended (to avoid generating overcorrection).

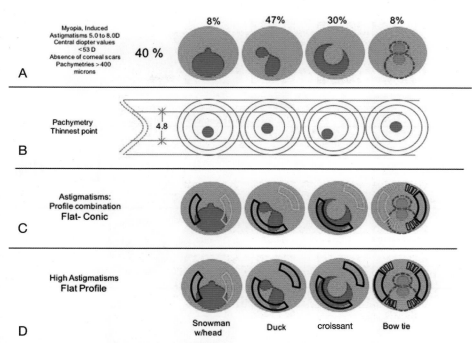

Fig. 24.17 (A) Topographic patterns of keratoconus stage II. (B) Location of the minimum corneal thickness. (C) Topographic patterns showing the treatment of low and moderate astigmatism. Flat segments are shown in *black* and conical segments in *yellow*. Snowman and bow-tie cases should be treated using segments of equal arc. For duck and croissant patterns, the primary segment (temporal-inferior) should have a greater arc than the secondary one (superior-nasal). (D) Topographic patterns associated with astigmatism greater than 4 D. These cases are treated with flat profile segments up to 150 microns, or conical profile segments up to 350 microns.

STAGE I

Fig. 24.16 demonstrates the most frequently topographic pattern of KC stage I according to Amsler-Krumeich classification. Stage I is usually treated with a single segment.

Fig. 24.16A depicts the clinical characteristics and keratometric values of stage 1 ectasia, as well as the percentage of appearance that is around 4% of all ectasias. Fig. 24.16B demonstrates the thinnest pachymetric points associated with the respective patterns and Fig. 24.16C lists treatments for mild asymmetries.

STAGE II

Fig. 24.17 summarizes stage II ectasias, which includes most of the cases that undergo ISCRs implantation, as they no longer improve with spectacle correction. Duck and croissant patterns are the most common pattterns in this stage.

STAGE III

Fig. 24.18 summarizes our understanding of the evolution of different topographic patterns.

Uncited References

17

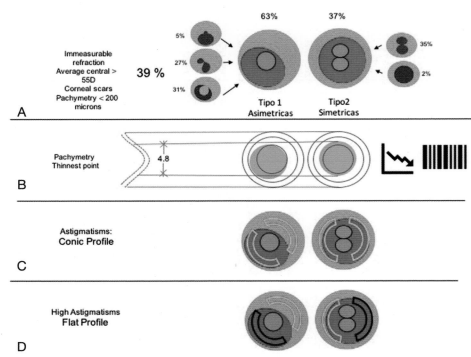

Fig. 24.18 (A) Topographic patterns of keratoconus stage III patterns presenting paracentrally cone with pachymetric thinning (snowman, duck, and croissant) usually evolve to a larger paracentral ectasia and bow-tie and nipple patterns shift to a more central symmetric ectasia. (B) Area commonly associated with the thinnest pachymetry. (C) Topographic patterns associated with mild and moderate astigmatism with conical segments. (D) Topographic patterns associated with astigmatism above 4 D. These cases are treated using a combination of flat profile segments preferably not exceeding 150 microns *(black)* and conical segments not exceeding 350 microns *(yellow)*.

References

1. Blavatskaia ED, Viazovskiĭ IA, Barsegian LG. Change in corneal curvature in intralamellar homotrans-plantation of discs of various diameter and thickness. *Oftalmol Zh.* 1967;22:123–128.
2. Intacs. Surgeon Training Manual for the correction of myopia. Pag 20 MK-US-50024-01-TOC/Rev.
3. Burris TE, Baker PC, Ayer CT, Loomas BE, Mathis ML, Silvestrini TA. Flattening of central corneal curvature with intrastromal corneal rings of increasing thickness: an eye-bank eye study. *J Cataract Refract Surg.* 1993;19(suppl):182–187.
4. Ferrara G, Torquetti L, Ferrara P, Merayo-Lloves J. Intrastromal corneal ring segments: visual outcomes from a large case series. *Clin Exp Ophthalmol.* 2012;40(5):433–439.
5. Krumeich JH, Daniel J, Knülle A. Live-epikeratophakia for keratoconus. *J Catarac Refract Surg.* 1998;24:456–463.
6. Albertazzi RG. Nueva Linea de Segmentos KCSolutions. *World Keratoconus Meeting;* 2019.
7. Albertazzi RG. Intracorneal implant and injector to treat corneal disorder. Patent Application Publication US 2019/0159888A1. May 30, 2019.
8. Albertazzi RG, ed Buenos Aires: Argentine Scientific Editions for the Keratoconus Society; 2010. Queratocono: pautas para su diagnostico y tratamiento. 144.

9. Blavatskaia ED. Intralamellar homoplasty for the purpose of relaxation of refraction of the eye. *Oftalmol Zh.* 1968;7:530–537.
10. Prisant O, Pottier E, Guedj T, Hoang Xuan T. Clinical outcomes of an asymmetric model of intrastromal corneal ring segments for the correction of keratoconus. *Cornea.* 2020;39(2):155–160.
11. Albertazzi R, Rao G, Ferlini L, et al. Combination of intracorneal ring segments (Ferrara & Intacts) in the care of patients with keratoconus. ARVO Meeting; 2013.
12. Alfonso JF, Lisa C, Merayo-Lloves J, Fernández-Vega Cueto L, Montés-Micó R. Intrastromal corneal ring implantation in paracentral keratoconus with coincident topographic and coma axis. *J Cataract Refract Surg.* 2012;38:1576–1582.
13. Refraction in Primary Corneal Ectasias, Keratoconus: Guidelines for its management, Consejo Argentino de Oftalmologia, en imprenta; 2020.
14. Barraquer JI. Keraomileusis and Keratophakia, Instituto Barraquer de Colombia, 1980.
15. Fernandez Vega-Cueto L. Classification of Keratoconus for its surgical correction with Ferrara -type intra corneal ring segments: Research work to qualify for the degree of Doctor of the University of Oviedo; April 2016.
16. Albertazzi RG. Methods and apparatus for treating keratoconus. United States Patent US 9,931,199 B2 Apr. 3, 2018.
17. Albertazzi RG. Treatment of Duck and Croissant patterns with combinations of profile. World Keratoconus Meeting; 2019-Elche.
18. Combinations of profiles in the treatment of primary ectasias, Keratoconus: Guidelines for its management, Consejo Argentino de Oftalmologia, in press; 2020.
19. Krumeich JH, Daniel J, Knülle A. Live-epikeratophakia for keratoconus. *J Cataract Refract Surg.* 1998;24:456–463.
20. Kling S, Marcos S. Finite-element modeling of intrastromal ring segment implantation into a hyperelastic cornea. *Invest Ophthalmol Vis Sci.* 2013;54(1):881–889.

CHAPTER 25

Intrastromal Corneal Ring Segments: Outcomes and Complications

Taíse Tognon ▪ Mauro Campos

KEY CONCEPTS

- Intrastromal corneal ring segments (ICRSs) reshape the cornea form by modifying its geometry, improving the patient's corneal surface and leading to a best vision in the majority of treated cases.
- ICRS implantation decreases the keratometric and refractive measures, reduces high order aberrations, and improves visual acuity.
- Success rates after ICRS implantation are high, depending on appropriate patient selection and adherence to suitable nomograms.
- ICRSs can be combined with other procedures, and some complications have been reported; however, it remains a safer surgery when compared with intraocular procedures.

Introduction

Intrastromal corneal ring segment (ICRS) implantation is a surgical technique developed to restore vision and postpone or avoid intraocular invasive procedures or corneal keratoplasty.[1] The rings act as elements that reshape corneal form by modifying its geometry, flattening the central area and decreasing irregular astigmatism, thereby improving the patient's corneal surface and leading to a best vision in the majority of the cases.[1-3] Vision rehabilitation is faster than after other corneal surgical procedures, presenting many fewer serious complications, and offering the specific advantages of not removing corneal tissue and minimizing epithelial changes.[4-7]

It is well documented that ICRS implantation leads to decreases in keratometric readings, spherical equivalent, and cylinder, reduces high order aberrations, and improves uncorrected visual acuity (UCVA) and best-corrected visual acuity (BCVA) in patients with hereditary or acquired corneal ectasias or irregular astigmatism.[2]

Success rates after ICRS implantation, as described in published articles, are high, depending on appropriate patient selection and adherence to suitable implantation nomograms.[2] Moreover, ICRS implantation can be combined with other procedures such as cross-linking.[8,9]

Outcomes

Corneal changes induced by ICRS implantation are responsible for visual, refractive, and keratometric improvement in patients with ectatic diseases. The procedure has an "orthopedic" function, regularizing the geometry of corneal tissue. In some patients, ring segments act as spacers, interfering with corneal collagen turnover, with consequent increases in the corneal pachymetry and corneal collagen remodeling.[3]

Most of the peer-reviewed scientific literature demonstrates a statistically significant central corneal flattening, improving both uncorrected and corrected visual acuity by reducing spherical equivalent and cylinder and by modifying corneal high order aberrations.[2] A better visual outcome is expected when the alignment of the refractive and keratometric axis angle is <15%.[2,10,11] All types and brands of ICRSs appear to be safe and effective (Table 25.1). ICRSs are effective even in patients older than 40 years, as demonstrated by Gatzioufas et al.[12] Keraring and Ferrara Ring are more effective in the treatment of keratoconus when compared with Intacs.[7] Piñero et al. demonstrated less astigmatism correction with Intacs and more prevalent symptoms of halos and glare.[13] These findings are related to the nature of the device, with fewer options of shapes and a larger diameter (which induces less corneal central flattening).[14]

Rates of success in upgrading vision are higher than 70% to 80% of treated patients.[2,15–18] However, Sakellaris et al. suggest that preoperative visual acuity is a prognostic factor, especially in keratoconus.[2] Some authors assert that poor preoperative visual acuity is a good prognostic factor for visual improvement, whereas others suggest that the procedure is less likely to achieve visual improvement in advanced keratoconus.[2] Today, these concepts are changing as new long arc ICRS models are launched by industry, acting more precisely in those challenging and advanced cases.

Regarding the arcs, long arc rings segments provide more spherical reduction and less astigmatic reduction, and the opposite occurs with short arc lengths.[3] The mainstay of success in ICRS surgery for keratoconus correction is the correct choice of ICRS, based on the manufacturer's nomogram.[19]

Both techniques for tunnel creation—exclusively manual (mechanical procedure) or using a femtosecond laser—are effective in producing the previously described corneal changes, and they provide similar visual and refractive outcomes.[19–21] More aberrations are described after the exclusively manual technique, which implies that corneal irregularity is not as well controlled with this method of surgical intervention.[20]

Surgeons differ in their preference of ICRS implantation depth. The majority prefer implants at a depth of 70% to 80%, considering the thinnest point of the channel in the exclusively manual technique and the thinnest point of total cornea in femto-assisted surgeries. Different depths of implantation are being studied; thus some authors suggest that a more superficial implantation may also be effective.[22]

In cases of progressive keratoconus, corneal collagen cross-linking can be performed before, after, or at the same surgical time as ICRS implantation. Such a combined procedure increases biomechanical rigidity and stability of the cornea and offers an additive effect to refractive and keratometric values.[2,23]

ICRS implantation in keratoconus has also been demonstrated to be useful for improving contact lens tolerance.[15,24,25] Procedures such as phakic intraocular lenses[26,27] and surface ablations[28] have also been described in combination with ICRS.

Despite adequate and exhaustive patient selection and suitable surgical planning and execution, the results of the surgery are unpredictable in some cases. Under such circumstances, corneal studies using biomechanics could be the key to better treatment choices in the near future.

Complications

Regardless of being considered a safer and a more stable procedure, some complications have been reported, not only in exclusively manual implantation but also when using a femtosecond laser to create the ring tunnel. Such complications have not been related to a specific group of patients or brand/manufacturer. Intraoperative or postoperative adverse effects have been reported, but the majority of intraoperative complications seemed to occur at the beginning of the learning curve and in the first years after the surgery.[29] The most prevalent reported complications are described later.

TABLE 25.1 ■ Visual/Refractive Outcomes and Complications of ICRS Implantation Reported in Different Studies

Authors[a]	Eyes Enrolled	ICRS Model	Mean Follow-Up (Months)	Visual Acuity Change	Refractive Change	Complications
Abdellah and Ammar[47]	38	Keraring	36	Mean UCVA improved from 0.93 to 0.63 logMAR and mean BCVA from 0.67 to 0.43 logMAR.	Preoperative MRSE −12.55 D to 9.62 D. Mean sphere measurements from −9.68 D to −7.45 D; mean cylinder from −5.82 D to −4.32 D. K_{max} changed from 53.82 D to 50.47 D; K_{min} from 48.83 D to 47.01 D; and K_{mean} from 51.29 D to 47.51 D.	Corneal neovascularization 14 cases (36.84%), corneal melting 10 cases (26.3%), and ring extrusion 12 cases (31.5%).
Alfonso et al.[68]	56	Keraring	6	BCVA improvement from 0.70 to 0.80 Snellen decimal scale. 15 eyes gained 1 line of BCVA, 9 eyes gained 2 lines, 7 eyes gained 3 lines; and 3 eyes gained 4 lines.	MRSE decreased from −3.10 D to −0.77 D.	5 eyes lost 1 line of corrected visual acuity; 17 eyes had unchanged BCVA. No other intraoperative or postoperative complications occurred.
Alfonso et al.[69]	219	Keraring	6	In author's patient classification stage 1, 52.16% of the eyes gained lines in BCVA evaluation, stage 2 65.48%, and stage 3 60%.	A significant decrease in MRSE after surgery was found for stages 1 and 2, but not for stage 3.	3.20% of the eyes lost 2 or more lines of BCVA.
Alió et al.[70]	13	Intacs	48	BCVA increased from 0.46 logMar (20/50 Snellen) preoperatively to 0.66 logMar (20/30 Snellen) postoperative.	MRSE improved from −5.40 D to −3.95 D; K_{max} decreased from 51.07 D to 47.69 D; and K_{mean} changed 3.13 D.	Extrusion in 7 eyes, excluded from statistical analysis. 4 eyes showed channel deposits, 2 eyes presented superficial vascularization.
Alió et al.[71]	25	Intacs	6	In group A, mean preoperative BCVA was 0.43 logMar (20/50 Snellen) and mean postoperative BCVA 0.82 logMar (20/20 Snellen). In group B, mean preoperative BCVA was 0.36 logMar (20/63 Snellen) and mean postoperative BCVA 0.24 logMar (20/80 Snellen).	Postoperative reduction in spherical dioptric power was 2.11 D and MRSE 2.81 D in group A, only significant in this group. Reduction in K_{mean} was 4.30 D in group A and 6.19 D in group B.	None described.

Continued on following page

TABLE 25.1 ■ **Visual/Refractive Outcomes and Complications of ICRS Implantation Reported in Different Studies** (Continued)

Authors	Eyes Enrolled	ICRS Model	Mean Follow-Up (Months)	Visual Acuity Change	Refractive Change	Complications
Alió et al.[72]	26	Intacs	12	BCVA improved from 20/63 to 20/32 Snellen in both groups studied (1 and 2).	MRSE decreased from −5.00 D to −1.73 D in group 1 and −5.50 D to −3.25 D in group 2.	Mild superficial corneal neovascularization observed in 3 eyes. Mild segment migration (1–3 mm) occurred in 7 of 26 eyes. 4 of 26 eyes developed severe segment migration and partial extrusion from the wound.
Al-Tuwairqi et al.[73]	44	Keraring and MyoRing	6	BCVA increased in group A (Keraring) but not in group B (MyoRing); however, 77% of the patients were satisfied in group A and 89% of group B 6 months after surgery.	MSRE decreased by 2.90 D and 3.60 D in groups A and B, respectively; K_{mean} reduced by 4.55 D in group A and 6.51 D in group B.	3 complications in group A: segment displacement repaired after 1 week, superficial movement of the segment (ring was removed), and infiltrative keratitis (ring was taken off). In group B, 1 eye underwent cross-linking owing to keratoconus progression.
Arantes et al.[74]	25	Ferrara Ring	12	BCVA improved from 0.33 to 0.20 logMAR.	MRSE reduced from −3.67 D to −0.71 D; 3.5 D reduction in K1, 1.53 D in K2, and 2.52 D in K_{mean}.	None described.
Boxer Wachler et al.[75]	74	Intacs	1	45% of the patients gained ≥2 lines in BCVA, 51% of 74 eyes had no change of BCVA, and 4% of 74 lost ≥2 lines.	MRSE decreased from −3.89 D to −1.46 D.	1 eye experienced a superficial channel dissection with anterior Bowman layer perforation. Segment migration and externalization was found in 1 eye.

Study	N	Device	Follow-up	BCVA/Visual Outcome	MRSE	Complications
Colin et al.[76]	10	Intacs	12	Gain of 2 lines in BCVA; improvement from 0.38 logMAR (20/50 Snellen scale) to 0.22 logMAR (20/32 Snellen scale).	MRSE changed 2.12 D and K_{max} decreased 4.60 D.	None described.
Colin[55]	57	Intacs	12	BCVA of 20/40 Snellen or better improved from 53% of patients preoperatively to 74% of patients.	MRSE improved to 3.1 D; K_{mean} changed in 3.70 D.	At the 6-month examination, 9 patients reported "moderate" or "severe" visual symptoms consisting of discomfort ($n = 1$), itching ($n = 1$), burning ($n = 1$), photophobia ($n = 1$), difficulty with night vision ($n = 1$), glare ($n = 3$), and fluctuating vision ($n = 1$). Dissatisfaction with visual symptoms was the reason for removal of the inserts in 7 eyes (12%).
Coskunseven et al.[77]	50	Keraring	12	BCVA was a gain of 1.3 lines (range, loss of 2 lines to a gain of 4 lines).	MRSE decreased from −5.62 D to −2.49 D.	Segment migration to the incision site was seen in 3 eyes (6%) at the first postoperative day.
Ertan et al.[38]	118	Intacs	12	73.7% of eyes gained lines in BCVA evaluation.	MRSE decreased from −7.57 D to −3.72 D; K_{mean} decreased from 51.56 D to 47.66 D.	Epithelial plugs at the incision site occurred in 15.2% of the eyes. 8.5% of the eyes presented granulomatous particles around the ring in the first 6 months, resolved using steroids drops.
Ertan et al.[78]	306	Intacs	4	15% and 10.7% gained lines of UCVA and BCVA, respectively.	MRSE decreased from −7.81 D to −4.72 D; K_{mean} decreased from 50.70 D to 47.91 D.	Segment extrusion occurred in 3 eyes 6 months after ICRS implantation.

Continued on following page

TABLE 25.1 ■ **Visual/Refractive Outcomes and Complications of ICRS Implantation Reported in Different Studies** (Continued)

Authors	Eyes Enrolled	ICRS Model	Mean Follow-Up (Months)	Visual Acuity Change	Refractive Change	Complications
Fahd et al.[79]	30	Intacs	6	BCVA improved from 20/42 to 20/27Snellen.	MRSE decreased from −2.24 D to −1.02 D; central K decreased from 49.14 D to 47.43 D.	Deposits in 7 eyes and 1 patient with transient foreign-body sensation and glare.
Cueto et al.[80]	58	Ferrara Ring	60	BCVA improved from 0.16 to 0.11 logMAR.	MRSE declined from −2.74 D to −1.42 D.	Loss of 2 lines in BCVA during first 6 months in 4 eyes. No intra- or postoperative complications.
Fernandez-Vega Cueto et al.[81]	409	Ferrara Ring	6	BCVA changed from 0.69 to 0.77 Snellen decimal scale.	MRSE declined from −4.16 D to −2.81 D; K_{max} decreased from 48.23 D to 46.31 D.	None described.
Ferrara et al.[3]	1073	Ferrara Ring	12	For group 1 of patients, UCVA increased to 20/80 Snellen and BCVA increased to 20/40 Snellen. For group 2 of patients, UCVA increased to 20/13 Snellen and BCVA increased to 20/60 Snellen.	For group 1 of patients, asphericity decreased to −0.35, MRSE decreased to −2.26 D, and K_{mean} decreased to 45.72 D. For group 2 of patients, asphericity decreased to −0.56, MRSE decreased to −4.14 D, and K_{mean} decreased to 48.10 D.	Undercorrection (needing implantation of additional segment) 16 eyes (1.49%), overcorrection (needing segment removal and reimplantation) 11 eyes (1.02%), extrusion 6 eyes (0.56%), malposition 4 eyes (0.37%), progressive corneal steepening 2 eyes (0.18%), and ring neovascularization 2 eyes (0.18%).
Heikal et al.[82]	30	Keraring	6	BCVA improved from 0.85 to 0.14 logMAR.	MRSE reduced from −5.43 D to −2.43 D; K_{max} decreased from 55.85 D to 44.05 D.	None described.

Study				Outcomes	Complications
Hellstedt et al.[83]	50	Intacs	12	Gain of lines of BCVA 76.70% in 6 months and both BCVA and UCVA improved throughout follow-up. Visual functioning index improved from 61.6 to 80.8, and the percentage of satisfaction with vision improved from 24.3% to 87.5% at 12 months. Mean change in spherical error of 2.67 D. Vector analysis of astigmatism correction showed that mean change in corneal astigmatism was 2.9 D at 6 months postoperatively.	In 8% of eyes, both Intacs segments were removed. In addition, 7 refractive adjustments in 7 eyes were performed successfully to improve visual and surgical outcome.
Israel et al.[84]	29	KERATACx Plus	6	BCVA improvement from 0.17 to 0.50 Snellen decimal scale. K1 decreased from 49.42 D to 45.05 D, K2 from 54.23 D to 48.93 D, and K_{mean} from 51.71 D to 46.88 D.	None described.
Jabbarvand et al.[85]	21	MyoRing	12	BCVA improved in group 1 from 0.26 to 0.24 logMar and in group 2 from 0.35 to 0.23 logMar. K_{max} improved in group 1 from 49.59 D to 44.16 D and in group 2 from 49.73 D to 44.77 D.	Transient sensation of foreign body in 4 patients in group 1 and 3 patients in group 2.
Jadidi et al.[86]	32	MyoRing	3	BCVA improvement from 0.47 to 0.22 logMAR.	MRSE improvement from −10.51 D to −1.32 D; reduction of 3.55 D in K_{mean}. None described.
Kanellopoulos et al.[42]	20	Intacs	12	BCVA improved from 20/37 to 20/22 Snellen.	MRSE improved from −5.33 D to −1.87 D; K_{mean} decreased from 49.50 D to 46.35 D. 1 case of anterior chamber perforation, 6 eyes had ring exposure secondary to corneal thinning over the implants postoperatively, and a dense corneal infiltrate developed in 1 patient at 7th month after surgery.

Continued on following page

TABLE 25.1 ■ Visual/Refractive Outcomes and Complications of ICRS Implantation Reported in Different Studie (Continued)

Authors	Eyes Enrolled	ICRS Model	Visual Acuity Change	Refractive Change	Mean Follow-Up (Months)	Complications
Kwitko and Severo[87]	51	Ferrara Ring	BCVA improved in 86.4% of eyes, was unchanged in 1.9%, and worsened in 11.7%. UCVA improved in 86.4% of eyes, was unchanged in 7.8%, and worsened in 5.8%.	MSRE was reduced from −6.08 D to −4.55 D and mean refractive astigmatism from −3.82 D to −2.16 D. K_{mean} reduced from 48.76 D to 43.17 D.	39	Intracorneal ring segment decentration occurred in 2 eyes (3.9%), segment extrusion in 10 eyes (19.6%), bacterial keratitis in 1 eye (1.9%) with segment extrusion, and disciform keratitis in 1 eye (1.9%).
Kymionis et al.[88]	36	Intacs	Preoperative UCVA was 20/50 Snellen or worse in all eyes; at the last follow-up examination, 10 (59%) of 17 eyes had UCVA of 20/50 Snellen or better. 6 eyes (35%) maintained preoperative BCVA, whereas the remaining 10 eyes (59%) experienced a gain of 1 up to 8 lines.	MSRE reduced from −5.54 D to −3.02 D. Mean change in keratometry 1.57 D.	60	1 eye lost 3 lines of BCVA.
Lisa et al.[89]	32	Keraring	BCVA improved from 0.67 to 0.80 Snellen decimal scale. Postoperatively, BCVA was better than 20/40 Snellen in 96.9% of eyes and 20/25 or better in 56.2% of eyes.	MRSE decreased from −1.93 D to −0.26 D; K_{max} decreased from 48.63 D to 44.98 D.	6	4 eyes lost 1 line in vision.
Lisa et al.[90]	43	Ferrara Ring	BCVA improved from 0.36 to 0.17 logMAR. The percentages of eyes with BCVA of 0.3 logMAR or better increased from 51.2% to 95.3%.	MRSE declined from −3.19 D to −1.88 D; K_{max} declined from 53.89 D to 51.27 D.	33	None described.

Study	N	Device	Follow-up	Visual outcome	Refractive/K outcome	Complications
Mirzaftab et al.[91]	30	Intacs	27.8 after surgery	BCVA improved from 20/40 to 20/32 Snellen.	K_{mean} decreased from 47.23 D to 45.66 D.	None described.
Miranda et al.[92]	36	Ferrara Ring	12	BCVA improved in 29 eyes (80.56%).	MRSE decreased from −7.29 D to −4.80 D.	Segment decentration in 1 eye (2.7%), asymmetric positioning in 2 eyes (5%), migration of the segments in 2 eyes (5%), segment extrusion in 5 eyes (13.8%), and bacterial keratitis in 1 eye (2.7%).
Moreira et al.[93]	10	Ferrara Ring	3	BCVA improved from 0.7 to 0.4 logMAR.	50% of eyes improved BCVA ≥0.5 logMAR.	In 2 patients, corneal perforation was observed. Segment externalization was found in 1 eye and 3 patients had segment migration.
Mounir et al.[29]	623	Keraring	48	BCVA improved from 0.79 to 0.72 logMAR in 18-month postoperative evaluation.	MRSE decreased from −10.86 D to −7.52 D in 18-month postoperative evaluation; K1 from 49.13 D to 46.88 D; K2 from 53.50 D to 49.83 D; and K_{mean} 51.31 D to 48.35 D.	Intraoperative complications occurred in 44 eyes (7.1%), and were represented by vacuum loss, incomplete or decentered tunnel creation, misdirection of the ring, perforation to anterior chamber, broken body, or orifice of the ring. Postoperative complications occurred in 35 eyes (5.6%): segment migration or extrusion, incision opacification, infectious keratitis, corneal melting, sterile keratitis, and steroid-induced glaucoma.

Continued on following page

TABLE 25.1 ■ **Visual/Refractive Outcomes and Complications of ICRS Implantation Reported in Different Studie** (Continued)

Authors	Eyes Enrolled	ICRS Model	Mean Follow-Up (Months)	Visual Acuity Change	Refractive Change	Complications
Muftuoglu et al.[94]	89	Keraring	6	BCVA improved from 0.35 to 0.07 logMAR.	MRSE changed from −4.54 D to −0.98 D; K_{mean} improved from 46.39 D to 42.64 D.	None described.
Nobari et al.[95]	15	MyoRing	10	BCVA improved from 0.39 to 0.19 logMAR.	MRSE decreased from −6.00 D to −0.70 D; K values decreased significantly (K_{max} 5.00 D, K_{min} 1.10 D, and K_{mean} 4.00 D).	Halo and glare in night vision in 1 patient.
Peña-García et al.[96]	127	Keraring	6	Studied patients were divided into grade 1 and 2 groups. Patients with grade 1 gained at least 1 line of BCVA in 30.77% of cases. BCVA remained unchanged in 46.15% of cases. In the best group, BCVA increased from 0.16 to 0.06 logMAR, but did not improve in the remaining cases.	Keratometry improved significantly in the best group; mean K2 power decreased by almost 3.00 D from preoperatively to 6 months postoperatively; K_{mean} also decreased by almost 3.00 D.	None described.
Rabinowitz et al.[16]	30	Intacs	12 mechanical group 6 femto-group	Improvement in BCVA (3.92 laser vs 1.63 mechanical group).	MRSE changed 2.96 D in mechanical group and 3.98 D in femto-group; K_{mean} change in mechanical group 2.52 D and 2.91 D in the other group.	No data.
Rocha et al.[97]	34	Ferrara Ring	6	BCVA improved from 0.51 to 0.18 logMAR.	MRSE decreased from −7.52 D to −3.61 D; K_{mean} decreased from 51.36 D to 47.19 D, K1 from 48.79 D to 45.69 D, and K2 from 54.25 D to 48.82 D.	None described.

Study	No.	Device	No.	BCVA	Refractive/Keratometric	Complications
Sadoughi et al.[98]	18	Keraring	4	BCVA improved from 0.39 to 0.26 logMAR.	MRSE decreased from −8.03 D to −3.01 D, K_{mean} decreased from 51.43 D to 47.42 D.	Ring deposits in 4 eyes, without visual impairments.
Sandes et al.[99]	58	Ferrara Ring	16	BCVA improved from 0.5 to 0.3 logMAR (20/60 to 20/40 Snellen).	Reduction in K_{mean} from 49.87 D to 47.34 D.	None described.
Shabayek and Alió[37]	21	Keraring	6	Improvements in BCVA from 0.54 to 0.71 Snellen decimal scale.	MRSE decreased by 2.28 D, K_{mean} decreased 2.24 D.	Localized infectious keratitis occurred in 1 eye (4.8%); incision opacification occurred in 8 eyes (38%).
Shetty et al.[25]	14	Intacs	12	At 6 months, UCVA improved from 0.05 to 0.16 Snellen decimal scale, and BCVA improved from 0.50 to 0.67 Snellen decimal scale.	Spherical refractive error improved from −6.68 D to −3.11 D, whereas cylindrical refractive error improved from −4.89 D to −3.64 D. MRSE reduced from −9.13 D to −4.93 D, and K_{mean} decreased from 53.01 D to 49.42 D.	1 eye (7.14%) developed superficial corneal vascularization 3 weeks postoperatively, directed toward the incision site. Vascularization resolved after suture removal and topical fluorometholone therapy.
Siganos et al.[100]	26	Ferrara Ring	6	BCVA improved from 0.37 to 0.60 Snellen decimal scale.	MRSE decreased from −6.91 D to −1.11 D.	In 2 eyes, the rings had to be removed early in the postoperative period, owing to superficial implantation of the rings and asymmetrical placement.
Stival et al.[101]	41	CornealRing	32	BCVA improved in group A (post-PRK ectasia) from 0.30 to 0.11 logMAR and in group B (post-LASIK ectasia) from 0.43 to 0.17 logMAR.	MRSE decreased from −2.97 D to −2.05 D in group A and −3.31 D to −2.42 D in group B; K_{max} decreased from 45.34 D to 43.74 D in group A and from 49.96 D to 47.55 D in group B.	None described.

Continued on following page

TABLE 25.1 ■ **Visual/Refractive Outcomes and Complications of ICRS Implantation Reported in Different Studies** (Continued)

Authors	Eyes Enrolled	ICRS Model	Mean Follow-Up (Months)	Visual Acuity Change	Refractive Change	Complications
Tognon et al.[18]	1222	Keraring	3	BCVA improved in all satisfied patients after surgery; in the majority of dissatisfied patients mean BCVA did not improve. Before the procedure, the distribution of patients according to visual impairment was not homogeneous, and the majority of the patients were in moderate visual impairment group (World Health Organization Classification for Visual Impairment). After the procedure, a larger number of the patients ascended to normal or mild visual impairment groups.	Not detailed.	67 surgical complications (external environment or anterior chamber perforation, late or early infection, late or early segment extrusion, and malposition/movement of the ICRS after procedure). 164 patients dissatisfied after ICRS implantation.
Torquetti et al.[102]	36	Ferrara Ring	120	BCVA improved from 0.45 to 0.29 logMAR; 66.7% of patients gained 2 or more lines of BCVA at 10 years.	K_{max} decreased from 54.99 D to 50.65 D.	Ring segment exchange required in 2 eyes and keratoplasty in 2 eyes.
Torquetti et al.[103]	37	Ferrara Ring	30	BCVA improved from 20/160 to 20/50 Snellen.	MRSE decreased from −4.64 D to −3.04 D; K_{mean} reduced from 49.33 D to 46.16 D.	None described.

First author		Ring type		BCVA/UCVA	MRSE/Keratometry	Complications
Torquetti et al.[104]	138	Ferrara Ring	6	BCVA improved from 20/100 to 20/40 Snellen; 2 or more lines of BCVA gained in 87% of eyes.	MRSE reduced from −7.02 D to −3.29 D; K1 reduced from 50.5 D to 46.0 D, K2 55.2 D to 49.0 D, and K_{mean} reduced from 53.3 D to 47.8 D.	4 cases of migration and 2 cases of intraoperative perforation; all cases were excluded from statistical analysis.
Vega-Estrada et al.[105]	18	Intacs and Keraring	69	Decimal BCVA changed from 0.59 to 0.68 in 6 months and to 0.63 in 5 years.	MRSE changed from −4.35 D to −2.10 D in 6 months and −4.79 D in 5 years.	None described.
Yildirim et al.[106]	8	Keraring	67	Improved BCVA from 0.69 to 0.29 logMAR.	MRSE decreased 5.7 D; K_{mean} decreased 2.1 D.	None described.
Zare et al.[44]	30	Intacs	6	Mean UCVA improved from 0.60 to 0.29 logMAR and mean BCVA from 0.25 to 0.13 logMAR.	MRSE improved from −6.93 D to −3.23 D and mean refractive cylinder from −4.65 D to −3.90 D. K_{mean} decreased from 49.84 D to 47.90 D.	3 eyes had ring exposure and 1 eye had bacterial keratitis and ring exposure.

[a]First authors only.

BCVA, Best-corrected visual acuity; *D,* diopter; *K,* keratometry; *K1,* flattest keratometry; *K2,* steeper keratometry; *max,* maximum; *min,* minimum; *mm,* millimeters; *MRSE,* mean refractive spherical equivalent; *n,* number; *Snellen and LogMAR,* validated charts for visual acuity; *UCVA,* uncorrected visual acuity; *%,* percentage.

INCISION AND EPITHELIAL COMPLICATIONS

Incision complications are most commonly related to the manual technique and may range from extending the incision to the visual axis (Fig. 25.1) or the limbus to inadequate healing of the incision site (Fig. 25.2).

To avoid the first complication, which is exclusively observed in the manual technique, proper anesthesia and fixation of the eyeball with tweezers is necessary. The patient must remain motionless during the execution of this surgical step.[30] Another consideration is the use of a millimeter diamond knife with frontal cut (not presenting cuts on its sides) and to initiate cutting toward the limbus, directing and controlling the force to the periphery of the cornea and not to the central region. Additional guidance would be to keep the diamond knife position exactly perpendicular to the cornea to avoid cuts of irregular depths.

Inadequate healing of the incision is also a complication related exclusively to the manual technique, caused by the manipulation of the instruments for creating the tunnel ring.[30] Significant scarring can lead to infection and extrusion or migration of the ring. Some authors suggest the use of prophylactic topical antibiotics and therapeutic contact lenses when epithelial irregularities are present. Another concerning matter is in the implantation of long arc ICRSs, where there may be difficulty in healing the incisions because of greater proximity of the ring.[31,32]

Persistent incisional gaping, stromal thinning, and corneal stromal edema around the incision (and channel) from excessive surgical manipulation are also recognized complications. The epithelial defect rate seems to be significantly higher when the channel is created exclusively by using the manual technique.[33] Some authors report that epithelial defects are the most common complication experienced by patients, especially during the first postoperative days. This usually subsides spontaneously within a few days.[34,35]

Epithelial ingrowth toward the tunnel may occur when the incision is not completely sealed, caused by the migration of superficial epithelial corneal cells into the ring tunnel. In some cases, this problem can be solved by increasing the frequency of topical steroid instillation,[36] and temporary sutures can be placed for wound closure when the incision site appears enlarged.[37] Epithelial plugs may also form at the incision site and are related to enlargement of wound edges and trauma at the incision site during implantation.[17,24,38]

DECENTRATION, ASYMMETRY BETWEEN THE RINGS, AND PROBLEMS RELATED TO TUNNEL CREATION

The first step in ring implant surgery is to mark the visual axis for centering the rings. This step can be challenging in some patients, especially those with advanced keratoconus because of the parallax effect. The Purkinje reflex is routinely used as a guide for marking. Nevertheless, advanced keratoconus patients or patients whose angle kappa is too wide may experience off-center markings, usually inferior and nasal, respectively.[30]

Decentration in ICRS implants may also occur as a result of the applanation of the femtosecond laser suction ring.[39] When the suction is complete, the mark made guided by the Purkinje reflex sometimes does not correspond to the pupil center, and surgeons can be misled. Optimal surgical planning involves marking the patient's optic center—not the pupillary center—under normal conditions, with no pupillary changes (miosis or mydriasis induced by medications) or interference from applanations. A mark made with a myopic pupil (process induced in ICRS implantation) acquires a more nasal and superior position, which does not represent the real position (Fig. 25.3).[30]

ICRSs may be positioned equidistant from the visual axis (Fig. 25.4 for an incorrect ICRS position). Creating the ring tunnel with a femtosecond laser makes the tunnel regular and circular in shape. When the tunnel is created manually, the circular motion with the employed instrument

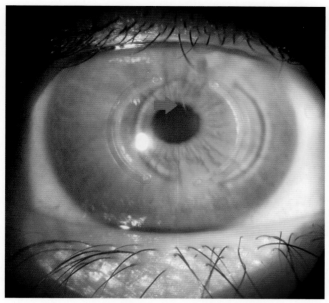

Fig. 25.1   Intrastromal corneal ring incision extended to the visual axis (indicated by the *arrow*).

tends to result in centripetal behavior. Therefore, in this technique, the surgeon must always correct the direction of the rotational movement, to create a rounded and symmetrical tunnel.

The femtosecond laser uses photodisruption to rapidly produce a more accurate predetermined depth and channel size.[17] Controversy exists over tunnel size nomograms with this technique, but more complications have been observed in narrow-channel methods than with use of wide channels.[17]

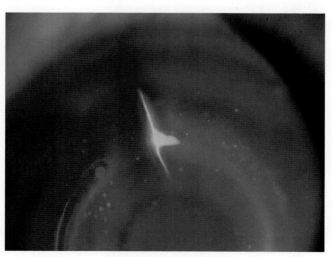

Fig. 25.2   Inadequate healing of the incision site evidenced by local fluorescein staining.

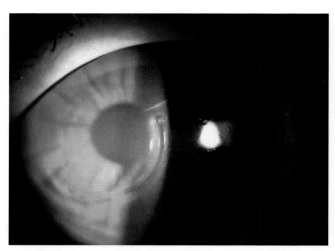

Fig. 25.3 Intrastromal corneal ring implantation decentered from visual axis.

Additional trauma to the incision (and channel) also results in increased keratocyte apoptosis, major tissue degradation, and, subsequently, an increased number of complications such as corneal melting.[7,40]

Incomplete tunnel creation arises mainly as a result of a low setting of the laser power used or lack of vacuum.[29] Incomplete tunnel creation caused by the insufficient energy levels of the laser can be minimized by increasing the energy levels or by decreasing spot separation.[41] In both cases, channels can be completed by using a mechanical spreader.[41]

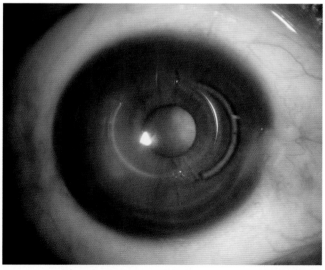

Fig. 25.4 Inadequate positioning and overlapping of the lower position of the rings, with adjacent edema/hydrops in one of the segments after anterior chamber perforation.

Galvanometer lag error (system malfunction) is also described in femtosecond laser–assisted surgeries and is a technical problem of the device located in the femtosecond memory system.[41] If the error remains after restarting the system, the incision can be made manually, or a new tunnel may be created next to the failed one.[41] To avoid galvo error during channel creation, it is important to maintain the vacuum during all steps.[41]

Both the femtosecond laser steps of docking and vacuum can be disrupted if the patient strains to close his/her eyes or moves their body/head, or when difficulties in positioning the device occur because of the patient's anatomical characteristics (restricted eye opening, deeper orbit, or prominent nose).

Implantation of inverted ring segments is another possible complication. It can be the result of surgeon inattention, ignorance of the ring anatomy and positioning during the surgical act, or inadvertent overlapping of the rings (Figs. 25.4 and 25.5). The correct apex-up orientation of the ring segments is essential for optimal results and should be checked before implantation.[29]

ANTERIOR CHAMBER DRILLING OR SUPERFICIAL ICRS POSITIONING

In the exclusively manual implantation technique, implantation that is too superficial or intrudes into the anterior chamber (see Fig. 25.4) occurs primarily because of pachymetry calculation errors or inadequate tunneling rotation.[30] Another point of concern is that during the tunnel creation, after the incision, the spreader instrument must reach the bottom of the incision. If this does not happen, a superficial channel can be created with the tunneling device. When inadequate strength is used, perforations into the anterior chamber may develop. Tunneling device rotation must always be parallel to the iris plane. If there is significant resistance while sliding this instrument, the channel is likely too superficial.[30]

The complications described earlier are less common when using femtosecond laser assistance, because the laser can deliver energy accurately to a precise depth in a programmed fashion.[41] Using this technique, endothelial perforation can be recognized intraoperatively as bubbles appearing in the anterior chamber. This can be caused by incorrect preoperative pachymetry or excessively deep channel creation.[41] The reference point for pachymetry in femtosecond-assisted surgery is different from that in manual surgery. In manual surgery, the thinnest point in the ring path is considered for calculation of the depth of the tunnel, whereas in femto surgery, the thinnest point of the pachymetry map is used. When anterior chamber perforation occurs, surgery must be postponed for at least 1 month, and a new channel should be created superficially (some authors defend 90 μm) to protect the endothelium.[41,42]

Shallow placement is caused by incorrect entry of the channel in a delayed ring implantation (after the bubbles produced by the femtosecond disappear) and can be recognized as resistance in the progression of the rings. The force and direction of the movements should be correct and carefully dosed, or the segments can be broken (see Fig. 25.5).[29,43]

MIGRATION, EXTRUSION OF THE RINGS, AND CORNEAL MELTING

Migration of ICRSs observed postoperatively may also be caused by segment dislocation provoked by external forces (such as when the patient rubs the eye, sleeps, or compresses the side of the operated eye). It can be avoided by providing the patient with acrylic protectors to be used in the early postoperative period. When the migration of the rings is symptomatic, they can be replaced and temporary sutures used in an attempt to keep them immobile.[44,45] Ring migration is considered an early indicator of extrusion.[29] Whenever the segment approaches the incision site,

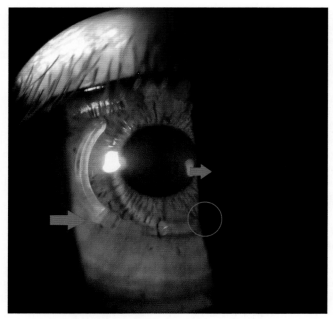

Fig. 25.5   Broken ring segments (indicated by the *arrow*) and inadvertent overlapped rings (indicated by the *circle*).

it should be closely observed; intervention is required in cases where the segment is within 0.5 mm of the incision site.[29]

Extrusion of the segments is reported even after several years of ring implantation.[46] Ozertürk et al. and Kubaloglu et al. argue that atopic patients are more predisposed to this type of complication.[34,35] Some authors have also cited superficial placement of the rings, or patients with very thin corneas or advanced keratoconus as causative factors for late extrusion.[34,41] Moreover, very thick rings in relation to the thinnest pachymetry are more related to extrusion.[45]

Extrusion caused by corneal melting may not be related to infections in some cases. Corneal melting is closely associated with the design of the rings. The rings place persistent pressure on the upper corneal stromal fibers through the segment-free tissues.[47] Reports have demonstrated that ICRSs contribute to keratocyte activation and keratocyte apoptosis, potentially leading to tissue degeneration and melting.[40] The keratocyte density appears to be decreased in the corneal stroma above and below the ring segments when compared with the density in other corneal areas, accompanied by epithelial hypoplasia overlying the ring segments.[40,48]

Some researchers have investigated the relationship between the material used in ICRSs (polymethyl methacrylate [PMMA]) and cases of melting and anterior stromal necrosis.[49] New segments, made with biologic rings (fashioned from human corneal donor tissue or xenograft corneal rings), have been more recently tested.[50–52]

Sterile inflammation around ICRSs is also a possible adverse effect leading to corneal melting and thinning.[53] The area of the most severe infiltrate typically surrounds the proximal end of the segment, closer to the entry incision.[53] These infiltrates should be differentiated from the typical white deposits on or near the segments (see later) and seem to disappear with segment removal.[53] Sterile keratitis and inflammation can be linked to rosacea, spring catarrh, and atopic/vernal keratoconjunctivitis.[29,54]

DEPOSITS SURROUNDING ICRSS, OPACIFICATION/SCARS, AND NEOVASCULARIZATION

The presence of intrastromal deposits that accumulate in the lamellar channel after implantation is not uncommon[24] and they are seen as white-yellow spiculated deposits surrounding the ICRS.[21,30,34,35,55] The incidence and density of these deposits increase with segment thickness and duration of implantation; the deposits consist of intracellular lipids such as cholesterol esters or triglycerides.[24,56] The presence of this material does not result in harm to the cornea or visual symptoms,[24,57] and no specific treatment has been reported.

Superficial corneal opacification coinciding with the incision site has occurred in large samples of ICRS-implanted cases.[37] After ICRS implantation, extracellular material can also be found in the lamellar channel, and this material has been referred to as acidophilic densification and/or channel haze.[58] In addition to that, hypocellular collagen scar and slightly edematous keratocytes may be found in the tunnel, as well as mild macrophage infiltration near the ICRS.[58] These findings are related to the abnormal scars and fibrosis observed in some patients.

Deep or superficial neovascularization invariably implies the need for ICRS removal.[30] Neovessels are attracted to the region as a result of chronic inflammation, sometimes subclinical, at the implant site. Neovascularization is also implicated in corneal melting and extrusion of the segments. It usually involutes after ring explants and topical corticosteroid treatment.

INFECTIOUS KERATITIS

This is one of the most feared complications and can be sight-threatening when associated with ICRSs (Fig. 25.6).[59] Reported rates in the literature describing this complication vary from 0.2% to 6.8%.[30,60]

A broad range of pathogens have been found in culture results: the most common is *Staphylococcus aureus*, followed by *Streptococcus viridians*, *Streptococcus pneumoniae*, *Pseudomonas* spp., *Nocardia* spp., and *Klebsiella* spp.; others are less common.[59,61] Reports of *Clostridium perfringens*,[62] *Staphylococcus epidermidis*,[62,63] *Acanthamoeba* spp.,[64,65] *Fusarium* spp.,[15] and *Aspergillus fumigatus*[66] can also be found in literature.

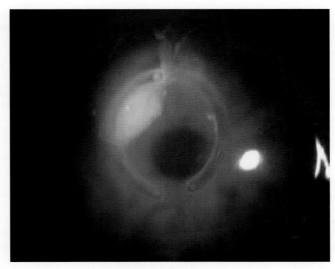

Fig. 25.6 Presence of infectious infiltrate in the upper area and incision, and incorrect corneal ring positioning.

The ocular surface is the probable source of these pathogens, but contamination of the wound, incision site, and channels postoperatively should be considered.[60] Inadequate preoperative cleaning of the eyelids and eyelashes, perpendicular and horizontal position incisions (all of which contribute to slow healing), superficial implantation of the ICRS, the presence of an intrastromal foreign body, history of eye trauma or immunosuppressive diseases, postoperative use of topical steroids, and therapeutic contact lenses are some risk factors.[30,60–62]

The most common symptoms are photophobia, redness, tearing, and decreased vision, although sometimes the diagnosis can be difficult.[60] Early diagnosis and intensive treatment of the most likely pathogen increases the success rate.

Because infection is a potential complication of any surgery, the chosen practice is to treat each eye on different days. Same-day implantation in both eyes followed by bilateral infection has been described.[61]

OTHER COMPLICATIONS

Some very common related adverse effects of ICRS implantation are glare, halos, and night reflexes.[6] In most of the cases, patients tolerated the earlier described adverse effects well when informed of them. Medications such as dilute pilocarpine or brimonidine can be prescribed where required until neuroadaptation occurs.[30]

Other complications described are chronic eye pain (caused by direct contact between the segment and corneal nerve), focal edema, photophobia, mild discomfort (diminishing over time), and fluctuation in distance vision.[2,49,67]

Some patients do not experience improvement in their vision and can be dissatisfied after the procedure, making ring explantation necessary at times.[2,33,53] In one major published case series that enrolled 1196 patients, 164 patients (13.71%) were not satisfied with the procedure after ICRS implantation.[18] The incidence of dissatisfaction has been decreasing over the years, thanks to mastery of the technique and more accurate nomograms.[3]

References

1. de Freitas Santos Paranhos J, Avila MP, Paranhos A Jr., Schor P. Evaluation of the impact of intracorneal ring segments implantation on the quality of life of patients with keratoconus using the NEI-RQL (National Eye Institute Refractive Error Quality of Life) instrument. *Br J Ophthalmol*. 2010;94(1):101–105.
2. Sakellaris D, Balidis M, Gorou O, et al. Intracorneal ring segment implantation in the management of keratoconus: an evidence-based approach. *Ophthalmol Ther*. 2019;8(suppl 1):5–14.
3. Ferrara G, Torquetti L, Ferrara P, Merayo-Lloves J. Intrastromal corneal ring segments: visual outcomes from a large case series. *Clin Exp Ophthalmol*. 2012;40(5):433–439.
4. Colin J, Velou S. Current surgical options for keratoconus. *J Cataract Refract Surg*. 2003;29(2):379–386.
5. Alio JL, Shabayek MH, Artola A. Intracorneal ring segments for keratoconus correction: long-term follow-up. *J Cataract Refract Surg*. 2006;32(6):978–985.
6. Hood CT. Complications of intracorneal implants in refractive surgery. *Int Ophthalmol Clin*. 2016;56(2):153–159.
7. Bautista-Llamas MJ, Sanchez-Gonzalez MC, Lopez-Izquierdo I, et al. Complications and explantation reasons in intracorneal ring segments (ICRS) implantation: a systematic review. *J Refract Surg*. 2019;35(11):740–747.
8. Al-Tuwairqi WS, Osuagwu UL, Razzouk H, Ogbuehi KC. One-year clinical outcomes of a two-step surgical management for keratoconus-topography-guided photorefractive keratectomy/cross-linking after intrastromal corneal ring implantation. *Eye Contact Lens*. 2015;41(6):359–366.
9. Coskunseven E, Jankov MR 2nd, Hafezi F, Atun S, Arslan E, Kymionis GD. Effect of treatment sequence in combined intrastromal corneal rings and corneal collagen crosslinking for keratoconus. *J Cataract Refract Surg*. 2009;35(12):2084–2091.
10. Vega-Estrada A, Alio JL. The use of intracorneal ring segments in keratoconus. *Eye Vis*. 2016;3:8.

11. Vega-Estrada A, Alio JL, Brenner LF, et al. Outcome analysis of intracorneal ring segments for the treatment of keratoconus based on visual, refractive, and aberrometric impairment. *Am J Ophthalmol.* 2013;155(3):575–584. e1.
12. Gatzioufas Z, Khine A, Elalfy M, et al. Clinical outcomes after Keraring implantation for keratoconus management in patients older than 40 years: a retrospective, interventional, cohort study. *Ophthalmol Ther.* 2018;7(1):95–100.
13. Piñero DP, Alió JL, El Kady B, Pascual I. Corneal aberrometric and refractive performance of 2 intrastromal corneal ring segment models in early and moderate ectatic disease. *J Cataract Refract Surg.* 2010;36(1):102–109.
14. Kaya V, Utine CA, Karakus SH, Kavadarli I, Yilmaz OF. Refractive and visual outcomes after Intacs vs Ferrara intrastromal corneal ring segment implantation for keratoconus: a comparative study. *J Refract Surg.* 2011;27(12):907–912.
15. Carrasquillo KG, Rand J, Talamo JH. Intacs for keratoconus and post-LASIK ectasia: mechanical versus femtosecond laser-assisted channel creation. *Cornea.* 2007;26(8):956–962.
16. Rabinowitz YS, Li X, Ignacio TS, Maguen E. INTACS inserts using the femtosecond laser compared to the mechanical spreader in the treatment of keratoconus. *J Refract Surg.* 2006;22(8):764–771.
17. Ertan A, Kamburoğlu G, Akgun U. Comparison of outcomes of 2 channel sizes for intrastromal ring segment implantation with a femtosecond laser in eyes with keratoconus. *J Cataract Refract Surg.* 2007;33(4):648–653.
18. Tognon T, Campos M, Wengrzynovski JP, et al. Indications and visual outcomes of intrastromal corneal ring segment implantation in a large patient series. *Clinics.* 2017;72(6):370–377.
19. Monteiro T, Alfonso JF, Franqueira N, Faria-Correira F, Ambrósio R Jr, Madrid-Costa D. Comparison of clinical outcomes between manual and femtosecond laser techniques for intrastromal corneal ring segment implantation. *Eur J Ophthalmol.* 2020;30(6):1246–1255.
20. Piñero DP, Alió JL, El Kady B, et al. Refractive and aberrometric outcomes of intracorneal ring segments for keratoconus: mechanical versus femtosecond-assisted procedures. *Ophthalmology.* 2009;116(9):1675–1687.
21. Izquierdo L Jr, Mannis MJ, Mejias Smith JA, Henriquez MA. Effectiveness of intrastromal corneal ring implantation in the treatment of adult patients with keratoconus: a systematic review. *J Refract Surg.* 2019;35(3):191–200.
22. Renesto ADC, Hirai FE, Campos M. Refractive and visual outcomes after Ferrara corneal ring segment implantation at a 60% depth in keratoconic eyes: case series. *Arq Bras Oftalmol.* 2019;82(6):488–494.
23. Renesto Ada C, Melo LA Jr, Sartori Mde F, Campos M. Sequential topical riboflavin with or without ultraviolet a radiation with delayed intracorneal ring segment insertion for keratoconus. *Am J Ophthalmol.* 2012;153(5):982–993.e3.
24. Piñero DP, Alio JL. Intracorneal ring segments in ectatic corneal disease—a review. *Clin Experiment Ophthalmol.* 2010;38(2):154–167.
25. Shetty R, Kurian M, Anand D, Mhaske P, Narayana KM, Shetty BK. Intacs in advanced keratoconus. *Cornea.* 2008;27(9):1022–1029.
26. Almodin EM, Camin FMA, Colallilo JMA. Two-staged treatment for advanced keratoconus in children. *Rev Bras Oftalmol.* 2018;77:159–163.
27. Ferreira TB, Guell JL, Manero F. Combined intracorneal ring segments and iris-fixated phakic intraocular lens for keratoconus refractive and visual improvement. *J Refract Surg.* 2014;30(5):336–341.
28. Coskunseven E, Jankov MR 2nd, Grentzelos MA, Plaka AD, Limnopoulou AN, Kymionis GD. Topography-guided transepithelial PRK after intracorneal ring segments implantation and corneal collagen CXL in a three-step procedure for keratoconus. *J Refract Surg.* 2013;29(1):54–58.
29. Mounir A, Radwan G, Farouk MM, Mostafa EM. Femtosecond-assisted intracorneal ring segment complications in keratoconus: from novelty to expertise. *Clin Ophthalmol.* 2018;12:957–964.
30. Ghanem VC, Lautert J, Ghanem RC. Complicações dos Implantes Intraestromais. In: Santhiago MR, ed. *Cirurgia Refrativa.* Rio de Janeiro: Cultura Médica; 2017:506.
31. Abd Elaziz MS, El Saebay Sarhan AR, Ibrahim AM, Elshafy Haggag HA. Anterior segment changes after femtosecond laser-assisted implantation of a 355-degree intrastromal corneal ring segment in advanced keratoconus. *Cornea.* 2018;37(11):1438–1443.
32. Vega-Estrada A, Chorro E, Sewelam A, Alio JL. Clinical outcomes of a new asymmetric intracorneal ring segment for the treatment of keratoconus. *Cornea.* 2019;38(10):1228–1232.
33. Giacomin NT, Mello GR, Medeiros CS, et al. Intracorneal ring segments implantation for corneal ectasia. *J Refract Surg.* 2016;32(12):829–839.

34. Ozertürk Y, Sari ES, Kubaloglu A, Koytak A, Piñero D, Akyol S. Comparison of deep anterior lamellar keratoplasty and intrastromal corneal ring segment implantation in advanced keratoconus. *J Cataract Refract Surg.* 2012;38(2):324–332.
35. Kubaloglu A, Sari ES, Cinar Y, et al. Comparison of mechanical and femtosecond laser tunnel creation for intrastromal corneal ring segment implantation in keratoconus: prospective randomized clinical trial. *J Cataract Refract Surg.* 2010;36(9):1556–1561.
36. Bali SJ, Chan C, Hodge C, Sutton G. Intracorneal ring segment reimplantation in keratectasia. *Asia-Pac J Ophthalmol.* 2012;1(6):327–330.
37. Shabayek MH, Alió JL. Intrastromal corneal ring segment implantation by femtosecond laser for keratoconus correction. *Ophthalmology.* 2007;114(9):1643–1652.
38. Ertan A, Kamburoğlu G, Bahadir M. Intacs insertion with the femtosecond laser for the management of keratoconus: one-year results. *J Cataract Refract Surg.* 2006;32(12):2039–2042.
39. Ertan A, Kamburoğlu G. Analysis of centration of Intacs segments implanted with a femtosecond laser. *J Cataract Refract Surg.* 2007;33(3):484–487.
40. Kugler LJ, Hill S, Sztipanovits D, Boerman H, Swartz TS, Wang MX. Corneal melt of incisions overlying corneal ring segments: case series and literature review. *Cornea.* 2011;30(9):968–971.
41. Coskunseven E, Kymionis GD, Tsiklis NS, et al. Complications of intrastromal corneal ring segment implantation using a femtosecond laser for channel creation: a survey of 850 eyes with keratoconus. *Acta Ophthalmol.* 2011;89(1):54–57.
42. Kanellopoulos AJ, Pe LH, Perry HD, Donnenfeld ED. Modified intracorneal ring segment implantations (INTACS) for the management of moderate to advanced keratoconus: efficacy and complications. *Cornea.* 2006;25(1):29–33.
43. Hamdi IM. Preliminary results of intrastromal corneal ring segment implantation to treat moderate to severe keratoconus. *J Cataract Refract Surg.* 2011;37(6):1125–1132.
44. Zare MA, Hashemi H, Salari MR. Intracorneal ring segment implantation for the management of keratoconus: safety and efficacy. *J Cataract Refract Surg.* 2007;33(11):1886–1891.
45. Kapitánová K, Nikel J. Femtosecond laser-assisted intrastromal corneal segment implantation—our experience. *Cesk Slov Oftalmol.* 2018;74(1):31–36.
46. Oatts JT, Savar L, Hwang DG. Late extrusion of intrastromal corneal ring segments: a report of two cases. *Am J Ophthalmol Case Rep.* 2017;8:67–70.
47. Abdellah MM, Ammar HG. Femtosecond laser implantation of a 355-degree intrastromal corneal ring segment in keratoconus: a three-year follow-up. *J Ophthalmol.* 2019;2019:6783181.
48. Samimi S, Leger F, Touboul D, Colin J. Histopathological findings after intracorneal ring segment implantation in keratoconic human corneas. *J Cataract Refract Surg.* 2007;33(2):247–253.
49. Bourges JL, Trong TT, Ellies P, Briat B, Renard G. Intrastromal corneal ring segments and corneal anterior stromal necrosis. *J Cataract Refract Surg.* 2003;29(6):1228–1230.
50. Kanellopoulos AJ, Vingopoulos F. Combining porcine xenograft intra-corneal ring segments and CXL: a novel technique. *Clinical Ophthalmology.* 2019;13:2521–2525.
51. Jarade E, Issa M, Chanbour W, Warhekar P. Biologic stromal ring to manage stromal melting after intrastromal corneal ring segment implantation. *J Cataract Refract Surg.* 2019;45(9):1222–1225.
52. Jacob S, Patel SR, Agarwal A, Ramalingam A, Saijimol AI, Raj JM. Corneal allogenic intrastromal ring segments (CAIRS) combined with corneal cross-linking for keratoconus. *J Refract Surg.* 2018;34(5):296–303.
53. Nguyen N, Gelles JD, Greenstein SA, Hersh PS. Incidence and associations of intracorneal ring segment explantation. *J Cataract Refract Surg.* 2019;45(2):153–158.
54. McAlister JC, Ardjomand N, Ilari L, Mengher LS, Gartry DS. Keratitis after intracorneal ring segment insertion for keratoconus. *J Cataract Refract Surg.* 2006;32(4):676–678.
55. Colin J. European clinical evaluation: use of Intacs for the treatment of keratoconus. *J Cataract Refract Surg.* 2006;32(5):747–755.
56. Ruckhofer J. [Clinical and histological studies on the intrastromal corneal ring segments (ICRSI, IntI(R))]. *Klinische Monatsblatter fur Augenheilkunde.* 2002;219(8):557–574.
57. Ruckhofer J, Twa MD, Schanzlin DJ. Clinical characteristics of lamellar channel deposits after implantation of Intacs. *J Cataract Refract Surg.* 2000;26(10):1473–1479.
58. Cao X, Ursea R, Shen D, Ramkumar HL, Chan CC. Hypocellular scar formation or aberrant fibrosis induced by an intrastromal corneal ring: a case report. *J Med Case Rep.* 2011;5:398.

59. Hofling-Lima AL, Branco BC, Romano AC, et al. Corneal infections after implantation of intracorneal ring segments. *Cornea.* 2004;23(6):547–549.
60. Tabatabaei SA, Soleimani M, Mirghorbani M, Tafti ZF, Rahimi F. Microbial keratitis following intracorneal ring implantation. *Clin Exp Optom.* 2019;102(1):35–42.
61. Chaudhry IA, Al-Ghamdi AA, Kirat O, Al-Swelmi F, Al-Rashed W, Shamsi FA. Bilateral infectious keratitis after implantation of intrastromal corneal ring segments. *Cornea.* 2010;29(3):339–341.
62. Bourcier T, Borderie V, Laroche L. Late bacterial keratitis after implantation of intrastromal corneal ring segments. *J Cataract Refract Surg.* 2003;29(2):407–409.
63. Shehadeh-Masha'our R, Modi N, Barbara A, Garzozi HJ. Keratitis after implantation of intrastromal corneal ring segments. *J Cataract Refract Surg.* 2004;30(8):1802–1804.
64. Levy J, Lifshitz T. Keratitis after implantation of intrastromal corneal ring segments (Intacs) aided by femtosecond laser for keratoconus correction: case report and description of the literature. *Eur J Ophthalmol.* 2010;20(4):780–784.
65. Slade DS, Johnson JT, Tabin G. Acanthamoeba and fungal keratitis in a woman with a history of Intacs corneal implants. *Eye Contact Lens.* 2008;34(3):185–187.
66. Shihadeh WA. Aspergillus fumigatus keratitis following intracorneal ring segment implantation. *BMC Ophthalmol.* 2012;12:19.
67. Neuffer MC, Panday V, Reilly C. Intrastromal corneal ring segments for post-LASIK ectasia complicated by persistent pain. *J Cataract Refract Surg.* 2010;36(2):336–339.
68. Alfonso JF, Lisa C, Merayo-Lloves J, Fernandez-Vega Cueto L, Montes-Mico R. Intrastromal corneal ring segment implantation in paracentral keratoconus with coincident topographic and coma axis. *J Cataract Refract Surg.* 2012;38(9):1576–1582.
69. Alfonso JF, Lisa C, Fernández-Vega L, Madrid-Costa D, Montés-Micó R. Intrastromal corneal ring segment implantation in 219 keratoconic eyes at different stages. *Graefes Arch Clin Exp Ophthalmol.* 2011;249(11):1705–1712.
70. Alió JL, Shabayek MH, Artola A. Intracorneal ring segments for keratoconus correction: long-term follow-up. *J Cataract Refract Surg.* 2006;32(6):978–985.
71. Alió JL, Shabayek MH, Belda JI, Correas P, Feijoo ED. Analysis of results related to good and bad outcomes of Intacs implantation for keratoconus correction. *J Cataract Refract Surg.* 2006;32(5):756–761.
72. Alió JL, Artola A, Hassanein A, Haroun H, Galal A. One or 2 Intacs segments for the correction of keratoconus. *J Cataract Refract Surg.* 2005;31(5):943–953.
73. Al-Tuwairqi WS, Osuagwu UL, Razzouk H, AlHarbi A, Ogbuehi KC. Clinical evaluation of two types of intracorneal ring segments (ICRS) for keratoconus. *Int Ophthalmol.* 2017;37(5):1185–1198.
74. Arantes JCD, Coscarelli S, Ferrara P, Araujo LPN, Avila M, Torquetti L. Intrastromal corneal ring segments for astigmatism correction after deep anterior lamellar keratoplasty. *J Ophthalmol.* 2017;2017:8689017.
75. Boxer Wachler BS, Christie JP, Chandra NS, Chou B, Korn T, Nepomuceno R. Intacs for keratoconus. *Ophthalmology.* 2003;110(5):1031–1040.
76. Colin J, Cochener B, Savary G, Malet F, Holmes-Higgin D. INTACS inserts for treating keratoconus: one-year results. *Ophthalmology.* 2001;108(8):1409–1414.
77. Coskunseven E, Kymionis GD, Tsiklis NS, et al. One-year results of intrastromal corneal ring segment implantation (KeraRing) using femtosecond laser in patients with keratoconus. *Am J Ophthalmol.* 2008;145(5):775–779.
78. Ertan A, Kamburoğlu G. Intacs implantation using a femtosecond laser for management of keratoconus: comparison of 306 cases in different stages. *J Cataract Refract Surg.* 2008;34(9):1521–1526.
79. Fahd DC, Alameddine RM, Nasser M, Awwad ST. Refractive and topographic effects of single-segment intrastromal corneal ring segments in eyes with moderate to severe keratoconus and inferior cones. *J Cataract Refract Surg.* 2015;41(7):1434–1440.
80. Cueto LFV, Lisa C, Madrid-Costa D, Merayo-Lloves J, Alfonso JF. Long-term follow-up of intrastromal corneal ring segments in paracentral keratoconus with coincident corneal keratometric, comatic, and refractive axes: stability of the procedure. *J Ophthalmol.* 2017;2017:4058026.
81. Fernandez-Vega Cueto L, Lisa C, Poo-Lopez A, Madrid-Costa D, Merayo-Lloves J, Alfonso JF. Intrastromal corneal ring segment implantation in 409 paracentral keratoconic Eyes. *Cornea.* 2016;35(11):1421–1426.
82. Heikal MA, Abdelshafy M, Soliman TT, Hamed AM. Refractive and visual outcomes after Keraring intrastromal corneal ring segment implantation for keratoconus assisted by femtosecond laser at 6 months follow-up. *Clin Ophthalmol.* 2017;11:81–86.

83. Hellstedt T, Makela J, Uusitalo R, Emre S, Uusitalo R. Treating keratoconus with Intacs corneal ring segments. *J Refract Surg.* 2005;21(3):236–246.
84. Israel M, Yousif MO, Osman NA, Nashed M, Abdelfattah NS. Keratoconus correction using a new model of intrastromal corneal ring segments. *J Cataract Refract Surg.* 2016;42(3):444–454.
85. Jabbarvand M, Hashemi H, Mohammadpour M, Khojasteh H, Khodaparast M, Hashemian H. Implantation of a complete intrastromal corneal ring at 2 different stromal depths in keratoconus. *Cornea.* 2014;33(2):141–144.
86. Jadidi K, Nejat F, Mosavi SA, et al. Full-ring intrastromal corneal implantation for correcting high myopia in patients with severe keratoconus. *Med Hypothesis Discov Innov Ophthalmol J.* 2016;5(3):89–95.
87. Kwitko S, Severo NS. Ferrara intracorneal ring segments for keratoconus. *J Cataract Refract Surg.* 2004;30(4):812–820.
88. Kymionis GD, Siganos CS, Tsiklis NS, et al. Long-term follow-up of Intacs in keratoconus. *Am J Ophthalmol.* 2007;143(2):236–244.
89. Lisa C, Garcia-Fernandez M, Madrid-Costa D, Torquetti L, Merayo-Lloves J, Alfonso JF. Femtosecond laser-assisted intrastromal corneal ring segment implantation for high astigmatism correction after penetrating keratoplasty. *J Cataract Refract Surg.* 2013;39(11):1660–1667.
90. Lisa C, Fernandez-Vega Cueto L, Poo-Lopez A, Madrid-Costa D, Alfonso JF. Long-term follow-up of intrastromal corneal ring segments (210-degree arc length) in central keratoconus with high corneal asphericity. *Cornea.* 2017;36(11):1325–1330.
91. Miraftab M, Hashemi H, Hafezi F, Asgari S. Mid-term results of a single intrastromal corneal ring segment for mild to moderate progressive keratoconus. *Cornea.* 2017;36(5):530–534.
92. Miranda D, Sartori M, Francesconi C, Allemann N, Ferrara P, Campos M. Ferrara intrastromal corneal ring segments for severe keratoconus. *J Refract Surg.* 2003;19(6):645–653.
93. Moreira H, de Oliveira CS, de Godoy G, Wahab SA. Anel Intracorneano de Ferrara em ceratocone [Ferrara's intracorneal ring in keratoconus]. *Arq Bras Oftalmol.* 2002;65:59–63.
94. Muftuoglu O, Aydin R. Kilic Muftuoglu I. Persistence of the cone on the posterior corneal surface affecting corneal aberration changes after intracorneal ring segment implantation in patients with keratoconus. *Cornea.* 2018;37(3):347–353.
95. Nobari SM, Villena C, Jadidi K. Full-ring intracorneal implantation in corneas with pellucid marginal degeneration. *Iran Red Crescent Med J.* 2015;17(12):e28974.
96. Peña-García P, Alió JL, Vega-Estrada A, Barraquer RI. Internal, corneal, and refractive astigmatism as prognostic factors for intrastromal corneal ring segment implantation in mild to moderate keratoconus. *J Cataract Refract Surg.* 2014;40(10):1633–1644.
97. Rocha GADN, Ferrara de Almeida Cunha P, Torquetti Costa L, Barbosa de Sousa L. Outcomes of a 320-degree intrastromal corneal ring segment implantation for keratoconus: results of a 6-month follow-up. *Eur J Ophthalmol.* 2020;30(1):139–146.
98. Sadoughi MM, Einollahi B, Veisi AR, et al. Femtosecond laser implantation of a 340-degree intrastromal corneal ring segment in keratoconus: short-term outcomes. *J Cataract Refract Surg.* 2017;43(10):1251–1256.
99. Sandes J, Stival LRS, de Avila MP, et al. Clinical outcomes after implantation of a new intrastromal corneal ring with 140-degree of arc in patients with corneal ectasia. *Int J Ophthalmol.* 2018;11(5):802–806.
100. Siganos D, Ferrara P, Chatzinikolas K, Bessis N, Papastergiou G. Ferrara intrastromal corneal rings for the correction of keratoconus. *J Cataract Refract Surg.* 2002;28(11):1947–1951.
101. Stival LR, Nassaralla BR, Figueiredo MN, Bicalho F, Nassaralla Junior JJ. Intrastromal corneal ring segment implantation for ectasia after refractive surgery. *Arq Bras Oftalmol.* 2015;78(4):212–215.
102. Torquetti L, Ferrara G, Almeida F, et al. Intrastromal corneal ring segments implantation in patients with keratoconus: 10-year follow-up. *J Refract Surg.* 2014;30(1):22–26.
103. Torquetti L, Ferrara G, Almeida F, Cunha L, Ferrara P, Merayo-Lloves J. Clinical outcomes after intrastromal corneal ring segments reoperation in keratoconus patients. *Int J Ophthalmol.* 2013;6(6):796–800.
104. Torquetti L, Cunha P, Luz A, et al. Clinical outcomes after implantation of 320 degrees-arc length intrastromal corneal ring segments in keratoconus. *Cornea.* 2018;37(10):1299–1305.
105. Vega-Estrada A, Alió JL, Plaza-Puche AB. Keratoconus progression after intrastromal corneal ring segment implantation in young patients: five-year follow-up. *J Cataract Refract Surg.* 2015;41(6):1145–1152.
106. Yildirim A, Cakir H, Kara N, Uslu H. Long-term outcomes of intrastromal corneal ring segment implantation for post-LASIK ectasia. *Cont Lens Anterior Eye.* 2014;37(6):469–472.

CHAPTER 26

Corneal Cross-Linking: History, Physiology, and Techniques

Theo G. Seiler ■ Theo Seiler

KEY CONCEPTS

- Corneal cross-linking (CXL) is a photopolymerization process using riboflavin as initiator or photo mediator.
- In the cornea, oxygen and energy (ultraviolet light) are consumed during this process, riboflavin is degraded, free radicals (reactive oxygen species) are formed, and cross-links are formed as new covalent bonds within the extracellular matrix.
- This chapter highlights the whole process in detail and discusses the experimental and clinical studies related to CXL.

Basic Parameters

Corneal cross-linking (CXL) is a photopolymerization process using riboflavin as initiator or photomediator. Photopolymerization initiators are used in many fields to generate photocurable composites. Within these composites, polymerization is triggered by an irradiation interacting with the photomediator, for example, with ultraviolet (UV) light. This leads to altered physical properties of the composites such as solubility, viscosity, and elasticity. In particular, the phenomenon in which a liquid state changes into a solid state is most useful and is applied to surface-treating techniques in fields including painting, printing inks, dental materials, and lithography, among others.

In the cornea and in particular in the extracellular matrix, the composites are represented by collagen and proteoglycans. Using riboflavin as initiator, which is stimulated by near UV light with a wavelength of approximately 365 nm, polymerization does not occur, because the third adjunct, oxygen,[1] is missing. Although the detailed steps of the process are not fully understood yet,[2] we can summarize by stating that (1) oxygen and energy (UV light) are consumed during the process, (2) riboflavin is degraded,[2] (3) free radicals (reactive oxygen species) are formed, and (4) cross-links are formed as new covalent bonds within the extracellular matrix.[3] (For more details, see the paper of Hayes et al.[3])

The first ingredient of CXL is riboflavin.

In a deepithelialized cornea, the intrastromal gradient of riboflavin was measured by two-photon microscopy[4] after application of 0.1% riboflavin solutions in either 20% dextran or 1.1% hydroxypropyl methylcellulose (HPMC) for 10 or 30 minutes (Fig. 26.1). The results appear similar and are in accordance with the mathematical diffusion equation indicating a one-directional passive diffusion process. As riboflavin experiences only minor photodegradation, the effective loss of riboflavin happens mainly by diffusion across the endothelium into the aqueous.

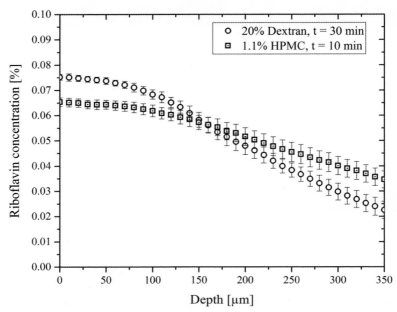

Fig. 26.1 Intrastromal riboflavin concentrations measured by two-photon microscopy after 0.1% riboflavin imbibition either in hydroxypropyl methylcellulose (*HPMC*; 10 minutes, *squares*) or in dextran (30 minutes, *circles*) solution.

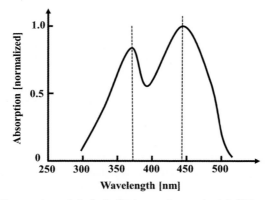

Fig. 26.2 Absorption spectrum of riboflavin. Peaks are at approximately 365 and 440 nm.

The riboflavin diffuses not through endothelial cells but passes through intercellular spaces.[5] This is one reason why, during the irradiation only every 5 minutes, riboflavin drops have to be applied. The riboflavin film acts as protection for more posterior structures (additional UV absorption) and prevents corneal dehydration.[6] It is not clear whether all riboflavin molecules act as reaction partners for CXL or whether a fraction of riboflavin molecules build dimers that would not act as photomediators.[2] This would mean that the "active" riboflavin concentration is significantly smaller than 0.1%.

The second component of CXL is UV light of 365 nm in wavelength, which was selected based on the absorption spectrum of riboflavin (Fig. 26.2). The second absorption maximum is at 440 nm, which, however, was avoided owing to the potential hazard of blue light for the retina.

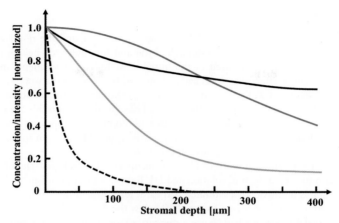

Fig. 26.3 Normalized intrastromal gradients of riboflavin *(red line)*, available ultraviolet (UV) light *(blue line)*, and oxygen before UV irradiation *(black line)* and during UV irradiation *(interrupted black line)* with 3 mW/cm².

UV light is absorbed by riboflavin according to Lambert-Beer's law (exponential decay). However, as the concentration of riboflavin decreases with depth in the cornea, the gradient of the light intensity flattens toward the endothelium (Fig. 26.3, *blue line*). In total, approximately 90% of the UV light is absorbed in the riboflavin-soaked cornea.[7] In principle, it is one photon that lifts the riboflavin molecule into an excited singlet or triplet state and, therefore, only the number of photons counts for the efficiency regarding CXL. Holding the radiant exposure constant at 5.4 J/cm², the number of photons hitting the cornea is identical in cases of 3 mW/cm² for 30 minutes, 9 mW/cm² for 10 minutes, or 30 mW/cm² for 3 minutes, and all these combinations should provide identical results. However, for many biological systems, this rule (Bunsen-Roscoe law) does not hold, and in particular, for CXL it has been shown to be invalid.[8,9]

The third ingredient is oxygen, which participates in radical formation and in the chemical bonding process. The gradient of oxygen in the deepithelialized corneal stroma without crosslinking decreases only minimally: at the Bowman's layer level, it equals atmospheric pressure (21% of volume) decreasing to 17% at 100 microns and to 14% at 300 microns.[10] Again, the oxygen diffuses passively into the cornea, and the gradient is flatter compared with the riboflavin gradient because of the much smaller size of the O_2 molecule and its faster diffusion (see Fig. 26.3, *black line*).

The situation changes dramatically once UV light initiates the CXL process (see Fig. 26.3, *black interrupted line*). Whereas the riboflavin gradient and the UV decay remain practically unchanged, the oxygen concentration decreases within 20 seconds and to less than 3% at 100-microns depth at an irradiance of 3 mW/cm² and to 1% at 9 mW/cm². With irradiances higher than 9 mW/cm², oxygen falls beyond the measurement sensitivity of the sensor (1%).[10] When the depletion process is faster and extinguishes oxygen more completely, the irradiance is higher. With 3 mW/cm² even at 200-micron depth, the equilibrium oxygen concentration (during CXL) is at 1.5%, which means that there is still some oxygen to support radical formation.[10] This result is clearly not achieved when using 18 mW/cm² or more. Compared with riboflavin and UV light, the oxygen gradient is now by far the steepest (see Fig. 26.3) and determines, therefore, the depth of CXL. As a consequence, oxygen represents a kind of bottleneck parameter that limits the efficiency of CXL, and this may be the reason the Bunsen-Roscoe law is not valid for irradiances higher than 9 mW/cm².

A new technical approach employing an oxygen concentration of >95% over the cornea tries to counteract this bottleneck and, indeed, under such a hyperoxygenation even with 9 mW/cm², there is a measurable oxygen concentration of 1.2% at a depth of 300 microns.[10]

Experimental Studies

For electron microscopy of the cornea, aldehyde fixatives are used, and the result is a rigid and clear piece of tissue looking like glass. Glutaraldehyde and formaldehyde belong to the group of cross-linking fixatives and were used in the initial cross-linking experiments in Dresden in the 1990s. The stiffening effect was spectacular; however, the side effects were also significant. Another approach was the use of sugar solutions, which are known to produce advanced glycation end products (AEGs) in biologic tissues. These cross-links are also responsible for complications in diabetes mellitus. The Boston group tried another photomediator approach (rose bengal and green light),[11] which delivered significant stiffening of the cornea. However, in animal experiments side effects such as prolonged epithelial healing occurred.

After 5 years of experimental work in Dresden in the late 1990s, it was clear that the technique of riboflavin (0.1%) in dextran solution and UV light was most promising.[12] Riboflavin is a natural vitamin and is not toxic. In a saturated cornea, at least 90% of the UV light is absorbed, so the residual UV irradiance is at least a factor of 10 below the damage thresholds of iris, lens, and retina.[13] In the pre-LED era, we had to use a mercury vapor lamp and band filters delivering 3 mW/cm^2 at the cornea level. In rabbit experiments, we learned that a radiant exposure of 5.4 J/cm^2 killed keratocytes approximately 300 microns deep and the endothelial cells showed neither apoptosis nor necrosis.[14,15] Based on theoretical calculations of the riboflavin concentration at the level of the endothelium (again: diffusion equation), the UV damage threshold of the endothelium was determined, which corresponded to the irradiance at corneal depth at approximately 330 microns. Including safety margins, we concluded that the cornea prior to CXL should have a minimal thickness of at least 400 microns. Recently, we discovered that the solution of the diffusion equation was overly pessimistic and that the measured riboflavin concentration at the endothelium level is at least a factor of two smaller, which implies a revision of the 400-micron rule.[5]

Wollensak who joined the group only in the late 90-ties discovered that crosslinked cornea is more resistant against digesting enzymes16, which plays a role during corneal melting. Native pig corneal buttons were digested in trypsin solution within 2 days, whereas in cross-linked corneas, the process took 5 days and more.

Clinical Studies

The first clinical application of CXL was anti-melting treatment in four eyes with therapy-refractory corneal melting. Three of the four corneas healed, and in only one eye was a keratoplasty à chaud necessary.[17] As many of these melting processes create ulcers localized in the periphery of the cornea, this application has become the domain of customized CXL, and we mostly use ring segment irradiation patterns (Fig. 26.4). During this treatment, the 400-micron rule is clearly violated but sacrificing endothelium of a small limited area in this circumstance is considered reasonable.

For many years, the Dresden protocol (epi-off, 0.1% riboflavin, 3 mW/cm^2 for 30 minutes, normal oxygenation) was the standard and was used in hundreds of thousands of keratoconus and post-LASIK ectasia eyes. The procedure is simple, inexpensive, and successful in halting progression in more than 90% of the cases, and it has a low complication rate of 3% and less.[18] At 1 month after surgery, at the slit lamp[19] but observed even better in anterior segment optical coherence tomography (OCT) imaging,[20] a demarcation line is visible in the stroma, and this line is believed to indicate the depth of cell death.[21]

The most frequent complication of the treatment is sterile infiltrates (Fig. 26.5A), which occur after up to 10% of the operations. The infiltrates may present as single peripheral lesions with no impact on visual acuity or as multiple lesions (see Fig. 26.5B) inducing transient visual loss. The fact that the infiltrates occur on the first day after surgery makes the diagnosis and therapy easy. For many years, the complication of continuous flattening was underestimated, and it may occur

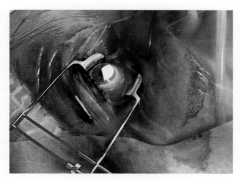

Fig. 26.4 Corneal cross-linking with a ring segment pattern.

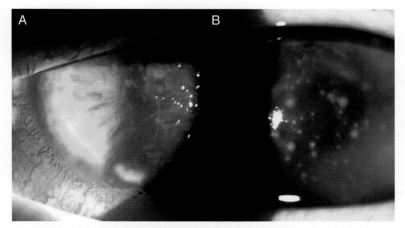

Fig. 26.5 Typical peripheral sterile infiltrate (A) and atypical multifocal sterile infiltrate (B).

in up to 4% of the cases.[22] Herpes simplex virus (HSV) or other viruses may be activated by CXL and can lead to severe intraocular inflammations.[23] Patients with ocular HSV or significantly reduced corneal sensitivity in their history should receive prophylactic antiviral therapy. Deep stromal scars may occur but generally clarify over the years. Severe complications such as infections and ulcerations are rare and may require keratoplasty.

Although the Dresden protocol was successful, it was, and is, an inconvenient surgery. It is inconvenient for the patient because of the epithelial removal and its side effects and inconvenient for the physician because it is a time-consuming procedure. In 2005, Kanellopoulos proposed using higher irradiances to shorten the irradiation time (assuming that the Bunsen-Roscoe law would apply). The term "accelerated CXL" was coined for any shorter irradiation, and currently irradiances from 3 mW/cm^2 up to 30 mW/cm^2 are available. Clinical observation documented that the higher the irradiance, the shallower the CXL depth (measured via the demarcation line in the OCT)[24,25] and, therefore, the Bunsen-Roscoe law is not applicable to CXL. Also, experimental studies demonstrated that accelerated CXL resulted in less biomechanical stiffening.[8] However, as we have no in vivo instrument to measure biomechanics reliably, we do not know how much stiffening an individual keratoconus cornea requires. Based on the oxygen availability in the stroma, we cannot recommend an irradiance of more than 9 mW/cm^2 in an atmospheric oxygen environment.[10]

The question of whether to remove the epithelium has become a war of faith and market shares, especially in the United States. Why not save the epithelium and avoid pain and postoperative complications such as infections? The difficulty with epi-on CXL is two-fold: (1) the epithelium represents a diffusion barrier for riboflavin and (2) the epithelium consumes substantial parts of the oxygen and may limit the rediffusion. Several proposals to overcome the barrier for riboflavin resulted in "epi-on drops" that did not work very well and yielded high failure rates after 2 years, especially in young patients.[26] Improved preparations claimed to work better; however, the recipes were never disclosed and, therefore, the results could not be confirmed. One meta-analysis compared the literature on epi-on versus epi-off CXL and found that the early postoperative vision favors epi-on and the depth of the demarcation line and stabilization rate favors epi-off.[27] These results are not surprising, as we have learned that it is the oxygen that determines the CXL depth and that intact epithelium consumes up to 50% of the oxygen diffusing into the cornea.[28] To avoid too shallow CXL depths, Kamaev and Friedman proposed to enrich the atmosphere with oxygen. Promising studies on supplemental oxygen showed biomechanically, as well as physiologically, that the poor oxygen balance under epi-on conditions can be compensated for,[2,29] and prospective studies are enrolled. It will take at least 2 years until such techniques are verified clinically.

Another topic, that is still under debate is the combination of customized laser ablation and CXL. Once transepithelial photorefractive keratectomy (PRK) is completed, there exists an erosion that can be used as an entrance port for riboflavin and oxygen. This approach saves the patient one pain episode and the risk of infection. Ten years ago, Krueger and Kanellopoulos[30] and Kymionis et al.[31] published promising results, which were later refuted. Moraes et al. presented a retrospective study that showed an improvement in uncorrected vision and in topography; however, they also found a loss of corrected vision of more than two lines in 25% of the cases.[32] The authors concluded that this procedure should be approached with caution and may not be as safe as initially thought. Reviewing our own cases of simultaneous CXL and transepithelial PRK, we can confirm the findings of Moraes et al. and have stopped using the simultaneous treatment regimen.

References

1. Richoz O, Hammer A, Tabibian D, Gatzioufas Z, Hafezi F. The biomechanical effect of corneal collagen cross-linking (CXL) with riboflavin and UV-A is oxygen dependent. *Transl Vis Sci Technol*. 2013;2:6.
2. Kamaev P, Friedman MD, Sherr E, Muller D. Photochemical kinetics of corneal cross-linking with riboflavin. *Invest Ophthalmol Vis Sci*. 2012;53:2360–2367.
3. Hayes S, Kamma-Lorger CS, Boote C, et al. The effect of riboflavin/UVA collagen cross-linking therapy on the structure and hydrodynamic behaviour of the ungulate and rabbit corneal stroma. *PLoS One*. 2013;8:e52860.
4. Ehmke T, Seiler TG, Fischinger I, Ripken T, Heisterkamp A, Frueh BE. Comparison of corneal riboflavin gradients using dextran and HPMC solutions. *J Refract Surg*. 2016;32:798–802.
5. Seiler TG, Batista A, Frueh BE, Koenig K. Riboflavin concentrations at the endothelium during corneal cross-linking in humans. *Invest Ophthalmol Vis Sci*. 2019;60:2140–2145.
6. Wollensak G, Aurich H, Wirbelauer C, Sel S. Significance of the riboflavin film in corneal collagen crosslinking. *J Cataract Refract Surg*. 2010;36(1):114–120.
7. Seiler TG, Fischinger I, Senfft T, Schmidinger G, Seiler T. Intrastromal application of riboflavin for corneal crosslinking. *Invest Ophthalmol Vis Sci*. 2014;55:4261–4265.
8. Hammer A, Richoz O, Arba Mosquera S, Tabibian D, Hoogewoud F, Hafezi F. Corneal biomechanical properties at different corneal cross-linking (CXL) irradiances. *Invest Ophthalmol Vis Sci*. 2014;55(5):2881–2884.
9. Wernli J, Schumacher S, Spoerl E, Mrochen M. The efficacy of corneal cross-linking shows a sudden decrease with very high intensity UV light and short treatment time. *Invest Ophthalmol Vis Sci*. 2013;54(2):1176–1180.
10. Seiler TG, Komninou MA, Nambiar MH, Schuerch K, Frueh BE, Büchler P. Oxygen kinetics during corneal crosslinking with and without supplementary oxygen. *Am J Ophthalmol*. 2021;223:368–376.

11. Zhu H, Alt C, Webb RH, Melki S, Kochevar IE. Corneal crosslinking with rose bengal and green light: efficacy and safety evaluation. *Cornea.* 2016;35(9):1234–1241.
12. Seiler T, Spoerl E, Huhle M, Kamouna A. Conservative therapy of keratoconus by enhancement of collagen cross-links [ARVO Abstract]. Invest Ophthalmol Vis Sci. 1996;37:4671.
13. Spoerl E, Mrochen M, Sliney D, *Trokel S, Seiler T. Safety of UVA*-riboflavin cross-linking of the cornea. *Cornea.* 2007;26(4):385–389.
14. Wollensak G, Spörl E, Reber F, Pillunat L, Funk R. Corneal endothelial cytotoxicity of riboflavin/UVA treatment in vitro. *Ophthalmic Res.* 2003;35:324–328.
15. Wollensak G, Spoerl E, Wilsch M, Seiler T. Endothelial cell damage after riboflavin-ultraviolet-A treatment in the rabbit. *J Cataract Refract Surg.* 2003;29:1786–1790.
16. Spoerl E, Wollensak G, Seiler T. Increased resistance of crosslinked cornea against enzymatic digestion. *Curr Eye Res.* 2004;29(1):35–40.
17. Schnitzler E, Spörl E, Seiler T. Irradiation of cornea with ultraviolet light and riboflavin administration as a new treatment for erosive corneal processes, preliminary results in four patients. *Klin Monbl Augenheilkd.* 2000;217(3):190–193.
18. Koller T, Mrochen M, Seiler T. Complication and failure rates after corneal crosslinking. *J Cataract Refract Surg.* 2009;35(8):1358–1362.
19. Seiler T, Hafezi F. Corneal cross-linking-induced stromal demarcation line. *Cornea.* 200:25(9):1057–1059.
20. Doors M, Tahzib NG, Eggink FA, Berendschot TT, Webers CA, Nuijts RM. Use of anterior segment optical coherence tomography to study corneal changes after collagen cross-linking. *Am J Ophthalmol.* 2009;148(6):844–851.e2.
21. Mazzotta C, Traversi C, Baiocchi S, et al. Corneal healing after riboflavin ultraviolet-A collagen cross-linking determined by confocal laser scanning microscopy in vivo: early and late modifications. *Am J Ophthalmol.* 2008;146(4):527–533.
22. Noor IH, Seiler TG, Noor K, Seiler T. Continued long-term flattening after corneal cross-linking for keratoconus. *J Refract Surg.* 2018;34(8):567–570.
23. Eberwein P, Auw-Hädrich C, Birnbaum F, Maier PC, Reinhard T. Corneal melting after cross-linking and deep lamellar keratoplasty in a keratoconus patient. *Klin Monbl Augenheilkd.* 2008;225(1):96–98.
24. Mazzotta C, Hafezi F, Kymionis G, et al. In vivo confocal microscopy after corneal collagen crosslinking. *Ocul Surf.* 2015;13(4):298–314.
25. Asgari S, Hashemi H, Hajizadeh F, et al. Multipoint assessment of demarcation line depth after standard and accelerated cross-linking in central and inferior keratoconus. *J Curr Ophthalmol.* 2018;30(3):223–227.
26. Caporossi A, Mazzotta C, Paradiso AL, Baiocchi S, Marigliani D, Caporossi T. Transepithelial corneal collagen crosslinking for progressive keratoconus: 24-month clinical results. *J Cataract Refract Surg.* 2013;39(8):1157–1163.
27. Kobashi H, Rong SS, Ciolino JB. Transepithelial versus epithelium-off corneal crosslinking for corneal ectasia. *J Cataract Refract Surg.* 2018;44(12):1507–1516.
28. Freeman RD. Oxygen consumption by the component layers of the cornea. *J Physiol.* 1972;225:15–32.
29. Hill J, Liu C, Deardorff P, et al. Optimization of oxygen dynamics, UV-A delivery, and drug formulation for accelerated epi-on corneal crosslinking. *Curr Eye Res.* 2020;45(4):450–458.
30. Krueger RR, Kanellopoulos AJ. Stability of simultaneous topography-guided photorefractive keratectomy and riboflavin/UVA cross-linking for progressive keratoconus: case reports. *J Refract Surg.* 2010;26(10):S827–S832.
31. Kymionis GD, Kontadakis GA, Kounis GA, et al. Simultaneous topography-guided PRK followed by corneal collagen cross-linking for keratoconus. *J Refract Surg.* 2009;25(9):S807–S811.
32. Moraes RLB, Ghanem RC, Ghanem VC, Santhiago MR. Haze and visual acuity loss after sequential photorefractive keratectomy and corneal cross-linking for keratoconus. *J Refract Surg.* 2019;35(2):109–114.

CHAPTER 27

Corneal Cross-Linking: Results and Complications

Emilio A. Torres-Netto ■ Mark Hillen ■ Farhad Hafezi

KEY CONCEPTS

- The standard epithelium-off corneal cross-linking (CXL) protocol has the greatest body of evidence supporting its safety and efficacy in treating keratoconus and corneal ectasias.
- The patient's age at the time of performing CXL and collagen turnover time are decisive factors in the clinical response.
- The dependency of the CXL photochemical reaction on oxygen may explain unsatisfactory results of certain newer CXL protocols, such as epithelial-preserving (epi-on) CXL techniques.
- Standard epithelium-off CXL is usually associated with a transient mild haze that does not affect vision.

Keratoconus is a common cause of severe visual impairment in childhood and adolescence worldwide, with a published prevalence of between 1:50 and 1:2000.[1,2] It is a progressive disease that usually presents as corneal thinning that weakens the cornea and is associated with the development of a cone-like protrusion that leads to low vision. In 1997 Spörl et al.[3] proposed a new technique to increase the biomechanical stiffness of the cornea: corneal cross-linking (CXL). Between 1998 and 2003, CXL was established in Dresden and Zurich, and it brought, for the first time, the possibility of halting the progressive natural course of keratoconus.[4] After approximately two decades, hundreds of PubMed-listed publications involving the term "corneal cross-linking" are now available, and CXL has become the standard of care for treating keratoconus and related corneal ectatic disorders in over 120 countries.[5,6]

The stability of the cornea and its shape are closely linked to its biomechanical properties.[7] In keratoconus and other ectatic eye diseases, the biomechanical strength of the cornea is significantly reduced,[8,9] and CXL is a surgical means of increasing the biomechanical resistance in these compromised corneas.[10]

CXL involves de-epithelialization of the cornea, then soaking of the corneal stroma with a photosensitizer (vitamin B_2, riboflavin), followed by ultraviolet (UV)-A-irradiation. The standard epithelium-off CXL protocol, the "Dresden protocol,"[4] comprises a total UV-A fluence of 5.4 J/cm² using a 3 mW/cm² irradiation for 30 minutes and is the protocol that has the greatest body of evidence supporting its efficacy in treating corneal ectasias.

Clinical Results

Several studies have shown that CXL successfully stops the progression of keratoconus[11] and can also arrest postsurgical corneal ectasia.[12] In 2003 the first clinical results—an analysis of 23 eyes with a maximum follow-up of 4 years—were published. In this inaugural series, CXL stopped disease progression in all eyes and even improved vision in more than 60%. Long-term results have confirmed these initial findings.[13] Today, CXL has been successfully used in clinical practice for more than 15 years, and reports from multiple countries have shown that CXL has significantly reduced the total number of corneal transplantations needed for keratoconus patients,[14,15] since CXL can arrest disease progression at a stage before corneal transplantation becomes necessary.

Although a detailed description is beyond the scope of this book, CXL can also be used to treat postoperative ectasias[16] and other forms of peripheral corneal thinning disorders, such as pellucid marginal degeneration (PMD).[17,18] In both situations, there are reports that CXL has successfully been used to prevent disease progression.[16–18]

DECISIVE FACTORS IN THE CLINICAL RESPONSE

The speed of disease progression in keratoconus can vary greatly. Some of the risk factors linked to changes in corneal biomechanics and topography include early age,[19,20] thyroid hormone variations,[21,22] eye-rubbing habits,[23] pregnancy,[21,24–26] and the use of medications such as estrogen regulators.[27] Moreover, it is hypothesized that such factors may also alter the ability of CXL to stabilize keratoconus over time. It is believed, however, that two elements would be most relevant in this regard: the age of the patient at the time of performing the CXL[20,28] and the collagen turnover time.[29]

Cross-linking is considered a natural process that occurs with age not only in the cornea but also in other ocular structures, such as the lens.[30] In the cornea, the diameter of the corneal fibrils increases over time because of age-dependent glycosylation.[30] This means that the cornea becomes progressively stiffer, broadly decreasing the likelihood of keratoconus progression as people grow older. A further relevant point that may be related to the long-term stability of CXL is the CXL-induced delay in corneal collagen turnover.[28] Collagen turnover usually declines with age.[29] Estimates of collagen turnover time vary from 3 to 7 years, but this process could be delayed by at least 12 to 24 months by CXL due to CXL-induced changes such as increased resistance of corneal collagen and matrix components to enzymatic degradation.[28]

EMERGING PROTOCOLS

Since the introduction and adoption of the standard-of-care Dresden protocol, a number of other approaches to cross-linking the cornea have emerged. The Dresden protocol requires 30 minutes of UV-A irradiation, and the first modifications made were to try and make the total procedure faster—in other words, accelerated CXL. In theory, this is supported by the Bunsen-Roscoe law of reciprocity, which states that an equivalent photochemical effect could be achieved with any combination of intensity and illumination time, if one maintains the total fluence. This would suggest that 30 minutes of 3 mW/cm² illumination for 30 minutes would give an equivalent effect to 30 mW/cm² for 10 minutes. However, the Bunsen-Roscoe law fails to hold true, as decreasing effects on corneal strength are seen as illumination intensity increases and intensity time decreases, and our group was the first to show that the photochemical cross-linking reaction also requires another molecule that has a restricted availability within the corneal stroma: oxygen.[31–33]

To better understand the effect of accelerated CXL on the cornea, the biomechanical effect of cross-linking under different combinations of irradiation times and UV intensity (with the same total fluence) was studied. The stiffening effect was significantly lower when the procedure was accelerated, with 9 mW/cm² energy being delivered for 10 minutes resulting in a significantly lower stiffening effect than that achieved with the Dresden protocol, and this decrease in effect was even more pronounced when 18 mW/cm² of UV-A energy was applied for 5 minutes.[34] Similarly, more distinct changes in gene transcription were observed with Dresden protocol cross-linking compared with accelerated CXL protocols.[35] This tendency for accelerated CXL to produce a weaker effect than the Dresden protocol has also been observed clinically,[36] with mixed results being observed when using faster CXL protocols.[37]

The dependence of the CXL photochemical reaction on oxygen may also explain some of the more unsatisfactory results of newer cross-linking protocols under development or already in clinical use, such as CXL with epithelium-preserving techniques ("epi-on" CXL).[31,32,38–42] The epithelium is removed in the Dresden protocol because it forms an effective barrier for riboflavin penetration into the collagen-rich corneal stroma where the cross-linking reaction needs to take place. Even if an epi-on technique managed to provide adequate riboflavin saturation of the stroma, leaving the epithelium in place results in not only a ~20% attenuation of UV energy that reaches the stroma, but the epithelium also limits the diffusion of oxygen into the stroma.[43] This is in part because the corneal epithelium has a high oxygen requirement, consuming approximately 10 times more oxygen than the stroma.[44] For this reason, even if transepithelial techniques could improve the diffusion of riboflavin into the stroma,[45] they cannot influence the speed of oxygen diffusion. These factors may explain why numerous transepithelial CXL protocols evaluated in the past have not been able to halt keratoconus progression as effectively as the Dresden protocol.[38–40]

ROOM FOR IMPROVEMENT

The Dresden protocol was developed with an abundance of caution. UV-A energy can damage corneal endothelial cells, so the protocol was designed with wide safety margins to avoid this; hence the UV-irradiation settings and the requirement for a minimum corneal thickness of 400 μm. However, as more is known about the safety profile of CXL, as well as what is involved in the photochemical reaction, some of those parameters are being altered to improve the efficacy of the accelerated and epithelial-sparing cross-linking protocols. Although the studies examining this are in their infancy, and we still lack an ideal clinical metric for examining the true efficacy of CXL (we currently rely on a number of relatively suboptimal measurements such as refraction, corneal topography, and a number of air puff tonometry corneal deflection-related measurements), we are beginning to see some promising initial results.

Accelerated protocols that deliver a higher total fluence are now achieving functional outcomes that are close to those of the Dresden protocol.[46] Pulsed-light protocols have been developed that enable oxygen to diffuse into the stroma during the UV-A off-period (rather than being consumed in the on-period) and pilot studies of these enhanced-fluence pulsed-light iontophoresis protocols have shown—with the caveat of a currently short follow-up period—that they may be able to overcome relevant limitations of transepithelial protocols and achieve effective keratoconus stabilization rates.[47] At present, however, more studies are needed to evaluate and validate such results in both the medium and long term.

Another approach, customized CXL, uses different energies applied unevenly in different locations on the same cornea and has displayed (again, over a short follow-up period) a stronger corneal regularization effect than standard cross-linking protocols.[48]

Important advances have also been made in the treatment of thin corneas.[33,49] A new, individualized CXL modality has been introduced by our group as a way to cross-link each cornea based on the individual.[50] The "sub400" experimental protocol takes into account the diffusion of oxygen and applies different energies according to each patient's individual intraoperative corneal thickness.[33,49,50] This has allowed us to treat corneas below 400 μm without using methods to artificially increase the corneal thickness such as swelling with hyperosmolar riboflavin or contact lenses (which introduce another factor that can increase the variability of outcomes).

SHORT- AND LONG-TERM RESULTS

A longitudinal evaluation of the first 130 patients with keratoconus who underwent Dresden protocol CXL found that 1 year after cross-linking, the anterior keratometry (K) of the corneal apex decreased by a mean of 2.68 D in 62% of the eyes, and stability (a variation ≤0.50 D) was found in 17% of the eyes.[51] Fig. 27.1 exemplifies typical corneal remodeling after just over a year in a patient after standard epithelium-off CXL. Similarly, the maximum K value decreased by an average of 1.46 D in 56% of the eyes, whereas 30% of eyes remained stable topographically after 1 year of follow-up.[52] Interestingly, even with some patients being lost to follow-up, the same series showed a flattening in K apex value by an average of 4.84 D after 3 years in 78% of the 33 eyes analyzed.[52]

Until 2020, only one study had been published that encompassed clinical results up to 10 years after CXL using standard epithelium-off Dresden protocol in adults. The maximum K, minimum K, and K apex values were significantly reduced 10 years after and corrected distance visual acuity (CDVA) significantly improved by an average of 0.14 logMAR.[13] This analysis was performed in 34 eyes, and only one eye (3%) had permanent corneal scar with reduced visual acuity. Although other persistent anterior stromal opacities were found in 13 eyes (38%), these did not affect best-corrected visual acuity (BCVA). Of the entire series, two eyes (6.25%) failed the treatment and required a repeat CXL procedure because of an increase in keratometry values, at 5 and 10 years after the initial procedure.[13]

An unpublished joint study data from the ELZA Institute (Dietikon, Switzerland), the IROC Institute (Zurich, Switzerland), and the Center for Applied Biotechnology and Molecular Medicine at the University of Zurich also showed that topographic readings tend to decrease significantly over time, and despite such changes, corrected visual acuity remained stable in a 10-year follow-up period.[53] In this retrospective series, preliminary data show a failure rate of around 10% at 10 years after the procedure.[53]

As with adults, standard epithelium-off CXL has also been shown to be safe and effective in providing keratoconus stability in pediatric patients.[28] As expected, the rate of progression in pediatric patients was up to 24% in 10 years,[28] showing that although CXL can slow down KC progression and improve functional performance,[28] age is a decisive factor and younger patients should be followed closely.

Complications

Over the 20-plus years since its creation and development, CXL has transformed from an experimental technique to the global standard of care for treating keratoconus. Progressive forms of keratoconus now have a stabilizing treatment, and visual impairments due to progressive corneal steepening and thinning—as well as other surgical complications such as keratoplasty—have been prevented during the period since CXL was introduced to the clinic. Although safe for both children and adults, CXL can still present a certain profile of complications or unexpected responses.

EARLY POSTOPERATIVE

A mild haze (that does not affect vision) usually appears after CXL. For this reason, there is debate as to whether haze should be viewed as a normal finding in CXL or considered as a complication that could potentially cause loss of visual quality.

The primary safety considerations with CXL focus on the corneal endothelium and stem cells present in the limbus, lens, and retina. Originally, one of the major concerns was potential endothelial damage caused by UV irradiation: 400 μm of corneal minimum thickness was required to protect eye structures, as a result of riboflavin shielding. A threshold of 0.35 mW/cm² of corneal endothelium UV irradiation would lead to cell death by apoptosis,[54] putting corneal homeostasis and transparency at stake. Although this limit might be overestimated according to new evaluations,[55] most of the few reported cases of endothelial dysfunction after CXL arose because surgeons failed to respect the protocol to measure corneal thickness immediately before UV

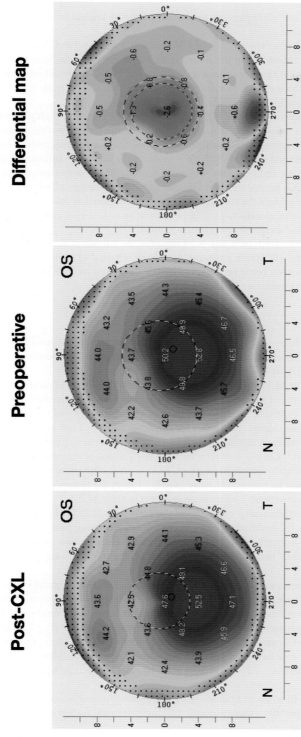

Fig. 27.1 Image of the anterior sagittal curvature using a Scheimpflug imaging device, showing a typical effect after performing standard epithelium-off corneal cross-linking (CXL). The left image represents corneal curvature after CXL; the central image represents preoperative topography; and the image on the right shows differential map between both images, displaying central flattening of 2.6 D after 1.3 years.

irradiation.[12] In both pediatric and adult patients, long-term follow-up studies have not reported endothelial cell changes or failures.[13,28]

Richoz et al. investigated whether the amount of UV irradiation delivered in CXL can affect corneal limbal stem cells.[56] They showed that irradiating with double the standard fluence (10.8 J/cm²) on the limbus, altered neither the regenerative capacity of the limbal epithelial cells nor the expression pattern of the putative stem cell marker p63, suggesting that CXL can be used safely, even in eccentric irradiation situations as in PMD.[56]

Another relevant point concerns epithelial cell removal. Although currently highly effective, the CXL treatment protocol is invasive and may be painful, since the most effective treatment occurs when the epithelium is removed.[57] Photoactivated chromophore for keratitis corneal cross-linking (PACK-CXL) has been used successfully for the treatment of keratitis[58] and has the ability to reduce the microbial load, depending on the total fluence used,[59] to a lesser or greater degree. Therefore at the end of each CXL procedure, the irradiated corneal surface has a lower microbial load,[59] which would potentially protect the surface from infections acquired at this point in time. However, the persistence of epithelial defects poses a postoperative risk of contracting a corneal infection in cases where the open surface is not properly handled.[60,61]

Other unexpected responses to CXL have also been reported. As a result of cellular immunity to staphylococcal antigens, peripheral sterile infiltrates have been reported as complications after CXL.[61,62] Finally, herpes reactivation could be triggered by UV light even in individuals with no apparent history of clinical herpes virus ocular infections.[61]

LATE POSTOPERATIVE

There are distinctive forms of haze after CXL. As mentioned earlier, a transient mild haze that does not affect visual quality is observed in most patients. However, haze can also become permanent. In these cases, this is usually associated with corneal flattening.[63]

In a retrospective assessment of 127 patients, approximately 9% developed clinically significant persistent haze at 12 months of follow-up.[64] Advanced keratoconus with decreased corneal thickness, higher keratometry values, or a reticular pattern of stromal *microstriae* (as seen by *in vivo* confocal microscopy) are considered risk factors for the development of late and permanent haze.[61,64,65] Interestingly, eyes with haze associated with massive corneal remodeling may not have visual acuity negatively affected.[63] On the contrary, visual acuity can improve, even in eyes with moderate haze and flattening of up to almost 10 D after CXL.[63] Corneal flattening in highly aberrated corneas preoperatively may be potentially more beneficial than the formation of the haze itself, and despite the haze, some patients display improvements in their BCVA.[63]

In a minority of cases, corneal flattening can occur in the early years after CXL, and this usually stabilizes after 1 to 3 years.[52] Nevertheless, cases of continuous flattening have recently been reported—even after up to 12 years after CXL.[66] Interestingly, such cases had no stromal opacity other than transient stromal haze,[67] hence this process differs from the standard long-term behavior of corneas after CXL.

Ectasia progression after treatment is considered to be a CXL failure and could be viewed as a long-term potential complication; however, because of the phenomenon of corneal collagen turnover one could also interpret this as a spontaneous process that occurs once keratocytes have been renewed after many years have passed. A failure rate of 7.6% was reported after 12 months in a study that prospectively evaluated 117 eyes.[68] This study identified that high preoperative maximum K was a significant risk factor for failure.[68] For context, long-term follow-up studies available report a failure rate between 6.25% and 10% after 10 years of CXL using the standard epithelium-off protocol.[13,53]

Questions can be raised as to when to evaluate whether re–cross-linking would be necessary and which protocol to use, especially owing not only to long-term reactivation of progression, but also to immediate treatment failures occurring as early as 6 months after the procedure.[69,70] Although there is no consensus, 6 months after CXL seems to be an adequate time to reconsider a new procedure, in the rare event of a treatment failure. Moreover, repeating CXL very early after the first procedure is unlikely to increase corneal stiffness any further, as has been shown in *in vivo* studies.[71] Finally, it is interesting to mention that there is an absence of complete agreement between corneal imaging devices, especially in highly aberrated keratoconic corneas.[72] There remains the lack of an ideal metric for comparing and monitoring patients using topographers and tomographers available on the market today,[46,72] although technologies like optical coherence tomography-based devices may help better assess the success in the future.

References

1. Torres Netto EA, Al-Otaibi WM, Hafezi NL, et al. Prevalence of keratoconus in paediatric patients in Riyadh, Saudi Arabia. *Br J Ophthalmol*. 2018;102(10):1436–1441. doi:10.1016/s0002-9394(02)02220-1.
2. Kennedy RH, Bourne WM, Dyer JA. A 48-year clinical and epidemiologic study of keratoconus. *Am J Ophthalmol*. 1986;101(3):267–273. doi:10.1016/0002-9394(86)90817-2.
3. Spörl E, Huhle M, Kasper M, Seiler T. [Increased rigidity of the cornea caused by intrastromal cross-linking]. *Ophthalmologe*. 1997;94(12):902–906. doi:10.1007/s003470050219.
4. Wollensak G, Spoerl E, Seiler T. Riboflavin/ultraviolet-a-induced collagen crosslinking for the treatment of keratoconus. *Am J Ophthalmol*. 2003;135(5):620–627. doi:10.1016/s0002-9394(02)02220-1.
5. Gomes JA, Rapuano CJ, Belin MW, Ambrósio Jr. R. Group of Panelists for the Global Delphi Panel of Keratoconus and Ectatic Diseases. Global Consensus on Keratoconus Diagnosis. *Cornea*. 2015;34(12):e38–e39. doi:10.1097/ICO.0000000000000623.
6. Randleman JB, Khandelwal SS, Hafezi F. Corneal cross-linking. *Surv Ophthalmol*. 2015;60(6):509–523. doi:10.1016/j.survophthal.2015.04.002.
7. Steinberg J, Katz T, Mousli A, et al. Corneal biomechanical changes after crosslinking for progressive keratoconus with the corneal visualization Scheimpflug technology. *J Ophthalmol*. 2014;2014:579190. doi:10.1155/2014/579190.
8. Ortiz D, Piñero D, Shabayek MH, Arnalich-Montiel F, Alió JL. Corneal biomechanical properties in normal, post-laser in situ keratomileusis, and keratoconic eyes. *J Cataract Refract Surg*. 2007;33(8):1371–1375. doi:10.1016/j.jcrs.2007.04.021.
9. Andreassen TT, Simonsen AH, Oxlund H. Biomechanical properties of keratoconus and normal corneas. *Exp Eye Res*. 1980;31(4):435–441. doi:10.1016/s0014-4835(80)80027-3.
10. Hayes S, Kamma-Lorger CS, Boote C, et al. The effect of riboflavin/UVA collagen cross-linking therapy on the structure and hydrodynamic behaviour of the ungulate and rabbit corneal stroma. *PLoS One*. 2013;8(1):e52860. doi:10.1371/journal.pone.0052860.
11. Wollensak G, Spörl E, Seiler T. [Treatment of keratoconus by collagen cross linking]. *Ophthalmologe*. 2003;100(1):44–49. doi:10.1007/s00347-002-0700-3.
12. Hafezi F, Kanellopoulos J, Wiltfang R, Seiler T. Corneal collagen crosslinking with riboflavin and ultraviolet A to treat induced keratectasia after laser in situ keratomileusis. *J Cataract Refract Surg*. 2007;33(12):2035–2040. doi:10.1016/j.jcrs.2007.07.028.
13. Raiskup F, Theuring A, Pillunat LE, Spoerl E. Corneal collagen crosslinking with riboflavin and ultraviolet-A light in progressive keratoconus: ten-year results. *J Cataract Refract Surg*. 2015;41(1):41–46. doi:10.1016/j.jcrs.2014.09.033.
14. Sandvik GF, Thorsrud A, Råen M, Østern AE, Sæthre M M, Drolsum L. Does corneal collagen cross-linking reduce the need for keratoplasties in patients with keratoconus?. *Cornea*. 2015;34(9):991–995. doi:10.1097/ICO.0000000000000460.
15. Godefrooij DA, Gans R, Imhof SM, Wisse RP. Nationwide reduction in the number of corneal transplantations for keratoconus following the implementation of cross-linking. *Acta Ophthalmol*. 2016;94(7):675–678. doi:10.1111/aos.13095.
16. Richoz O, Mavrakanas N, Pajic B, Hafezi F. Corneal collagen cross-linking for ectasia after LASIK and photorefractive keratectomy: long-term results. *Ophthalmology*. 2013;120(7):1354–1359. doi:10.1016/j.ophtha.2012.12.027.

17. Hassan Z, Nemeth G, Modis L, Szalai E, Berta A. Collagen cross-linking in the treatment of pellucid marginal degeneration. *Indian J Ophthalmol.* 2014;62(3):367–370. doi:10.4103/0301-4738.109523.
18. Spadea L. Corneal collagen cross-linking with riboflavin and UVA irradiation in pellucid marginal degeneration. *J Refract Surg.* 2010;26(5):375–377. doi:10.3928/1081597X-20100114-03.
19. Bailey AJ, Paul RG, Knott L. Mechanisms of maturation and ageing of collagen. *Mech Ageing Dev.* 1998;106(1-2):1–56. doi:10.1016/s0047-6374(98)00119-5.
20. Chatzis N, Hafezi F. Progression of keratoconus and efficacy of corneal collagen cross-linking in children and adolescents. *J Refract Surg.* 2012;28(11):753–758. doi:10.3928/1081597X-20121011-01.
21. Tabibian D, de Tejada BM, Gatzioufas Z, et al. Pregnancy-induced changes in corneal biomechanics and topography are thyroid hormone related. *Am J Ophthalmol.* 2017;184:129–136. doi:10.1016/j.ajo.2017.10.001.
22. Lee R, Hafezi F, Randleman JB. Bilateral keratoconus induced by secondary hypothyroidism after radioactive iodine therapy. *J Refract Surg.* 2018;34(5):351–353. doi:10.3928/1081597X-20171031-02.
23. McMonnies CW, Boneham GC. Keratoconus, allergy, itch, eye-rubbing and hand-dominance. *Clin Exp Optom.* 2003;86(6):376–384. doi:10.1111/j.1444-0938.2003.tb03082.x.
24. Bilgihan K, Hondur A, Sul S, Ozturk S. Pregnancy-induced progression of keratoconus. *Cornea.* 2011;30(9):991–994. doi:10.1097/ICO.0b013e3182068adc.
25. Hoogewoud F, Gatzioufas Z, Hafezi F. Transitory topographical variations in keratoconus during pregnancy. *J Refract Surg.* 2013;29(2):144–146. doi:10.3928/1081597X-20130117-11.
26. Mackensen F, Paulus WE, Max R, Ness T. Ocular changes during pregnancy. *Dtsch Arztebl Int.* 2014;111(33–34):567–575. doi:10.3238/arztebl.2014.0567.
27. Torres-Netto EA, Randleman JB, Hafezi NL, Hafezi F. Late-onset progression of keratoconus after therapy with selective tissue estrogenic activity regulator. *J Cataract Refract Surg.* 2019;45(1):101–104. doi:10.1016/j.jcrs.2018.08.036.
28. Mazzotta C, Traversi C, Baiocchi S, et al. Corneal collagen cross-linking with riboflavin and ultraviolet A light for pediatric keratoconus: ten-year results. *Cornea.* 2018;37(5):560–566. doi:10.1097/ICO.0000000000001505.
29. Malik NS, Moss SJ, Ahmed N, Furth AJ, Wall RS, Meek KM. Ageing of the human corneal stroma: structural and biochemical changes. *Biochim Biophys Acta.* 1992;1138(3):222–228. doi:10.1016/0925-4439(92)90041-k.
30. Dahl BJ, Spotts E, Truong JQ. Corneal collagen cross-linking: an introduction and literature review. *Optometry.* 2012;83(1):33–42. doi:10.1016/j.optm.2011.09.011.
31. Richoz O, Hammer A, Tabibian D, Gatzioufas Z, Hafezi F. The biomechanical effect of corneal collagen cross-linking (CXL) with riboflavin and UV-A is oxygen dependent. *Transl Vis Sci Technol.* 2013;2(7):6. doi:10.1167/tvst.2.7.6.
32. Torres-Netto EA, Kling S, Hafezi N, Vinciguerra P, Randleman JB, Hafezi F. Oxygen diffusion may limit the biomechanical effectiveness of iontophoresis-assisted transepithelial corneal cross-linking. *J Refract Surg.* 2018;34(11):768–774. doi:10.3928/1081597X-20180830-01.
33. Kling S, Richoz O, Hammer A, et al. Increased biomechanical efficacy of corneal cross-linking in thin corneas due to higher oxygen availability. *J Refract Surg.* 2015;31(12):840–846. doi:10.3928/1081597X-20151111-08.
34. Hammer A, Richoz O, Mosquera S, Tabibian D, Hoogewoud F, Hafezi F. Corneal biomechanical properties at different corneal collagen cross-linking (CXL) irradiances. *Invest Ophthalmol Vis Sci.* 2014;55(5):2881–2884. doi:10.1167/iovs.13-13748.
35. Kling S, Hammer A, Netto EAT, Hafezi F. Differential gene transcription of extracellular matrix components in response to in vivo corneal crosslinking (CXL) in rabbit corneas. *Transl Vis Sci Technol.* 2017;6(6):8. doi:10.1167/tvst.6.6.8.
36. Ng AL, Chan TC, Cheng AC. Conventional versus accelerated corneal collagen cross-linking in the treatment of keratoconus. *Clin Experiment Ophthalmol.* 2016;44(1):8–14. doi:10.1111/ceo.12571.
37. Hashemi H, Miraftab M, Seyedian MA, et al. Long-term results of an accelerated corneal cross-linking protocol (18 mW/cm) for the treatment of progressive keratoconus. *Am J Ophthalmol.* 2015;160(6):1164–1170.e1. doi:10.1016/j.ajo.2015.08.027.
38. Gatzioufas Z, Raiskup F, O'Brart D, Spoerl E, Panos GD, Hafezi F. Transepithelial corneal cross-linking using an enhanced riboflavin solution. *J Refract Surg.* 2016;32(6):372–377. doi:10.3928/1081597X-20160428-02.

39. Soeters N, Wisse RP, Godefrooij DA, Imhof SM, Tahzib NG. Transepithelial versus epithelium-off corneal cross-linking for the treatment of progressive keratoconus: a randomized controlled trial. *Am J Ophthalmol.* 2015;159(5):821–828.e823. doi:10.1016/j.ajo.2015.02.005.

40. Caporossi A, Mazzotta C, Paradiso AL, Baiocchi S, Marigliani D, Caporossi T. Transepithelial corneal collagen crosslinking for progressive keratoconus: 24-month clinical results. *J Cataract Refract Surg.* 2013;39(8):1157–1163. doi:10.1016/j.jcrs.2013.03.026.

41. Zhang ZY, Zhang XR. Efficacy and safety of transepithelial corneal collagen crosslinking. *J Cataract Refract Surg.* 2012;38(7):1304. author reply 1304–1305. doi:10.1016/j.jcrs.2012.05.012.

42. Seiler T, Randleman JB, Vinciguerra P, Hafezi F. Corneal crosslinking without epithelial removal. *J Cataract Refract Surg.* 2019;45(6):891–892. doi:10.1016/j.jcrs.2019.01.042.

43. Kolozsvari L, Nogradi A, Hopp B, Bor Z. UV absorbance of the human cornea in the 240- to 400-nm range. *Invest Ophthalmol Vis Sci.* 2002;43(7):2165–2168.

44. Freeman RD. Oxygen consumption by the component layers of the cornea. *J Physiol.* 1972;225(1):15–32. doi:10.1113/jphysiol.1972.sp009927.

45. Mastropasqua L, Nubile M, Calienno R, et al. Corneal cross-linking: intrastromal riboflavin concentration in iontophoresis-assisted imbibition versus traditional and transepithelial techniques. *Am J Ophthalmol.* 2014;157(3):623–630.e621. doi:10.1016/j.ajo.2013.11.018.

46. Lang PZ, Hafezi NL, Khandelwal SS, Torres-Netto EA, Hafezi F, Randleman JB. Comparative functional outcomes after corneal crosslinking using standard, accelerated, and accelerated with higher total fluence protocols. *Cornea.* 2019;38(4):433–441. doi:10.1016/j.jcrs.2013.03.026.

47. Mazzotta C, Bagaglia SA, Vinciguerra R, Ferrise M, Vinciguerra P. Enhanced-fluence pulsed-light iontophoresis corneal cross-linking: 1-year morphological and clinical results. *J Refract Surg.* 2018;34(7):438–444. doi:10.3928/1081597X-20180515-02.

48. Seiler TG, Fischinger I, Koller T, Zapp D, Frueh BE, Seiler T. Customized corneal crosslinking - one year results. *Am J Ophthalmol.* 2016;166:14–21. doi:10.3928/1081597X-20161206-01.

49. Kling S, Hafezi F. An algorithm to predict the biomechanical stiffening effect in corneal cross-linking. *J Refract Surg.* 2017;33(2):128–136. doi:10.3928/1081597X-20161206-01.

50. Abdshahzadeh H, Gilardoni F, Torres-Netto EA, Kling S, Hafezi N, Hafezi F. Individualized corneal-crosslinking in ultra-thin corneas - 2 year follow-up. Paper presented at: European Society for Cataract and Refractive Surgery (ESCRS)2020; Marrakech, Morocco.

51. Spoerl E, Raiskup-Wolf F, Kuhlisch E, Pillunat LE. Cigarette smoking is negatively associated with keratoconus. *J Refract Surg.* 2008;24(7):S737–S740. doi:10.3928/1081597X-20080901-18.

52. Raiskup-Wolf F, Hoyer A, Spoerl E, Pillunat LE. Collagen crosslinking with riboflavin and ultraviolet-A light in keratoconus: long-term results. *J Cataract Refract Surg.* 2008;34(5):796–801. doi:10.1016/j.jcrs.2007.12.039.

53. Torres-Netto EA, Seiler T, Adamcik S, Gilardoni F, Abdshahzadeh H, Hafezi F. Corneal cross-linking for progressive keratoconus: 10-year outcomes. Paper presented at: European Society for Cataract and Refractive Surgery (ESCRS)2020; Marrakech, Morocco.

54. Spoerl E, Hoyer A, Pillunat LE, Raiskup F. Corneal cross-linking and safety issues. *Open Ophthalmol J.* 2011;5:14–16. doi:10.2174/1874364101105010014.

55. Seiler TG, Batista A, Frueh BE, Koenig K. Riboflavin concentrations at the endothelium during corneal cross-linking in humans. *Invest Ophthalmol Vis Sci.* 2019;60(6):2140–2145. doi:10.1167/iovs.19-26686.

56. Richoz O, Tabibian D, Hammer A, Majo F, Nicolas M, Hafezi F. The effect of standard and high-fluence corneal cross-linking (CXL) on cornea and limbus. *Invest Ophthalmol Vis Sci.* 2014;55(9):5783–5787. doi:10.1167/iovs.14-14695.

57. O'Brart DPS. Corneal collagen crosslinking for corneal ectasias: a review. *Eur J Ophthalmol.* 2017;27(3):253–269. doi:10.5301/ejo.5000916.

58. Knyazer B, Krakauer Y, Tailakh MA, et al. Accelerated corneal cross-linking as an adjunct therapy in the management of presumed bacterial keratitis: a cohort study. *J Refract Surg.* 2020;36(4):258–264. doi:10.3928/1081597X-20200226-02.

59. Kling S, Hufschmid FS, Torres-Netto EA, et al. High fluence increases the antibacterial efficacy of PACK cross-linking. *Cornea.* 2020;39(8):1020–1026. doi:10.1097/ICO.0000000000002335.

60. Steinwender G, Pertl L, El-Shabrawi Y, Ardjomand N. Complications from corneal cross-linking for keratoconus in pediatric patients. *J Refract Surg.* 2016;32(1):68–69. doi:10.3928/1081597X-20151210-03.

61. Dhawan S, Rao K, Natrajan S. Complications of corneal collagen cross-linking. *J Ophthalmol.* 2011;2011:869015. doi:10.1155/2011/869015.

62. Angunawela RI, Arnalich-Montiel F, Allan BD. Peripheral sterile corneal infiltrates and melting after collagen crosslinking for keratoconus. *J Cataract Refract Surg.* 2009;35(3):606–607. doi:10.1016/j.jcrs.2008.11.050.

63. Hafezi F, Koller T, Vinciguerra P, Seiler T. Marked remodelling of the anterior corneal surface following collagen cross-linking with riboflavin and UVA. *Br J Ophthalmol.* 2011;95(8):1171–1172. doi:10.1136/bjo.2010.184978.

64. Raiskup F, Hoyer A, Spoerl E. Permanent corneal haze after riboflavin-UVA-induced cross-linking in keratoconus. *J Refract Surg.* 2009;25(9):S824–S828. doi:10.3928/1081597X-20090813-12.

65. Caporossi A, Mazzotta C, Baiocchi S, Caporossi T. Long-term results of riboflavin ultraviolet A corneal collagen cross-linking for keratoconus in Italy: the Siena eye cross study. *Am J Ophthalmol.* 2010;149(4):585–593. doi:10.1016/j.ajo.2009.10.021.

66. Noor IH, Seiler TG, Noor K, Seiler T. Continued long-term flattening after corneal cross-linking for keratoconus. *Journal of Refractive Surgery.* 2018;34(8):567–570. doi:10.3928/1081597X-20180607-01.

67. de Almeida Ferreira G, Coral Ghanem V, Coral Ghanem R. Late progressive corneal flattening, haze and visual loss after eccentric crosslinking for pellucid marginal degeneration. *Am J Ophthalmol Case Rep.* 2020;18:100621. doi:10.1016/j.ajoc.2020.100621.

68. Koller T, Mrochen M, Seiler T. Complication and failure rates after corneal crosslinking. *J Cataract Refract Surg.* 2009;35(8):1358–1362. doi:10.1016/j.jcrs.2009.03.035.

69. Akkaya Turhan S, Aydin FO, Toker E. Clinical results of repeated corneal collagen cross-linking in progressive keratoconus. *Cornea.* 2020;39(1):84–87. doi:10.1097/ico.0000000000002128.

70. Hafezi F, Tabibian D, Richoz O. Additive effect of repeated corneal collagen cross-linking in keratoconus. *J Refract Surg.* 2014;30(10):716–718. doi:10.3928/1081597X-20140903-03.

71. Tabibian D, Kling S, Hammer A, Richoz O, Hafezi F. Repeated cross-linking after a short time does not provide any additional biomechanical stiffness in the mouse cornea in vivo. *J Refract Surg.* 2017;33(1):56–60. doi:10.3928/1081597X-20161006-02.

72. Piccinini AL, Golan O, Torres-Netto EA, Hafezi F, Randleman JB. Corneal higher-order aberrations measurements: comparison between Scheimpflug and dual Scheimpflug-Placido technology in keratoconic eyes. *J Cataract Refract Surg.* 2019;45(7):985–991. doi:10.1016/j.jcrs.2019.02.005.

CHAPTER 28

Corneal Collagen Cross-Linking in Pediatric Patients with Keratoconus

Maria A. Henriquez

KEY CONCEPTS

Patients at risk of progression

- Younger age (less than 17 years old)
- Maximum keratometry greater than 55 D at time of diagnosis
- Family history
- Connective tissue disorders, Down syndrome, Leber congenital amaurosis
- Eye rubbing
- Inflammation.

Keratoconus in a child

- More aggressive and active
- Progresses rapidly
- Already at advanced stages when diagnosed.

Transepithelial CXL versus epi-off CXL

- TE-CXL is an option that minimizes the risks associated with epithelial debridement.
- Both can halt the progression of keratoconus
- Epi-off corneal cross-linking (CXL) shows higher flattening effect and slower progression rate after procedure.

Introduction

Keratoconus (KC) is an illness that affects corneas in the first three decades of life.[1,2] KC may progress aggressively and rapidly in the pediatric population. Unfortunately it is diagnosed at advanced stages in a significant percentage of cases. Almost 30% of cases are diagnosed when the disease is at stage IV,[1–4] and advanced KC cases progress more rapidly and severely.[5] When KC is diagnosed in a child, it is usually more severe and with greater risk of progression than when it is first diagnosed in an adult. Management in the child should, therefore, be more aggressive.

In a review of 2650 patients that required corneal transplantation over a 13-year follow-up period that, ectasia and thinning represented the most common indications for corneal transplantation.[6] Collagen corneal cross-linking (CXL) should be considered early in children, to avoid a corneal transplantation as there is a higher incidence of complications, such as allograft rejection and glaucoma, in this population.[7,8] It is, therefore, important to halt the progression of KC in the child, given that more than 80% of the pediatric KC patients progress without treatment, compared with the 20% to 35% who progress after CXL.[5,9,10]

In a hypothetical model, an analysis of cost-effectiveness showed early CXL demonstrated superiority when compared with penetrating keratoplasty. The 10-year effect after early treatment with CXL would provide a net increase in quality-adjusted life years and an increase in cost-effectiveness ratios compared with standard management.[11]

CXL in Children

Corneal collagen cross-linking was approved for progressive KC and post-LASIK ectasia in 2016. It is currently the only US Food and Drug Administration (FDA)-approved treatment available to halt the progression of KC, but it has not been approved in children. However, to date, there are at least 20 published articles documenting the use of CXL in children with more than 10 years follow-up. The application of CXL in the child should be preceded by a careful assessment of risks and benefits based on the principles of the Declaration of Helsinki.

Epi-Off CXL (Dresden Protocol)

The Dresden protocol, also called standard epi-off CXL, is used in adults and children. The corneal epithelium is removed manually or with a laser over the central 9 mm; riboflavin solution is then applied every 5 minutes for 30 minutes, and finally an ultraviolet A (UVA) irradiation is performed for 30 minutes (3 mW/cm^2) in conjunction with continued riboflavin application. The riboflavin used for this procedure is the so-called isotonic riboflavin that is composed of 0.1% riboflavin and 20% dextran. However, when corneal thickness is less than 350 to 400 μm, hypotonic riboflavin can be used in children as well. This procedure has provided excellent results, with the longest registered follow-up available in the literature.

In the vast majority of the studies, uncorrected and/or best-corrected visual acuity (UCVA and BCVA, respectively) demonstrated statistically significant improvement. KC stabilization was achieved in nearly 65% to 100% of the cases, and there was a mean reduction in keratometric readings of 1 to 2 diopters (D). Table 28.1 shows the results of studies using epi-off CXL in children.

Henriquez et al, published results of the epi-off procedure with follow-up of up to 5 years, in 46 eyes of 46 patients under 18 years of age (range 10–17), and found that KC was stopped in 100% of cases, with an average reduction in mean keratometry of 3.18 +/- 5.17 D and significant improvement in the BCVA.[30] In a prospective study of 47 keratoconic patients younger than 18 years old, with a follow-up of 10 years, Mazzotta et al.[4] found KC stability in nearly 80% of the patients. There was significant improvement in the UCVA, BCVA, and maximum keratometry readings from the sixth month of treatment until the eighth year of follow-up. After the eighth postoperative year, they noted that the maximum keratometry improvement had lost its statistical significance. Only 4.35% of the patients needed a corneal graft due to KC progression.

Based on the current literature, we can say that CXL is effective in halting the progression of KC at least at 8 years of follow-up.

Transepithelial CXL

Transepithelial corneal collagen cross-linking (TE-CXL), usually termed epi-on CXL, has been used in children in the same way as it is used in adults.[16,24,27,29–36] It is based on the use of a specially formulated riboflavin solution that enhances passage through intact epithelium, thereby avoiding the need for epithelial debridement. The theoretical basis of TE-CXL lies in the use of a hydrophilic macromolecule such as riboflavin that penetrates intact corneal epithelium, avoiding the need for epithelial debridement.

TABLE 28.1 ■ Standard Epi-Off CXL in Pediatric Patients

Author, Year	Age (Years)	No Eyes	Follow-Up (Months)	Significant Improvement	Significant Worsening K Readings	Irradiation Time/Energy	Adverse Effects	Comparative Study	Randomized Study
Chatzis and Hafezi,[1] 2012	9–19	46	26.3	BCVA	No	30' (3 mW/cm²)	No	No	No
Caporossi et al.,[13] 2012	10–18	77	36	K, asymmetry index	No	30' (3 mW/cm²)	No	Subgroup analysis	No
Vinciguerra et al.,[14] 2012	9–18	40	24	UCVA, BCVA, coma and spherical aberrations	No	30' (3 mW/cm²)	No	No	No
Zotta et al.,[15] 2012	11–16	8	36	VA	No	30' (3 mW/cm²)	No	No	No
Magli et al.,[16] 2013	12–18	19	12	K, SAI, I-S, IHA, AE	No	30' (3 mW/cm²)	Corneal edema	Epi-off vs. TE-CXL	No
Viswanathan et al.,[17] 2014	8–17	25	20	K	No	30' (3 mW/cm²)	No	No	No
McAnena and O'Keefe,[18] 2015	13–18	25	12	BCVA	No	4' (30 mw/cm²)	No	No	No
Uçakhan et al.,[19] 2016	10–18	40	48	BCVA, K$_{max}$	No	30' (3 mW/cm²)	No	No	No
Wise et al.,[20] 2016	11–18	39	12	No	No	30' (3 mW/cm²)	No	No	No
Godefrooij et al.,[21] 2016	11–17	54	12	BCVA, K	No	30' (3 mW/cm²)	No	No	No
Ulusoy et al.,[22] 2016	<18	28	17	BCVA, K	No	10' (9 mW/cm²)	No	Subgroup analysis	No
Sarac et al.,[23] 2016	9–17	72	24	UCVA	No	30' (3 mW/cm²)	No	Subgroup analysis	No

Continued on following page

TABLE 28.1 ■ Standard Epi-Off CXL in Pediatric Patients (Continued)

Author, Year	Age (Years)	No Eyes	Follow-Up (Months)	Significant Improvement	Significant Worsening K Readings	Irradiation Time/Energy	Adverse Effects	Comparative Study	Randomized Study
Henriquez et al.,[24] 2017	12–15	25	12	BCVA	No	30' (3 mW/cm^2)	No	TE accelerate vs. epi-off	No
Padmanabhan et al.,[25] 2017	8–18	194	42	BCVA, topographic ast	No	30' (3 mW/cm^2)	No	No	No
Zotta et al.[26] 2017	10–17	20	91	K, topographic cylinder	No	30' (3 mW/cm^2)	No	No	No
Eraslan et al.,[27] 2017	12–18	18	24	BCVA, K	No	30' (3 mW/cm^2)	No	Epi-on vs. epi-off	No
Henriquez et al.,[12] 2018	10–17	26	36	BCVA	No	30' (3 mW/cm^2)	No	No	No
Mazzotta et al.,[4] 2018	<18	62	120	UCVA, BCVA	No	30' (3 mW/cm^2)	No	No	
Sarac et al.,[28] 2018	10–17	87	24	UCVA (accelerate CXL)	No	30' (3 mW/cm^2) and 10' (9 mW/cm^2)	Corneal haze	Mechanical vs. PTK epithelial removal	No
Buzzonetti et al.[29] 2019	9–18	20	36	BCVA	No	30' (3 mW/cm^2)	20% corneal haze, resolved without sequelae	I-CXL TE vs. epi-off CXL	No
Henriquez et al.,[30] 2020	10–17	46	60	BCVA, cylinder, K, asphericity	No	30' (3 mW/cm^2)	No	TE accelerate vs. epi-off	No

AE, Anterior elevation; Ast, astigmatism; BCVA, best-corrected visual acuity; CXL, corneal cross-linking; I, iontophoretic; IHA, index of height asymmetry; I-S, inferior-superior symmetry index; K, keratometries; Kmax, maximum keratometry; PTK, phototherapeutic keratectomy; SAI, surface asymmetry index; TE, transepithelial; UCVA, uncorrected visual acuity.

In children, trometamol and sodium, ethylenediaminetetraacetic acid (EDTA), and benzalkonium chloride have been used in association with riboflavin as enhancing substances with no associated adverse effects. Table 28.2 shows the results of the studies using TE-CXL in children.

TE-CXL is a promising procedure for the pediatric population, because it avoids de-epithelization, resulting in more rapid recovery, less pain on the first postoperative day, and fewer complications.[16] In selected cases, there is no need for general anesthesia, since corneal de-epithelization is not performed, and there is significantly less stress for the patient. There is, nonetheless, limited literature available to claim similar effectiveness between TE-CXL and epi-off procedures.[16,24,27,29,30]

Our group recently published the results of a prospective, nonrandomized study including 78 eyes of patients younger than 18 years old, in which accelerated epi-on TE-CXL (5 minutes of irradiation at 18 mW/cm^2) was applied in 32 eyes compared with a standard epi-off CXL in 46 eyes with a follow-up of 1 and 5 years.[33] We found no significant changes in the UCVA at 1-year and 5-year follow-up in both groups. Epi-off CXL halted the progression of KC in 100% of the cases, compared with 90.63% of the cases in the accelerated TE-CXL. In the epi-off group, there was no loss of BCVA lines. However, in the accelerated TE-CXL group, there was a loss of BCVA lines in three of the three eyes that progressed. For the epi-off group, flat, steep, and maximum keratometry did not demonstrate significant changes at 1-year postoperatively. However, at 5 years, all patients demonstrated significant flattening. For the accelerated TE-CXL group, flat, steep, maximum, and mean keratometry did not demonstrate significant changes at 1-year or 5-years postoperation.[33] The rate of patients with flattening of the maximum keratometry greater than or equal to 2 D at 5 years postoperative was 43.47% in the epi-off group and 12.5% in the accelerated TE-CXL group. Fig. 28.1 shows a case after accelerated transepithelial CXL that experienced an increase in maximum keratometry of 3 D at 5 years of follow-up.

Magli et al.,[16] in a comparative nonrandomized study, found no significant differences between epi-off and TE-CXL (irradiation time 30 minutes/3 mW/cm^2) in terms of minimum and maximum keratometry, astigmatism, anterior elevation at the thinnest location and at the apex, at 1 year of follow-up.

Unfortunately, to date, there is no randomized published literature that demonstrates the superiority of one procedure over the other in children. In adults, there is a single randomized study that shows superiority of the epi-off procedure for halting the progression of KC at 24 months when compared with TE-CXL. The riboflavin used in the TE-CXL group was composed of riboflavin 0.25%, hydroxypropyl methylcellulose (HPMC) 1.2%, benzalkonium chloride 0.01% (Peschke MedioCross TE, Peschke Trade GmbH, Hünenberg, Switzerland), instilled every 2 minutes for the duration of a 60-minute treatment alternated every other minute with instillation of topical proparacaine 0.5% containing benzalkonium chloride 0.01%. Subjects in the epi-off CXL group demonstrated a greater improvement in keratometry compared with subjects in the TE-CXL group, but no statistically significant difference in BCVA between groups.[37]

Further evaluation with long-term follow-up is necessary to evaluate both procedures in children. However, currently both procedures are capable of halting the progression of KC. Epi-off CXL performs at a significantly higher degree of efficacy and with a greater flattening effect than accelerated TE-CXL procedure.

There are cases where corneal debridement is a significant challenge in the pediatric patient, for example, in younger children and in those with developmental delay or when general anesthesia is not available. Moreover, the fact that epi-off CXL appears to be more effective in flattening keratometry reading when compared with TE-CXL should be considered, for example, in cases with steeper corneas that would benefit from greater flattening effects, and in patients with mild KC where stabilization of the K readings or lower flattening effects are desired.

TABLE 28.2 ■ Transepithelial Corneal Collagen Cross-Linking in Pediatric Patients

Author, Year	Age	No Eyes	Follow-Up (Months)	Significant Improvement	Significant Worsening K Readings	Irradiation Time (Energy)	Adverse Effects	Riboflavin Used	Comparative Study	Randomized Study
Buzzonetti and Petrocelli,[31] 2012	8–18	13	18	BCVA	Yes	30' (3 mW/cm²)	No	Ricrolin TE[a]	No	No
Magli et al.,[16] 2013	12–18	14	12	K, AE, corneal SI	No	30' (3 mW/cm²)	No	Ricrolin TE; Sooft[b]	Epi-off vs. TE-CXL	No
Salman,[32] 2013	13–18	22	12	UDVA, K apex, AE, TP	No	30' (3 mW/cm²)	Epithelial defect, transient hyperemia mild foreign-body sensation	TE riboflavin[c]	TE-CXL vs. conservative treatment	No
Buzzonetti et al.,[33] 2015	10–18	14	15	BCVA	No	9'(10 mW/cm²)	No	Ricrolin+[b]	No	No
Salman,[34] 2016	<18	22	12	UCVA, K_{max}, peak 1, peak 2	No	30' (3 mW/cm²)	No	Ricrolin TE Sooft[b]	No	No
Magli et al.,[35] 2016	11–18	13	18	UCVA, BCVA, ISV, KI	No	9' (10 mW/cm²)	No	Ricrolin+ Sooft	I-TE-CXL general vs. topic anesthesia	No
Henriquez et al.,[24] 2017	8–16	36	12	None	No	5' (18 mW/cm²)	No	TE riboflavin[d]	Epi-off vs. accelerate TE-CXL	No
Eraslan et al.,[27] 2017	12–18	18	24	BCVA	Yes	30' (3 mW/cm²)	No	TE riboflavin[d]	Epi-off vs. epi-on	No

TABLE 28.2 ■ Transepithelial Corneal Collagen Cross-Linking in Pediatric Patients (Continued)

Author, Year	Age	No Eyes	Follow-Up (Months)	Significant Improvement	Significant Worsening K Readings	Irradiation Time (Energy)	Adverse Effects	Riboflavin Used	Comparative Study	Randomized Study
Tian et al.,[36] 2018	14.44 ± 1.98	18	12	None	No	5' 20" (365-nm UV-A light and 45 mW/cm² (pulsed mode)	No	ParaCel solution^e/VibeX Xtra solution^d	No	No
Buzzonetti et al.,[29] 2019	9–18	20	36	No	Yes	9'(10 mW/cm²)	45% superficial punctate	Ricrolin+^a	I-TE-CXL vs. epi-off CXL	No
Henriquez et al.,[30] 2020	8–16	32	60	Asphericity, BCVA	No	5' (18 mW/cm²)	No	TE riboflavin^d	Epi-off vs. accelerate TE	No

[a] Enhanced riboflavin solution: 0.1% riboflavin containing trometamol (tris-hydroxymethylaminomethane) and sodium EDTA as excipients.
[b] Ricrolin+; Sooft: a hypoosmolar riboflavin 0.1% dextran-free solution enriched with ethylenediaminetetraacetic acid and tromethamine.
[c] Transepithelial riboflavin: 0.1% riboflavin + ethylenediaminetetraacetic acid (EDTA) disodium salt.
[d] Transepithelial riboflavin solution: 0.25% hydroxypropyl methylcellulose, 1.2% hydroxypropyl methylcellulose, and 0.01% benzalkonium chloride (MedioCross TE; Peschke Medio-Haus Medizinprodukte GmbH).
[e] ParaCel solution: 0.25% riboflavin-5-phosphate, hydroxylpropyl methylcellulose, NaCl, ethylenediaminetetraaceticacid, Tris, and benzalkonium chloride. VibeX Xtra solution: riboflavin phosphate 2.80 mg/mL and NaCl, Avedro, Inc.

AE, Anterior elevation; *BCVA,* best-corrected visual acuity; *epi-off,* epithelium off; *I,* iontophoretic; *ISV,* index of surface variance; *K,* keratometry; *KI,* keratoconus index; *Max,* maximum, *Peak 1,* amplitude of the first peak (mmHg); *Peak 2,* amplitude of the second peak (mmHg) del ORA (Ocular Response Analyzer); *SI,* surface index; *TE,* transepithelial; *TP,* thinnest point.

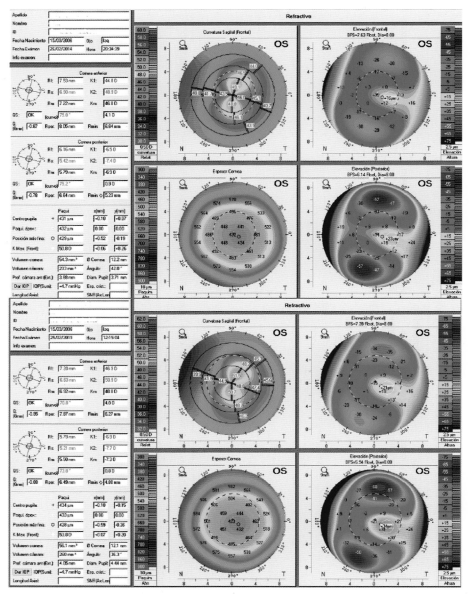

Fig. 28.1 Progression of case after accelerated transepithelial corneal cross-linking at 5 years of follow-up having a K$_{max}$ increase of 3 D.

IONTOPHORESIS

Iontophoresis is a method that can be used in addition to TE-CXL, to facilitate the penetration of riboflavin through an intact tissue in the presence of a low-intensity electric field. The low-intensity electric flow allows the penetration of riboflavin into the cornea in only 5 minutes versus the 30 minutes required by passive imbibition. Table 28.2 demonstrates the results of iontophoresis in association with CXL in children. The riboflavin used for this type of procedure is designed specifically for iontophoresis (I-CXL) and commonly uses two enhancers: ethylenediaminetetraacetic acid and tromethamine. The results of this procedure differ in currently available studies. In a comparative study using iontophoretic TE-CXL versus epi-off CXL Buzzonetti and Petrocelli[31] found significant worsening of the keratometry reading in the iontophoresis TE-CXL group at 3 years of follow-up. Magli et al.,[35] however, at 18 months of follow-up, found a significant improvement in the UCVA, BCVA, the index of surface variance, and the KC index using I-CXL, but no significant changes on K readings.

ACCELERATED CORNEAL COLLAGEN CROSS-LINKING

Accelerated CXL uses a different energy and UVA irradiation exposure time to shorten the duration of the procedure. In 10 minutes of irradiation, this method uses 9 mW/cm and in 5 minutes of irradiation it uses 18 mW/cm. Both have been used in children in association with epi-off (Dresden protocol) or TE-CXL (see Tables 28.1 and 28.2). Different results between authors have been published to date; some found significant improvement in keratometry readings using 10 or 5 minutes of irradiation,[16,33] with follow-up to 18 months. However, others did not find significant improvement in either variable[29,30] with up to 5 years of follow-up. Sarac et al.,[28] in a comparative study using standard epi-off and accelerated epi-off CXL, found significant improvement in UCVA in the accelerated epi-off group at 24 months of follow-up. Our group reported the results of a comparative study using accelerated TE-CXL versus epi-off CXL and found that despite no differences at 1 year of follow-up, at 5 years of follow-up there were significant differences in terms of keratometric flattening and pachymetry.[30]

Despite the interest in this modality of CXL for children, which, by shortening the irradiation period from 30 minutes to 5 minutes, makes the procedure easier and avoids general anesthesia, randomized studies are necessary to determine its efficacy in stopping the progression of KC in children.

COMPLICATIONS AFTER CXL

Corneal collagen cross-linking is a safe procedure. Loss of lines of vision is usually related to treatment failure and, therefore, to disease progression. This occurs in approximately 20% to 35% of cases. If we remember that the progression of KC in children without treatment is approximately 80% of the cases, we may conclude that CXL is an acceptable risk. Long-term studies have showed its safety in terms of endothelial cell count and macular thickness at 5 and 10 years of follow-up.[25,30,38]

The most common adverse effect found after CXL is haze that can occur in up to 20% of cases. However, this haze is a temporary adverse effect that resolves without sequelae with the use of topical corticosteroids. Other adverse effects include epithelial defects, transient hyperemia, mild foreign-body sensation, and superficial punctate keratitis. Many of these are associated with de-epithelialization performed during the epi-off procedure. Tables 28.1 and 28.2 show the adverse effects associated with CXL in children.

Despite its safety as a procedure, there are several reports of microbial/herpetic keratitis, which are shown in Table 28.3; most of them have been reported after accelerated CXL followed by epi-off procedure. Despite the fact that microbial keratitis is the most feared complication, it should not be the reason for avoiding CXL in a child.

If we do not perform CXL in a child, there is an implicit risk of progression, and potentially, the need of a corneal transplant, with its attendant complications including glaucoma and a significantly higher incidence of rejection than in adults.[6–8]

TABLE 28.3 ■ Clinical Features of Published Case Reports of Microbial Keratitis in Pediatric Patients

Author, Year	Age (Years), Sex	CXL Protocol	CDVA at Presentation	Time After the CXL (Days)	Organism	Final CDVA
Sharma et al.,[39] 2010	19, female	Epi-off CXL (3 mW/cm² × 30 min)	HM	1	Pseudomona. aureginosa	20/200
Shetty et al.,[40] 2014	18, male	Epi-off CXL (3 mW/cm² × 30 min)	NA	3	Staphylococcus. aureus	20/30
Al-Qarni and AlHarbi,[41] 2015	18, male	Epi-off CXL (3 mW/cm² × 30 min)	NA	7	Herpes. simplex	20/25
Rana et al.[42] 2015	19, female	TE Acc CXL (9 mW/cm² × 10 min)	NA	3	Staphylococcus aureus	NA
	18, male	Epi-off Acc CXL (9 mW/cm² × 10 min)	NA	5	Methicillin resistant S. taphylococcus aureus	20/70
Kodavoor et al.,[43] 2015	15, male	Acc CXL (30 mW/cm² × 3 min)	20/400	3	Staphylococcus aureus	20/40
Maharana et al.,[44] 2018	14, male	Acc CXL (18 mW/cm² × 6 min)	6/18	3	Staphylococcus epidermidis	6/18
	17, male	Acc CXL (18 mW/cm² × 6 min)	CF	2	Mucor spp.	6/36
	14, male	Acc CXL (18 mW/cm² × 6 min)	1/60	2	Staphylococcus aureus	6/18
	8, male	Acc CXL (18 mW/cm² × 6 min)	CF	1	NA	1/60
	11, female	Acc CXL (18 mW/cm² × 6 min)	6/60	3	Staphylococcus epidermidis	2/60
	11, female	Acc CXL (18 mW/cm² × 6 min)	CF	3	Alternaria spp.	3/60
	11, male	Acc CXL (18 mW/cm² × 6 min)	CF	4	NA	CF

Acc CXL, Accelerated cross-linking; BCVA, best-corrected visual acuity; CF, counting fingers; CXL, corneal collagen cross-linking; HM, hand motion; TE-CXL, transepithelial CXL; Y, year.

WHEN TO PERFORM CORNEAL COLLAGEN CROSS-LINKING IN CHILDREN

The indication for CXL is "progressive" KC. It is, therefore, necessary to document progression before the procedure. There are, nonetheless, certain cases, where waiting for progression is riskier than performing CXL without documented progression.

An individualized analysis of risk factors for KC progression should be performed in each child. Among the risk factors that cannot be controlled are age (younger than 17 years old), maximum keratometry greater than 55 D at the time of diagnosis, genetic factors, connective tissue disorders (such as Ehlers-Danlos syndrome), Down syndrome, Leber congenital amaurosis, trisomy 21, and Turner syndrome.[45,46]

Among the risk factors that can be controlled are inflammation[47] and eye rubbing,[48] the latter of which has been associated with progression. It is, therefore, important to emphasize the avoidance of eye rubbing after treatment.

Our capacity to control the risk factors for progression has to be included in the management plan when we are deciding if CXL is the next step in management. We recommend analysis and categorization of the patient into high or low risk for progression, waiting for documented progression in cases where close follow-up is possible and not waiting for documented progression in cases where a modifiable risk factor cannot be controlled and/or a close follow-up is impossible.

CXL IN CHILDREN WITH DEVELOPMENTAL DELAYS OR INABILITY TO COOPERATE

Corneal collagen CXL can be performed under topical anesthesia, just as it is done in an adult. However, there are cases where topical anesthetics are not feasible. In these situations, such as developmental delay or inability to cooperate with topical anesthesia because of younger age, general anesthesia is required. Case series performing CXL with general anesthesia have proved its effectiveness and reported no complications.[35,49]

Standard postoperative care after CXL includes a bandage contact lens over the operated eye to prevent any shearing from the eyelids. In cases where bandage contact lens removal in the clinic is impossible, a pressure patch or bandage of fibrin glue and amniotic membrane can be employed.[49]

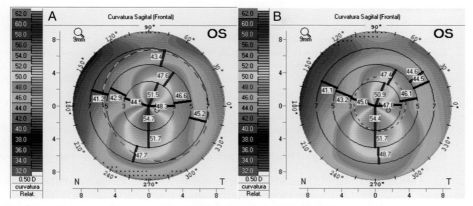

Fig. 28.2 Keratoconus (KC) stabilization 5 years after accelerated transepithelial corneal cross-linking in a patient with severe KC. (A) Preoperative curvature map, (B) postoperative curvature map.

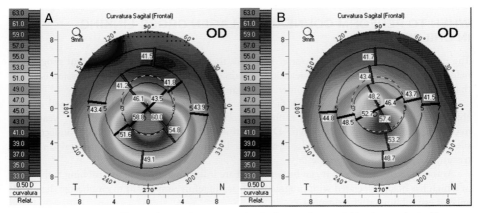

Fig. 28.3 Keratoconus (KC) stabilization after 5 years of epi-off corneal cross-linking in a patient with severe KC. (A) Preoperative curvature map, (B) postoperative curvature map.

CXL IN ADVANCED KERATOCONUS IN CHILDREN

Advanced KC does not represent a contraindication to CXL in children. Furthermore, it is an ideal option to avoid corneal transplantation, as long as the BCVA is better than 20/60 (Snellen) and the inclusion criteria for endothelial safety are met.

Effectiveness has been demonstrated in these types of KC. Furthermore, several studies show that having a high maximum keratometry at the time of diagnosis is a risk factor for KC progression.[42] A high maximum keratometry before CXL is also a positive factor for having greater corneal flattening. Fig. 28.2 shows a case of advanced KC having transepithelial CXL and Fig. 28.3 illustrates a case of advanced KC having epi-off CXL.

In conclusion, corneal collagen cross-linking is a safe and effective treatment to halt the progression of KC in children and should be considered in this population.

Acknowledgment

Cristóbal Moctezuma, MD and Jose Lievano for English grammar corrections.
Gustavo Hernandez, for bibliographic search.

References

1. Chatzis N, Hafezi F. Progression of keratoconus and efficacy of corneal collagen cross-linking in children and adolescents. *J Refract Surg*. 2012;28(11):753–758.
2. Léoni-Mesplié S, Mortemousque B, Touboul D, et al. Scalability and severity of keratoconus in children. *Am J Ophthalmol*. 2012;154(1):56–62.
3. Ertan A, Muftuoglu O. Keratoconus clinical findings according to different age and gender groups. *Cornea*. 2008;27(10):1109–1113.
4. Mazzotta C, Traversi C, Baiocchi S, et al. Corneal collagen cross-linking with riboflavin and ultraviolet A light for pediatric keratoconus: ten-year results. 2018;0(0):7.
5. Perez-Straziota C, Gaster RN, Rabinowitz YS. Corneal cross-linking for pediatric keratoconus review. *Cornea*. 2018;37(6):802–809.
6. Zhu A, Prescott C. Recent surgical trends in pediatric corneal transplantation: a 13-year review. *Cornea*. 2019;38(5):546–552.
7. Aasuri MK, Garg P, Gokhle N, Gupta S. Penetrating keratoplasty in children. *Cornea*. 2000;19(2):140–144.
8. Comer RM, Daya SM, O'Keefe M. Penetrating keratoplasty in infants. *AAPOS*. 2001;5(5):285–290.
9. McAnena L, Doyle F, O'Keefe M. Cross-linking in children with keratoconus: a systematic review and meta-analysis. *Acta Ophthalmol*. 2017;95(3):229–239.

10. Mukhtar S, Ambati BK. Pediatric keratoconus: a review of the literature. *Int Ophthalmol.* 2018;38(5):2257–2266.
11. Godefrooij DA, Mangen MJ, Chan E, et al. Cost-effectiveness analysis of corneal collagen crosslinking for progressive keratoconus. *Ophthalmology.* 2017;124(10):1485–1495.
12. Henriquez MA, Villegas S, Rincon M, et al. Long-term efficacy and safety after corneal collagen cross-linking in pediatric patients: three-year follow-up. *Eur J Ophthalmol.* 2018;28(4):415–418.
13. Caporossi A, Mazzotta C, Baiocchi S, et al. A. Riboflavin-UVA-induced corneal collagen cross-linking in pediatric patients. *Cornea.* 2012;31(3):227–231.
14. Vinciguerra P, Albé E, Frueh BE, Trazza S, Epstein D. Two-year corneal cross-linking results in patients younger than 18 years with documented progressive keratoconus. *Am J Ophthalmol.* 2012;154(3):520–526.
15. Zotta P, Moschou K, Diakonis V, et al. Corneal collagen cross-linking for progressive keratoconus in pediatric patients: a feasibility study. *J Refract Surg.* 2012;28(11):793–799.
16. Magli A, Forte R, Tortori A, et al. Epithelium-off corneal collagen cross-linking versus transepithelial cross-linking for pediatric keratoconus. *Cornea.* 2013;32(5):597–601.
17. Viswanathan D, Kumar NL, Males JJ. Outcome of corneal collagen crosslinking for progressive keratoconus in paediatric patients. *Biomed Res Int.* 2014;2014:1–5.
18. McAnena L, O'Keefe M. Corneal collagen crosslinking in children with keratoconus. *JAAPOS.* 2015;19(3):228–232.
19. Uçakhan ÖÖ, Bayraktutar BN, Saglik A. Pediatric corneal collagen cross-linking: long-term follow-up of visual, refractive, and topographic outcomes. *Cornea.* 2016;35(2):7.
20. Wise S, Diaz C, Termote K, Dubord PJ, McCarthy M, Yeung SN. Corneal crosslinking in pediatric patients with progressive keratoconus. *Cornea.* 2016;35:1441–1443.
21. Godefrooij DA, Soeters N, Imhof SM, Wisse RP Corneal Cross-Linking for Pediatric Keratoconus: Long-Term Results. Cornea. 2016;35(7):954–958
22. Ulusoy DM, Goktas E, Duru N, et al. Accelerated corneal crosslinking for treatment of progressive keratoconus in pediatric patients. *Eur J Ophthalmol.* 2016;27:319–325.
23. Sarac O, Caglayan M, Cakmak HB, Cagil N. Factors influencing progression of keratoconus 2 years after corneal collagen cross-linking in pediatric patients. *Cornea.* 2016;35:1503–1507.
24. Henriquez MA, Rodríguez AM, Izquierdo L. Accelerated epi-on versus standard epi-off corneal collagen cross-linking for progressive keratoconus in pediatric patients. *Cornea.* 2017;36(12):1503–1508.
25. Padmanabhan P, Rachapalle Reddi S, Rajagopal R, et al. Corneal collagen cross-linking for keratoconus in pediatric patients—long-term results. *Cornea.* 2017;36(2):138–143.
26. Zotta PG, Diakonis VF, Kymionis GD, Grentzelos M, Moschou KA. Long-term outcomes of corneal cross-linking for keratoconus in pediatric patients. *J AAPOS.* 2017;21(5):397–401.
27. Eraslan M, Toker E, Cerman E, Ozarslan D. Efficacy of epithelium-off and epithelium-on corneal collagen cross-linking in pediatric keratoconus. *Eye & Contact Lens.* 2016;0:1–7.
28. Sarac O, Kosekahya P, Caglayan M, Tanriverdi B, Taslipinar A. Mechanical versus transepithelial phototherapeutic keratectomy epithelial removal followed by accelerated corneal crosslinking for pediatric keratoconus: long-term results. *J Cataract Refract Surg.* 2018;44:827–835.
29. Buzzonetti L, Petrocelli G, Valente P, et al. Ontophoretic transepithelial collagen cross-linking versus epithelium-off collagen cross-linking in pediatric patients: 3-year follow-up. *Cornea.* 2019;38(7):859–863.
30. Henriquez MA, Hernandez G, Camargo J, Izquierdo Jr L. Accelerated epi-on vs standard epi-off corneal collagen cross-linking for progressive keratoconus in pediatric patients: five years of follow-up. *Cornea.* 2020;39(12):1493–1498.
31. Buzzonetti L, Petrocelli G. Transepithelial corneal cross-linking in pediatric patients: early results. *J Refract Surg.* 2012;28(11):763–767.
32. Salman AG. Transepithelial corneal collagen crosslinking for progressive keratoconus in a pediatric age group. *J Cataract Refract.* 2013;39(8):1164–1170.
33. Buzzonetti L, Petrocelli G, Valente P, Iarossi G, Ardia R, Petroni S. Iontophoretic transepithelial corneal cross-linking to halt keratoconus in pediatric cases: 15-month follow-up. *Cornea.* 2015;34(5):4.
34. Salman AG. Corneal biomechanical and anterior chamber parameters variations after 1-year of transepithelial corneal collagen cross-linking in eyes of children with keratoconus. *Middle East Afr J Ophthalmol.* 2016;23(1):129.

35. Magli A, Chiariello Vecchio E, Carelli R, Piozzi E, Di Landro F, Troisi S. Pediatric keratoconus and iontophoretic corneal crosslinking: refractive and topographic evidence in patients underwent general and topical anesthesia, 18 months of follow-up. *Int Ophthalmol.* 2016;36(4):585–590.

36. Tian M, Jian W, Sun L, Shen Y, Zhang X, Zhou X. One-year follow-up of accelerated transepithelial corneal collagen cross-linking for progressive pediatric keratoconus. *BMC Ophthalmol.* 2018;18(1):75.

37. Rush SW, Rush RB. Epithelium-off versus transepithelial corneal collagen crosslinking for progressive corneal ectasia: a randomised and controlled trial. *Br J Ophthalmol.* 2017;101(4):503–508.

38. Henriquez MA, Izquierdo L Jr, Bernilla C, Zakrzewski PA, Mannis M. Riboflavin/ultraviolet A corneal collagen cross-linking for the treatment of keratoconus: visual outcomes and Scheimpflug analysis. *Cornea.* 2011;30(3):281–286.

39. Sharma N, Maharana P, Singh G, Titiyal JS. Pseudomonas keratitis after collagen crosslinking for keratoconus: case report and review of literature. *J Cataract Refract Surg.* 2010;36(3):517–520.

40. Shetty R, Kaweri L, Nuijts RM, Nagaraja H, Arora V, Kumar RS. Profile of microbial keratitis after corneal collagen crosslinking. *Biomed Res Int.* 2014;2014:340509.

41. Al-Qarni A, AlHarbi M. Herpetic keratitis after corneal collagen cross-linking with riboflavin and ultraviolet-A for keratoconus. *Middle East Afr J Ophthalmol.* 2015;22(3):389–392.

42. Rana M, Lau A, Aralikatti A, Shah S. Severe microbial keratitis and associated perforation after corneal crosslinking for keratoconus. *Cont Lens Anterior Eye.* 2015;38(2):134–137.

43. Kodavoor SK, Sarwate NJ, Ramamurhy D. Microbial keratitis following accelerated corneal collagen cross-linking. *Oman J Ophthalmol.* 2015;8(2):111–113.

44. Maharana PK, Sahay P, Sujeeth M, et al. Microbial keratitis after accelerated corneal collagen cross-linking in keratoconus. *Cornea.* 2018;37(2):162–167.

45. Gordon-Shaag A, Millodot M, Kaiserman I, et al. Risk factors for keratoconus in Israel: a case-control study. *Ophthalmic Physiol Opt.* 2015;35(6):673–681.

46. Ferdi AC, Nguyen V, Gore DM, Allan BD, Rozema JJ, Watson SL. Keratoconus natural progression: a systematic review and meta-analysis of 11 529 eyes. *Ophthalmology.* 2019;126(7):935–945.

47. Shetty R, Sureka S, Kusumgar P, Sethu S, Sainani K. Allergen-specific exposure associated with high immunoglobulin E and eye rubbing predisposes to progression of keratoconus. *Indian J Ophthalmol.* 2017;65(5):399–402.

48. Henriquez MA, Cerrate M, Hadid MG, Cañola-Ramirez LA, Hafezi F, Izquierdo L Jr. Comparison of eye-rubbing effect in keratoconic eyes and healthy eyes using Scheimpflug analysis and a dynamic bidirectional applanation device. *J Cataract Refract Surg.* 2019;45(8):1156–1162.

49. Ahmad TR, Pasricha ND, Rose-Nussbaumer J, T Oatts J, M Schallhorn J, Indaram M. Corneal collagen cross-linking under general anesthesia for pediatric patients with keratoconus and developmental delay. *Cornea.* 2020;39(5):546–551.

CHAPTER 29

Corneal Laser Surgery for Keratoconus

Shady Awwad ■ Luis Izquierdo Jr.

KEY CONCEPTS

- Corneal laser surgery for keratoconus has become possible, thanks to the advent of corneal cross-linking and major improvements in customized excimer laser ablation algorithms.
- Laser surgery can be performed via various modalities, such as topography-guided and corneal wavefront–guided photorefractive keratectomy (PRK), ocular wavefront–guided PRK, and transepithelial phototherapeutic keratectomy.
- The main target is to fix relevant corneal aberrations rather than refractive errors, to keep stromal ablations to a minimum and avoid excessive biomechanical insult, haze formation, and refractive surprises.

Introduction

Corneal laser surgery for keratoconus has become possible, thanks to the advent of corneal cross-linking (CXL) and major improvements in customized excimer laser ablation algorithms. Reviled and revered by surgeons across the globe, this procedure has been the subject of controversy and fierce debates since 2009. A close, objective review of this procedure identifies its strengths, realistic goals, and limitations, and delineates surgical and clinical strategies. The target of corneal laser surgery in keratoconus is visual rehabilitation: improving corrected distance visual acuity (CDVA) and visual symptoms. It is especially useful when rigid gas permeable lenses are not an option, whether because of clinical or social intolerance. Laser treatments should not aim to eliminate or minimize spectacles dependence but should focus on improving corneal aberrations.

Procedure Planning

In planning for the procedure, the surgeon should keep in mind that the main issues in any customized excimer laser treatment are overcorrection, induction of refractive errors, epithelial and stromal healing, biomechanical adjustment, stromal haze, and, especially for keratoconus, biomechanical integrity. There are many reasons for overcorrection, including inputting a refractive correction that has higher-order aberrations (HOAs) embedded in it, such as spherical aberration and coma, among others. Hence, HOAs and corneal irregularities might be treated twice. Additionally, a larger stromal ablation to offset corneal irregularities entails greater chances to impact the refractive error and can lead to a larger biomechanical adjustment that can also affect the final refractive outcome. Additionally, the deeper the stromal ablation, the higher the chance of developing corneal haze. The latter is not uncommon in irregular eyes, especially in eyes with concomitant or previous procedures such as CXL.[1-4] Finally, ablating too deeply might affect the biomechanical integrity of the cornea and reverse any

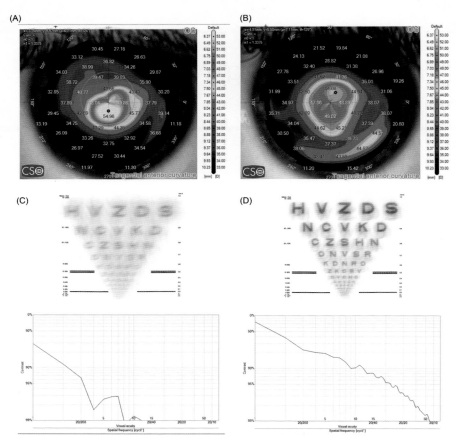

Fig. 29.1 (A) Instantaneous curvature topography map of an eye with advanced keratoconus with a previous corneal ring segment implanted inferotemporally. (B) Postoperative topography after combined ocular wavefront–guided photorefractive keratectomy with corneal cross-linking performed based on a pyramidal aberrometer with high dynamic range and focusing mainly on the higher-order aberrations and not on the concomitant myopic component, resulted in a much more regular cornea. (C) Preoperative simulated optical quality and contrast sensitivity by spatial frequency. (D) Postoperative optical quality simulation, showing major improvement.

benefit from a previous or concomitant cross-linking procedure. It has been shown that ablating a total of 50 μm was overall safe and did not result in ectasia progression, either simultaneously or sequentially with cross-linking.[3] This was further revisited and confirmed 10 years after the procedure.[5] However, this number should be regarded as a maximum to avoid rather than a safety allowance. The general rule in customized ablations for keratoconus eyes should be the less, the better. The target is to fix relevant corneal aberrations rather than refractive errors, so the less the stromal ablation, the less the chance of refractive overcorrection, induced refractive errors or aberrations, corneal haze, or ectasia progression. The eye can always be revisited when more tissue is spared, and lower-order aberrations (LOAs) can be "outsourced" to spectacles, soft contact lenses, or phakic intraocular lenses (IOLs; Fig. 29.1).

Treatment Modalities

Many methodologies are used to perform customized corneal ablation: ocular wavefront–guided (OWG), topography-guided (TG), and phototherapeutic keratectomy (PTK) treatments. OWG treatment aims to correct the aberrations of the whole eye and has the advantage of directly deriving and treating the refractive error from the measured wavefront. However, pupil size often limits treatment, as the ablation profile must be extrapolated outside the boundary margins, and a small optical zone treatment in keratoconus fails to address the irregular corneal changes that typically extend to the midperiphery. The latter concept of a large optical zone reflects the new trend in treating corneal irregularities in keratoconus and is a sharp departure from the small optical zone initially advocated in the Athens protocol.[3]

Additionally, traditional aberrometers have low dynamic range and suffer from aliasing when it comes to measuring highly aberrated wavefronts, typically encountered in keratoconus eyes. The advent of pyramidal aberrometers has made it possible to measure complex ocular wavefront patterns, including those of eyes with corneal ectasia, and they can be used to formulate accurate and reliable treatment profiles.

TG ablations measure the very surface affected by the disease in a highly predictable and accurate way. Corneal wavefront–guided (CWG) treatment is a spin-off of the TG method but relies on decomposition of the topography into a wavefront map. By doing so, it provides a way to select and deselect aberrations to be treated, allowing for decreased tissue ablation volume and depth while treating the relevant aberrations in a specific eye. Both modalities suffer from the fact that refraction is estimated and never measured directly. More importantly, topography is based on the anterior curvature, which is partially offset by the posterior curvature, sitting on a negative refractive meniscus. Treating the total corneal wavefront (ray-traced sum of anterior and posterior) might provide a better functional treatment and save on tissue ablation. It has already been shown that OWG treatments ablate up to 44% less tissue than CWG ablations, planned on the same eyes using the same excimer platform (Schwind Amaris).[6] This difference probably represents the effect of the posterior corneal curvature, which is embedded in OWG treatment profiles. Whether total CWG or OWG treatment more accurately addresses the corneal aberrations is yet to be determined, as overcorrecting total corneal aberrations by performing an anterior CWG ablation might be offset by an inherent undercorrection of the target aberrations. All the above treatments can be performed via a transepithelial approach.

Finally, PTK, which is usually reserved for irregularly irregular corneas, can be used in the keratoconus eye to ablate the epithelium and shave tissue from the cone where the epithelium is thinnest. This would result in partial treatment of coma and ensures minimal tissue ablation.[7–9] This treatment modality is useful in severe keratoconus with not much stromal tissue to ablate. It is also useful in mild keratoconus with relatively good CDVA, in which slight acuity boosting with minimal tissue ablation is desired. In addition, this modality can be especially useful when there is clear discrepancy in epithelial thickness in a decentered cone, and where a transepithelial photorefractive keratectomy (PRK) approach might lead to excessive ablation over the cone, often resulting in "double treatment" of the coma and other components (Fig. 29.2).

Corneal Laser Ablation and Cross-Linking: Sequential Versus Combined

Another debate in therapeutic refractive surgery for keratoconus is when to perform customized ablation: in conjunction with CXL or after CXL treatment. Although many surgeons take sides, it appears that, based on the literature, little evidence is available to fully endorse one over the other, especially as randomized controlled studies are lacking. Instead, clinical experience shows that either can be performed, depending on patient selection and the ultimate goal of the physician for a particular patient.

The advantage of combined treatment is that the patient does not have to undergo two procedures, neither do they have to wait for a substantial amount of time to ensure stability before undergoing customized treatment, which is designed to improve the CDVA. Additionally, ablating the Bowman's layer improves riboflavin penetration in the cornea, providing deeper cross-linking. Disadvantages of combined treatment are that major changes in corneal curvature and refraction can develop in some patients, and these are typically unaccounted for by customized treatments.[10] Sequential treatments have the advantage of treating the cornea after it stabilizes and eliminating major refractive surprises. However, they ablate the most anterior cross-linked

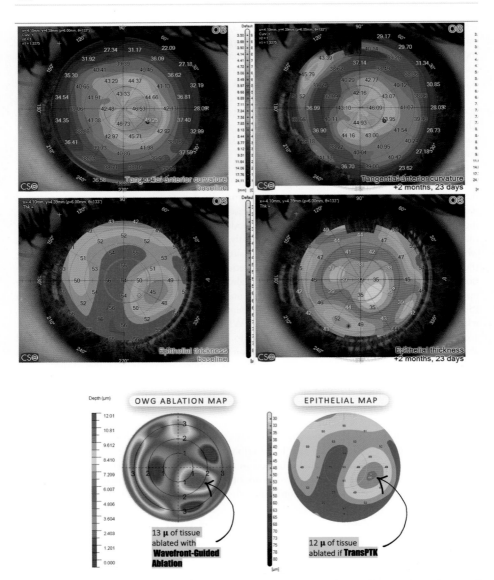

Fig. 29.2 (A) Instantaneous curvature topography and epithelial map of a cornea with mild-to-moderate decentered cone. Transepithelial phototherapeutic keratectomy was performed instead of a customized photorefractive keratectomy (PRK). The postoperative curvature and epithelial map is shown on the *right* side, with major improvement of curvature and epithelial symmetry. (B) The ablation map seen on the *left* side of the diagram shows a planned wavefront–guided PRK ablation of 13 μm on the cone. The epithelial map, on the *right* side, shows a difference of 11 to 12 μm between the center and the cone. Hence, a transepithelial PRK with central ablation set to 53 μm (central epithelial thickness) would shave 11 to 12 μm from the cone, very similar to PRK ablation. Hence, the effect would be expected to be similar between the two modalities. A transepithelial PRK approach, however, would have resulted in about 25 μm ablation on the cone, with potential "double treatment" of the coma.

and stiffest tissue. Additionally, patients with subpar CDVA must wait for at least 6 months, and sometimes years, to stabilize post-CXL before undergoing a procedure geared toward improving their vision. It makes more sense to perform combined treatment in patients suffering from large amounts of HOAs and poorer CDVA, and as long as customized ablation is geared to improving HOAs and not LOAs, any major change in corneal flattening post-CXL would not negate the initial treatment and can be taken care of with phakic IOLs, spectacles, and soft contact lenses (Fig. 29.3A). However, it makes sense that eyes with minimal HOAs and relatively good CDVA should be cross-linked first, and then later undergo customized ablation, if needed (Fig. 29.3B).

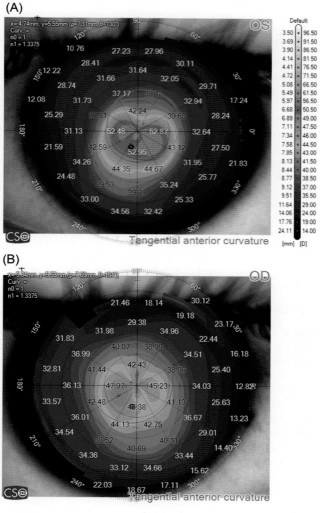

Fig. 29.3 (A) Instantaneous curvature topography map of an eye with advanced keratoconus. Combined photorefractive keratectomy (PRK) and cross-linking is warranted, targeting the higher-order aberrations and treating only concomitant embedded lower-order aberrations. (B) Instantaneous curvature topography map of an eye with mild-to-moderate keratoconus. Cross-linking is better performed first, with subsequent follow-up to monitor stability. When the latter is achieved, customized PRK could be performed, if judged necessary based on the visual, refractive, and topographical findings.

By doing so, there may be a chance for the patient to improve both in terms of HOAs and LOAs, even if the former was the main target of treatment. It is important to keep in mind that the stromal ablation rate in sequential procedures is lower than in virgin eyes by about 12%, as has been shown by Richoz et al.[11] This should be taken into consideration when planning PRK on previously cross-linked eyes.

A PTK-assisted epithelial removal, preferably guided by optical coherence tomography (OCT)–derived epithelial maps, can also be used to shave the cone and achieve partial coma treatment with minimal tissue ablation and refractive change. This can be an alternative for advanced cases with thin corneas or for mild keratoconus when minimal treatment is needed to avoid refractive change or haze induction.

Postoperative Stromal Haze

The development of corneal haze post cross-linking has been well documented,[10,12,13] but it seems to occur more when performed with PRK, whether simultaneously or sequentially. There is, nonetheless, some controversy around which one produces more haze.[1–3,12,15] Although Kanellopoulos et al. have reported more haze in the sequential group,[3] several studies claim severe haze developing in the simultaneous procedure,[1,2] which is at odds with other reports claiming minimal to mild haze.[4–5,6,12,15] The haze is sometimes late in onset, in which case it is typically deep,[1,6,16] similar to that reported to rarely occur with cross-linking alone.[12]

A possible reason for the discrepancy in haze among studies might be the amount of tissue ablated, as this seems to be directly proportional to the amount of haze induced. Another reason is the concomitant use of mitomycin C (MMC). Studies reporting minimal haze did not use MMC at all,[6,14,15] or used it for a maximum of 20 seconds,[3,5,16] whereas a study reporting severe haze described using MMC for 40 seconds.[2] Awwad and co-workers have described have described marked haze developing after CXL with MMC as opposed to CXL alone, as analyzed by a machine learning algorithm evaluating corneal haze using OCT.[17] It is possible that the combined cidal action of MMC and CXL on the keratocyte population releases a large surge of cytokines and chemokines, which can induce haze.

Outsourcing Aberrations Treatments

The surgeon's mantra in planning corneal laser ablation in keratoconus should be "the less, the better." Hence, debulking large aberrations using intrastromal corneal ring segments (ICRS) or corneal allogenic intrastromal ring segments (CAIRS) allows for a finer treatment with the excimer laser, achieving fewer refractive surprises, less haze induction, and better biomechanical integrity (Fig. 29.4).[18,19] In addition, outsourcing LOAs to phakic IOLs, soft contact lenses, and spectacles allows most of the ablated tissue to be invested in correcting HOAs and, hence, better CDVA.[19] This concept allows treatment of only LOAs such as sphere or cylinder that are embedded in the treatment plan aiming to correct HOAs (Fig. 29.5). By sticking to this approach, planning large optical zones will result in deeper ablation. However, planning additional spherocylindrical treatments on top of the basic treatment plan aimed at HOAs with embedded LOAs will significantly increase ablation depth, especially when larger optical zones are planned. This explains why the original Athens protocol adopted small optical zones of 5.5 mm, as the treatment targeted both LOAs and HOAs. By treating only the embedded spherocylindrical component in the ablation profile targeting HOAs, larger optical zones can be planned without an increase in ablation depth (Fig. 29.6).

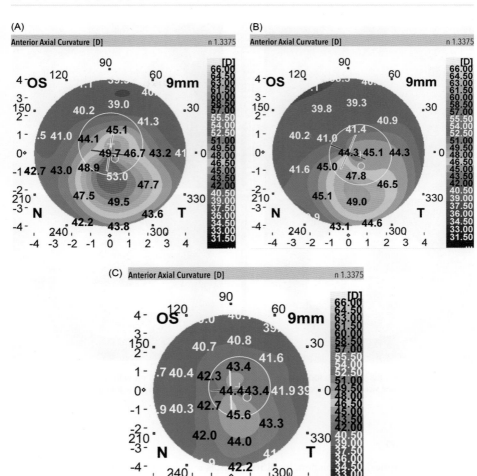

Fig. 29.4 (A) Axial corneal curvature map of the left eye of a keratoconus patient with asymmetrical disease and anisometropia. (B) Postoperative axial curvature of the same eye after implantation of a corneal ring segment. As can be seen, the ring segment failed to adequately address the coma component of the topography and the central cornea became significantly flatter, reducing the myopic component and hence the anisometropia. This was done without investing into precious stromal tissue. (C) Axial curvature map showing appreciable regularization after a corneal wavefront–guided PRK was performed to treat higher-order aberrations.

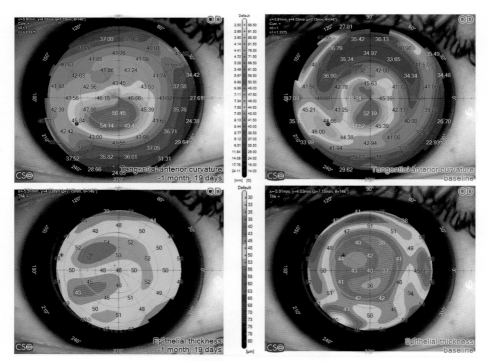

Fig. 29.5 Instantaneous curvature topography and epithelial map of a cornea with moderate to advanced keratoconus. Corneal wavefront–guided treatment was performed with minimal tissue ablation, resulting in a more regular cornea.

Conclusion

In conclusion, corneal laser ablation, in all its forms, is a mainstay in the refractive therapeutic armamentarium of keratoconus management. Proper patient selection and judicious choice of treatment strategy customized to the patient's eyes and needs while targeting HOAs with minimal tissue ablation, in close alliance with other surgical and clinical modalities, are vital to achieving safe and efficacious results.

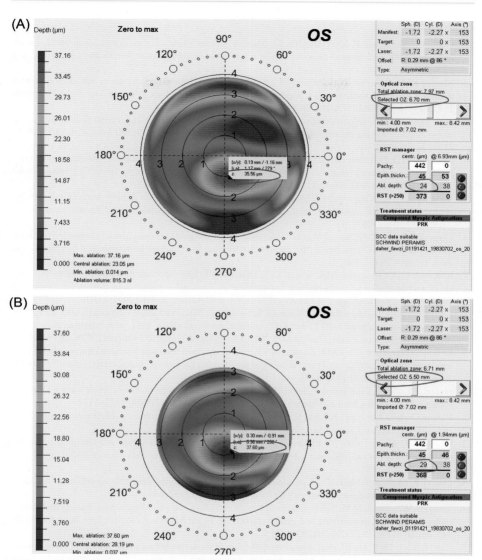

Fig. 29.6 (A) Ablation planning display for ocular wavefront–guided treatment, showcasing a minimum depth treatment of higher-order aberrations. The spherocylindrical treatment displayed in the *right upper* corner is the "embedded" lower-order aberration ablation within the ablation. It is the refractive error the laser would correct while tackling the higher-order aberrations. (B) Hence, the previously selected optical zone of 6.70 mm would yield equal, if not less, ablation depth than an ablation zone of 5.50 mm. This does not hold true if the clinician adds additional sphere or cylinder value to match the patient's refraction; then, a larger optical zone would significantly increase ablation depth.

References

1. Güell JL, Verdaguer P, Elies D, Gris O, Manero F. Late onset of a persistent, deep stromal scarring after PRK and corneal cross-linking in a patient with forme fruste keratoconus. *J Refract Surg.* 2014;30(4):286–288.
2. Moraes RLB, Ghanem RC, Ghanem VC, Santhiago MR. Haze and visual acuity loss after sequential photorefractive keratectomy and corneal cross-linking for keratoconus. *J Refract Surg.* 2019;35(2):109–114. doi:10.3928/1081597X-20190114-01.
3. Kanellopoulos AJ. Comparison of sequential vs same-day simultaneous collagen cross-linking and topography-guided PRK for treatment of keratoconus. *J Refract Surg.* 2009;25(9):S812–S818. doi:10.3928/10 81597X-20090813-10.
4. Kymionis GD, Portaliou DM, Diakonis VF, et al. Posterior linear stromal haze formation after simultaneous photorefractive keratectomy followed by corneal collagen cross-linking. *Invest Ophthalmol Vis Sci.* 2010;51(10):5030–5033. doi:10.1167/iovs.09-5105.
5. Kanellopoulos AJ, Vingopoulos F, Sideri AM. Long-term stability with the Athens protocol (topography-guided partial PRK combined with cross-linking) in pediatric patients with keratoconus. *Cornea.* 2019;38(8):1049–1057.
6. Gore DM, Leucci MT, Anand V, et al. Combined wavefront-guided transepithelial photorefractive keratectomy and corneal crosslinking for visual rehabilitation in moderate keratoconus. *J Cataract Refract Surg.* 2018;44(5):571–580.
7. Kymionis GD, Grentzelos MA, Kounis GA, Diakonis VF, Limnopoulou AN, Panagopoulou SI. Combined transepithelial phototherapeutic keratectomy and corneal collagen cross-linking for progressive keratoconus. *Ophthalmology.* 2012;119(9):1777–1784. doi:10.1016/j.ophtha.2012.03.038.
8. Grentzelos MA, Liakopoulos DA, Siganos CS, Tsilimbaris MK, Pallikaris IG, Kymionis GD. Long-term comparison of combined t-PTK and CXL (Cretan protocol) versus CXL with mechanical epithelial debridement for keratoconus. *J Refract Surg.* 2019;35(10):650–655. doi:10.3928/1081597X-20190917-01.
9. Kymionis GD, Grentzelos MA, Kankariya VP, et al. Long-term results of combined transepithelial phototherapeutic keratectomy and corneal collagen crosslinking for keratoconus: Cretan protocol. *J Cataract Refract Surg.* 2014;40(9):1439–1445.
10. Hafezi F, Koller T, Vinciguerra P, Seiler T. Marked remodelling of the anterior corneal surface following collagen cross-linking with riboflavin and UVA. *Br J Ophthalmol.* 2011;95(8):1171–1172.
11. Richoz O, Arba Mosquera S, Kling S, et al. Determination of the excimer laser ablation rate in previously cross-linked corneas. *J Refract Surg.* 2014;30(9):628–632.
12. Dhaini AR, Abdul Fattah M, El-Oud SM, Awwad ST. Automated detection and classification of corneal haze using optical coherence tomography in patients with keratoconus after cross-linking. *Cornea.* 2018;37(7):863–869.
13. Omary R, Shehadeh-Mashor R. Late onset of persistent, deep stromal haze after corneal cross-linking in a patient with keratoconus. *Canadian J Ophthalmol.* 2017;52(2):e81–e83.
14. Tuwairqi WS, Sinjab MM. Safety and efficacy of simultaneous corneal collagen cross-linking with topography-guided PRK in managing low-grade keratoconus: 1-year follow-up. *J Refract Surg.* 2012;28(5):341–345. doi:10.3928/1081597X-20120316-01.
15. Lee H, Kang DSY, Ha BJ, et al. Visual rehabilitation in moderate keratoconus: combined corneal wavefront-guided transepithelial photorefractive keratectomy and high-fluence accelerated corneal collagen cross-linking after intracorneal ring segment implantation. *BMC Ophthalmology.* 2017;17(1):270.
16. Kanellopoulos AJ, Vingopoulos F, Sideri AM. Long-term stability with the Athens protocol (topography-guided partial PRK combined with cross-linking) in pediatric patients with keratoconus. *Cornea.* 2019;38(8):1049–1057.
17. Awwad ST, Chacra L, Helwe C, et al. Mitomycin C application after corneal cross-linking for keratoconus increases stromal haze. *J Refract Surg.* 2020;37(2):83–90.
18. Al-Tuwairqi W, Sinjab MM. Intracorneal ring segments implantation followed by same-day topography-guided PRK and corneal collagen CXL in low to moderate keratoconus. *J Refract Surg.* 2013;29(1):59–63.
19. Coskunseven E, Sharma DP, Grentzelos MA, Sahin O, Kymionis GD, Pallikaris I. Four-stage procedure for keratoconus: ICRS implantation, corneal cross-linking, toric phakic IOL implantation, and topography-guided photorefractive keratectomy. *J Refract Surg.* 2017;33(10):683–689.

CHAPTER 30

Phakic Intraocular Lenses

Nuno Moura-Coelho ▦ Merce Morral ▦ Felicidad Manero ▦ Daniel Elies ▦ José Güell

KEY CONCEPTS

- Both anterior and posterior chamber phakic intraocular lenses (PIOL) are safe and effective options for visual rehabilitation in patients with stable, mild-moderate keratoconus (KC).
- In cases of progressive KC, corneal cross-linking (CXL) should be performed to halt the progression of the disease, prior to considering PIOL implantation. The timing between CXL and PIOL implantation should be individualized, usually after confirmed topographic and refractive stabilization.
- Intrastromal corneal ring segment (ICRS) implantation may be combined with PIOL implantation for correction of moderate-high refractive error in eyes with nonadvanced KC and significant irregular astigmatism.
- Phakic IOLs are safe and effective in correcting postkeratoplasty ametropia in KC eyes in the mid/long term.

Introduction

The two most important goals in the management of keratoconus (KC) are halting disease progression and visual rehabilitation.[1] Visual rehabilitation in KC patients is a challenge, usually requiring a stepwise approach: first stabilizing the disease if progression is present; then regularizing the corneal shape; and, finally, correcting the spherocylindrical error.[2,3] Phakic intraocular lenses (PIOLs) have been increasingly used for the correction of moderate-high levels of myopia and regular astigmatism in KC eyes, and reduction of the refractive difference between both eyes. By reducing the degree of anisometropia, PIOLs improve binocularity, as retinal images become more similar. In addition, PIOLs provide a larger image size compared with spectacles.[4] Finally, PIOLs in KC eyes do not affect the corneal surface, unlike other strategies such as intrastromal corneal ring segments (ICRSs) or photorefractive keratectomy (PRK).[4]

Studies of PIOLs in eyes with KC include anterior chamber (AC) iris-claw PIOLs and posterior chamber (PC) PIOL (Table 30.1). In appropriately selected patients with KC, PIOL implantation has shown a good efficacy index (postoperative uncorrected distance visual acuity [UDVA]/preoperative corrected distance visual acuity [CDVA] ratio), as well as a good safety index (postoperative CDVA/preoperative CDVA ratio), with low rates of complication (Tables 30.2 and 30.3).[2,3,5] Iris-claw AC PIOLs (Artisan and Artiflex, Ophtec BV, Groningen, The Netherlands) are fixated anteriorly to the iris by enclavation, effectively correcting spherocylindrical error. In our experience, advantages of the iris-claw concept include centration, fixation, positioning in the AC, and respect for the anatomy of the anterior segment.[6,7] We use Toric Artiflex in most cases of stable, mild-to-moderate KC, and only consider the polymethyl methacrylate (PMMA) Artisan PIOL if spherical power is less than −14.50 D and/or cylinder power is greater than 5.00 D. Aiming for emmetropia or slight undercorrection results in significant improvement of cylinder

TABLE 30.1 ■ Characteristics of Iris-Claw and Posterior Chamber Phakic Intraocular Lenses

	Trademark	Material/Design	Optic	Overall Diameter (mm)	Power (D)	IOL Power Calculation
Iris-Claw						
Nonfoldable	Artisan	Single-piece CQ UV PMMA	5.0–6.0 mm diameter	8.5	Myopia −3.00 D to −23.50 D (0.50 D increments)	Van der Heijde formula (based on patient's refractive error, AC depth, and keratometry)
					Hyperopia +2.00 D to +12.00 D (0.50 D increments)	
	Artisan Toric	Single-piece CQ UV PMMA	Spherical anterior surface and spherocylindrical posterior surface	8.5	Sphere +12.00 D to −23.50 D	
			5.0 mm diameter		Torus 1.00 D to 7.50 D	
Foldable	Artiflex Myopia	CQ UV PMMA haptics + polysiloxane optic	Foldable, 6.0-mm optic	8.5	Myopia −2.00 D to −14.50 D (0.50 D increments)	
	Artiflex Toric	CQ UV PMMA haptics + polysiloxane optic	Foldable, 6.0-mm optic, spherical anterior surface and spherocylindrical posterior surface	8.5	Sphere −2.00 D to −14.50 D	
					Torus 1.00 D to 5.00 D	
Posterior Chamber						
	EVO Visian (ICL and Toric ICL)	Rectangular, single-block lens with plate-haptic design	Foldable, convex-concave, collamer (porcine scleral tissue-derived hydrophilic, biocompatible material)	12.1, 12.6, 13.2, and 13.7	Sphere −0.50 D to −20.00 D	Power determined using manufacturer's software; TICL power calculation by manufacturer, using astigmatism decomposition method
			4.9–5.8 mm diameter		Torus 0.50 D to 6.00 D	

AC, Anterior chamber; ICL, implantable collamer lens; IOL, intraocular lens; PMMA, polymethyl methacrylate; TICL, toric implantable collamer lens.

and manifest refraction, as well as significant improvement in both UDVA and CDVA in eyes with stable, nonadvanced KC. Most patients gain ≥1 lines of CDVA (Table 30.2). The Visian ICL (EVO Visian ICL, STAAR Surgical Co., Monrovia, CA, USA) is a PC PIOL with a superior postoperative visual performance and with high safety and effectiveness profiles for the correction of moderate-high ametropia.[8–10] Long-term visual and refractive stability has been demonstrated after implantable collamer lens (ICL) implantation in eyes with stable, mild-to-moderate KC, with most eyes reaching UDVA ≥20/40, and a high percentage of eyes reaching UDVA in the 20/25 to 20/20 range (see Table 30.3).[10]

Patient Selection

Potential candidates for PIOL implantation include patients with stable or stabilized mild-moderate KC who have moderate-high ametropia and who do not have satisfactory best-corrected visual acuity (BCVA) (Fig. 30.1). The term "satisfactory BCVA" has been adopted to differentiate patients who achieve good corrected vision but are unable to tolerate or wear optical correction for long periods of time, including contact lenses (CL).[1] Exclusion criteria for PIOL implantation include low endothelial cell counts (ECC), according to patient age and for each PIOL; short AC depth; abnormal iris or pupil function; and a scotopic pupil size >6.00 mm (Box 30.1). Preoperative CDVA should be ≥20/50, as keratoplasty may achieve superior visual outcomes in these cases.[11] It has been suggested that KC patients with ECC of 2000 cells/mm² or slightly below may still be candidates for PIOL implantation,[11–13] as a measure to delay or prevent the need for penetrating keratoplasty (PK). However, with the increasing experience with deep anterior lamellar keratoplasty (DALK) and given the advantages of DALK over PK in KC, our group usually excludes patients with ECC <2300 cells/mm² for PIOL implantation, as these patients may fare better with DALK. In cases of documented progression, halting disease progression must be addressed before considering PIOL implantation either by corneal cross-linking (CXL) or by corneal transplantation (DALK or PK) (see Chapter 8).[1] Commonly used criteria to determine progression include clinical and topo-tomographic parameters (Box 30.2); consistent changes over two consecutive examinations spaced 6 to 12 months apart are needed to determine progression. However, no clear definition of progression is available.[1]

In patients with stable, nonadvanced KC and with low CDVA and/or high irregular astigmatism, ICRS implantation should be considered before PIOL implantation. Although a number of tomographic indices allow quantification of irregular astigmatism, clinically significant irregular astigmatism is considered if CDVA with spectacles is ≤1 Snellen line worse than CDVA with rigid gas-permeable CL.[14,15]

Combined Corneal Cross-Linking Plus Phakic Intraocular Lens Implantation

In progressive KC, PIOL implantation alone would not provide stable refractive results in the mid/long term. CXL is the only technique with proven effect on halting progression of KC.[2] CXL can be combined with other treatments for visual rehabilitation, including sequential or simultaneous CXL + topography-guided PRK (Athens protocol),[16] combined transepithelial phototherapeutic keratectomy + CXL,[17] combined CXL + ICRS, and combined CXL + PIOL.

Combined CXL + PIOL implantation is a safe and effective strategy in eyes with progressive KC with moderate-high refractive error, regular astigmatism, and good CDVA, providing stabilization of the cone, as well as visual and refractive improvements comparable to those of non-KC eyes for up to 3 years after surgery (Table 30.4).[2,18] However, there is still no consensus on the appropriate interval between CXL and PIOL implantation. The minimum interval between CXL and PIOL implantation should be individualized. In our experience, after a minimum of 3 months

TABLE 30.2 ■ Reported Outcomes and Complications of Iris-Claw Anterior Chamber Phakic Intraocular Lens Implantation in Keratoconus

Preoperative Data

Author	Publication (Year)	Eyes (n)	UDVA (logMAR)	CDVA (logMAR)	Sphere (D)	Cylinder (D)	RSE (D)	ECC (cells/mm²)
Budo et al.[11]	2005	6	N/R	0.32 ± 0.13	−12.00 ± 10.14	−3.75 ± 1.28	−13.88 ± 10.22	N/R
Moshirfar et al.[33]	2006	2	CF in all patients	0.25 ± 0.05	−13.50 ± 1.80	3.80 ± 1.30	−11.63 ± 2.40	1904.5 ± 114.5
Venter[12]	2009	18	N/R	0.13 ± 0.13	−4.64 ± 2.74	−3.07 ± 20.4	−6.17 ± 2.39	2644 ± 401
Kato et al.[13]	2011	36	1.39 ± 0.42	N/R	N/R	2.44 ± 2.25	−8.38 ± 3.42	N/R
Sedaghat et al.[34]	2011	16	CF in all patients	0.21 ± 0.14	−12.5 ± 4.61	−2.95 ± 4.06	−13.90 ± 4.61	N/R

Postoperative Data

Follow-Up (Months)	UDVA (logMAR)	CDVA (logMAR)	%UDVA ≥20/40	%Gain CDVA ≥1 lines	%Eyes CDVA loss ≥2 lines	Sphere (D)	Cylinder (D)	RSE (D)	%eyes RSE ± 0.50 D	%eyes RSE ± 1.00 D	ECL (%)	Complications	SI	EI
6	N/R	0.17 ± 0.09	N/R	83.3%	0.0%	0.38 ± 0.79	−1.16 ± 1.24	−0.21 ± 1.13	20%	66.67%	N/R	Mild glare (33.3%)	1.49	N/R
2 and 12	0.25 ± 0.05	0.20 ± 0.00	100%	50.0%	0.0%	−0.13 ± 0.13	3.13 ± 1.13	1.43 ± 0.69	0.00%	50.00%	<4%	None reported	1.13 ± 0.13	2.40 ± 0.74
6-12	0.12 ± 0.09	0.00 ± 0.05	100%	72.0%	0.0%	−0.03 ± 0.47	−0.86 ± 0.55	−0.46 ± 0.60	61.10%	83.30%	6.30%	KC progression (5.6%)	1.38 ± 0.48	1.07 ± 0.41
12	0.02 ± 0.21	N/R	N/R	38.9%	0.0%	N/R	0.62 ± 0.69	−0.42 ± 0.89	63.60%	83.60%	N/R	Wound recession requiring resuturing (2.8%)	1.16 ± 0.31	0.87 ± 0.31
14.2 ± 7.8	0.15 ± 0.13	0.11 ± 0.10	100%	68.8%	0.0%	−0.03 ± 1.81	−2.08 ± 1.04	−0.90 ± 1.90	33.30%	53.30%	N/R	Sterile uveitis requiring oral corticosteroid (12.5%)	1.36 ± 0.43	1.19 ± 0.37

CDVA, Corrected distance visual acuity; CF, counting fingers; D, diopters; ECC, endothelial cell count; ECL, endothelial cell loss; EI, efficacy index (postoperative UDVA/preoperative CDVA ratio); KC, keratoconus; N/R, not reported; RSE, refractive spherical equivalent; SI, safety index (postoperative CDVA/preoperative CDVA ratio); UDVA, uncorrected distance visual acuity.

Preoperative Data

Author	Publication (Year)	Eyes (n)	UDVA (log-MAR)	CDVA (log-MAR)	Sphere (D)	Cylinder (D)	RSE (D)	ECC (cells/mm²)	Follow-Up (Months)
Kamiya et al.[35]	2008	2	1.28	0.05	-9.00 ± 1.00	-4.38 ± 1.63	-11.19 ± 1.84	2541.5 ± 715.5	3.00
Alfonso et al.[36]	2008	25	N/R	0.15 ± 0.15	-8.54 ± 4.15	-1.24 ± 1.19	-9.13	N/R	12.00
Alfonso et al.[37]	2010	30	N/R	0.12 ± 0.10	-3.64 ± 3.27	-3.48 ± 1.24	-5.38 ± 3.26	2525 ± 414	12.00
Kamiya et al.[8]	2011	27	1.51 ± 0.20	-0.11 ± 0.08	N/R	-3.03 ± 1.58	-10.11 ± 2.46	2734 ± 482	6.00
Hashemian et al.[38]	2013	22	N/R	0.23	-3.59 ± 2.59	-2.77 ± 0.99	-4.98 ± 2.63	N/R	6.00
Kamiya et al.[10]	2014	21	1.46 ± 0.15	-0.07 ± 0.07	N/R	-3.21 ± 1.56	-9.70 ± 2.33	2793 ± 455	36.00
Hashemian et al.[26]	2018	23	All eyes were in the CF range	0.24 ± 0.14	-3.78 ± 2.64	-3.14 ± 1.58	-5.35 ± 2.80	2713 ± 250	60.00

Postoperative Data

UDVA (logMAR)	CDVA (logMAR)	%UDVA ≥20/40	%Gain ≥1 line CDVA	%Loss ≥2 lines CDVA	Sphere (D)	Cylinder (D)	RSE (D)	%RSE within ± 0.50 D	%RSE within ± 1.00 D	%ECL	Complications	SI	EI
0.07 ± 0.03	-0.08 ± 0.08	100.0%	100%	0%	0.13 ± 0.38	-1.13 ± 0.13	-0.44 ± 0.44	50%	100%	N/R	None reported	1.38 ± 0.13	0.95 ± 0.05
0.17 ± 0.19	0.12 ± 0.12	96.0%	20%	0%	-0.08 ± 0.23	-0.46 ± 0.72	-0.32 ± 0.55	84%	100%	N/R	None reported	1.05	0.98
0.09 ± 0.11	0.07 ± 0.08	96.7%	97%	0%	0.09 ± 0.34	0.41 ± 0.61	-0.08 ± 0.37	86.7%	100%	2.61%	None reported	1.16	1.07
-0.09 ± 0.16	-0.15 ± 0.09	100.0%	48%	0%	N/R	-0.56 ± 0.75	0.10 ± 0.43	85%	96%	4.40%	None reported	1.12 ± 0.18	1.01 ± 0.25
0.15	0.10	86.4%	77%	0%	0.28 ± 0.42	-1.25 ± 0.65	-0.33 ± 0.51	68.2%	90.9%	N/R	None reported	1.40 ± 0.32	1.24 ± 0.34
-0.06 ± 0.11	-0.12 ± 0.09	100.0%	53%	0%	N/R	-0.62 ± 0.79	-0.02 ± 0.53	67%	86%	4.40%	PIOL rotation requiring repositioning (5%)	N/R	N/R
N/R	0.06 ± 0.09	100.0%	83%	0%	0.00 ± 0.76	-1.56 ± 1.53	-0.78 ± 1.31	N/R	N/R	7.88%	PIOL rotation requiring repositioning (21.7%)	1.58	1.33

CDVA, Corrected distance visual acuity; D, diopters; ECC, endothelial cell count; ECL, endothelial cell loss; EI, efficacy index (postoperative UDVA/preoperative CDVA ratio); N/R, not reported; PIOL, phakic intraocular lens; RSE, refractive spherical equivalent; SI, safety index (postoperative CDVA/preoperative CDVA ratio); UDVA, uncorrected distance visual acuity.

following CXL, we consider PIOL implantation once both manifest refraction and tomography scans are stable at two different time points at least 2 months apart (Fig. 30.2). Both Izquierdo et al. and our group have found that combined CXL + iris-claw PIOL implantation significantly improved UDVA and CDVA, with high predictability of the refractive error in addition to a good safety profile.[7,18] Combined CXL + ICL implantation has shown similar outcomes in terms of effectiveness and safety in the long term.[9] A recent study showed that the combined Athens protocol and PIOL implantation was also safe and effective.[19]

Combined Intrastromal Corneal Ring Segment Plus Phakic Intraocular Lens Implantation

ICRSs are safe, reversible, and effective in improving vision in patients with KC, correcting mild-moderate refractive error, and improving optical quality. However, the magnitude of these effects is highly variable,[3] and a number of patients have significant refractive errors that require additional optical aids to achieve good visual performance. ICRS implantation can be combined with PIOL implantation to correct moderate-high spherocylindrical errors, providing significant visual and refractive improvement (Table 30.5 and Fig. 30.3A), with satisfactory long-term efficacy and safety profiles.[20] However, to date there is no consensus regarding the appropriate timing between ICRS and PIOL implantation. Most authors suggest that ICRS implantation should be first performed to correct gross corneal shape, followed by CXL to halt progression (if needed), and finally PIOL for correction of myopia and astigmatism.[3] One study found no significant differences between simultaneous versus sequential ICRS + PIOL implantation.[21]

Phakic Intraocular Lenses After Keratoplasty in Keratoconic Eyes

PK and more recently DALK have shown a long track record of safety and effectiveness in the treatment of advanced KC. However, keratoplasty in this setting usually results in high ametropia and consequent anisometropia, which hinders visual rehabilitation, even in clear corneal grafts. Strategies for the management of postkeratoplasty ametropia include conservative approaches (optical correction with spectacles or CL) and surgical interventions (either extraocular or intra-ocular). PIOL implantation is an alternative to correct postkeratoplasty ametropia in KC eyes (Table 30.6 and Fig. 30.3B). At least 6 months should be given after suture removal, and stable refraction confirmed with two observations spaced at least 2 months apart before considering PIOL implantation in these cases. The first report on the outcomes of iris-claw PIOL in PK eyes showed significant improvement in UDVA from 1.39 ± 0.44 to 0.55 ± 0.35 logMAR, and an 88.8% reduction in mean cylindrical error.[22] The first report on the outcomes of ICL following PK in keratoconic eyes demonstrated good 2-year efficacy and safety indices and good refractive outcomes (97.3% of eyes falling within ± 1.00 D of the predicted refraction).[23] Malheiro et al. have reported the longest follow-up data on iris-claw PIOL for the correction of post-DALK ametropia.[24] In eyes with 5-year follow-up, safety and efficacy indices were 1.26 and 1.02, respectively.[24]

Complications of Phakic Intraocular Lens in Keratoconus

Side effects associated with PIOLs include glare and halos, significant residual refractive error, pupil ovalization, pigment dispersion, intraocular pressure elevation, lens deposits and cataractogenesis, PIOL dislocation requiring repositioning, and increased rate of EC loss (%ECL). We refer the reader to a comprehensive review on PIOL-related complications.[25]

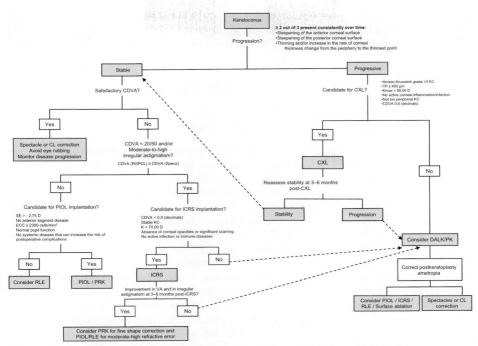

Fig. 30.1 Proposed decision tree for the management of keratoconus. *CDVA,* Corrected distance visual acuity; *CL,* contact lens; *CXL,* corneal cross-linking; *DALK,* deep anterior lamellar keratoplasty; *ECC,* endothelial cell count; *ICRS,* intrastromal corneal ring segments; *KC,* keratoconus; *PIOL,* phakic intraocular lens; *PK,* penetrating keratoplasty; *PRK,* photorefractive keratectomy; *RGPCL,* rigid gas-permeable contact lens; *RLE,* refractive lens exchange; *SE,* refractive spherical equivalent; *TP,* thinnest point in corneal pachymetry; *VA,* visual acuity. (Adapted from Güell et al.[2] and Gore et al.[3])

The data on complications of PIOL implantation in KC eyes are relatively scarce. Although most studies have not reported complications, reported rates of ICL rotation requiring reposition-ing have been reported in 5% to 21% of eyes.[10,26] It has been suggested that the enclavation system of iris-claw PIOL prevents potential rotation and provides increased stability compared with PC

BOX 30.1 ■ **Exclusion Criteria for Phakic Intraocular Lens Implantation in Patients With Keratoconus**

1. Progressive keratoconus
2. BSCVA <20/50 and/or significant irregular astigmatism
3. Significant corneal opacity
4. ECC <2300 cells/mm²
5. Shallow AC depth (<3.00 mm for Artisan/Artiflex, <3.2 mm for ICL)
6. Abnormal pupil function, or scotopic pupil >6.0 mm
7. Anterior segment disease (e.g., herpetic keratitis, recurrent or chronic uveitis, cataract)
8. Systemic disease that may increase risk of postoperative complications (atopy, diabetes mellitus, autoimmune disorder, connective tissue disease)

AC, Anterior chamber; *BSCVA,* best spectacle-corrected visual acuity; *ECC,* endothelial cell count; *ICL,* implantable collamer lens.

BOX 30.2 ■ Clinical and Corneal Topo-tomographic Parameters Frequently Used to Determine Progression of Keratoconus[3,14]

1. Increase in mean keratometry ≥0.75 D
2. Increase in SimK ≥1.00 D
3. Change in manifest refractive spherical equivalent (RSE) ≥0.50 D
4. Changes in manifest cylinder ≥ 1.00 D
5. Decrease in corneal pachymetry ≥ 25 μm

PIOLs; however, conclusive evidence is lacking. A retrospective analysis comparing the outcomes and stability of Artiflex and ICL in eyes with primary stable KC found similar safety indices between both types of PIOL, but a nonstatistically significant higher efficacy index with iris-claw PIOL.[4] Of note, there was a tendency toward undercorrection in the PC PIOL group, whereas most patients in the iris-claw PIOL group were close to emmetropia.[4] Finally, one PC PIOL eye (but no iris-claw PIOL eyes) required IOL repositioning because of spontaneous rotation.[4]

Accelerated endothelial cell loss (ECL) is a particular concern with PIOLs. Recent studies have found that 4- to 5-year %ECL is similar across angle-supported PIOL, iris-claw AC PIOL, and PC PIOLs, ranging from 7.8% to 13%.[27,28] Differences in %ECL between the ICL V4c and V4b models may be nonsignificant.[29] The American Academy of Ophthalmology has issued recommendations stating that specular microscopy should be performed preoperatively and at the 6-, 12-, 24-, and 36-month postoperative intervals.[30] In eyes with %ECL ≥20% or an ECC <1500 cells/mm², additional visits with a 4- to 6-month interval are recommended, and in these cases PIOL explantation may be considered if a %ECL ≥1% per year is documented.[30] In light of recent studies showing that %ECL occurs linearly in the long term, annual assessment should be considered.[27,28,31]

In eyes with stable, early KC, iris-claw PIOLs have shown a relatively low rate of complications; importantly, no cases of significant %ECL requiring IOL explantation have been reported in this setting (see Table 30.2). Reported %ECL following ICL implantation in stable nonadvanced KC ranges from 4.4% to 8.9% at 3 years,[10,32] and a recent study reported a 7.9% ECL at 5 years.[26] ECL following ICL implantation in eyes with KC has been reported in some studies and may be <5% within the first 6 to 12 postoperative months (see Tables 30.3 and 30.4).

The increased %ECL after PIOL implantation is a particularly severe risk in PK eyes. Initial reports suggested an additional yearly 6% to 7% ECL risk in these eyes.[22] However, their findings likely reflect the heterogeneity of the study group. Other reports of PIOL implantation for postkeratoplasty ametropia have reported variable %ECL, ranging from 5.7% to 10.6% at 1 to 2 years (see Table 30.6). Importantly, only one case of significant %ECL requiring PIOL explantation has been reported in published studies of PIOL postkeratoplasty in keratoconic eyes.[24]

Conclusion

The current management of KC eyes includes a number of different strategies, including CXL, ICRS implantation, surface ablation techniques, PIOL implantation, refractive lens exchange, and keratoplasty. One or more of these approaches can be used in combination to halt progression of the ectasia and for visual rehabilitation. However, despite the effort of many cornea specialists and cornea-focused societies, there is not yet a clear worldwide consensus on how and when to use them. Still today, most refractive errors in KC eyes are managed conservatively with spectacles and/or CL. In some cases of unsatisfactory CDVA with a stable refraction and without any contraindications, PIOLs might be considered for the correction of the spherical error and/or the regular component of the astigmatism, with good safety and efficacy profiles. PIOL implantation is also a valid option to correct postkeratoplasty ametropia.

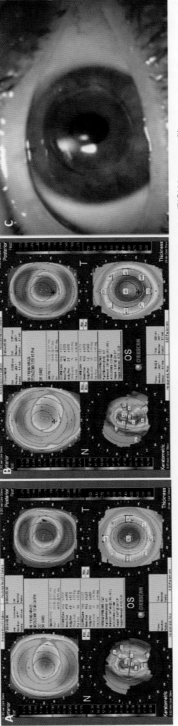

Fig. 30.2 Sequential corneal cross-linking (CXL) and phakic intraocular lens implantation (PIOL) in an eye with progressive keratoconus (KC). (A) Corneal topography before CXL documenting KC progression. Corrected distance visual acuity (CDVA) was 20/80 (refraction was SPH −4.50 D CYL −4.50 D x 160°), and keratometry was 53.9/46.8 D. (B) Corneal topography following CXL, showing flattening of the cone (keratometry 49.4/45.6 D); CDVA was 20/60. (C) Slit-lamp photography after CXL + PIOL implantation, CDVA improved to 20/40 (refraction was CYL −0.50 D x 140°). (From Güell JL, Morral M, Barbany M, et al. Role of corneal cross-linking and phakic intraocular lens implantation in progressive keratoconus. *Int J Kerat Ect Cor Dis.* 2018;7(1):26–30.)

TABLE 30.4 ■ **Reported Outcomes and Complications of Combined Corneal Cross-Linking and Phakic Intraocular Lens Implantation in Keratoconus**

Preoperative Data

Author	Publication (Year)	Eyes (n)	PIOL	UDVA (logMAR)	CDVA (logMAR)	Sphere (D)	Cylinder (D)	RSE (D)
Izquierdo et al.[7]	2011	11	Artiflex	1.40 ± 0.40	0.14 ± 0.06	−5.70 ± 1.21	−1.32 ± 0.86	−6.36 ± 1.09
Kymionis et al.[39]	2011	1	Visian ICL	CF	0.7	−10	−5	−12.5
Güell et al.[18]	2012	17	Artiflex	N/R	0.10 ± 0.09	−5.25	−3.54 ± 1.39	−6.99 ± 3.20
Fadlallah et al.[40]	2013	16	Visian ICL	1.67 ± 0.49	0.15 ± 0.06	−8.56 ± 3.90	2.64 ± 1.28	−7.24 ± 3.53
Shafik Shaheen et al.[32]	2014	16	Visian ICL	N/R	0.56 ± 0.13 (decimals)	−6 ± 4.0	−5 ± 1.5	−8.5 ± 4.0
Antonios et al.[41]	2014	30	Visian ICL	1.57 ± 0.50	0.17 ± 0.08	−8.37 ± 3.89	2.95 ± 1.40	−6.96 ± 3.68
Doroodgar et al.[9]	2017	40	Visian ICL	1.28 ± 0.37	N/R	N/R	N/R	N/R
Emerah et al.[42]	2019	14	Visian ICL	0.77 ± 0.20	0.18 ± 0.10	−3.7 ± 1.9	−2.3 ± 1.6	−4.48 ± 2.25

Postoperative Data

Follow-Up (Months)	UDVA (logMAR)	CDVA (logMAR)	Spherical Error (D)	Cylinder (D)	Final RSE (D)	%RSE within ± 0.50 D
6	0.16 ± 0.06	0.04 ± 0.05	−0.27 ± 0.52	−0.91 ± 0.61	−0.727 ± 0.66	45.5%
3	0.3	0.2	−0.25	−0.5	−0.5	100.0%
36.9 ± 15.0	0.17 ± 0.13	0.10 ± 0.09	0.06 ± 0.26	−0.62 ± 0.39	−0.22 ± 0.33	82.4%
12	0.17 ± 0.06	0.12 ± 0.04	−1.47 ± 0.99	1.16 ± 0.64	−0.89 ± 0.76	75.0%
36	N/R	0.88 ± 0.18 (decimals)	0.00 ± 0.18	−0.05 ± 0.14	Final RSE < −0.25	100.0%
12	0.17 ± 0.06	0.11 ± 0.05	−1.36 ± 0.94	1.03 ± 0.60	−0.83 ± 0.76	N/R
48	0.11 ± 0.13	−0.14 ± 0.13	N/R	Mean change = 2.79 ± 1.78	Mean change = 7.44 ± 4.75	82.5%
6	0.15 ± 0.10	0.15 ± 0.10	−0.20 ± 0.50	−0.60 ± 0.50	Final RSE decreased 74% from preoperative	65% of eyes within ± 0.75 D

CDVA, Corrected distance visual acuity; *CF*, counting fingers; *CXL*, corneal cross-linking; *D*, diopters; *Kmax*, maximum keratometry; *Kmin*, minimum keratometry; *ECC*, endothelial cell count; *ECL*, endothelial cell loss; *EI*, efficacy index (postoperative UDVA/preoperative CDVA ratio); *N/R*, not reported; *PIOL*, phakic intraocular lens; *RSE*, refractive spherical equivalent; *SI*, safety index (postoperative CDVA/preoperative CDVA ratio); *UDVA*, uncorrected distance visual acuity.

Post-CXL, Pre-PIOL Data

K_{max}/K_{min} (D)	ECC (cells/mm²)	CDVA	RSE (D)	Cylinder (D)	K_{max}/K_{min} (D)	ECC (cells/mm²)	Time Between CXL and PIOL (Months)
48.20 ± 3.47 / 43.94 ± 2.92	2759.6 ± 159.8	1.16 ± 0.46	−5.90 ± 1.14	−1.30 ± 0.67	46.93 ±3.49 / 44.17 ± 1.64	2739.1 ± 157.0	6
63.51 / 57.24	N/R	0.5	−14.25	−4.5	61.72/57.17	N/R	12
46.11 ± 1.17/43.29 ± 1.17	2847	0.10 ± 0.09	−6.93 ± 3.09	−3.51 ± 1.93	46.17 ± 1.26 /43.60 ± 1.26	2868	3.9 ± 0.7
52.59±4.79/ 46.00±3.58	N/R	0.15 ± 0.06	−7.16 ± 3.58	2.45 ± 1.19	51.33 ± 4.41 / 46.02 ± 2.99	N/R	6
N/R	2850	N/R	N/R	N/R	N/R	N/R	12
53.08 ± 5.17 / 46.52 ± 3.72	N/R	0.15 ± 0.06	−6.81 ± 3.48	2.74 ± 1.33	52.01 ± 4.87/46.23 ± 3.21	N/R	6
N/R	N/R	0.19 ± 0.11	−7.55 ± 4.22	−3.57 ± 1.56	N/R	2426.6 ± 107.6	≥12
N/R	N/R	71.4% of eyes had CXL before ICL implantation					

%RSE within ± 1.00 D	%eyes UDVA ≥ 20/40	%eyes gain ≥ 1 lines CDVA	%eyes loss ≥ 2 lines CDVA	%ECL	Complications
63.6%	100.0%	63.6%	0%	3.3%	Mild haze (18.1%)
100.0%	100.0%	100.0%	0%	N/R	None reported
94.1%	94.1%	30.0%	0.0%	0.1%	Mild giant cell reaction (11.7%)
87.5%	81.0%	N/R	0%	N/R	None reported
100.0%	81% had UDVA ≥ 20/25	N/R	0.0%	8.89%	None reported
63.3%	60% had UDVA ≥ 20/30	43.0%	0.0%	N/R	None reported
97.1%	100.0%	82.5%	0.0%	≤5%	None reported
85.0%	N/R	42.9%	0%	N/R	None reported

TABLE 30.5 ■ **Reported Outcomes and Complications of Combined Intrastromal Corneal Ring Segment and Phakic Intraocular Lens Implantation in Keratoconus.**

Preoperative Data

Author	Eyes (n)	Protocol	PIOL	UDVA (logMAR)	CDVA (logMAR)	Sphere (D)	Cylinder (D)
Colin and Velou[43]	1	ICRS + PIOL	Nuvita	1.70	0.15	−9	−4.5
El-Raggal et al.[44]	8	ICRS + PIOL	Verisyse	0.03 ± 0.01 (decimals)	0.55 ± 0.16 (decimals)	−10.81 ± 1.31	2.81 ± 0.53
Coskunseven et al.[45]	3	ICRS + PIOL	Vision ICL	CF	0.70 ± 0.22	−16.17 ± 1.31	−4.58 ± 1.71
Kamburoğlu et al.[46]	2	ICRS + PIOL	Artisan	CF	0.55 ± 0.15	−9.5 ± 0.5	−5.5 ± 0.0
Alfonso et al.[47]	40	ICRS + PIOL + corneal relaxing incisions	ICL	0.11 ± 0.05 (decimals)	0.56 ± 0.23 (decimals)	−7.56 ± 7.27	J0 −1.15 ± 1.12 / J45 0.25 ± 1.71
Moshirfar et al.[21]	12	Simultaneous ICRS + PIOL	Verisyse	2.13 ± 0.23	0.26 ± 0.23	−11.94 ± 3.80	2.98 ± 0.99
	7	Sequential ICRS + PIOL	Verisyse	1.96 ± 0.38	0.43 ± 0.19	−13.04 ± 4.78	4.00 ± 2.59
Kurian et al.[48]	10	PIOL ± ICRS ± CXL	Vision ICL	0.07 ± 0.04 (decimals)	0.82 ± 0.25 (decimals)	−5.58 ± 3.00	−3.28 ± 2.04
Navas et al.[20]	11	ICRS + PIOL	Vision ICL	N/R			
Dirani et al.[49]	11	ICRS + CXL + PIOL	Vision ICL	1.47 ± 0.38	0.50 ± 0.22	−11.61 ± 3.33	3.81 ± 1.15
Coskunseven et al.[50]	14	ICRS + CXL + PIOL	Vision ICL	0.01 ± 1.3 lines	0.14 ± 2.40 lines	N/R	−4.73 ± 1.32
Ferreira et al.[51]	21	ICRS + PIOL	Artisan/ Artiflex	2.0 ± 0.0	0.31 ± 0.13	−9.14 ± 6.87	−3.25 ± 1.20
Abdelmassih et al.[52]	16	ICRS + CXL+PIOL	Vision ICL	1.06	0.42 ± 0.16	−9.25 ± 3.22	3.83 ± 1.23

					After ICRS Implantation (±CXL)				
RSE (D)	Kmax/Kmin (D)	ECC (cells/mm²)	UDVA	CDVA	RSE (D)	Cylinder (D)	Kmax/Kmin (D)	ECC (cells/mm²)	Time Between ICRS (± CXL) and PIOL (Months)
−11.25	N/R	N/R	1.30	0.20	−9.13	−1.75	N/R	2720	N/R
−12.18 ± 1.09	52.89 ± 0.92 / 47.85 ± 1.10	N/R	0.04 ± 0.03 (decimals)	0.65 ± 0.09 (decimals)	−10.28 ± 1.62	−1.75 ± 0.33	49.35 ± 1.26 / 44.56 ± 1.48	N/R	6
−18.46 ± 2.17	58.53 ± 0.58 / 54.43 ± 1.99	2179.3 ± 56.0	N/R	0.37 ± 0.05	−13.71 ± 1.88	−2.58 ± 0.82	N/R	N/R	8.7 ± 1.9
−12.25 ± 0.50	52.55 ± 0.75 / 48.45 ± 0.25	N/R	0.85 ± 0.15	0.35 ± 0.15	−8.88 ± 0.13	−4.75 ± 0.25	49.2 ± 1.1 / 45.5 ± 0.9	3117.5 ± 122.5	N/R
−9.67 ± 6.96	48.95 ± 4.77 / 45.03 ± 3.33	N/R	0.18 ± 0.14 (decimals)	0.68 ± 0.25 (decimals)	−7.88 ± 6.44	J0 −0.68 ± 0.55 / J45 0.11 ± 0.68	N/R	N/R	6
N/R	Mean K = 46.58 ± 2.11	N/R			N/A				
N/R	Mean K = 47.59 ± 3.73	N/R	1.94 ± 0.31	0.29 ± 0.17	N/R	3.25 ± 2.58	Mean K = 46.65 ± 3.34	N/R	
−7.21 ± 2.25	N/R	1 eye required ICRS, 3 required CXL, and 2 eyes required CXL + ICRS							
			1.31 ± 0.37	0.29 ± 0.14	−10.52 ± 5.88	−2.95 ± 1.35	Mean K = 51.87 ± 5.39	N/R	≥12 months
−9.70 ± 3.10	57.41 ± 6.32 / 48.51 ± 4.26	N/R	1.13 ± 0.50	0.29 ± 0.23	−7.65 ± 3.23	4.06 ± 1.58	54.01 ± 4.75 / 45.19 ± 3.98	N/R	≥6 months after CXL
−16.40 ± 3.56	60.57 ± 2.14 / 56.16 ± 2.40	N/R	0.06 ± 4.3 lines	0.47 ± 1.00 lines	−9.67 ± 2.79	−2.09 ± 1.31	54.61 ± 2.74 / 53.54 ± 2.24	N/R	8.4
10.76 ± 6.86	48.21 ± 4.7 / 45.24 ± 4.7	2513 ± 265	0.93 ± 0.63	0.37 ± 0.18			N/R		18.23 (range 6–48)
	N/R		0.76	0.26				N/R	≥6 months after CXL

Continued on following page

TABLE 30.5 ■ Reported Outcomes and Complications of Combined Intrastromal Corneal Ring Segment and Phakic Intraocular Lens Implantation in Keratoconus (Continued)

Postoperative Data

Follow-Up (Months)	UDVA (log-MAR)	CDVA (logMAR)	Spherical Error (D)	Cylinder (D)	Final RSE (D)	%RSE within ± 0.50 D	%RSE within ± 1.00 D
6	0.50	0.10	−1.25	−1.75	−2.13	0	0
24	0.59 ± 0.06 (decimals)	0.74 ± 0.09 (decimals)	−0.28 ± 0.98	1.81 ± 0.42	−1.19 ± 0.89	37.5%	75.0%
4.0 ± 1.4	0.43 ± 0.09	0.27 ± 0.05	−0.08 ± 0.24	−1.00 ± 0.20	−0.58 ± 0.33	33.3%	100.0%
5	0.25 ± 0.05	0.15 ± 0.00	−1.00 ± 0.50	−1.00 ± 0.50	−1.50 ± 0.25	0.0%	0.0%
6	0.50 ± 0.27 (decimals)	0.73 ± 0.20 (decimals)	N/R	J0 −0.22 ± 0.70 J45 0.02 ± 0.66	−1.20 ± 1.33	45.0%	65.0%
19 ± 6	0.40 ± 0.20	0.14 ± 0.09	−0.79 ± 1.00	2.06 ± 1.21	0.16 ± 1.08	50.0%	83.3%
36 ± 21	0.53 ± 0.15	0.43 ± 0.19	−1.64 ± 1.31	2.07 ± 1.03	−0.61 ± 1.28	14.3%	42.9%
6	0.59 ± 0.37 (decimals)	0.93 ± 0.14 (decimals)	0.43 ± 1.03	−1.73 ± 1.59	−0.44 ± 1.21	30.0%	70.0%
38.2 ± 18.7	0.14 ± 0.04	0.16 ± 0.08	−0.06 ± 0.46	−1.22 ± 0.65	−0.68 ± 0.45	18.0%	55.0%
6	0.27 ± 0.20	0.19 ± 0.11	−1.50 ± 1.06	1.84 ± 0.35	−0.58 ± 1.01	54.5%	63.6%
12	0.45 ± 1.10	0.57 ± 0.70 lines	N/R	−0.93 ± 0.31	−0.80 ± 1.02	N/R	50.0%
12	0.25 ± 0.22	0.13 ± 0.13	0.14 ± 0.45	−1.2 ± 1.18	−0.46 ± 0.80	61.9%	90.5%
24	0.33	0.16	−2.11 ± 1.63 (at 6 months)	2.47 ± 1.62 (at 6 months)	N/R	50.0%	69.0%

CDVA, Corrected distance visual acuity; *CF,* counting fingers; *CXL,* corneal cross-linking; *D,* diopters; *Kmax,* maximum keratometry; Kmin, minimum ke *Kmax,* maximum keratometry; *ECC,* endothelial cell count; *ECL,* endothelial cell loss; *EI,* efficacy index (postoperative UDVA/preoperative CDVA ratio); *ICRS,* intrastromal corneal ring segment; *Kmax,* maximum keratometry; *Kmin,* minimum keratometry; *N/R,* not reported; *PIOL,* phakic intraocular lens; *RSE,* refractive spherical equivalent; *SI,* safety index (postoperative CDVA/preoperative CDVA ratio); *UDVA,* uncorrected distance visual acuity; *CF,* counting fingers.

%eyes UDVA ≥ 20/40	%eyes gain ≥ 1 lines CDVA	%eyes loss ≥ 2 lines CDVA	%ECL	Complications
0%	100%	0%	2.90%	None reported
100.0%	N/R	0%	N/R	Slight increase in cylindrical error after PIOL (mean change 0.06 D)
33.3%	100.0%	0.0%	N/R	None reported
100.0%	100.0%	0.0%	2.9%	None reported
N/R	70.0%	2.5% of eyes after ICRS	N/R	None reported
41.7%	50.0%	0.0%	N/R	None reported
14.3%	100.0%	0.0%	N/R	None reported
100.0%	40.0%	0%	N/R	None reported
81.8%	82.0%	0%	N/R	None reported
63.7%	N/R	0.0%	N/R	None reported
64.0%	100.0%	21.0%	N/R	None reported
63.1%	85.7%	0%	8.0%	None reported
93.8%	81.0%	0.0%	N/R	None reported

TABLE 30.6 ■ Reported Outcomes and Complications of Phakic Intraocular Lens Implantation Following Keratoplasty in Keratoconic Eyes

Preoperative Data

Author	Publication (Year)	Type of Corneal Transplant	Phakic IOL	Time Between Transplant and PIOL Implantation (Months)	Eyes (n)	UDVA (logMAR)
Tahzib et al.[22]	2006	PK	Artisan	30.8 ± 28.2	36 (14% KC)	1.39 ± 0.44
Alfonso et al.[53]	2009	PK	Visian ICL	40.2 ± 28.1	15	N/R
Akcay et al.[54]	2009	PK	Visian ICL	Unspecified	1	0.82
Iovieno et al.[55]	2013	PK or DALK	Visian ICL	52.0 ± 27.5	7	1.18 ± 0.40
Al-Dreihi et al.[56]	2013	DALK	Artisan	18	1	0.40
Tiveron et al.[57]	2017	DALK	Artisan/Artiflex	All patients >18 months post-DALK	24	1.05 ± 0.35
Qin et al.[58]	2017	DALK	Visian ICL	All patients > 18 months post-DALK	9	0.74 ± 0.21
Malheiro et al.[24]	2019	DALK	Artisan/Artiflex	35.7	11	1.27

Postoperative Data

UDVA (logMAR)	CDVA (logMAR)	%UDVA ≥20/40	%Gain ≥1 line CDVA	%Loss ≥2 lines CDVA	Sphere (D)	Cylinder (D)	RSE (D)	%RSE within ± 0.50 D	%RSE within ± 1.00 D
0.55 ± 0.35	0.26 ± 0.24	27.80%	N/R	8.30%	−0.03 ± 1.23	−2.00 ± 1.53	−1.03 ± 1.20	N/R	N/R
0.47 ± 0.34	0.23 ± 0.18	46.7%	46.7%	0.0%	−0.53 ± 0.90	−0.85 ± 1.02	−0.96 ± 1.08	66.6	80
0.10	0.00	100.0%	100.0%	0.0%	0.75	−0.5	0.5	100	100
0.20 ± 0.15	0.05 ± 0.08	85.7%	N/R	0.0%	−0.53 ± 0.75	−1.74 ± 0.84	−0.33 ± 0.54	85.7% within ± 0.75 D of emmetropia	
0.10	0.10	100.0%	100.0%	0.0%	0.00	−1.00	−0.50	100%	100%
0.18 ± 0.15	0.14 ± 0.13	88.0%	54.0%	0.0%	0.09 ± 0.72	−0.66 ± 0.61	−0.23 ± 0.74	71	92%
0.14	0.05	100.0%	100.0%	0.0%	−0.13 ± 0.21	−0.42 ± 0.18	−0.35 ± 0.24	81.8	100%
0.22	0.08	45.4% had UDVA ≥ 20/25	63.6%	0.0%	−0.55 ± 0.82	−1.00 ± 0.95	−1.02 ± 1.07	45.4	64%

CDVA, Corrected distance visual acuity; *CXL,* corneal cross-linking; *DALK,* deep anterior lamellar keratoplasty; *ECC,* endothelial cell count; *ECL,* endothelial cell loss; *EI,* efficacy index (postoperative UDVA/preoperative CDVA ratio); *N/R,* not reported; *PIOL,* phakic intraocular lens; *PK,* penetrating keratoplasty; *RSE,* refractive spherical equivalent; *SI,* safety index (postoperative CDVA/preoperative CDVA ratio); *UDVA,* uncorrected distance visual acuity.

CDVA (logMAR)	Sphere (D)	Cylinder (D)	RSE (D)	ECC (cells/mm²)	Follow-Up (Months)	%ECL	Complications	SI	EI
0.26 ± 0.17	0.34 ± 4.36	−7.06 ± 2.01	−3.19 ± 4.31	N/R	28.5 ± 12.5	30.4 ± 32.0 %	BSCVA loss ≥2 lines (8.3%); haptic dislocation requiring repositioning (2.8%); corneal decompensation (2.8%)	N/R	N/R
0.33 ± 0.22	−7.08 ± 4.34	−3.45 ± 1.63	−8.81 ± 4.14	1660 ± 427	24	8.07%	None reported	1.58	1.02
0.40	−8	−1.75	−8.88	2326.00	12	9.84%	None reported	N/R	N/R
0.09 ± 0.11	−5.89 ± 3.43	−4.39 ± 0.95	−8.09 ± 3.77	N/R	12.8 ± 8.8	N/R	None reported	0.55	2.19
0.18	4.75	−5	2.25	2043	12	10.57%	None reported	N/R	N/R
0.21 ± 0.16	−2.26 ± 3.06	−4.92 ± 1.55	−4.73 ± 2.59	2632.3 ± 357.6	12	6.10%	None reported	1	0.93
0.24 ± 0.11	−3.31	−3.39	−5	2521.2	24	5.66%	None reported	1.2	0.98
0.16	−4.14 ± 4.87	−7.41 ± 3.61	−8.02 ± 4.63	2318	36	13.1 ± 8.6 %	Significant %ECL with indication for PIOL explantation (9.1%)	1.21	0.97

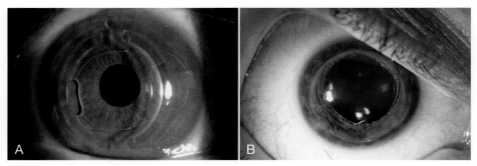

Fig. 30.3 (A) Slit-lamp photography of an iris-claw anterior chamber phakic intraocular lens implantation following intrastromal corneal ring segment implantation in an eye with keratoconus. (B) Slit-lamp photography of an iris-claw anterior chamber phakic intraocular lens implantation for the correction of postkeratoplasty ametropia following penetrating keratoplasty in a keratoconic eye.

References

1. Gomes JA, Tan D, Rapuano CJ, et al. Global consensus on keratoconus and ectatic diseases. *Cornea.* 2015;34:359–369.
2. Güell JL, Morral M, Barbany M, et al. Role of corneal cross-linking and phakic intraocular lens implantation in progressive keratoconus. *Int J Kerat Ect Cor Dis.* 2018;7(1):26–30.
3. Gore DM, Shortt AJ, Allan BD. New clinical pathways for keratoconus. *Eye.* 2013;27(3):329–339.
4. Alió JL, Peña-García P, Abdulla GF, Zein G, Abu-Mustafa SK. Comparison of iris-claw and posterior chamber collagen copolymer phakic intraocular lenses in keratoconus. *J Cataract Refract Surg.* 2014;40(3):383–394.
5. Vastardis I, Sagri D, Fili S, Wölfelschneider P, Kohlhaas M. Current trends in modern visual intraocular lens enhancement surgery in stable keratoconus: a synopsis of do's, don'ts and pitfalls. *Ophthalmol Ther.* 2019;8(suppl 1):33–47.
6. Güell JL, Vázquez M, Malecaze F, et al. Artisan toric phakic intraocular lens for the correction of high astigmatism. *Am J Ophthalmol.* 2003;136:442–447.
7. Izquierdo L, Henriquez MA, McCarthy M. Artiflex phakic intraocular lens implantation after corneal collagen cross-linking in keratoconic eyes. *J Refract Surg.* 2011;27:482–487.
8. Kamiya K, Shimizu K, Kobashi H, et al. Clinical outcomes of posterior chamber toric phakic intraocular lens implantation for the correction of high myopic astigmatism in eyes with keratoconus: 6-month follow-up. *Graefes Arch Clin Exp Ophthalmol.* 2011;249(7):1073–1080.
9. Doroodgar F, Niazi F, Sanginabadi A, et al. Comparative analysis of the visual performance after implantation of the toric implantable collamer lens in stable keratoconus: a 4-year follow-up after sequential procedure (CXL+TICL implantation). *BMJ Open Ophthalmol.* 2017;2(1):e000090.
10. Kamiya K, Shimizu K, Kobashi H, et al. Three-year follow-up of posterior chamber toric phakic intraocular lens implantation for the correction of high myopic astigmatism in eyes with keratoconus. *Br J Ophthalmol.* 2015;99:177–183.
11. Budo C, Bartels MC, van Rij G. Implantation of Artisan toric phakic intraocular lenses for the correction of astigmatism and spherical errors in patients with keratoconus. *J Refract Surg.* 2005;21(3):218–222.
12. Venter J. Artisan phakic intraocular lens in patients with keratoconus. *J Refract Surg.* 2009;25(9):759–764.
13. Kato N, Toda I, Hori-Komai Y, Sakai C, Arai H, Tsubota K. Phakic intraocular lens for keratoconus. *Ophthalmology.* 2011;118(3):605–605.e2.
14. . Cataract. ESASO Course Series. In: Güell JL, ed.; 2013. *Basel: Karger.* 3:100–115.
15. Alió J, Vega-Estrada A, Sanz-Díez P, Peña-García P, Durán-García ML, Maldonado M. Keratoconus Management Guidelines. *Int J Kerat Ect Cor Dis.* 2015;4(1):1–39.
16. Kanellopoulos AJ. Comparison of sequential vs same-day simultaneous collagen cross-linking and topography-guided PRK for treatment of keratoconus. *J Refract Surg.* 2009;25(9):S812–S818.
17. Kymionis GD, Grentzelos MA, Kankariya VP, Pallikaris IG. Combined transepithelial phototherapeutic keratectomy and corneal collagen crosslinking for ectatic disorders: Cretan protocol. *J Cataract Refract Surg.* 2013;39:1939.

18. Güell JL, Morral M, Malecaze F, Gris O, Elies D, Manero F. Collagen crosslinking and toric iris-claw phakic intraocular lens for myopic astigmatism in progressive mild to moderate keratoconus. *J Cataract Refract Surg.* 2012;38(3):475–484.
19. Assaf A, Kotb A. Simultaneous corneal crosslinking and surface ablation combined with phakic intraocular lens implantation for managing keratoconus. *Int Ophthalmol.* 2015;35:411–419.
20. Navas A, Tapia-Herrera G, Jaimes M. Implantable collamer lenses after intracorneal ring segments for keratoconus. *Int Ophthalmol.* 2012;32(5):423–429.
21. Majid M, Fenzl CR, Meyer JJ, Neuffer MC, Espandar L, Mifflin M. Simultaneous and sequential implantation of Intacs and Verisyse phakic intraocular lens for refractive improvement in keratectasia. *Cornea.* 2011;30:158–163.
22. Tahzib NG, Nuijts RM, Wu WY, Budo CJ. Long-term study of Artisan phakic intraocular lens implantation for the correction of moderate to high myopia: ten-year follow-up results. *Ophthalmology.* 2007;114(6):1133–1142.
23. Alfonso JF, Lisa C, Abdelhamid A, Montés-Micó R, Poo-López A, Ferrer-Blasco T. Posterior chamber phakic intraocular lenses after penetrating keratoplasty. *J Cataract Refract Surg.* 2009;35:1166–1173.
24. Malheiro L, Coelho J, Neves MM, Gomes M, Oliveira L. Phakic intraocular lens implantation after deep anterior lamellar keratoplasty: retrospective case series analysis with long-term follow-up. *Clin Ophthalmol.* 2019;13:2043–2052.
25. Kohnen T, Kook D, Morral M, Güell JL. Phakic intraocular lenses: part 2: results and complications. *J Cataract Refract Surg.* 2010;36(12):2168–2194.
26. Hashemian SJ, Saiepoor N, Ghiasian L, et al. Long-term outcomes of posterior chamber phakic intraocular lens implantation in keratoconus. *Clin Exp Optom.* 2018;101(5):652–658.
27. Güell JL, Morral M, Gris O, Gaytan J, Sisquella M, Manero F. Five-year follow-up of 399 phakic Artisan-Verisyse implantation for myopia, hyperopia, and/or astigmatism. *Ophthalmology.* 2008;115(6):1002–1012.
28. Jonker S, Berendschot TT, Ronden AE, Saelens IEY, Bauer NJC, Nuijts R. Five-year endothelial cell loss after implantation with Artiflex myopia and Artiflex toric phakic intraocular lenses. *Am J Ophthalmol.* 2018;194:110–119.
29. Goukon H, Kamiya K, Shimizu K, Igarashi A. Comparison of corneal endothelial cell density and morphology after posterior chamber phakic intraocular lens implantation with and without central hole. *Br J Ophthalmol.* 2017;101:1461–1465.
30. MacRae S, Holladay JT, Hilmantel G, et al. Special Report: American Academy of Ophthalmology Task Force Recommendations for Specular Microscopy for Phakic Intraocular Lenses. *Ophthalmology.* 2017;124:141–142.
31. Jonker S, Berendschot TT, Ronden AE, Saelens IEY, Bauer NJC, Nuijts R. Long-term endothelial cell loss in patients with Artisan myopia and Artisan toric phakic intraocular lenses: 5- and 10-year results. *Ophthalmology.* 2018;125(4):486–494.
32. Shafik Shaheen M, El-Kateb M, El-Samadouny MA, Zaghloul H. Evaluation of a toric implantable collamer lens after corneal collagen crosslinking in treatment of early-stage keratoconus: 3-year follow-up. *Cornea.* 2014;33(5):475–480.
33. Moshirfar M, Grégoire FJ, Mirzaian G, Whitehead GF, Kang PC. Use of Verisyse iris-supported phakic intraocular lens for myopia in keratoconic patients. *J Cataract Refract Surg.* 2006;32(7):1227–1232.
34. Sedaghat M, Ansari-Astaneh MR, Zarei-Ghanavati M, Davis SW, Sikder S. Artisan iris-supported phakic IOL implantation in patients with keratoconus: a review of 16 eyes. *J Refract Surg.* 2011;27(7):489–493.
35. Kamiya K, Shimizu K, Ando W, Asato Y, Fujisawa T. Phakic toric implantable collamer lens implantation for the correction of high myopic astigmatism in eyes with keratoconus. *J Refract Surg.* 2008;24(8):840–842.
36. Alfonso JF, Palacios A, Montés-Micó R. Myopic phakic STAAR collamer posterior chamber intraocular lenses for keratoconus. *J Refract Surg.* 2008;24(9):867–874.
37. Alfonso JF, Fernández-Vega L, Lisa C, Fernandes P, González-Méijome JM, Montés-Micó R. Collagen copolymer toric posterior chamber phakic intraocular lens in eyes with keratoconus. *J Cataract Refract Surg.* 2010;36(6):906–916.
38. Hashemian SJ, Soleimani M, Foroutan A, Joshaghani M, Ghaempanah J, Jafari ME. Toric implantable collamer lens for high myopic astigmatism in keratoconic patients after six months. *Clin Exp Optom.* 2012;96:225–232.

39. Kymionis GD, Grentzelos MA, Karavitaki AE, Paraskevi Z, Yoo SH, Pallikaris IG. Combined corneal collagen cross-linking and posterior chamber toric implantable collamer lens implantation for keratoconus. *Ophthalmic Surg Lasers Imaging.* 2011;42:e22–e25.

40. Fadlallah A, Dirani A, El Rami H, Cherfane G, Jarade E. Safety and visual outcome of Visian toric ICL implantation after corneal collagen cross-linking in keratoconus. *J Refract Surg.* 2013;29(2):84–89.

41. Antonios R, Dirani A, Fadlallah A, et al. Safety and visual outcome of Visian Toric ICL implantation after corneal collagen cross-linking in keratoconus: up to 2 years of follow-up. *J Ophthalmol.* 2015;2015:514834.

42. Emerah SH, Sabry MM, Saad HA, Ghobashy WA. Visual and refractive outcomes of posterior chamber phakic IOL in stable keratoconus. *Int J Ophthalmol.* 2019;12(5):840–843.

43. Colin J, Velou S. Implantation of Intacs and a refractive intraocular lens to correct keratoconus. *J Cataract Refract Surg.* 2003;29:832–834.

44. El-Raggal TM, Abdel Fattah AA. Sequential Intacs and Verisyse phakic intraocular lens for refractive improvement in keratoconic eyes. *J Cataract Refract Surg.* 2007;33:966–970.

45. Coskunseven E, Onder M, Kymionis GD, et al. Combined Intacs and posterior chamber toric implantable collamer lens implantation for keratoconic patients with extreme myopia. *Am J Ophthalmol.* 2007;144:387–389.

46. Kamburoğlu G, Ertan A, Bahadir M. Implantation of Artisan Toric phakic intraocular lens following Intacs in a patient with keratoconus. *J Cataract Refract Surg.* 2007;33(3):528–530.

47. Alfonso JF, Lisa C, Fernández-Vega L, Madrid-Costa D, Poo-López A, Montés-Micó R. Intrastromal corneal ring segments and posterior chamber phakic intraocular lens implantation for keratoconus correction. *J Cataract Refract Surg.* 2011;37(4):706–713.

48. Kurian M, Nagappa S, Bhagali R, Shetty R, Shetty BK. Visual quality after posterior chamber phakic intraocular lens implantation in keratoconus. *J Cataract Refract Surg.* 2012;38(6):1050–1057.

49. Dirani A, Fadlallah A, Khoueir Z, Antoun J, Cherfan G, Jarade E. Visian toric ICL implantation after intracorneal ring segments implantation and corneal collagen crosslinking in keratoconus. *Eur J Ophthalmol.* 2013;24:338–344.

50. Cockunseven E, Sharma DP, Jankov MR, Kymionis GD, Richoz O, Hafezi F. Collagen copolymer toric phakic intraocular lens for residual myopic astigmatism after intrastromal corneal ring segment implantation and corneal collagen crosslinking in a 3-stage procedure for keratoconus. *J Cataract Refract Surg.* 2013;39:722–729.

51. Ferreira TB, Güell JL, Manero F. Combined intracorneal ring segments and iris-fixated phakic intraocular lens for keratoconus refractive and visual improvement. *J Cataract Refract Surg.* 2014;30(5):336–341.

52. Abdelmassih Y, El-Khoury S, Chelala E, Slim E, Cherfan C, Jarade E. Toric ICL implantation after sequential intracorneal ring segments implantation and cornel cross-linking in keratoconus: 2-year follow-up. *J Refract Surg.* 2017;33(9):610–616.

53. Alfonso JF, Lisa C, Abdelhamid A, Montés-Micó R, Poo-López A, Ferrer-Blasco T. Posterior chamber phakic intraocular lenses after penetrating keratoplasty. *J Cataract Refract Surg.* 2009;35:1166–1173.

54. Akcay L, Kaplan AT, Kandemir B, et al. Toric intraocular Collamer lens for high myopic astigmatism after penetrating keratoplasty. *J Cataract Refract Surg.* 2009;35:2161–2163.

55. Iovieno A, Guglielmetti S, Capuano V, Allan BD, Maurino V. Correction of postkeratoplasty ametropia in keratoconus patients using a toric implantable Collamer lens. *Eur J Ophthalmol.* 2013;23:361–367.

56. Al-Dreihi MG, Louka BI, Anbari AA. Artisan iris-fixated toric phakic intraocular lens for the correction of astigmatism after deep anterior lamellar keratoplasty. *Digit J Ophthalmol.* 2013;19:39–41.

57. Tiveron MC, Alió Del Barrio JL, Kara-Junio N, et al. Outcomes of toric iris-claw phakic intraocular lens implantation after deep anterior lamellar keratoplasty for keratoconus. *J Refract Surg.* 2017;33:538–544.

58. Qin Q, Yang L, He Z, Huang Z. Clinical application of TICL implantation for ametropia following deep anterior lamellar keratoplasty for keratoconus: a CONSORT-compliant article. *Medicine (Baltimore).* 2017;96(8):e6118.

CHAPTER 31

Lamellar Keratoplasty in Keratoconus

Rajesh Fogla ■ Enrica Sarnicola

KEY CONCEPTS

- Lamellar keratoplasty is often required for advanced keratoconus when contact lens wear is no longer comfortable or an ideal fit cannot be achieved.
- Regional pachymetry and anterior segment optical coherence tomography (OCT) assessment preoperatively are essential to help decide on surgical technique.
- Cannula-assisted, sequential air injection technique for big bubble (BB) bubble deep anterior lamellar keratoplasty (DALK) appears to be safe and effective, if scars do not involve the Descemet membrane (DM). The viscobubble technique is an alternate option for primary surgery or rescue technique for failed air injection.
- Manual techniques should ensure a smooth residual bed with thickness less than 80 microns for optimal visual outcome.
- Femtosecond laser and intraoperative anterior segment OCT can provide further assistance to surgical techniques and help improve outcomes.
- Early recognition of complications and appropriate management can eliminate the need for conversion to penetrating keratoplasty (PKP).

Introduction

Advanced cases of keratoconus often require surgical intervention to restore corneal anatomy and improve vision. Although there is no precise definition for advanced disease, most specialists would agree that a keratoconus patient is eligible for corneal transplant when spectacle or contact lens correction is insufficient, continued contact lens wear is intolerable, and visual acuity has reduced to unacceptable levels.[1]

Traditionally, penetrating keratoplasty (PK) has been performed for advanced keratoconus with a higher success rate of graft survival than for other indications.[2] Since 2002, lamellar keratoplasty (LK), especially deep anterior lamellar keratoplasty (DALK), has emerged as an alternative procedure to PK.[3,4] DALK allows surgical replacement of the recipient's corneal stroma, preserving healthy Descemet membrane (DM) and endothelium, and is the ideal surgery for eyes affected by keratoconus that need a transplant. This technique offers substantial advantages compared with PK, primarily the avoidance of endothelial rejection and longer graft survival, which is particularly important in young patients with a long life expectancy.[3–5] In a study of DALK performed for different preoperative diagnoses in over 660 eyes, with a mean follow-up of 4.5 years (range 0.5–10 years), the average graft survival rate has been reported as 99.3% (range 98.5%–100%).[6] The Cornea Donor Study Group has demonstrated that, even in the absence of rejection, substantial endothelial cell loss occurs following PK, with a 76% endothelial cell loss from baseline after 10 years.[7] On the contrary, the endothelial cell density (ECD) after DALK suffers from a small loss only during the first 6 months postoperatively but then remains stable.[6,8] Visual outcomes of DALK are comparable to PK if the surgical technique provides a smooth interface with minimal host residual stromal thickness.[4,9]

Moreover, the DALK procedure is extraocular, carries a lower risk of endophthalmitis and expulsive hemorrhage, and allows earlier tapering of steroids with a decreased risk of secondary glaucoma and cataract. DALK also offers better wound integrity, which is very useful in patients with intellectual disability in which PK has a higher incidence of postoperative complications.[1,4]

Classification

The goal of LK is to replace the affected stroma, preserving healthy host endothelium. Various LK surgical techniques have been described in the literature, including manual dissection, microkeratome-assisted, excimer laser, and femtosecond laser-assisted LK (Box 31.1). The majority of anterior lamellar keratoplasty (ALK) techniques remove only 70% to 80% of host stroma, leaving behind >100 microns of residual host stroma. Wide variations in these techniques, along with suboptimal long-term visual outcomes compared with PK, did not make them popular worldwide. Currently, DALK is the most frequently performed surgery for advanced keratoconus. In this technique 85% to 90% of host stroma is removed by lamellar dissection, leaving behind a smooth interface, minimal residual stroma, and healthy DM and endothelium, and is replaced by full-thickness donor corneal tissue devoid of DM. Various DALK techniques have been described to create a good optical graft-host interface, including layer-by-layer manual dissection and stromal injection of air/fluid/viscoelastic material.

Although agreement is not yet unanimous, DALK is broadly classified in the literature as descemetic DALK (dDALK), in which the dissection is achieved up to the DM, and as pre-descemetic DALK (pdDALK), in which a small amount of posterior stroma is left intact along with the DM.[10] The majority of articles in the literature show that visual recovery after pdDALK is slower (2–5 years of follow-up) but comparable with dDALK when the residual recipient bed thickness is less than 80 microns and is homogeneous in its thickness.[9] However, dDALK techniques are

---

BOX 31.1 ■ Classification of Anterior Lamellar Keratoplasty Procedures

1. **Superficial Anterior Lamellar Keratoplasty (SALK)**

   Level: dissection <200 microns of anterior stroma
   Technique: microkeratome-assisted or femtosecond laser–assisted
   Apposition: sutureless

2. **Anterior Lamellar Keratoplasty (ALK)/Midstromal ALK**

   Level: dissection 200–400 microns of stroma
   Technique: manual/microkeratome-assisted or femtosecond laser–assisted
   Apposition: sutures required

3. **Deep Anterior Lamellar Keratoplasty (DALK)**

   Level: dissection >400 microns of stroma
   pdDALK—pre-Descemetic DALK (minimal residual stroma with PDL and DM)
   dDALK—Descemetic DALK (DM along with PDL)
   Technique: stromal air/viscoelastic injection/manual near DM dissection
   Apposition: sutures required.

DM, Descemet membrane; *PDL*, pre-Descemet layer.

usually preferred because they are largely considered faster and more reliable, making the surgeon confident to have performed optimal stromal removal with a good visual prognosis (see Box 31.1).

The recent description of Dua's layer, also called pre-Descemetic layer (PDL), has demonstrated that what was often thought to be a DM-endothelium surgical exposure in fact also includes a very thin layer of stroma.[11] Taking this finding into consideration, a new nomenclature for DALK has been proposed recently.[12]

DALK Techniques

Several techniques have been employed to achieve deep stromal dissections.[13,14] However, the most common of these techniques are air injection—big bubble (BB),[15] viscodissection,[16,17] manual layer by layer,[18] and stromal peeling.[19]

BIG BUBBLE TECHNIQUE

The BB technique was originally described by Anwar and Teichmann in 2002, and it is probably the most popular DALK technique.[15] This technique involves injection of air into deep corneal stroma to create a plane of separation between the stroma and DM, surgically seen as formation of a circular air-pocket that is referred to as a "big bubble."

There are three types of bubble formation (Fig. 31.1). Type 1 BB is well circumscribed, with white margins and a diameter measuring up to 8.5 mm. It starts in the center and enlarges circumferentially toward the periphery, and it is quite resistant (Fig. 31.2). It is the most common type of bubble, and its posterior wall is formed by endothelium, DM, and PDL.[11] Type 2 BB has clear margins and its diameter can measure up to 10.5 mm. It is usually eccentric in location, starting in the periphery and enlarging centrally (see Fig. 31.2). This rare type of bubble cleaves off the DM from the stroma and is very fragile.[11] Type 3 BB consists of mixed types of bubble: BB type 1 and one or more smaller type 2 bubbles.[11]

With the original BB technique, a trephine is used to perform a partial thickness corneal trephination at about 60% to 80% depth. A 27- or 30-gauge needle, attached to an air-filled syringe, is then inserted deep into the paracentral stroma through the bottom of the trephination groove and is advanced, with the bevel facing downward and parallel to the DM, for 3 to 4 mm. Air is injected with formation of BB (Fig. 31.3). A type 1 BB formation occurs in 60% to 70% of cases.[20] Paracentesis is performed to normalize the intraocular pressure (IOP). Subsequently, anterior keratectomy is performed followed by deflation of BB by creating a small opening at the center of the anterior wall using a sharp blade. The remaining corneal stromal layers are lifted with an iris spatula, severed with a blade, and excised using scissors.[15] The residual stroma is divided into four quadrants to facilitate easy removal. Any residual peripheral adhesions between the stroma and PDL are separated using a blunt dissector prior to excision. Scissors designed for a stromal excision, in which the lower blade is slightly longer than the upper blade, allow removal of tissue in a safe manner. Donor corneal tissue, usually of the same diameter as host trephine, is punched out, followed by removal of DM. The donor tissue is secured into position using an interrupted, continuous, or combined technique with 10-0 nylon (Fig. 31.4). Postoperative medications include topical corticosteroids, antibiotics, and lubricants. Topical steroids are continued with a tapering dosage for 4 to 6 months, along with lubricants for an extended duration of time. The corneal graft clears rapidly with healthy endothelial cell counts (Fig. 31.5).

One should be extremely careful with type 2 BB, given the high risk of spontaneous DM rupture, and even consider not opening the bubble and instead performing a manual dissection technique to near DM. The type 2 bubble spontaneously resolves in the early postoperative period.[21,22]

The deeper the air is injected, the higher are the chances of creating a BB.[23] Therefore several modifications of the original technique have been described that attempt to increase the bubble success rate.

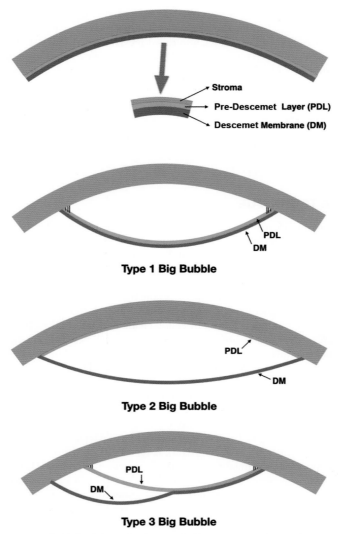

Fig. 31.1 Schematic diagram of different types of big bubble.

Cannula Big Bubble

Bottom port blunt-tipped cannulas for air injection have been described by several surgeons; these reduce the risk of intraocular perforation, compared with a sharp needle. Anterior lamellar keratectomy to debulk 40% to 50% of stroma facilitates deeper placement of the cannula and also allows faster deflation of the BB. A pointed dissector (Fogla Pointed Dissector, Storz Ophthalmics, MO) is used to make an initial track in the peripheral stroma at the base of trephination. A 27-gauge blunt-tipped, bottom port, air injection cannula (Fogla 27G Air Injection Cannula, Storz Ophthalmics, MO) is attached to a 5 mL air-filled syringe. The tip of this cannula is introduced into the peripheral stromal track and moved toward the central/paracentral cornea for 3 to 4 mm using a wiggling motion. Air is then injected using a firm continuous pressure

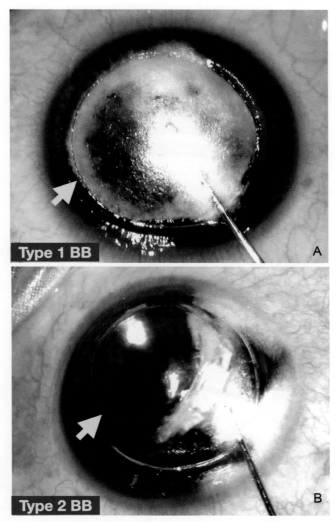

Fig. 31.2 Intraoperative photographs of type 1 and type 2 big bubble *(BB)*. *Yellow arrow* marks the edge of the BB.

until the formation of BB is noted. Paracentesis is performed to normalize the IOP and reduce counter resistance from the aqueous in a closed anterior chamber (AC). Air is gradually injected to increase the bubble size. Once increasing resistance is felt again, air injection is discontinued. Using this modified technique, Fogla was able to increase the success rate of BB from 69% to over 95%.[5,20] The advantages of using a blunt-tipped bottom port cannula have been confirmed by several studies.[24,25]

Pachy-Bubble

Intraoperative corneal thickness measurement to create a pachymetry-guided intrastromal air injection to increase the rate of BB formation has been described. After an initial partial trephination

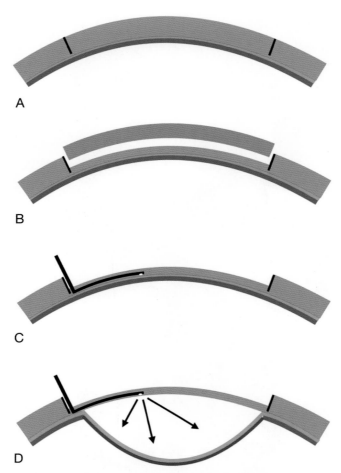

Fig. 31.3 Schematic diagram of Anwar's big bubble technique using stromal air injection.
A) partial depth trephination, B) Anterior lamellar keratectomy , C) introduction of air injection cannula, D) Air injection to create big bubble

to approximately 60% to 70% of corneal thickness, intraoperative corneal thickness measurements
using ultrasound pachymetry are taken 0.8-mm internally from the trephination groove in the 11 to
1 o'clock position. In this area, a 2-mm incision is made, parallel to the groove, with a micrometer
diamond knife, calibrated to 90% depth of the thinnest measurement. The incision is then opened
with toothed forceps and widened superficially with a 15-degree blade. The deep stroma is exposed,
and an initial stromal track is made with an iris spatula, close to the DM. A bottom port blunt-tipped
cannula attached to an air-filled syringe is inserted into the deep stromal track and advanced toward
the central or paracentral cornea, and it is used to create a BB.[26] Subsequent surgical steps are similar.

Bubble Size Optimization

Once the type 1 BB is initiated, its expansion is limited by counterpressure from aqueous humor
in a closed AC.[27] This is felt as increased resistance to air injection for BB expansion following
its initiation. Because of this, the BB often fails to reach the margin of trephination, and if air
injection is continued forcefully for further expansion, there is a risk of rupture of the BB. For
a BB smaller than the trephination diameter, manual dissection of the residual stroma between

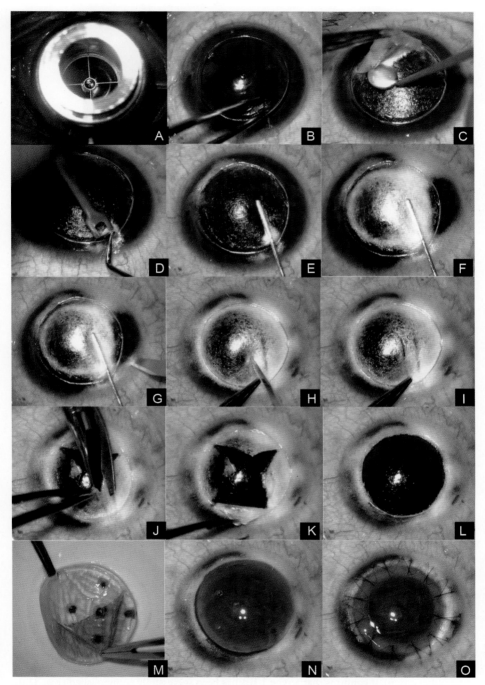

Fig. 31.4 Intraoperative photographs of big bubble (BB) deep anterior lamellar keratoplasty. (A and B) Deep trephination; (C) anterior lamellar keratectomy; (D) stromal track using pointed dissector; (E) placement of bottom port, blunt-tipped cannula; (F) stromal air injection and type 1 BB formation; (G) paracentesis to lower intraocular pressure; (H and I) BB deflation; (J–L) residual stromal removal; (M) Descemet membrane peel from donor button; (N) placement of donor on host bed; and (O) donor secured using 10-0 nylon sutures.

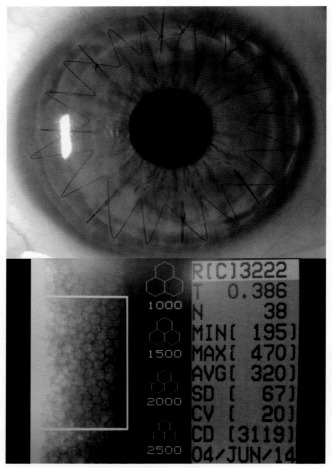

R[C]3222
T   0.386
N   38
MIN[195]
MAX[470]
AVG[320]
SD [67]
CV [20]
CD [3119]
04/JUN/14

1000
1500
2000
2500

Fig. 31.5 Postoperative slit-lamp photograph showing a clear corneal graft following deep anterior lamellar keratoplasty, with good endothelial cell counts on specular microscopy.

the outer edge of the BB and trephination margin is required for optimal graft-host apposition, which can sometimes lead to unwanted microperforations. To avoid this, a sequential air injection technique can be performed, in which a paracentesis is performed after initiation of the BB, to lower the IOP and reduce counterpressure to bubble expansion. A repeat air injection now allows BB expansion with lower resistance, helping achieve an ideal size reaching up to or beyond the trephination margin.

Small Bubble Test

Stromal emphysema can occur following air injection and may hinder visualization of the BB. A simple test has been described, in which a small air bubble is injected into the AC via a limbal paracentesis.[28,29] If the small air bubble remains in the peripheral AC (usually with a sausage configuration), it confirms that a type 1 BB has been successfully accomplished (Fig. 31.6). Alternatively, if the small bubble is located centrally beneath the opaque corneal stroma, this would suggest that a type 1 BB has not been obtained. Sometimes corneal emphysema, especially after multiple air injection attempts, may make it difficult to visualize the small bubble test. The

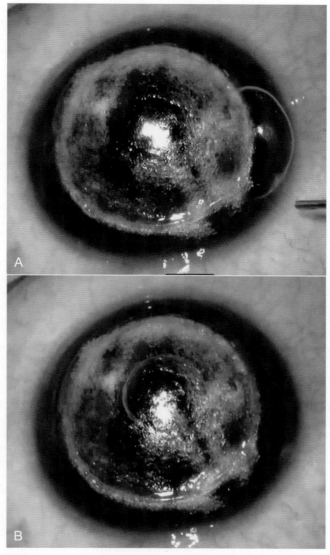

Fig. 31.6 Intraoperative photographs of small bubble test. (A) Small bubble remains in periphery when type 1 big bubble (BB) is present. (B) Small bubble moves to the center following deflation of BB.

presence of a BB can be ascertained by releasing aqueous via paracentesis to lower IOP. If a BB has formed, the cornea would have a protruding central dome shape, besides having a firm consistency to touch compared with the softer, flatter peripheral cornea.

Bubble Deflation

The technique to open the BB described by Anwar and Teichmann is associated with a known risk of DM perforation.[15] Goshe et al. refined the BB opening technique, advising to coat the stroma overlying the BB with a cohesive viscoelastic prior to entering the BB.[30] A 1.0- to 1.5-mm incision is then created with a 1.0-mm diamond blade/sharp knife, using only the tip of the blade in a "lifting" motion. This limits the escape of air, preventing a sudden collapse of the bubble while entering with a sharp blade. Viscoelastic can be injected into the bubble to maintain space and facilitate easy removal of the overlying residual stromal tissue. To further limit the escape of air from the BB during its opening, a 2.2-mm keratotome can be applied in a horizontal plane for entry, instead of the lifting-motion cut using a sharp knife.

VISCOBUBBLE

In 1999 Melles et al. described a technique that employed the injection of an ophthalmic visco-elastic device (OVD) to create a viscobubble and separate DM from the corneal stroma.[16] This bubble mimics the behavior of the type 1 BB seen with air injection. In this technique, a 27-gauge needle or blunt-tipped bottom port cannula, attached to a viscoelastic-filled syringe, is inserted into the corneal stroma as close to the DM as possible. To visualize the depth of corneal incision and lamellar dissection during surgery, Melles proposed the creation of an air-to-endothelium interface by filling the AC with air, which then behaves as a convex mirror. A dark nonreflec-tive band can be seen between the tip of the blade and its reflection, representing the nonincised corneal tissue between the blade and the air-to-endothelium interface. This dark band becomes thinner as the blade is advanced into deeper stromal layers. The needle/cannula is advanced in this plane, and when the tip appears to touch its reflection, the OVD can be injected to create the viscobubble. The formation of the viscobubble is outlined by a typical golden ring reflex. After the corneal pocket filled with the OVD has been created, a suction trephine can be centered over the anterior corneal surface. Trephination is performed until viscoelastic is seen to escape from the pocket through the trephine incision. The overlying stroma is excised and the recipient bed is thoroughly irrigated to remove all the OVD.[16]

Some surgeons prefer to debulk the cornea before attempting the viscobubble, to enhance the chances of injecting the OVD as close as possible to the DM. The use of a cohesive OVD is preferred, because it is easier to remove and reduces the risk of a postoperative double AC.[17] The viscobubble has also been suggested as a rescue bubble technique, after failed air injection: air-viscobubble (AVB).[31] When air dissection does not result in the formation of a BB, superficial keratectomy is performed with a crescent blade and a new deeper tunnel is created into the stroma by using a blunt spatula/pointed dissector. Viscobubble though a blunt-tipped bottom port can-nula is tried as a second strategy to separate DM from the corneal stroma. In a case series of 507 eyes affected by keratoconus, this combined technique (AVB) increased the percentage of bubble formation by 12%, bringing the total cases of successful bubble formation to 94%.[25] When the BB fails, the cornea is generally pneumatized and offers many pathways of less resistance to air compared with the pre-Descemet space (i.e., leakage of air through the stroma, the trabecular meshwork, or the trephination groove). Because of its high viscosity, an OVD does not easily escape, creating a much higher intrastromal pressure, increasing the chances of bubble formation and probably also increasing the pressure inside the small stromal bubbles (from the failed BB attempt) that spontaneously merge to form a large DM detachment.[31]

MANUAL DISSECTION DALK

Despite being technically more challenging, manual dissection techniques are still valid options. They are mainly adopted in cases in which air- or viscodissection fails or is not indicated because of previous hydrops or deep stromal scars involving DM.

Peeling Technique

Malbran and Stefani described this easy and rapid manual technique in 1972, and it still repre-sents a useful option, especially in eyes with keratoconus.[19] After performing initial trephination, the inner stromal edges are raised using a Paufique knife and are then grasped securely with forceps, which are used to pull the stromal tissue to peel it from underlying deeper layers.[19] Once the proper plane of 85% to 90% depth is reached, peeling off the stroma without applying excessive force is relatively easy, especially in the area of the cone of keratoconus in which the deeper lamellae have the lowest adhesion. This technique usually creates a recipient bed that is very deep, smooth, and regular in its thickness.

Some modifications of the original techniques have been proposed. Performing a partial debulking and using dedicated blunt-tipped forceps (Fogla stromal pocket forceps, Storz Ophthalmics, MO) or a blunt-tipped spatula (Sarnicola DALK spatula, ASICO, IL) to try to find an appropriate deep plane in the peripheral cornea all around the trephination groove, may facilitate the peeling of the stroma. The peeling of the stroma may by aided by a semisharp dissector (Fogla lamellar dissector, Storz Ophthalmics, MO), which may be particularly helpful in the presence of an intraoperative DM rupture, to limit the force of the peeling and the risk of enlarging the rupture.

Layer-by-Layer Manual Dissection

Dry manual dissection is one of the oldest described DALK techniques, which gained attention again when Tsubota et al. applied the cataract surgery principle of "divide-and-conquer" to corneal transplantation.[18] After the initial trephination, to facilitate lamellar dissection, the recipient cornea is divided into four quadrants at approximately 70% of corneal depth. This division is then continued until a deep, smooth, and regular plane is exposed. "Layer-by-layer" manual dissection usually results in a pdDALK, as baring the DM is challenging.

This technique has a high risk of intraoperative perforation, especially while performing deeper dissections close to DM. Reducing the IOP by evacuating some aqueous through a peripheral paracentesis and wetting the stroma with some balanced salt solution to avoid dessication might help to reduce this risk. Injecting air or fluid into the stroma to create emphysema can be helpful to determine the depth of the stromal dissection, as described by Archila in 1985 and by Sugita and Kondo in 1997.[32,33] New technological tools such as intraoperative anterior segment optical coherence tomography (AS-OCT)[34] or a handheld pachymeter may be helpful to assess the residual stromal bed and the need for further dissection. An irregular stromal bed with thickness >80 microns is likely to impact the visual outcome of DALK with the manual dissection technique.

Pachymetry-Assisted Manual DALK

Pachymetry-guided use of a diamond knife to initiate the plane of manual dissection for stromal removal has been successful in performing a pdDALK.[35,36] After a circular mark is made at the desired trephine diameter, intraoperative pachymetry is performed at the site of planned incision using a diamond knife. The diamond knife is set at a depth of 30 microns less than the pachymetry reading and used to make a 2.0-mm incision just internal to the trephination mark, at 11 to 12 o'clock position. The dissection plane is initiated at the base of the cut, followed by using curved medium-sized fine blade scissors to extend the incision on either side circumferentially. An open centripetal lamellar dissection is performed using lamellar dissectors.

MICROKERATOME-ASSISTED ALK

Microkeratome-assisted ALK, also known as automated therapeutic lamellar keratoplasty (ATLK), involves the use of an automated microkeratome to perform anterior lamellar dissection of both the donor and recipient cornea. Being automated, the resultant bed is usually very smooth. However, this technique is usually not successful in performing an ideal lamellar dissection in thin corneas with areas of elevation, such as in advanced keratoconus. Semiautomated LK, a procedure that combines manual recipient bed lamellar dissection with automated donor preparation using a microkeratome, seems to be a safe and effective technique.[37] It combines the benefits of smooth microkeratome lamellar dissection of the donor with customized lenticule thickness and diameter together with a manual lamellar dissection technique for the recipient, providing encouraging visual outcomes that show continuing improvement with time.

Busin et al. have also reported successful outcomes for DALK using a microkeratome-prepared large-diameter (9 mm) donor, along with baring of PDL only in the central 6 mm of the recipient bed.[38]

FEMTOSECOND-ASSISTED ALK

The use of femtosecond lasers in DALK allows corneal-shaped wound creation in a precise manner instead of manual trephination and, in addition, the ability to create a plane for air injection at a desired depth in the corneal stroma.[39,40] Stromal removal is performed using the BB technique or near-DM manual dissection techniques. The shaped wound configuration has the advantage of better donor host apposition, with increased surface area contact, resulting in faster wound healing, greater tectonic stability, earlier suture removal, and possibly reduced astigmatism (Fig. 31.7). The predefined stromal track facilitates air injection close to DM with improved rates of BB formation.[41]

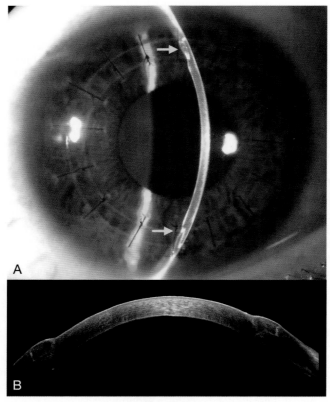

Fig. 31.7 Postoperative slit-lamp photograph of a femtosecond laser-assisted deep anterior lamellar keratoplasty. Note the mushroom configuration of the edges (yellow arrows) (A), clearly seen on anterior segment optical coherence tomography image (B).

Use of zigzag or mushroom-shaped edge configuration has been described for DALK cases with successful outcomes.

General Surgical Tips

PREOPERATIVE PLANNING

Surgical planning involves a detailed slit-lamp evaluation to assess the extent of corneal involvement. Regional pachymetry can be performed using corneal tomography, anterior segment optical coherence tomography (OCT), or ultrasound pachymeter, and this information is used for performing a planned depth trephination.[5] Anterior segment OCT is also used preoperatively to identify any involvement of DM with scar tissue[5,42] (Fig. 31.8). In such cases, air injection is avoided owing to increased risk of perforations and instead manual dissection techniques should be performed for DALK.

ANESTHESIA

Retrobulbar or peribulbar anesthesia using a relatively long-lasting drug such as bupivacaine in combination with lidocaine is often adequate. However, an additional lid block should be applied to avoid blinking during delicate phases of the surgery. Application of a Honan balloon or digital massage for a few minutes to obtain a soft eye is desirable. General anesthesia may be advisable

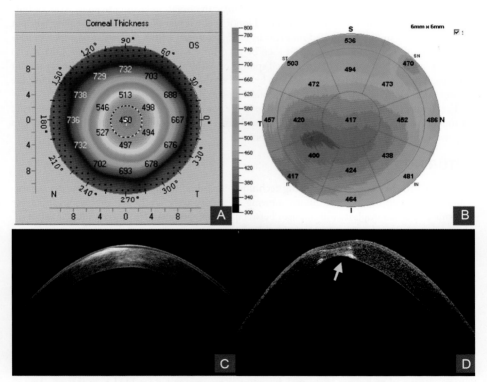

Fig. 31.8 Preoperative assessment. Regional pachymetry using tomography (A), or anterior segment optical coherence tomography (AS-OCT) (B). Corneal assessment with AS-OCT shows (C) scar tissue only in the anterior cornea and (D) stromal scar involving the Descemet membrane *(yellow arrow)*.

for young or noncompliant patients, in cases with language barriers, or in difficult cases with prolonged surgical time.

TREPHINATION

The size of the trephination varies according to the corneal diameter and the extent of corneal pathology. However, it should be large enough to excise the entire cone. Marking the center of the host cornea will ensure adequate centration of trephination. Vacuum trephines are available that allow (1) preset depth (Moria); (2) a measured cut depth of 60 microns with each quarter turn (Katena/Jedmed/Surgistar); or (3) a centering device along with a preset depth handheld trephine (Coronet). Preoperative pachymetry assessment is used for planning the host trephination.[5] The depth of the trephination is checked to ensure appropriate depth is achieved. A 15-degree blade may be used to deepen the trephination groove if the depth is found to be inadequate.

Femtosecond laser trephination (for both donor and recipient) has the unique ability to create a variety of complex incisions, such as zigzag/mushroom configurations, which allow better apposition of donor tissue with host cornea, with a larger surface area of graft-host junction.[39,40]

DONOR PREPARATION

Donor cornea preparation can be performed using trephine of the surgeon's choice (with/without suction). Preparation is done from the endothelial side; care should be taken to ensure there is no fluid under the tissue, to avoid slippage and to perform proper centration prior to carrying out the donor punch. Centration is essential to avoid eccentric trephination leading to an oval donor button with higher postoperative astigmatism.[43] Donor tissue is placed in a storage medium without peeling the DM until the required moment in DALK surgery. In the rare event of intraoperative macroperforation, the donor tissue can then be used for PK. For DALK, the donor DM has to be gently stripped off using a dry weck cell sponge or with fine nontooth forceps, taking care not to damage the stroma. Trypan blue dye can be used to stain DM and aid peeling; roughening the donor endothelium with a swab makes the staining stronger.[44]

For keratoconus, the preferred donor size is the same as the recipient trephination to avoid postoperative myopia. However, in very advanced cases of keratoconus, oversizing by 0.25 mm can help avoid occurrence of folds in the posterior layer.

SUTURING TECHNIQUES

Similar to PK, the options for suturing technique include interrupted, continuous, or a combination of interrupted and continuous suturing. A comparative study has shown no difference in terms of postkeratoplasty astigmatism between running, interrupted, and combined sutures.[45] However, interrupted sutures have some evident advantages, such as easier management of postoperative astigmatism and selective removal in case of infected or loose stitches without the need for replacing the suture. Intraoperative suture adjustment using a Maloney keratometer can help minimize postoperative astigmatism.

Intraoperative Complications

Intraoperative complications in DALK usually involve a microperforation or a macroperforation (more than one-quarter of cornea). Inadvertent entry into the AC from full-thickness trephination involving one or more clock hours can occur during initial trephination. In these cases, DALK can still be performed, following a temporary repair of the full-thickness AC entry using interrupted sutures. A manual technique of stromal dissection is recommended for DALK in this situation.

Intraoperative microperforation of the posterior layer can occur during various stages of DALK surgery. However, in the majority of these cases, DALK can still be completed successfully and a conversion to PK can be avoided. The rate of PK conversion ranges between 0% and 60% and is often related to surgeon experience and the effective management of intraoperative DM ruptures.[46,47] DALK recovery techniques are designed to avoid conversion to PK and to bestow all the advantages of this technique on the patients.

A number of principles guide the repair of DM ruptures:

1. A midsize air bubble can be placed in the AC to tamponade the break and prevent leakage of fluid onto the stromal surface, which can hamper visualization during further dissection. The lid speculum can be adjusted to minimize external pressure on the eye.

2. Manual stromal dissection should be initiated from the opposite quadrant and a smooth host bed must be maintained to ensure optimal graft-host apposition. The area of microperforation is approached only at the end of dissection.

3. If air keeps leaking through the perforation, a temporary suture can be placed through the stromal tissue to secure the break and allow further stromal dissection.

4. Appropriate suture tension should be maintained while securing the donor, as tight sutures can flatten the donor, which in turn can press on the recipient bed and prevent proper apposition of the rupture, keeping it patent. A 0.25-/0.5-mm oversized donor can be used in this situation to overcome this problem.

5. A large air bubble can be placed in the AC to tamponade the break in the postoperative period thus avoiding a double AC. To avoid pupillary block, an intraoperative inferior peripheral iridectomy can be performed via an inferior limbal paracentesis, or the pupillary dilation must be maintained in the postoperative period.

6. Postoperative monitoring is still essential to rule out any pupillary block and prevention of a fixed dilated pupil (Urrets-Zavalia syndrome), especially in phakic patients.

7. Ruptures occurring in the superior half have a reduced risk of postoperative double AC as the tamponade is maintained for a longer duration with normal positioning. Hence, for perforations occurring in the lower half, 20% sulfur hexafluoride (SF6) can be used instead of air to provide longer tamponade, along with positioning of the head to ensure optimal tamponade.

Some studies have shown that DM ruptures and their management during DALK are associated with higher endothelial cell loss when compared with uneventful DALK. However, preserving the patient's own endothelium is better than an allograft, even at the cost of a greater endothelial cell loss.[48-50]

Postoperative Complications

DOUBLE ANTERIOR CHAMBER

Double AC, or pseudo-AC, results from a break in the DM with continuous flow of aqueous on both sides of the DM. This complication can be largely avoided by using air or gas intraoperatively to tamponade the break (Fig. 31.9). Small, localized areas of shallow detachment may resolve spontaneously in a few days, but large areas may persist for weeks. Surgical intervention is recommended for large detachments, to avoid potential damage to the endothelium and scarring. Management includes rebubbling using air or 20% SF6 via a limbal paracentesis, ensuring that injection is performed into the AC and not into the interface.

Residual viscoelastic material in the interface may also be responsible for causing a double AC, with or without a DM break. In the presence of a DM rupture, after the rebubbling, it is advisable to separate the donor from the recipient momentarily along the trephination groove to promote the drainage of the viscoelastic material.

In cases where the DM is intact, a simple interface wash can be performed for a nonresolving double AC to ensure removal of viscoelastic material.

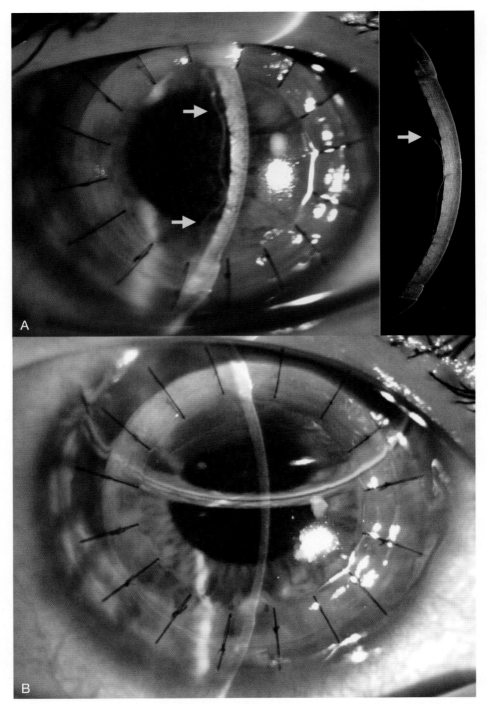

Fig. 31.9 Postoperative slit-lamp photographs. (A) Detachment of posterior layer *(yellow arrows)* with double anterior chamber (AC), seen clearly on anterior segment optical coherence tomography. (B) Good resolution following air bubble injection into AC with clear cornea.

Decision making for DALK procedure in Keratoconus.

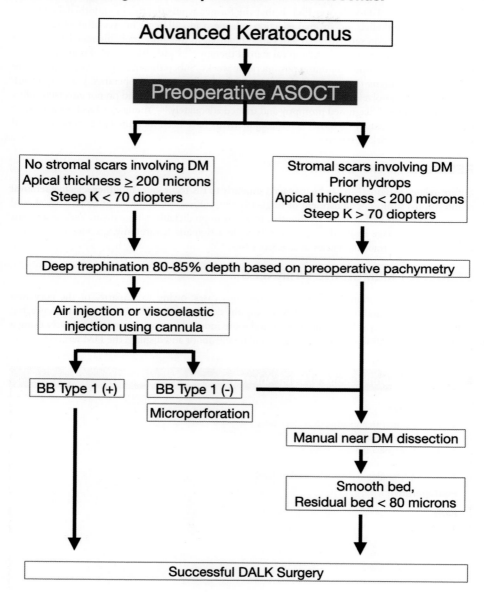

Fig. 31.10 Flowchart of decision-making for deep anterior lamellar keratoplasty (*DALK*) procedure in keratoconus. *ASOCT,* Anterior segment optical coherence tomography; *BB,* big bubble; *DM,* Descemet membrane; *K,* keratometry.

REJECTION

A clear advantage of DALK over PKP is that the former avoids the risk of endothelial rejection. Epithelial, subepithelial, and stromal rejection episodes can still occur in eyes after DALK. Discrepancies in rejection rates (0%–20% of cases) reported in literature probably may be explained by different lengths of prophylactic topical steroid therapy.[3,51] Epithelial rejection is an early complication occurring within the initial postoperative weeks. Subepithelial and stromal rejection are delayed complications that generally happen within the first two postoperative years. Rejection episodes usually resolve with short-term use of topical corticosteroids and do not adversely affect graft performance if diagnosed promptly and treated adequately.[3,13] Young age, black race, manual trephination, and history of vernal keratoconjunctivitis have been identified as factors associated with an increased risk of rejection.[51]

RESIDUAL ASTIGMATISM

Suture-related astigmatism can be managed similarly to PK techniques by either selective removal of interrupted sutures or adjustment of single running sutures.[52] Complete suture removal should not be performed earlier than 12 months, to avoid unpredictable astigmatism. Various options described to manage residual astigmatism include astigmatic keratotomy, excimer laser procedures, and toric intraocular lenses in selective cases.[53–58]

DESCEMET MEMBRANE WRINKLES

DM wrinkles may occur in advanced keratoconus cases, owing to disparity of the curvature between the donor and the recipient. Oversizing the donor graft may limit this inconvenience, but it also causes a higher spherical equivalent and more induced myopia. Interrupted sutures using a gradual pressure technique can help to manipulate the donor and displace the DM wrinkles in the

---

BOX 31.2 ■ Complications of Deep Anterior Lamellar Keratoplasty

Intraoperative
1. Full-thickness trephination (few clock hours)
2. Failed air injection for type 1 BB
3. Type 2 or type 3 BB formation
4. Microperforation
5. Macroperforation (>25% of corneal surface)

Postoperative

Early
1. Double anterior chamber
2. Non-healing epithelial defect
3. Interface keratitis
4. Folds or wrinkles in DM

Late
1. Epithelial/stromal rejection
2. High astigmatism
3. Interface vascularization/lipid keratopathy/epithelial ingrowth
4. Recurrence of keratoconus
5. Traumatic dehiscence of graft-host junction

BB, Big bubble; *DM*, Descemet membrane.

periphery, to decrease the occurrence of the folds in the central cornea and avoid a negative effect on visual acuity (VA). However, DM wrinkles tend to disappear or at least to decrease, over time.[59]

RARE COMPLICATIONS

Rare complications reported in the literature include suture-related complications, dry eye syndrome, microbial infections, transmission of donor-to-host infections, recurrence of keratoconus, epithelial ingrowth, and glaucoma.[3,60]

In conclusion, LK plays an important role in the management of advanced keratoconus to restore normal corneal anatomy and improve eyesight. Decision-making for ideal DALK technique includes preoperative assessment using anterior segment OCT (Fig. 31.10). Surgeons should be aware of the possible complications associated with the DALK procedure (Box 31.2) to ensure optimal management for a good final visual outcome.

References

1. Parker JS, van Dijk K, Melles GR. Treatment options for advanced keratoconus: a review. *Surv Ophthalmol*. 2015;60(5):459–480.
2. Lim L, Pesudovs K, Coster DJ. Penetrating keratoplasty for keratoconus: visual outcome and success. *Ophthalmology*. 2000;107(6):1125–1131.
3. Reinhart WJ, Musch DC, Jacobs DS, Lee WB, Kaufman SC, Shtein RM. Deep anterior lamellar keratoplasty as an alternative to penetrating keratoplasty a report by the American Academy of Ophthalmology. *Ophthalmology*. 2011;118(1):209–218.
4. Tan DT, Dart JK, Holland EJ, Kinoshita S. Corneal transplantation. *Lancet*. 2012;379(9827):1749–1761.
5. Fogla R. Deep anterior lamellar keratoplasty in the management of keratoconus. *Indian J Ophthalmol*. 2013;61(8):465–468.
6. Sarnicola V, Toro P, Sarnicola C, Sarnicola E, Ruggiero A. Long-term graft survival in deep anterior lamellar keratoplasty. *Cornea*. 2012;31(6):621–626.
7. Group Writing Committee for the Cornea Donor Study Research, JH Lass, Benetz BA, et al. Donor age and factors related to endothelial cell loss 10 years after penetrating keratoplasty: specular microscopy ancillary study. *Ophthalmology*. 2013;120(12):2428–2435.
8. Shimazaki J, Shimmura S, Ishioka M, Tsubota K. Randomized clinical trial of deep lamellar keratoplasty vs penetrating keratoplasty. *Am J Ophthalmol*. 2002;134(2):159–165.
9. Ardjomand N, Hau S, McAlister JC, et al. Quality of vision and graft thickness in deep anterior lamellar and penetrating corneal allografts. *Am J Ophthalmol*. 2007;143(2):228–235.
10. Sarnicola V, Toro P, Gentile D, Hannush SB. Descemetic DALK and predescemetic DALK: outcomes in 236 cases of keratoconus. *Cornea*. 2010;29(1):53–59.
11. Dua HS, Faraj LA, Said DG, Gray T, Lowe J. Human corneal anatomy redefined: a novel pre-Descemet's layer (Dua's layer). *Ophthalmology*. 2013;120(9):1778–1785.
12. Sarnicola E, Sarnicola C, Cheung AY, Holland EJ, Sarnicola V. Surgical corneal anatomy in deep anterior lamellar keratoplasty: suggestion of new acronyms. *Cornea*. 2019;38(4):515–522.
13. Luengo-Gimeno F, Tan DT, Mehta JS. Evolution of deep anterior lamellar keratoplasty (DALK). *Ocul Surf*. 2011;9(2):98–110.
14. Arenas E, Esquenazi S, Anwar M, Terry M. Lamellar corneal transplantation. *Surv Ophthalmol*. 2012;57(6):510–529.
15. Anwar M, Teichmann KD. Big-bubble technique to bare Descemet's membrane in anterior lamellar keratoplasty. *J Cataract Refract Surg*. 2002;28(3):398–403.
16. Melles GR, Lander F, Rietveld FJ, Remeijer L, Beekhuis WH, Binder PS. A new surgical technique for deep stromal, anterior lamellar keratoplasty. *Br J Ophthalmol*. 1999;83(3):327–333.
17. Shimmura S, Shimazaki J, Omoto M, Teruya A, Ishioka M, Tsubota K. Deep lamellar keratoplasty (DLKP) in keratoconus patients using viscoadaptive viscoelastics. *Cornea*. 2005;24(2):178–181.
18. Tsubota K, Kaido M, Monden Y, Satake Y, Bissen-Miyajima H, Shimazaki J. A new surgical technique for deep lamellar keratoplasty with single running suture adjustment. *Am J Ophthalmol*. 1998;126(1):1–8.
19. Malbran E, Stefani C. Lamellar keratoplasty in corneal ectasias. *Ophthalmologica*. 1972;164(1):50–58.

20. Fogla R, Padmanabhan P. Results of deep lamellar keratoplasty using the big-bubble technique in patients with keratoconus. *Am J Ophthalmol*. 2006;141(2):254–259.
21. Goweida MB, Ragab AM, Liu C. Management of type 2 bubble formed during big bubble deep anterior lamellar keratoplasty. *Cornea*. 2019;38(2):189–193.
22. Gujar P. Type 2 big bubble deep anterior lamellar keratoplasty-serial anterior segment optical coherence tomography documentation showing resolution of bubble in the postoperative period. *Indian J Ophthalmol*. 2017;65(10):1017–1018.
23. Pasricha ND, Shieh C, Carrasco-Zevallos OM, et al. Needle depth and big-bubble success in deep anterior lamellar keratoplasty: an ex vivo microscope-integrated OCT study. *Cornea*. 2016;35(11):1471–1477.
24. Sarnicola V, Toro P. Blunt cannula for descemetic deep anterior lamellar keratoplasty. *Cornea*. 2011;30(8):895–898.
25. Sarnicola E, Sarnicola C, Sabatino F, Tosi GM, Perri P, Sarnicola V. Cannula DALK versus needle DALK for keratoconus. *Cornea*. 2016;35(12):1508–1511.
26. Ghanem RC, Ghanem MA. Pachymetry-guided intrastromal air injection ("pachy-bubble") for deep anterior lamellar keratoplasty. *Cornea*. 2012;31(9):1087–1091.
27. Bhullar PK, Carrasco-Zevallos OM, Dandridge A, et al. Intraocular pressure and big bubble diameter in deep anterior lamellar keratoplasty: an ex-vivo microscope-integrated OCT with heads-up display study. *Asia Pac J Ophthalmol (Phila)*. 2017;6(5):412–417.
28. Fontana L, Parente G, Tassinari G. Simple test to confirm cleavage with air between Descemet's membrane and stroma during big-bubble deep anterior lamellar keratoplasty. *J Cataract Refract Surg*. 2007;33(4):570–572.
29. Parthasarathy A, Por YM, Tan DT. Using a "small bubble technique" to aid in success in Anwar's "big bubble technique" of deep lamellar keratoplasty with complete baring of Descemet's membrane. *Br J Ophthalmol*. 2008;92(3):422.
30. Goshe J, Terry MA, Shamie N, Li J. Ophthalmic viscosurgical device-assisted incision modification for the big-bubble technique in deep anterior lamellar keratoplasty. *J Cataract Refract Surg*. 2011;37(11):1923–1927.
31. Muftuoglu O, Toro P, Hogan RN, et al. Sarnicola air-visco bubble technique in deep anterior lamellar keratoplasty. *Cornea*. 2013;32(4):527–532.
32. Archila EA. Deep lamellar keratoplasty dissection of host tissue with intrastromal air injection. *Cornea*. 1984;3(3):217–218.
33. Sugita J, Kondo J. Deep lamellar keratoplasty with complete removal of pathological stroma for vision improvement. *Br J Ophthalmol*. 1997;81(3):184–188.
34. De Benito-Llopis L, Mehta JS, Angunawela RI, Ang M, Tan DT. Intraoperative anterior segment optical coherence tomography: a novel assessment tool during deep anterior lamellar keratoplasty. *Am J Ophthalmol*. 2014;157(2):334–341.e3.
35. Rama P, Knutsson KA, Razzoli G, Matuska S, Viganò M, Paganoni G. Deep anterior lamellar keratoplasty using an original manual technique. *Br J Ophthalmol*. 2013;97(1):23–27.
36. Vajpayee RB, Maharana PK, Sharma N, Agarwal T, Jhanji V. Diamond knife-assisted deep anterior lamellar keratoplasty to manage keratoconus. *J Cataract Refract Surg*. 2014;40(2):276–282.
37. Yuen LH, Mehta JS, Shilbayeh R, Lim L, Tan DT. Hemi-automated lamellar keratoplasty (HALK). *Br J Ophthalmol*. 2011;95(11):1513–1518.
38. Busin M, Leon P, Nahum Y, Scorcia V. Large (9 mm) deep anterior lamellar keratoplasty with clearance of a 6-mm optical zone optimizes outcomes of keratoconus surgery. *Ophthalmology*. 2017;124(7):1072–1080.
39. Farid M, Steinert RF. Femtosecond laser-assisted corneal surgery. *Curr Opin Ophthalmol*. 2010;21(4):288–292.
40. Chamberlain WD. Femtosecond laser-assisted deep anterior lamellar keratoplasty. *Curr Opin Ophthalmol*. 2019;30(4):256–263.
41. Buzzonetti L, Laborante A, Petrocelli G. Standardized big-bubble technique in deep anterior lamellar keratoplasty assisted by the femtosecond laser. *J Cataract Refract Surg*. 2010;36(10):1631–1636.
42. Borderie VM, Touhami S, Georgeon C, Sandali O. Predictive factors for successful type 1 big bubble during deep anterior lamellar keratoplasty. *J Ophthalmol*. 2018;2018:4685406.
43. Nanavaty MA, Vijjan KS, Yvon C. Deep anterior lamellar keratoplasty: a surgeon's guide. *J Curr Ophthalmol*. 2018;30(4):297–310.

44. Sarnicola E, Sarnicola C, Sarnicola V. Deep anterior lamellar keratoplasty: surgical technique, indications, clinical results and complications. In: Güell JL, ed. *Cornea*. Basel: ESASO Course Series, Karger; 2015:81–101.
45. Javadi MA, Naderi M, Zare M, Jenaban A, Rabei HM, Anissian A. Comparison of the effect of three suturing techniques on postkeratoplasty astigmatism in keratoconus. *Cornea*. 2006;25(9):1029–1033.
46. Smadja D, Colin J, Krueger RR, et al. Outcomes of deep anterior lamellar keratoplasty for keratoconus: learning curve and advantages of the big bubble technique. *Cornea*. 2012;31(8):859–863.
47. Kubaloglu A, Sari ES, Unal M, et al. Long-term results of deep anterior lamellar keratoplasty for the treatment of keratoconus. *Am J Ophthalmol*. 2011;151(5):760–767.e1.
48. Den S, Shimmura S, Tsubota K, Shimazaki J. Impact of the Descemet membrane perforation on surgical outcomes after deep lamellar keratoplasty. *Am J Ophthalmol*. 2007;143(5):750–754.
49. Leccisotti A. Descemet's membrane perforation during deep anterior lamellar keratoplasty: prognosis. *J Cataract Refract Surg*. 2007;33(5):825–829.
50. Sarnicola V, Sarnicola E, Sarnicola C. Recovery techniques in DALK. In: Holland M, ed. *Cornea*. 4th ed.. Elsevier: Health Sciences Division; 2016.
51. Gonzalez A, Price MO, Feng MT, Lee C, Arbelaez JG, Price FW. Immunologic rejection episodes after deep anterior lamellar keratoplasty: incidence and risk factors. *Cornea*. 2017;36(9):1076–1082.
52. Shimazaki J, Shimmura S, Tsubota K. Intraoperative versus postoperative suture adjustment after penetrating keratoplasty. *Cornea*. 1998;17(6):590–594.
53. Javadi MA, Feizi S, Mirbabaee F, Rastegarpour A. Relaxing incisions combined with adjustment sutures for post-deep anterior lamellar keratoplasty astigmatism in keratoconus. *Cornea*. 2009;28(10):1130–1134.
54. Acar BT, Utine CA, Acar S, Ciftci F. Laser in situ keratomileusis to manage refractive errors after deep anterior lamellar keratoplasty. *J Cataract Refract Surg*. 2012;38(6):1020–1027.
55. Al-Dreihi MG, Louka BI, Anbari AA. Artisan iris-fixated toric phakic intraocular lens for the correction of high astigmatism after deep anterior lamellar keratoplasty. *Digit J Ophthalmol*. 2013;19(2):39–41.
56. Pedrotti E, Sbabo A, Marchini G. Customized transepithelial photorefractive keratectomy for iatrogenic ametropia after penetrating or deep lamellar keratoplasty. *J Cataract Refract Surg*. 2006;32(8):1288–1291.
57. Leccisotti A. Photorefractive keratectomy with mitomycin C after deep anterior lamellar keratoplasty for keratoconus. *Cornea*. 2008;27(4):417–420.
58. Mimouni M, Kreimei M, Sorkin N, et al. Factors associated with improvement in vision following femtosecond astigmatic keratotomy in post keratoplasty keratoconus patients. *Am J Ophthalmol*. 2020;219:59–65.
59. Shi W, Li S, Gao H, Wang T, Xie L. Modified deep lamellar keratoplasty for the treatment of advanced-stage keratoconus with steep curvature. *Ophthalmology*. 2010;117(2):226–231.
60. Feizi S, Javadi MA, Rezaei Kanavi M. Recurrent keratoconus in a corneal graft after deep anterior lamellar keratoplasty. *J Ophthalmic Vis Res*. 2012;7(4):328–331.

CHAPTER 32

Penetrating Keratoplasty in Keratoconus

Milad Modabber ■ Mark Mannis

KEY CONCEPTS

- Despite the increasing popularity of deep anterior lamellar keratoplasty (DALK), penetrating keratoplasty (PK) remains an important modality in the surgical management of advanced keratoconus, particularly in cases of deep stromal scarring and/or history of corneal hydrops.
- PK provides excellent graft survival and acceptable visual outcomes. However, visual rehabilitation can be prolonged, owing to high postoperative astigmatism or anisometropia.
- Femtosecond laser for trephination in PK theoretically enables better apposition, faster wound healing, and patterns of trephination not achievable with conventional trephines.
- DALK eliminates the risk of endothelial graft rejection, resulting in improved long-term graft survival, comparable visual outcomes, reduced endothelial cell loss, and decreased need for postoperative steroids. The procedure is, however, more technically challenging, and interface haze remains a concern.

Introduction

Historically, for almost a century, penetrating keratoplasty (PK), in which the entire thickness of the cornea is replaced by a donor corneal tissue, has been the gold standard surgical approach for the treatment of advanced keratoconus.[1,2] In contemporary practice, however, deep anterior lamellar keratoplasty (DALK)—in which the superficial corneal layers are removed, leaving only the host Descemet layer and endothelium intact—is increasingly becoming the preferred primary surgical option, currently representing 10% to 20% of all transplants for keratoconus.[3,4] PK, nonetheless, has a significant role in the surgical management of advanced keratoconus, especially where there is deep stromal scarring or a history of corneal hydrops, and in the less common scenario of coexisting endothelial dysfunction, such as Fuchs endothelial dystrophy.[1,5]

INDICATIONS

Longitudinal data show that keratoconus is one of the most common indications for PK. In a review of data from the years 1980 to 2014, keratoconus was the leading indication for PK in many regions of the globe (Europe, Australia, the Middle East, Africa, and South America).[6] In North America, keratoconus represented the third most common indication for PK (approximately 14% of cases), following pseudophakic bullous keratopathy/aphakic bullous keratopathy and regrafts.[6] Along with regional variabilities in the incidence of keratoconus, this difference can also be attributed partially to the availability of less invasive surgical options in the developed world.

Although PK is the most common surgical option in advanced keratoconus, most patients do not ultimately require penetrating surgery.[7] A study of keratoconus subjects followed for 48 years reported that fewer than 20% of patients underwent PK.[8] Another study of 1065 keratoconus subjects found that only 12% required PK over an 8-year follow-up period.[9] Reported indications for PK include the presence of corneal scarring, best-corrected visual acuity (BCVA) worse than 20/40 with contact lens correction, keratometry steeper than 55 diopters (D), corneal astigmatism greater than 10 D, early age of keratoconus development, poor contact lens tolerance, and non-clearing corneal hydrops.[10–12]

TECHNIQUE

PK techniques for the treatment of keratoconus have evolved over the years. However, a recent review concluded that there was no evidence of superiority for any specific technique.[13] The pattern of graft suturing (interrupted, single, combined interrupted and running, or double running) does not appear to influence ultimate BCVA.[14,15] The effect of graft sizing, although the subject of controversy, is likely modest.[15–17] The type of mechanical trephine used has also not been shown to influence visual outcome, although the use of femtosecond laser trephination may enable better wound healing and faster visual rehabilitation with earlier suture removal (see section later).

Graft sizing has been controversial, with various studies reporting slightly better (or worse) results with oversized versus same-sized grafts.[15–19] Postkeratoplasty myopia can be reduced by using donor tissue that is the same size as the recipient trephination.[20–22] Some have suggested undersizing the donor to further flatten the postoperative corneal contour.[23] These maneuvers have to be undertaken with caution, since reducing donor size in an eye with a relatively short axial length may result in significant postoperative hyperopia. In addition, if undersizing the donor, the surgeon must take extreme care in coaptation of the wound to avoid leaks. Moreover, the flattened corneal contour can complicate postoperative contact lens fitting.

"Recurrent" keratoconus has been observed at a rate of 12% over 25 years.[24–26] Recurrence in the donor graft is commonly the result of an error in technique, related to incomplete excision of the cone. The iron (Fleischer) ring, found at the base of the cone, can be used as a reference when planning graft size and should be excised fully.

POSTOPERATIVE MANAGEMENT

Postoperative suture adjustment may play an important role in visual rehabilitation following PK. The timing of first suture removal is debated but can be initiated when wound healing is evidenced (typically at 3–6 months postoperatively). If corneal astigmatism is satisfactory with sutures in place (typically equal or lower than 3.00 D), sutures can remain unless there are other indications for removal, such as suture breakage, infection, vascularization, marked perisutural fibrosis, patient discomfort, or graft rejection. Loose interrupted sutures provide no structural support and are a risk for graft infection. They should, therefore, be removed. This can generally be done without endangering wound integrity (Fig. 32.1).

Postoperative suture removal can cause large and unpredictable swings in the degree of astigmatism, regardless of the type of suture used.[27–30] In the interrupted suture technique, one can attempt to titrate the astigmatic effect through sequential suture removal.[30] Alternatively, adjusting the tension of a continuous suture at the slit lamp, in the first 48 to 72 hours postkeratoplasty, can be employed to reduce corneal astigmatism, albeit with the inherent risk of suture breakage. Once all sutures have been removed, however, the measured astigmatism tends to remain relatively stable.[2]

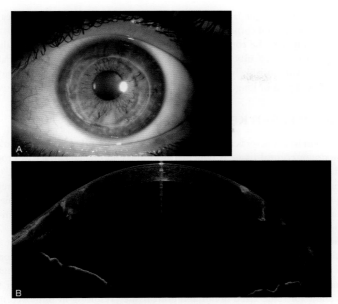

Fig. 32.1   (A) Clear penetrating graft status post suture removal. (B) Anterior segment of a penetrating graft in situ. (Image courtesy Luis Izquierdo.)

OUTCOMES

PK provides excellent outcomes in terms of graft clarity, exceeding 90% at 1 year. Graft survival following PK for keratoconus is also quite high, with a survival rate of 97% at 5 years, 89% to 92% at 10 years, and 49% at 20 years.[24,31–33] This does suggest, however, that a young keratoconic patient with a PK may require more than one graft over a lifetime. Subsequent grafts may have a shorter survival than the first graft.[2] Risk factors for PK failure in this setting include previous graft failure, glaucoma, synechia formation, corneal neovascularization, aphakia, and pseudophakia.

The definition of successful PK continues to evolve. Beyond maintaining a clear cornea, a successful refractive result also needs to be considered. PK offers good vision in the long term but visual rehabilitation may be slow, owing to high postoperative astigmatism or anisometropia.[34] After PK for advanced keratoconus, the final uncorrected visual acuity (UCVA) ranges from 20/50 to 20/100.[14,17,35–39] Contact lenses can improve BCVA to 20/25 or better, with 67% to 96% of patients seeing at least 20/40 at 1 year postoperatively.[14,17,18,35,39,40–47]

The visual gains post-PK may occasionally recede over time owing to progressive donor-recipient misalignment or recurrence of keratoconus, with resultant irregular astigmatism in the graft.[48–51] This period of gradual worsening vision tends to begin around 10 years after first suture removal.[52] Moreover, recurrence of keratoconus, occurring in 12% at 25 years, can also confound long-term visual outcomes.[24]

There are significant challenges in the postoperative management of the keratoconus patient undergoing PK. These include suture and wound-healing problems, progression of disease in the recipient rim, allograft reaction in a generally younger population, and persistent high or irregular astigmatism.[2] In addition, all penetrating grafts are at risk of dehiscence with trauma.

Although primary graft failure following PK is quite rare, allograft rejection affects 13% to 31% of eyes within the first 3 years after surgery, with a mean onset of 8 to 15 months.[53–55] Risk factors for graft rejection include larger-sized grafts, the number of previous corneal transplants, and the presence of peripheral corneal neovascularization.[2]

Ultimately, patients must be counseled on the goals of transplantation and realistic expectations for postoperative visual acuity, as well as about the modalities for correction. Patients should be advised that they will most likely require spectacles or contact lenses to attain best vision, and it often takes at least 1 year or longer to achieve stable BCVA.

FEMTOSECOND LASER KERATOPLASTY

Manual trephination in PK is vertical, with little variation in wound construction. In conventional PKP, when the donor corneal tissue is punched from the endothelial surface, it produces a graft with an anterior diameter of 0.2 to 0.3 mm smaller than the posterior diameter.[56,57] Moreover, vacuum trephines can lead to incomplete/oblique cuts.[58] This may result in an irregular donor-host junction, anteroposterior and rotational misalignment of the donor-host corneal interfaces, and slow and asymmetric postoperative wound healing.[59] This, in turn, can result in regular and/or irregular astigmatism that may influence final visual outcome.

The introduction of the femtosecond laser in PK for trephination of both donor and recipient tissues theoretically enables better apposition and faster wound healing. Femtosecond laser incisions produce precise and reproducible trephination of the donor and recipient buttons, avoiding the aforementioned disparities produced by the manual techniques.[58] Moreover, femtosecond laser incisions allow for same-sized donor and graft tissues, resulting in improved natural alignment, a watertight seal, less suture tension, and less induced astigmatism.[58]

The femtosecond laser also allows for patterns and angles of incisions not achievable with conventional trephines. The variations in wound configurations include top hat, mushroom, zigzag, and christmas tree, among others.[58,60] These shaped incisions have been associated with a stronger wound profile, presumed faster donor-recipient junction wound healing, earlier suture removal, less surgically induced corneal astigmatism, and earlier visual rehabilitation.[61]

Laboratory investigations have demonstrated significantly higher resistance to wound leakage in laser-fashioned incisions compared with the traditional vertical trephination (240.69 vs. 38.11 mmHg, respectively).[62] Ignacio et al. also observed that femtosecond-created incisions in a top-hat shape led to a seven-fold increase in resistance to wound leakage and less astigmatism.[63]

Clinically, femtosecond-assisted PK has been associated with better visual outcomes, including earlier stabilization of UCVA and BCVA, and lower astigmatism compared with conventional PK.[58] More rapid wound healing, as evidenced by fibrosis along incisions and suture tracks, enabled earlier suture removal.[64]

PK VERSUS DALK

DALK has become the preferred surgical procedure for keratoconic eyes that are free of deep corneal scarring or hydrops. DALK involves a staged dissection of the stroma down to the level of the Descemet membrane followed by transplantation of an endothelium-denuded donor tissue. However, it is technically more challenging and time-consuming than PK, and several techniques have been introduced, including Anwar's big bubble technique and injection of intracameral air, to improve surgical success.[65–70]

In DALK, the host Descemet membrane and endothelium are preserved. This eliminates the risk of endothelial immunogenic graft rejection, although stromal and epithelial rejection can still occur.[5] In turn, DALK entails improved long-term graft survival, reduced endothelial cell loss, and a decreased need for postoperative steroid treatment with its associated complications (cataract, glaucoma). Mitigated risk of rejection also enables for larger grafts. Moreover, given that the procedure remains extraocular, the risk of endophthalmitis is theoretically lessened.

Graft survival after DALK is better than that of penetrating graft PK.[75–77] In the largest reported series, an average DALK graft survival rate of 99.3% was observed over a mean follow-up period of 4.5 years.[77] Visual and refractive outcomes comparing DALK to PK are similar, specifically in cases of DALK where minimal (equal or lower than 20 microns) or no residual host stroma remains.[15,78] Retention of thicker (greater than 30 microns) stromal tissue in DALK can result in significant haze at the graft-host tissue interface and reduce long-term visual outcomes. Interface haze has been reported in 0.7% of cases.[79] Indeed, a single-center comparative study demonstrated equivalent or better visual acuity in eyes following DALK using the big bubble technique when compared with PK. However, visual outcomes were inferior when DALK was performed via manual pre-Descemet dissection.[80]

A recent Cochrane meta-analysis was conducted comparing outcomes in PK versus DALK in keratoconus patients. Only two randomized controlled trials, both conducted in Iran, were included, with a total of 111 participants. Although the quality of evidence was limited, the data indicated that rejection rates were lower in DALK than in PK (odds ratio: 0.33, 95% confidence interval: 0.14–0.81).[14,15,81] No evidence was found to support a difference in outcomes with regard to postoperative BCVA, graft survival, final UCVA, or keratometric outcomes.[15] The authors felt that there was insufficient evidence to determine which technique led to superior outcomes.

Reinhart et al. also reviewed the literature comparing DALK and PK for any indication (not specifically for keratoconus) and found the two techniques to be comparable in terms of visual and refractive measurements.[79] Shi et al. found greater improvement in BCVA with PK, but no significant differences in refractive measurements, and a significantly lower likelihood of rejection with DALK.[82] In terms of postoperative astigmatism, no significant differences have been observed between eyes undergoing PK compared with DALK, with mean astigmatism of 4.00 to 5.00 D.[15] This is not surprising given that both techniques have similar suturing requirements for securing the donor tissue.

Overall, DALK appears to deliver visual and refractive outcomes comparable to those of PK. With the preservation of host endothelial cells, DALK is associated with lower rejection rates and better graft survival. Conversely, the more technically demanding and time-consuming DALK procedure has contributed to a slower uptake than might have otherwise been expected.

Conclusion

PK remains an important surgical modality for advanced keratoconus, offering excellent graft survival and reasonable visual outcomes. The evolving role of femtosecond laser in PK is promising but warrants further investigation.

References

1. Castroviejo R. Keratoplasty for the treatment of keratoconus. *Trans Am Ophthalmol Soc.* 1948;46:127–153.
2. Parker JS, van Dijk K, Melles GRJ. Treatment options for advanced keratoconus: a review. *Surd Ophthalmic.* 2015;60:459–480.
3. Boimer C, Lee K, Sharpen L, Mashour RS, Slomovic AR. Evolving surgical techniques of and indications for corneal transplantation in Ontario from 2000 to 2009. *Can J Ophthalmol.* 2011;46:360–366.
4. Reddy JC, Hammersmith K, Nagra PK, Rapuano CJ. The role of penetrating keratoplasty in the era of selective lamellar keratoplasty. *Int Ophthalmol Clin.* 2013;53:12.
5. Cassidy D, Beltz J, Jhanji V, Loughnan MS. Recent advances in corneal transplantation for keratoconus. *Clin Exp Optom.* 2013;96:165–172.
6. Matthaei M, Sandhaeger H, Hermel M, et al. Changing indications in penetrating keratoplasty: a systematic review of 34 years of global reporting. *Transplantation.* 2017;101(6):1387–1399.
7. Romero-Jiméneza M, Santodomingo-Rubidob J, Wolffsohn JS. Keratoconus: a review. *Contact Lens Ant Eye.* 2010;33:157–166.

8. Kennedy RH, Bourne WM, Dyer JA. A 48-year clinical and epidemiologic study of keratoconus. *Am J Ophthalmol.* 1986;101:267–273.
9. Gordon MO, Steger-May K, Szczotka-Flynn L, et al. Baseline factors predictive of incident penetrating keratoplasty in keratoconus. *Am J Ophthalmol.* 2006;142:923–930.
10. Sray WA, Cohen EJ, Rapuano CJ, Laibson PR. Factors associated with the need for penetrating keratoplasty in keratoconus. *Cornea.* 2002;21:784–786.
11. Tuft SJ, Moodaley LC, Gregory WM, Davison CR, Buckley RJ. Prognostic factors for the progression of keratoconus. *Ophthalmology.* 1994;101:439–447.
12. Adelman RA, Afshari NA. Risk factors for progression to penetrating keratoplasty in patients with keratoconus. *Am J Ophthalmol.* 2005;140:607–611.
13. Frost NA, Wu J, Lai TF, Coster DJ. A review of randomized controlled trials of penetrating keratoplasty techniques. *Ophthalmology.* 2006;113(6):942–949.
14. Javadi MA, Naderi M, Zare M, Jenaban A, Rabei HM, Anissian A. Comparison of the effect of three suturing techniques on postkeratoplasty astigmatism in keratoconus. *Cornea.* 2006;25(9):1029–1033.
15. Keane M, Coster D, Ziaei M, Williams K. Deep anterior lamellar keratoplasty versus penetrating keratoplasty for treating keratoconus. *Cochrane Database Syst Rev.* 2014;7:CD009700.
16. Jaycock PD, Jones MN, Males J, et al. Outcomes of same-sizing versus oversizing donor trephines in keratoconic patients undergoing first penetrating keratoplasty. *Ophthalmology.* 2008;115(2):268–275.
17. Goble RR, Hardman Lea SJ, Falcon MG. The use of the same size host and donor trephine in penetrating keratoplasty for keratoconus. *Eye (Lond).* 1994;8:311–314.
18. Choi JA, Lee MA, Kim MS. Long-term outcomes of penetrating keratoplasty in keratoconus: analysis of the factors associated with final visual acuities. *Int J Ophthalmol.* 2014;7:517–521.
19. Heidemann DG, Sugar A, Meyer RF, Musch DC. Oversized donor grafts in penetrating keratoplasty. A randomized trial. *Arch Ophthalmol.* 1985;103:1807–1811.
20. Wilson SE, Bourne WM. Effect of recipient-donor trephine size disparity on refractive error in keratoconus. *Ophthalmology.* 1989;96(3):299–305.
21. Perry HD, Foulks GN. Oversize donor buttons in corneal transplantation surgery for keratoconus. *Ophthalmic Surg.* 1987;18(10):751–752.
22. Spadea L, Bianco G, Mastrofini MC, et al. Penetrating keratoplasty with donor and recipient corneas of the same diameter. *Ophthalmic Surg Lasers.* 1996;27(6):425–430.
23. Girard LJ, Eguez I, Esnaola N, et al. Effect of penetrating keratoplasty using grafts of various sizes on keratoconic myopia and astigmatism. *J Cataract Refract Surg.* 1988;14(5):541–547.
24. Pramanik S, Musch DC, Sutphin JE, Farjo AA. Extended long-term outcomes of penetrating keratoplasty for keratoconus. *Ophthalmology.* 2006;113(9):1633–1638.
25. Kremer I, Eagle RC, Rapuano CJ, et al. Histologic evidence of recurrent keratoconus seven years after keratoplasty. *Am J Ophthalmol.* 1995;119(4):511–512.
26. Belmont SC, Muller JW, Draga A, et al. Keratoconus in a donor cornea. *J Refract Corneal Surg.* 1994;10(6):658.
27. Mader TH, Yuan R, Lynn MJ, et al. Changes in keratometric astigmatism after suture removal more than one year after penetrating keratoplasty. *Ophthalmology.* 1993;100:119–126.
28. Musch DC, Meyer RF, Sugar A. The effect of removing running sutures on astigmatism after penetrating keratoplasty. *Arch Ophthalmol.* 1988;106:488–492.
29. Yilmaz S, Ali Ozdil M, Maden A. Factors affecting changes in astigmatism before and after suture removal following penetrating keratoplasty. *Eur J Ophthalmol.* 2007;17:301–306.
30. Burk LL, Waring GO 3rd, Radjee B, et al. The effect of selective suture removal on astigmatism following penetrating keratoplasty. *Ophthalmic Surg.* 1988;19:849–854.
31. Jensen LB, Hjortdal J, Ehlers N. Long-term follow-up of penetrating keratoplasty for keratoconus. *Acta Ophthalmol.* 2010;88:347–351.
32. Kelly TL, Coster DJ, Williams KA. Repeat penetrating corneal transplantation in patients with keratoconus. *Ophthalmology.* 2011;118:1538–1542.
33. Thompson RW Jr, MO Price, Bowers PJ, et al. Long-term graft survival after penetrating keratoplasty. *Ophthalmology.* 2003;110:1396–1402.
34. Mohammadpour M, Heidari Z, Hashemi H. Updates on managements for keratoconus. *J Current Ophthalmol.* 2018;30:110–124.
35. Buzard KA, Fundingsland BR. Corneal transplant for keratoconus: results in early and late disease *J Cataract Refract Surg.* 1997;23:398–406.

36. Cheng YY, Visser N, Schouten JS, et al. Endothelial cell loss and visual outcome of deep anterior lamellar keratoplasty versus penetrating keratoplasty: a randomized multicenter clinical trial. *Ophthalmology.* 2011;118:302–309.
37. Fontana L, Parente G, Sincich A, et al. Influence of graft-host interface on the quality of vision after deep anterior lamellar keratoplasty in patients with keratoconus. *Cornea.* 2011;30:497–502.
38. Jaycock PD, Jones MN, Males J, et al. UK Transplant Ocular Tissue Advisory Group and Contributing Ophthalmologists. Outcomes of same-sizing versus oversizing donor trephines in keratoconic patients undergoing first penetrating keratoplasty. *Ophthalmology.* 2008;115:268–275.
39. Sutton G, Hodge C, McGhee CN. Rapid visual recovery after penetrating keratoplasty for keratoconus. *Clin Experiment Ophthalmol.* 2008;36:725–730.
40. Al-Mohaimeed MM. Penetrating keratoplasty for keratoconus: visual and graft survival outcomes. *Int J Health Sci (Qassim).* 2013;7:67–74.
41. Brierly SC, Izquierdo L Jr, Mannis MJ. Penetrating keratoplasty for keratoconus. *Cornea.* 2000;19:329–332.
42. Kim MH, Chung TY, Chung ES. A retrospective contralateral study comparing deep anterior lamellar keratoplasty with penetrating keratoplasty. *Cornea.* 2013;32:385–389.
43. Lim L, Pesudovs K, Coster DJ. Penetrating keratoplasty for keratoconus: visual outcome and success. *Ophthalmology.* 2000;107:1125–1131.
44. Olson RJ, Pingree M, Ridges R, et al. Penetrating keratoplasty for keratoconus: a long-term review of results and complications. *J Cataract Refract Surg.* 2000;26:987–991.
45. Price FW Jr, Whitson WE, Marks RG. Progression of visual acuity after penetrating keratoplasty. *Ophthalmology.* 1991;98:1177–1185.
46. Severinsky B, Behrman S, Frucht-Pery J, et al. Scleral contact lenses for visual rehabilitation after penetrating keratoplasty: long term outcomes. *Cont Lens Anterior Eye.* 2014;37:196–202.
47. Silbiger JS, Cohen EJ, Laibson PR. The rate of visual recovery after penetrating keratoplasty for keratoconus. *CLAO J.* 1996;22:266–269.
48. Langenbucher A, Naumann GO, Seitz B. Spontaneous long-term changes of corneal power and astigmatism after suture removal after penetrating keratoplasty using a regression model. *Am J Ophthalmol.* 2005;140:29–34.
49. Lim L, Pesudovs K, Goggin M, et al. Late onset post-keratoplasty astigmatism in patients with keratoconus. *Br J Ophthalmol.* 2004;88:371–376.
50. Noble BA, Ball JL. Late onset post-keratoplasty astigmatism in patients with keratoconus. *Br J Ophthalmol.* 2004;88:317.
51. Raecker ME, Erie JC, Patel SV, et al. Long-term keratometric changes after penetrating keratoplasty for keratoconus and Fuchs endothelial dystrophy. *Am J Ophthalmol.* 2009;147:227–233.
52. de Toledo JA, de la Paz MF, Barraquer RI, et al. Long-term progression of astigmatism after penetrating keratoplasty for keratoconus: evidence of late recurrence. *Cornea.* 2003;22:317–323.
53. Wagoner MD, Ba-Abbad R. King Khaled Eye Specialist Hospital Cornea Transplant Study Group. Penetrating keratoplasty for keratoconus with or without vernal keratoconjunctivitis. *Cornea..* 2009;28:14–18.
54. Williams KA, Ash JK, Pararajasegaram P, et al. Long-term outcome after corneal transplantation. Visual result and patient perception of success. *Ophthalmology.* 1991;98:651–657.
55. Wisse RP, van den Hoven CM, Van der Lelij A. Does lamellar surgery for keratoconus experience the popularity it deserves? *Acta Ophthalmol.* 2014;92:473–477.
56. Foulks GN, Perry HD, Dohlman CH. Oversize corneal donor grafts in penetrating keratoplasty. *Ophthalmology.* 1979;86:490–494.
57. Olson RJ. Variation in corneal graft size related to trephine technique. *Arch Ophthalmol.* 1979;97:1323–1325.
58. Shivanna Y, Nagaraja H, Kugar T, Shetty R. Femtosecond laser enabled keratoplasty for advanced keratoconus. *Ind J Ophthalmol.* 2013;61(8):469–472.
59. Farid M, Steinert RF, Gaster RN, Chamberlain W, Lin A. Comparison of penetrating keratoplasty performed with a femtosecond laser zig-zag incision versus conventional blade trephination. *Ophthalmology.* 2009;116:1638–1643.
60. Farid M, Steinert RF. Deep anterior lamellar keratoplasty performed with the femtosecond laser zig-zag incision for the treatment of stromal corneal pathology and ectatic disease. *J Cataract Refract Surg.* 2009;35(5):809–813.
61. Chan CC, Ritenour RJ, Kumar NL, Sansanayudh W, Rootman DS. Femtosecond laser-assisted mushroom configuration deep anterior lamellar keratoplasty. *Cornea.* 2010;29:290–295.

62. Steinert RF, Ignacio TS, Sarayba MA. "Top hat"-shaped penetrating keratoplasty using the femtosecond laser. *Am J Ophthalmol.* 2007;143:689–691.
63. Ignacio TS, Nguyen TB, Chuck RS, Kurtz RM, Sarayba MA. Top hat wound configuration for penetrating keratoplasty using the femtosecond laser: a laboratory model. *Cornea.* 2006;25:336–340.
64. Price Jr FW, MO Price. Femtosecond laser shaped penetrating keratoplasty: one-year results utilizing a top-hat configuration. *Am J Ophthalmol.* 2008;145:210–214.
65. Anwar M, Teichmann KD. Big-bubble technique to bare Desçemet's membrane in anterior lamellar keratoplasty. *J Cataract Refract Surg.* 2002;28:398–403.
66. Archila EA. Deep lamellar keratoplasty dissection of host tissue with intrastromal air injection. *Cornea.* 1984;3:217–218.
67. van Dooren BT, Mulder PG, Nieuwendaal CP, Beekhuis WH, Melles GRJ. Endothelial cell density after deep anterior lamellar keratoplasty (Melles technique). *Am J Ophthalmol.* 2004;137:397–400.
68. Anwar M, Teichmann KD. Deep lamellar keratoplasty: surgical techniques for anterior lamellar keratoplasty with and without baring of Desçemet's membrane. *Cornea.* 2002;21:374–383.
69. Sugita J, Kondo J. Deep lamellar keratoplasty with complete removal of pathological stroma for vision improvement. *Br J Ophthalmol.* 1997;81:184–188.
70. Jhanji V, Beltz J, Sharma N, Graue E, Vajpayee RB. "Double bubble" deep anterior lamellar keratoplasty for management of corneal stromal pathologies. *Int Ophthalmol.* 2011;31:257–262.
71. Terry M, Ousley P. Deep lamellar endothelial keratoplasty visual acuity, astigmatism, and endothelial survival in a large prospective series. *Ophthalmology.* 2005;112(9):1541–1548.
72. Watson S, Ramsay A, Dart J, et al. Comparison of deep lamellar keratoplasty and penetrating keratoplasty in patients with keratoconus. *Ophthalmology.* 2004;111:1676–1682.
73. Shimazaki J, Shimmura S, Ishioka M, et al. Randomized clinical trial of deep lamellar keratoplasty vs. penetrating keratoplasty. *Am J Ophthalmol.* 2002;134:159–165.
74. Romano V, Iovieno A, Parente G, et al. Long-term clinical outcomes of deep anterior lamellar keratoplasty in patients with keratoconus. *Am J Ophthalmol.* 2015;159(3):505–511.
75. Borderie VM, Sandali O, Bullet J, et al. Long-term results of deep anterior lamellar versus penetrating keratoplasty. *Ophthalmology.* 2012;119:249–255.
76. Sharma N, Kandar AK, Singh Titiyal J. Stromal rejection after big bubble deep anterior lamellar keratoplasty: case series and review of literature. *Eye Contact Lens.* 2013;39:194–198.
77. Sarnicola V, Toro P, Sarnicola C, Sarnicola E, Ruggiero A. Long-term graft survival in deep anterior lamellar keratoplasty. *Cornea.* 2012;31:621–626.
78. Ardjomand N, Hau S, McAlister JC, et al. Quality of vision and graft thickness in deep anterior lamellar and penetrating corneal allografts. *Am J Ophthalmol.* 2007;143:228–235.
79. Reinhart WJ, Musch DC, Jacobs DS, Lee WB, Kaufman SC, Shtein RM. Deep anterior lamellar keratoplasty as an alternative to penetrating keratoplasty: a report by the American Academy of Ophthalmology. *Ophthalmology.* 2011;118:209–218.
80. Han DC, Mehta JS, Por YM, Htoon HM, Tan DT. Comparison of outcomes of lamellar keratoplasty and penetrating keratoplasty in keratoconus. *Am J Ophthalmol.* 2009;148:744–751.
81. Razmju H, Shams M, Abtahi MA, Abtahi SH. Comparison of deep lamellar keratoplasty and penetrating keratoplasty in patients with keratoconus: a clinical trial study. *J. Isfahan Med. Sch.* 2011;29(144):798–802.
82. Shi JL, Feng YF, Yu JG, Wang QM. Meta-analysis of deep lamellar keratoplasty and penetrating keratoplasty for keratoconus. *CJEO.* 2012;30(10):926–931.

CHAPTER 33

Combined Procedures for Keratoconus

Maria A. Henriquez ■ Luis Izquierdo Jr. ■ Mark J. Mannis

KEY CONCEPTS

- A combined procedure is justified when a single procedure cannot achieve the same safety and efficacy.
- Inclusion and exclusion criteria for the individual procedures should be respected when two procedures are combined.
- The key indication for corneal collagen cross-linking is to halt the progression of corneal ectasia.
- Corneal cross-linking associated with refractive treatment offers stabilized ectasia and improved functional vision.
- No consensus exists on how many procedures and combinations of surgical approaches for the visual rehabilitation of eyes with keratoconus.
- Photorefractive keratectomy after any previous corneal procedure should be performed with care because of the risk of severe haze.

Until recently, treatment for keratoconus (KC) was focused on the correction of refractive error and corneal irregularity. Since corneal collagen cross-linking (CXL) has become a common treatment, halting progression of the disease has become a priority. Moreover, the excellent refractive results achieved with various refractive procedures in KC eyes have led us to employ combined treatments. When faced with a KC patient today, two issues should be addressed: (1) avoiding disease progression and (2) treating the refractive defect and corneal irregularity.

CXL-Plus

When the CXL procedure is associated with an adjuvant refractive treatment, it is referred to as CXL-plus. The combined procedure is a technique that can offer patients corneal stability (via CXL) together with improved functional vision via adjuvant treatments.

The key indication for CXL is to halt the to progression of KC.[1] Different CXL protocols use varying combinations of irradiance time and energy to maintain total fluence. Early studies used the standard Dresden protocol (3 mW/cm² for 30 minutes, total fluence 5.4 J/cm²), whereas accelerated protocols have used a power of up to 30 mW for durations as short as 3 minutes, with varying fluences and differing protocols. Most combined procedures for CXL-plus have used different protocols.

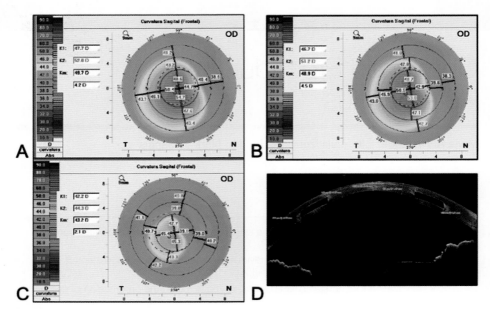

Fig. 33.1 Case example of a patient with keratoconus in whom corneal cross-linking (CXL) was performed first and an intracorneal ring segment (ICRS) implanted 6 months later: (A) preoperative curvature map, (B) curvature map 3 months after CXL, (C) curvature map after 6 months of ICRS and 13 months of CXL, and (D) anterior segment optical coherence tomography (MS39) showing the implanted ICRS.

CXL can be performed before, during, or after the combined procedure, and each approach has distinct advantages and disadvantages. However, the stability and predictability of the refractive results of cross-linking remain under study. Although the keratometric reduction is typically between 1 and 2 diopters (D), which is often reached 6 months to 1 year after the procedure, studies have reported progressive flattening as much as 10 years after CXL,[2] as well as an intense flattening effect of up to 14 D.[3]

CXL AND INTRASTROMAL CORNEAL RINGS

Intrastromal corneal rings (ICRs) are segments or rings inserted into the corneal stroma that flatten the central corneal curvature by exerting an arc-shortening effect while maintaining clarity in the central optic zone. They are frequently used to improve irregular astigmatism. ICRs do not stop the progression of KC[4]; hence they are used in combination with CXL. Fig. 33.1 shows the pre- and postoperative anterior curvature maps of a patient with CXL followed by ICRs implantation. Fig. 33.2 shows the slit-lamp photography of the same patient.

Several studies have suggested that CXL may exert an additive effect when combined with ICRs. Superior visual acuity, refraction, and keratometry readings have been reported for combined CXL and ICR implantation when compared with ICR insertion alone,[5–7] although this has not been consistently demonstrated in all studies.[8]

ICRS can be implanted on the same day that CXL is performed, either before or after cross-linking. Some studies have suggested that the sequence of implanting ICRs first and performing CXL second achieves superior results in terms of uncorrected visual acuity (UCVA), best-corrected visual acuity (BCVA), cylinder, and keratometric readings when compared with the reverse sequence.[9] Their hypothesis is that a cornea pretreated with CXL will not react to ICR

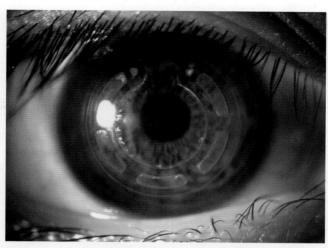

Fig. 33.2 Slit-lamp photography of the patient in Fig. 33.1 showing the implanted intracorneal ring segment. (The Keraring SG is a 330-degree segment consisting of two segments joined by several bridges to produce a double arch.)

implantation in the expected way or that its effect will be lessened by its application to a stiffer cornea. However, this is not a consistent finding. We have reported, in a previous study, reductions of up to 11 D when applying CXL first and ICRS 6 months later.[5]

Several studies comparing the three sequences claim superiority of the same-day procedure.

El-Raggal compared ICRS first versus same-day procedure and found similar improvements in terms of UCVA, BCVA, and refraction[10]; however, the reduction in keratometric values in the same-day procedure was significantly higher. Hashemi et al. evaluated the visual, refractive, and keratometric outcomes after three sequences: same-day, ICRS-first, and CXL-first, in a systematic review and meta-analysis.[11] The results showed that simultaneous surgery was superior to the CXL-first technique when comparing spherical refractive errors and flattest keratometry (K). Performing simultaneous surgery was also more effective than CXL-first and ICRS-first regarding change in steep-K, suggesting that simultaneous ICRS implantation and CXL may provide better outcomes than separated techniques, in terms of corneal shape.

Although the CXL-first sequence is considered less effective in keratometric reduction, it has other advantages. Performing CXL first may halt the disease progression, allowing the physician to choose a better suited and more constant solution from a wide range of surgical (ICRS, phakic intraocular lens [pIOL], etc.) and nonsurgical (contact lens, glasses) options based on the residual refractive error and the patient's needs.[12]

CXL AND PHAKIC INTRAOCULAR LENS

Izquierdo et al. first described the combination of CXL and iris-claw Artiflex pIOLs in 11 eyes with mild-to-moderate progressive KC and refractive astigmatism lower than 2.5 D with over 6 months of follow-up.[13] Kymionis et al. reported one case of combined CXL and toric posterior-chamber pIOLs.[14] The published data with follow-up of up to 5 years have shown that this combined procedure is safe and effective in halting the progression of KC and correcting the refraction-associated defects of progressive KC.[15-17]

Eyes that might be eligible for this combined procedure are those with progressive KC, moderate-to-high ametropia, absence of clinically significant irregular astigmatism, corrected distance

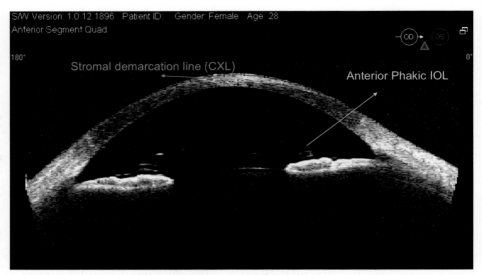

Fig. 33.3 Case example of a patient with keratoconus in whom corneal cross-linking (*CXL*) was performed (*red arrow* indicates the demarcation line) and iris-claw phakic intraocular lens (*pIOL*) was implanted 6 months later (*yellow arrow* indicates the pIOL).

visual acuity (CDVA) of 20/50 or better, a clear cornea, thinnest pachymetry >400 μm, central anterior chamber depth (ACD) >3.2 mm measured from the corneal epithelium to the anterior surface of the crystalline lens, central endothelial cell count >2300 cells/mm², normal iris and pupil function, and scotopic pupil <6.0 mm. Fig. 33.3 shows a patient with iris-claw pIOL and CXL.

CXL is typically performed first and is followed by an interval of 3 to 6 months before the pIOL implantation, to achieve refractive stability. Refraction is considered stable when the results of two consecutive manifest refractions and topographies, separated by at least 1 month, are stable. pIOLs should not be implanted after CXL until CDVA has reached at least the preoperative values, which also avoids errors in the pIOL power calculation caused by the flattening effect of the CXL.

This combined procedure seems to be as safe as pIOL implantation alone in terms of endothelial cell loss, with no substantial decrease in endothelial cell density at 5 years of follow-up.[15] This might be expected, because endothelial cell loss is related to ACD, and KC eyes generally have a deeper anterior chamber than normal myopic eyes.

CXL AND PHOTOREFRACTIVE KERATECTOMY

Combined topography-guided photorefractive keratectomy (PRK) and standard or accelerated CXL improve corneal irregularity and also treat refractive error, facilitating visual rehabilitation in KC.[16,17] The PRK can be performed before, during, or after CXL. Fig. 33.4 shows the pre- and postoperative anterior curvature maps of a patient who had CXL first and PRK 6 months later.

In sequential CXL and PRK, CXL is performed first, and PRK is performed after corneal stability is achieved, typically at 6 months. Notably, when topography-guided PRK is performed after a CXL procedure, some of the cross-linked anterior cornea is removed by ablation.

Same-day simultaneous customized topography-guided PRK and CXL (referred to by some as the Athens protocol) includes topography-guided PRK followed immediately by CXL (3 mW/cm²) for 30 minutes, using 0.1% topical riboflavin sodium phosphate. Simultaneous topography-guided PRK and CXL is associated with greater improvement in visual acuity, greater

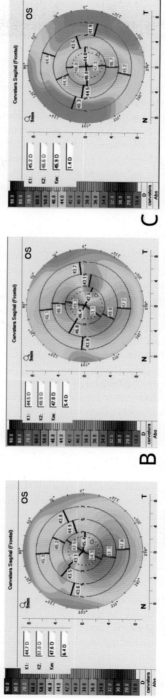

Fig. 33.4 Case example of a patient with keratoconus in whom corneal cross-linking (CXL) was performed first and photorefractive keratectomy (PRK) was performed 6 months later. (A) Preoperative curvature map, (B) curvature map 5 months after CXL, and (C) curvature map after 6 months of PRK.

mean reduction in spherical equivalent refraction and keratometry, and less corneal haze compared with sequential CXL and PRK. Typically, ablation no greater than 50 μm and laser treatment for undercorrection of both sphere and cylinder by at least 30% are recommended in anticipation of the refractive effect of CXL (corneal flattening).[18]

Long-term follow-up in adult patients with KC after this combined procedure suggests high safety and efficacy in terms of corneal ectasia and visual function. 94.4% of the eyes demonstrated stabilization of ectasia, and 3.5% showed progressive "overcorrection" or "hyperopic" shift at 10 years of follow-up.[19] This protocol was also used in children, reporting significant improvement in UCVA, BCVA, and keratometric readings at 4 years of follow-up. The study also demonstrated late-onset deep corneal haze (1 year after the procedure) observed in 5.12% of the patients.[20]

Despite the reported safety and effectiveness of these combined procedures, ectasia after PRK alone has been reported,[21] as well as progression of KC despite treatment with CXL.[22] Therefore corneal ablation procedures should be performed with caution, particularly with higher corrections, because the risk of triggering progressive corneal ectasia is increased when corneal laser ablations are performed in keratoconic eyes.

CXL AND PSEUDOPHAKIC IOL

CXL and IOL implantation is advised in unstable KC patients who require cataract surgery. When performing this type of combined procedure, certain issues should be considered and discussed thoroughly. Among them are proper intraocular lens (IOL) calculations, careful wound construction whether on the cornea or the sclera, toric versus conventional IOL implantation, and contact lens use in the form of rigid gas permeable or scleral lenses after cataract surgery.

IOL power calculations are difficult in KC eyes because of inaccurate keratometry measurements, longer axial length, deeper anterior chamber, and the role of posterior corneal curvature.[23-25] Therefore the severity, stability, and location of the KC can affect preoperative biometry and formulas that calculate the implanted lens power.

Surgical incisions must be created with caution. Clear corneal incisions may have delayed self-sealing and, therefore, sutures must be placed for adequate closure. The sutures should be located as close to the limbus as possible. Another alternative is a modified scleral incision with sutures.[26]

TRIPLE PROCEDURES

ICRs, CXL, and Phakic IOLs

Case series have reported the use of ICRs, CXL, and pIOLs to treat KC with extreme myopia and irregular astigmatism. ICR implantation is used to reduce irregular corneal astigmatism. CXL is used to stabilize the cornea, and posterior-chamber toric pIOLs are used to treat residual high myopic astigmatism. An interval of 4 to 6 weeks between procedures is recommended. Results have shown major improvement in UCVA and BCVA, as well as reduction in mean manifest refraction and spherical equivalent of up to 21 D.[27]

ICRs, CXL, and PRK/PTK

Sequential ICRs, CXL, and PRK have been used for mild-to-moderate KC in patients who have undergone ICR implantation. PRK for the treatment of residual mild refractive error is applied 6 months after sequential ICRS implantation and CXL in stable KC. After 12 months of follow-up, substantial improvement in uncorrected distance visual acuity (UDVA), CDVA, keratometry, and cylinder has been reported, with no patients losing lines of CDVA. Postoperative haze after 12 months of follow-up remained at 0% to 11% of the cases in various studies.[28-30]

Same-day phototherapeutic keratectomy (PTK), ICRS, and CXL procedures have been reported with a follow-up of 6 months, with significant improvement of UCVA, BCVA, and refraction. The advantage of this technique may be avoidance of ablation on previously cross-linked corneas and removal of cross-linked areas that affect the total volume of modified stroma needed to prevent further future progression.[31] It also avoids de-epithelialization twice in separate procedures. In terms of associated risks, one study reported that 2% of patients lost three lines of BCVA and 11% lost one line of BCVA.[32]

ICRs, CXL, and Toric Phakic IOLs

ICR implantation and CXL are performed sequentially in patients with moderate-to-severe KC with an interval of 4 weeks. Toric posterior-chamber pIOL implantation is performed at least 6 months after CXL. At 12 months of follow-up, substantial improvement in UDVA, CDVA, keratometry, and cylinder has been reported, with no complications.[33]

FOUR-STAGE PROCEDURE

ICRs, CXL, Phakic IOLs, and PRK

Case series studies have reported four-stage combined treatment of KC, including ICRs implantation followed by CXL, toric pIOL implantation, and topography-guided PRK. A minimum interval of 6 months is recommended between each stage. Reports after 12 months of follow-up indicate that the procedure is an effective and safe approach for corneal stabilization and improvement of functional vision in patients with KC, with substantial improvement in UCVA, refractive astigmatism, and spherical equivalent.[34]

ICRS AND REFRACTIVE PROCEDURE

Combined treatment of ICRS and PRK or pseudophakic/pIOLs for the correction of irregular astigmatism in KC has previously been reported.[35] However, these procedures are usually intended to correct cataract (in the case of pseudophakic IOL) or some residual refractive defect. With the improvement of ICRS nomograms and increased popularity of toric, phakic, and pseudophakic IOLs, these combinations are becoming obsolete and are only useful in specific cases. It is important to understand that these combination procedures do not stop the progression of KC and are therefore indicated only in nonprogressive KC.

REFERENCES

1. Kymionis GD, Grentzelos MA, Portaliou DM, et al. Corneal Collagen Cross-linking (CXL) Combined With Refractive Procedures for the Treatment of Corneal Ectatic Disorders: CXL Plus. *J Refract Surg.* 2014;30(8):566–576.
2. Mazzotta C, Traversi C, Baiocchi S, et al. Corneal Collagen Cross-Linking With Riboflavin and Ultraviolet A Light for Pediatric Keratoconus: Ten-Year Results. *Cornea.* 2018 May;37(5):560–566.
3. Santhiago MR, Giacomin NT, Medeiros CS, et al. Intense Early Flattening After Corneal Collagen Cross-linking. *J Refract Surg.* 2015;31(6):419–422.
4. Alio JL, Shabayek MH, Artola A. Intracorneal ring segments for keratoconus correction: long-term follow-up. *J Cataract Refract Surg.* 2006;32:978–985.
5. Henriquez MA, Izquierdo Jr L, Bernilla C, et al. Corneal collagen cross-linking before Ferrara intrastromal corneal ring implantation for the treatment of progressive keratoconus. *Cornea.* 2012;31:740–745.
6. Chan CCK, Sharma M, Boxer Wachler BS. Effect of inferior segment Intacs with and without C3-R on keratoconus. *J Cataract Refract Surg.* 2007;33:75–80.
7. Ertan A, Karacal H, Kamburo_glu G. Refractive and topographic results of transepithelial cross-linking treatment in eyes with Intacs. *Cornea.* 2009;28:719–723.
8. Legare ME, Iovieno A, Yeung SN, et al. Intacs with or without same-day corneal collagen cross-linking to treat corneal ectasia. *Can J Ophthalmol.* 2013;48:173–178.

9. Coskunseven E, Jankov M, Hafezi F, Atun S, et al. Effect of treatment sequence in combined intra-stromal corneal rings and corneal collagen cross-linking for keratoconus. *J Cataract Refract Surg.* 2009;35:2084–2091.

10. El-Raggal TM. Sequential versus concurrent Kerarings insertion and corneal collagen cross-linking for keratoconus. *Br J Ophthalmol.* 2011;95:37–41.

11. Hashemi H, Alvani A, Seyedian MA, et al. Appropriate Sequence of Combined Intracorneal Ring Implantation and Corneal Collagen Cross-Linking in Keratoconus: A Systematic Review and Meta-Analysis. *Cornea.* 2018;37(12):1601–1607.

12. Henriquez MA, Izquierdo Jr L. Reply: To PMID 22531433. *Cornea.* 2013;32(3):382.

13. Izquierdo Jr L, Henriquez MA, McCarthy M. Artiflex phakic intraocular lens implantation after corneal collagen cross-linking in keratoconic eyes. *J Refract Surg.* 2011;27:482–487.

14. Kymionis GD, Grentzelos MA, Karavitaki AE, et al. Combined corneal collagen cross-linking and posterior chamber toric implantable collamer lens implantation for keratoconus. *Ophthalmic Surg Lasers Imaging.* 2011;42:22–25.

15. Güell JL, Morral M, Malecaze F, et al. Collagen crosslinking and toric iris-claw phakic intraocular lens for myopic astigmatism in progressive mild to moderate keratoconus. *J Cataract Refract Surg.* 2012;38:475–484.

16. Kanellopoulos AJ, Binder PS. Collagen cross-linking (CCL) with sequential topography-guided PRK: a temporizing alternative for keratoconus to penetrating keratoplasty. *Cornea.* 2007;26(7):891–895.

17. Kymionis GD, Kontadakis GA, Kounis GA, et al. Simultaneous topography-guided PRK followed by corneal collagen crosslinking for keratoconus. *J Refract Surg.* 2009;25:807–811.

18. Kanellopoulos AJ. Comparison of sequential vs same-day simultaneous collagen cross-linking and topog-raphy-guided PRK for treatment of keratoconus. *J Refract Surg.* 2009;25:812–818.

19. Kanellopoulos AJ. Ten-Year Outcomes of Progressive Keratoconus Management With the Ath-ens Protocol (Topography-Guided Partial-Refraction PRK Combined With CXL). *J Refract Surg.* 2019;35(8):478–483.

20. Kanellopoulos AJ, Vingopoulos F, Sideri AM. Long-Term Stability With the Athens Protocol (Topog-raphy-Guided Partial PRK Combined With Cross-Linking) in Pediatric Patients With Keratoconus. *Cornea.* 2019;38(8):1049–1057.

21. Roszkowska AM, Sommario MS1, et al. Post photorefractive keratectomy corneal ectasia. *Int J Ophthal-mol.* 2017;10(2):315–317.

22. Henriquez MA, Izquierdo Jr L, Bernilla C, et al. Riboflavin/Ultraviolet A corneal collagen cross-linking for the treatment of keratoconus: visual outcomes and Scheimpflug analysis. *Cornea.* 2011;30(3):281–286.

23. Bozorg S, Pineda R. Cataract and keratoconus: minimizing complications in intraocular lens calculations. *Semin Ophthalmol.* 2014;29:376–379.

24. Alio´ JL, Pena-Garcia P, Abdulla Guliyeva F, et al. MICS with toric intraocular lenses in keratoconus: outcomes and predictability analysis of postoperative refraction. *Br J Ophthalmol.* 2014;98:365–370.

25. Tamaoki A, Kojima T, Hasegawa A, et al. Intraocular lens power calculation in cases with posterior kera-toconus. *J Cataract Refract Surg.* 2015;41:2190–2195.

26. Bourges JL. Cataract surgery in keratoconus with irregular astigmatism editor. In: Goggin M, ed. *Astig-matism – optics, physiology and management.* Croatia: InTech; 2012.

27. Coşkunseven E, Sharma DP, Jankov MR 2nd, et al. Collagen copolymer toric phakic intraocular lens for residual myopic astigmatism afterintrastromal corneal ring segment implantation and corneal collagen crosslinking in a 3-stageprocedure for keratoconus. *J Cataract Refract Surg.* 2013;39(5):722–729.

28. Kymionis GD, Grentzelos MA, Portaliou DM, et al. Photorefractive keratectomy followed by same-day corneal collagen crosslinking after intrastromal corneal ring segment implantation for pellucidmarginal degeneration. *J Cataract Refract Surg.* 2010;36:1783–1785.

29. Kremer I, Aizenman I, Lichter H, et al. Simultaneous wavefront-guided photorefractive keratectomy and corneal collagen crosslinkingafter intrastromal corneal ring segment implantation for keratoconus. *J Cataract Refract Surg.* 2012;38(10):1802–1807.

30. Iovieno A, Légaré ME, Rootman DB, et al. Intracorneal ring segments implantation followed by same-day photorefractive keratectomy and corneal collagen cross-linking in keratoconus. *J Refract Surg.* 2011;27(12):915–918.

31. Malta J, Soong H, Moscovici BK, et al. Two-year follow-up of corneal cross-linking and refractive surface ablation in patients with asymmetric corneal topography. *Br J Ophthalmol.* 2018;103:1136.

32. Rocha G, Ibrahim T, Gulliver E, et al. Combined Phototherapeutic Keratectomy, Intracorneal Ring Segment Implantation, and Corneal Collagen Cross-Linking in Keratoconus Management. *Cornea.* 2019;38(10):1233–1238.
33. Dirani A, Fadlallah A, Khoueir Z, et al. Visian toric ICL implantation after intracorneal ring segments implantation and corneal collagencrosslinking in keratoconus. *Eur J Ophthalmol.* 2014;24(3):338–344.
34. Coskunseven E, Sharma DP, Grentzelos MA, et al. Four-stage procedure for keratoconus: ICRS implantation, corneal cross-linking, toric phakic intraocular lens implantation, and topography-guided photorefractive keratectomy. *J Refract Surg.* 2017;33(1):683–689.
35. Lee SJ, Kwon HS, Koh IH. Sequential Intrastromal Corneal Ring Implantation and Cataract Surgery in a Severe Keratoconus Patient With Cataract. *Korean J Ophthalmol.* 2012;26(3):226–229.

CHAPTER 34

Alternative Surgical Techniques: Bowman's Layer Transplantation and Stromal Regenerating Techniques

Javier García-Montesinos ▓ Joaquín Fernández

KEY CONCEPTS

- Bowman's layer transplantation can be used for the treatment of patients with advanced keratoconus not eligible for corneal cross-linking or intrastromal corneal ring segments, effecting a reshaping and flattening of corneal curvature and improving contact lens tolerance in advanced keratoconus.
- Bowman's layer transplantation may stabilize and halt the progression of the disease in advanced keratoconus cases for the long-term prevention of further visual loss and may prevent or delay the need for corneal transplantation.
- Stromal regeneration through cell therapy may represent a future option to restore corneal thickness, shape, and transparency in keratoconus.
- Preliminary studies of stromal regeneration techniques have demonstrated safety and moderate efficacy in the treatment of advanced keratoconus.
- Laser-assisted crescent keratectomy may be a new surgical approach to improve corneal profile and reduce higher-order aberrations in eyes with keratoconus.

Introduction

Keratoconus is regarded as a corneal ectatic disease characterized by progressive central or paracentral protrusion and thinning of the cornea, leading to myopia and irregular astigmatism with reduced visual quality and acuity.[1,2]

The goal of the treatment is to arrest the progression of the disease and achieve visual rehabilitation. In the early stages of the disease, visual rehabilitation can be accomplished with success through optical correction of the refractive error with glasses or soft contact lenses. However, in more advanced cases, rigid contact lenses may be required to obtain a regular anterior optical surface, to compensate for high-order aberrations (HOAs) and provide better visual performance.[2,3]

For patients with moderate keratoconus who are intolerant of rigid contact lenses or who require better vision than with glasses, the implantation of intrastromal corneal ring segments (ICRSs) is an effective option for remodeling corneal shape and reducing the amount of spherical equivalent, astigmatism, and HOA.[2,4,5]

In cases of progression of the disease or high risk of progression (children and teenagers) corneal cross-linking (CXL) can stabilize the cornea and prevent vision loss.[6-8] However, in terms of efficacy and safety, the results of ICRS implantation or CXL in cases of advanced keratoconus with a thinner cornea are poor and the procedures are usually not indicated.[9-13]

The treatment for these advanced cases with very poor visual acuity (VA) and/or contact-lens intolerance is usually corneal transplantation, with either penetrating keratoplasty (PK) or deep anterior lamellar keratoplasty (DALK). Although corneal transplantation can provide efficient visual rehabilitation in the short term, long-term outcomes may be compromised by adverse events.[14-16]

Recently, a new surgical approach, Bowman's layer transplantation (BLT), has been introduced to treat progressive advanced keratoconus cases that are not good candidates for ICRS implantation or CXL or as an alternative to corneal transplantation with the intention to delay PK.

In addition, new approaches that regenerate the corneal stroma with cell-based therapy through different tissue engineering techniques and techniques to reshape corneal curvature through laser-assisted crescent keratectomy are being developed.

In this chapter, we will summarize the current available literature on BLT, stromal regeneration techniques, and laser crescent keratectomy.

Bowman's Layer Transplantation

The pathogenesis of keratoconus includes genetic, environmental, and mechanical factors. It is postulated that abnormally weak corneal collagen could lead to a progressive deformation and thinning of the cornea with mechanical factors such as eye rubbing, or overexpression of certain inflammatory factors.[1,17]

Bowman's layer (BL) is the second stratum of the cornea, between the basement membrane of the epithelium and the stroma. Previously considered a membrane, it is rather an acellular condensate of the anterior stroma, composed of highly compacted collagen type I and III fibrils. Its thickness is approximately 12 to 14 microns. BL does not have regenerative capacity and does not regenerate after trauma, surgical injury, or ablation with excimer laser.[18,19] It is present in primates, but not in other mammals, and its function remains unclear. It is thought that it protects the subbasal nerve plexus and the stroma against pathogens. It may play a role in modulating the epithelial-stromal wound healing process and it is considered as one of the strongest biomechanical layers of cornea.[19-22]

The first report in scientific literature on the use of isolated BLT was published by Lie et al. for the treatment of a case of recalcitrant haze after photorefractive keratectomy (PRK).[23]

BL appears to prevent excessive bulging of the cornea.[24] In fact, fragmentation and sectoral disappearance of BL are a pathognomonic feature in the histologic sections from keratoplasty of corneal specimens of patients with keratoconus.[1,2,25-27] That finding led these authors to study a variant of this technique to treat progressive advanced keratoconus. They theorized that a midstromal inlay of BL could partially restore corneal curvature with a flattening effect and at the same time stabilize the disease.[28]

DONOR TISSUE PREPARATION

Like other lamellar keratoplasty techniques, the graft is obtained prior to surgery. Graft tissue can be prepared from a corneoscleral button or a whole globe obtained less than 24 hours, with equivalent success.[29] Corneas not valid for PK or endothelial keratoplasty because of low endothelial cell count can be also used for harvesting the BL graft. Furthermore, corneoscleral buttons used to

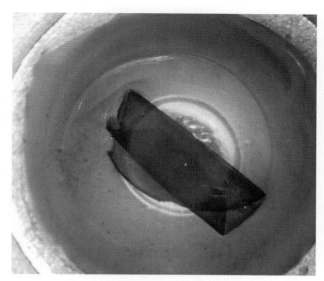

Fig. 34.1   Bowman's layer graft harvested and stained with trypan blue. (Courtesy Dr. Javier Giménez-Almenara.)

harvest Descemet membrane endothelial keratoplasty (DMEK) grafts can be used to obtain BL tissue for another patient, allowing expanded use of the donor tissue.[20,29,30]

The donor corneoscleral button is mounted on an artificial chamber and pressurized with balanced salt solution (BSS). Epithelium is removed completely with surgical sponges. A circular 360-degree superficial incision in the BL within the limbal corneal periphery is made using a 30-gauge needle, to access a peripheral plane of dissection. With McPherson forceps, the peripherical edge of BL is lifted, then BL is carefully peeled from anterior stroma, moving from the periphery to the center over the full 360 degrees (Fig. 34.1). Because of inherent elasticity of the tissue, BL graft spontaneously curls into a double or single roll with the epithelial border at the outside.[29] BL is usually trephined with a 9- to 11-mm corneal punch. The graft is submerged in 70% alcohol to eliminate any remaining epithelial cells. The BL inlay is then rinsed with BSS and stored in organ-culture medium at 31°C until implantation.[28–31]

Standardizing the harvesting of a thin BL graft is the most challenging step of the procedure. It is laborious and technically demanding, with a 30% failure rate.[29] Tearing of the BL during preparation or an unusually thick BL graft with additional stroma attached are the main reasons for discarding the tissue.[29] To help overcome this technical barrier, Parker et al. investigated the potential use of the femtosecond laser to prepare BL graft. Donor globes were mounted in a globe holder and, after de-epithelialization, the laser was programmed to make a superficial cut at a depth of 20 microns. However, grafts prepared using this method were statistically thicker than with the manual technique, owing to the presence of a variable amount of stromal residual tissue.[29,32] If the BL is dissected with additional stroma, visual quality and the clarity of the cornea can be affected postoperatively because of interface haze.[29]

SURGICAL TECHNIQUE

BLT consists of implanting a circular inlay of BL in the middle of the stroma of the recipient keratoconic cornea through a stromal pocket. This midstromal pocket can be made using the manual technique for lamellar dissection in DALK described by Melles et al.[33,34] or using a femtosecond laser.[24] The surgery can be done under topical, local, or general anesthesia.

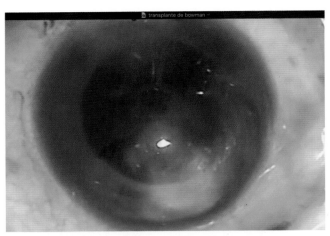

Fig. 34.2   Bowman's layer graft implanted into a manual midstromal pocket in an advanced keratoconus case. (Courtesy Dr. Javier Giménez-Almenara.)

In the manual technique, the anterior chamber is filled with air through a peripheral paracentesis. Then, the superior conjunctiva is opened and dissected and a superficial scleral incision of 5 mm in length, 1- to 2-mm outside the limbus, is made. With a set of dissection spatulas of specific design (Melles spatula set; DORC International BV, Zuidland, the Netherlands), the scleral incision is tunneled up to the superior cornea. A paracentesis is made, through which the anterior chamber is filled completely with air. The air-endothelium interface acts as a convex mirror that reflects images from the anterior and posterior corneal surfaces as a specular light reflex. The non-incised corneal tissue between the tip of the spatula and the light reflex from the air-endothelium interface is seen as a dark band directly surrounding the tip. In this way, one can control the depth of dissection, monitoring the width of this dark band to create the pocket at a depth of about 50% from limbus-to-limbus 360 degrees. When the midstromal pocket over a circumference of 8 to 9 mm in diameter is completed, the air in the anterior chamber is replaced by BSS. The BL graft is immersed again in 70% ethanol for 30 seconds, rinsed with BSS, and stained with trypan blue 0.06% for better visualization in the stroma. The BL roll is unfolded, inserted, and centered in the pocket through the scleral incision, helped by a glide (BD Visitec [Fichman]; Beaver-Visitec International, Waltham, MA) and a blunt spatula or a cannula with BSS (Fig. 34.2). Postoperative treatment includes topical antibiotics and steroid on a tapering dosage.[20,28–31]

Intraoperatively, a Descemet perforation during stromal dissection has been reported in 10% of cases (2/22 eyes). Management of this complication may include aborting the surgery and reattempting the dissection later when wound healing has occurred or proceeding with a consecutive PK.[20] Intraoperative anterior segment optical coherence tomography (iAS-OCT) can be used for better visualization of the dissection plane during the surgical procedure, even in the presence of corneal scarring, edema, or blood.[35]

To reduce the complication rate and make the stromal dissection in the host cornea easier, García de Oteyza et al. have introduced a variant of the surgical technique in which the stromal pocket is created by a femtosecond laser at a depth of 50%, instead of manually (Fig. 34.3). They reported two cases of grade IV keratoconus intolerant to contact lenses treated with BLT using this technique without complications. Both patients became contact lens tolerant with an improvement in best spectacle-corrected visual acuity (BSCVA) and best contact lens–corrected visual acuity (BCLVA), keratometry, and pachymetry values after surgery.[24]

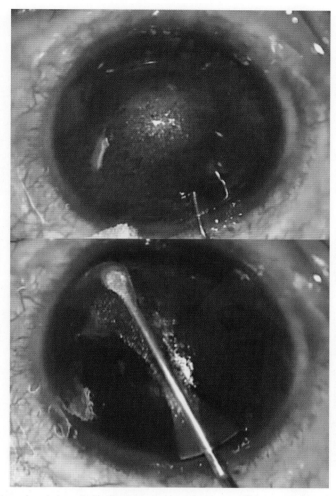

Fig. 34.3 Midstromal pocket created by femtosecond laser for Bowman's layer transplantation. (Courtesy Dr. Gonzalo García de Oteyza.)

CLINICAL OUTCOMES

van Dijk et al. were the first to report the results of BLT in 20 eyes with advanced progressive keratoconus with a follow-up to 5 to 7 years.[28,30,31,36] The outcomes of BLT are summarized in Table 34.1. A significant flattening effect of –4.1 diopter (D) in mean simulated keratometry (K_{mean}) and –6.9 D in maximum keratometry (K_{max}) was observed after BLT at 1 month, without significant changes thereafter up to 5 years.[30] This flattening effect seems more prominent in more advanced cases and with central cones.[31] BSCVA improved from 0.05 preoperatively to 0.13 postoperatively at 12 months, and was unchanged thereafter. Of the eyes, 85% gained Snellen lines of BSCVA or remained stable. BCLVA remained stable during follow-up; however, all patients tolerated rigid contact lenses better postoperatively, whereas most were intolerant before the surgery. Thinnest corneal thickness (TCT) showed an increase after surgery, whereas central corneal thickness (CCT) remained stable.[30] However, in 10% of cases (2/20 eyes), there was progressive

TABLE 34.1 ■ Outcomes of Bowman's Layer Transplantation

Authors	Study Type	Indication	Sample Size (Eyes/ Patients)	Mean Follow-Up (Months)	Stromal Pocket Dissection Technique	Main Outcome	Secondary Outcome	Complications
van Dijk et al. (2014)	Prospective	Progressive[a] advanced KC grades III and IV	10/9	16	Manual	Decrease in K_{mean} and K_{max}	Improvement in contact lens wearing.	None
van Dijk et al. (2015)	Prospective	Progressive[a] advanced KC grades III and IV	22/19	20	Manual	Decrease in K_{mean} and K_{max}	Improvement in contact lens wearing. Little increase in BSCVA.	Intraoperative perforation of Descemet membrane in two cases. Progressive steepening in two cases (10%).
Luceri et al. (2016)	Retrospective	Progressive[a] advanced KC grades III and IV	15/14	12	Manual	Decrease in anterior and posterior HOA RMS		Increase medium and posterior corneal backscattering
van Dijk et al. (2018)	Prospective	Progressive[a] advanced KC grades III and IV	20/17	60	Manual	Decrease in K_{mean} and K_{max}	Improvement in contact lens wearing. Little increase in BSCVA.	Progressive steepening in two cases (10%). Acute hydrops after 4.5 years in one case.
García de Oteiza et al. (2019)	Prospective	KC grade IV with intolerance to contact lenses	2/2	3	Femto second laser	Decreased simK1 and simK2. Contact lens tolerance.	Increased CCT and TCT	None

BSCVA, Best spectacle-corrected visual acuity; *CCT,* central corneal thickness; *HOA RMS,* high-order aberrations root-mean-square; *KC,* keratoconus; *Kmean,* mean keratometry; *Kmax,* maximum keratometry; *simK,* simulated keratometry; *TCT,* thinnest corneal thickness.
[a]Progression defined as ≥1 D change in simulated keratometry (simK) values, ≥2 D change in K_{max} value, or both.

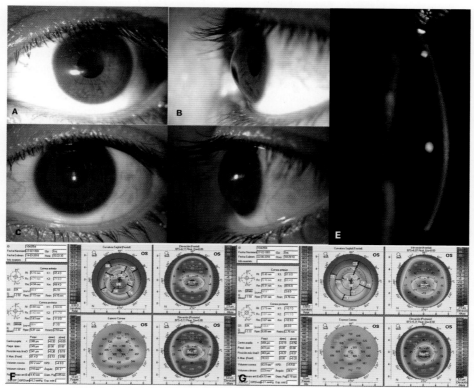

Fig. 34.4   Biomicroscopy details of a case of advanced keratoconus treated with Bowman's layer transplantation, shown preoperatively (A and B) and 3 months postoperatively (C and D). The Bowman's layer graft is viewed as a fine white line into the stroma (E). Preoperative and 3 months postoperative anterior curvature map, anterior and posterior elevation map, and pachymetry map (F and G); note the large flattening effect over the anterior curvature map. (Courtesy Dr. Gonzalo García de Oteyza.)

corneal steepening. Intraoperatively, two eyes were complicated by perforation of the Descemet membrane during manual dissection and were excluded from the analysis.[30,31] Three cases suffered an acute hydrops 4.5, 6, and 6.5 years after BLT without previous signs of progression but with a history of atopy and continuous eye rubbing.[21] No other complications such as adverse endothelial events or allograft rejection episodes were observed. Endothelial cell density remained stable after BTL for up to 5 years.[30,36]

At slit-lamp examination, the BL graft appears as a thin white line in the stroma (Fig. 34.4). Luceri et al. evaluated corneal densitometry and HOAs and found that anterior and posterior HOAs (especially spherical aberration) decreased significantly, whereas corneal backscattering involving mild and posterior layers of the cornea increased. However, these changes did not correlate with VA.[37]

DISCUSSION

Recently, the paradigm of the treatment of keratoconus may have shifted from contact lens fitting for as long as tolerated followed by corneal transplantation,[1] to ICRSs for contact lens–intolerant patients and CXL for progressive disease patients.[14,38]

Although keratoconus is one of the most successful indications for corneal transplantation, with a high graft survival rate,[1,39] issues with early and late complications can still jeopardize long-term visual outcomes, including endothelial failure, allograft rejection, suture- or wound healing–related complications, weakness to ocular trauma, steroid complications, worsening of preexisting ocular surface dysfunction, and high or irregular astigmatism.[14–16,21] This is of particular concern in young patients in whom the risk of rejection and other complications is higher.

Patients with severe thinning and/or steepening are not eligible for CXL or ICRS implantation but they benefit from well-fitted contact lenses. However, with progression of keratoconus, an alternative to corneal transplantation may be desirable in these cases. The ideal candidate for BTL is the patient with progressive or advanced keratoconus who is not eligible for either CXL or ICRS implantation owing to excessive thinning or steepening, but who still has subjective acceptable BCLVA. Therefore patients with severe central corneal scarring would be not good candidates for this technique.

The aim of BLT is to reinforce the thin and structurally weak keratoconic cornea, rendering it flatter and stiffer. BLT may arrest disease progression and reshape corneal curvature, thereby preserving, and in some cases restoring, the ability to wear a contact lens. The exact mechanism by which BLT achieves this is unclear. Some authors think that the BL graft itself may confer stiffness to the cornea, whereas others believe the wound healing response between host stroma and the BL graft may be responsible.

The wound healing effect after manual midstromal dissection without BL implantation was evaluated to determine if it would stabilize ectasia in progressive keratoconus. This procedure was effective in halting the disease in 50% of moderate cases (preoperative K_{max} < 60 D); however, none of the cases showed corneal flattening, and all the more advanced cases (preoperative K_{max} > 60 D) went on to progression.[40] This may imply that the BL graft is responsible for the flattening effect and can stabilize the ectasia in the more advanced cases.[20]

The advantage of BLT is that it is a minimally invasive, extraocular, sutureless procedure that avoids the primary intraoperative and suture-related complications of classic corneal transplantation. BLT has a theoretically negligible risk of allograft rejection, because the BL graft is an acellular tissue. Postoperative steroid can be tapered quickly, therefore minimizing steroid-related complications. Box 34.1 summarizes the main characteristics of BTL.

At time of writing, BLT is a relatively new technique with limited investigative data available. The studies published are from a single center with a small sample size, limited follow-up, and without comparison with other techniques or treatments. However, the reports of short- and midterm results show its efficacy in flattening the cornea and stabilizing progression in advanced keratoconus with a reported 5-year success rate of 84% and few postoperative complications.[30] Moreover, if corneal transplantation is required after BLT, the prognosis is not affected unless there has been an intraoperative Descemet membrane perforation in the primary procedure.

BLT is a new and promising technique for the surgical management of keratoconus. BLT may be regarded by corneal surgeons as a less invasive alternative technique to corneal transplantation or with the intention of delaying PK and rendering the eye with more advanced tolerance of contact lens correction. However, further research with a larger sample and longer follow-up is needed before introducing the technique for routine clinical practice.

Stromal Regeneration Techniques

The corneal stroma represents approximately 90% of corneal thickness. Its characteristics of transparency, stiffness, and refractive index, essential for the visual function of the cornea, are due to the disposition, microarchitecture, and biomechanics of the stromal lamellae.[41]

In keratoconus, corneas have been described with alterations in the organization and number of the stromal lamellae and collagen fibers, especially in the apex of the cone.[1,2,27,42] Moreover,

---

BOX 34.1 ■ Main Characteristics of Bowman's Layer Transplantation

Advantages	Disadvantages
Can stabilize advanced ectasia and preserve contact lens wearing	Steep learning curve in harvesting BL graft, midstromal manual dissection in thin KC corneas, and graft handling
Minimally invasive procedure	Surgical indication limited to advanced progressive ectasia with satisfactory BCLVA
Low risk for postoperative complications	Little or no improvement in BSCVA and BCLVA
Negligible risk of allograft rejection	Possibility of intraoperative complications during manual stromal dissection
Sutureless procedure	
Can use donor corneas not appropriate for PK or endothelial keratoplasty and corneas from anterior lamellae left behind from DMEK graft preparation	

BCLVA, Best contact lens–corrected visual acuity; *BSCVA,* best spectacle-corrected visual acuity; *BL,* Bowman's layer; *DMEK,* Descemet membrane endothelial keratoplasty; *KC,* keratoconus; *PK,* penetrating keratoplasty.

---

confocal microscopy studies have demonstrated a reduction in the number of keratocytes and stromal lamellae.[43] These tissue changes may contribute to the weakness of the keratoconus cornea, leading to biomechanical failure with progressive protrusion and thinning. An interesting approach to keratoconus would be to restore the normal corneal stromal collagen architecture, thickness, and cellularity.

Tissue engineering is a scientific discipline that seeks to enhance or replace a biological function through cells, biomaterials, and physical-chemical factors. The principle of these cellular therapies for regenerating the corneal stroma is to collect stem cells and implant them in the ectatic cornea, leading to their differentiation into adult keratocytes and the regeneration of the corneal stroma.[44]

Different types of mesenchymal stem cells have been used in stromal tissue engineering, among which we have corneal stromal stem cells, bone marrow mesenchymal stem cells, adipose-derived adult mesenchymal stem cells (ADASCs), umbilical cord mesenchymal stem cells, and embryonic stem cells.[44] Of these, ADASCs seem to be the ideal source for stromal regeneration techniques, since they have demonstrated the ability in vitro and in vivo to differentiate into adult keratocytes. Moreover, they can be easily extracted by liposuction from the patient, are autologous, and have high cell retrieval efficiency.[41,45]

Direct intrastromal injection of different types of stem cells through a stromal pocket has been tried in vivo in animal models, demonstrating the differentiation of these cells into adult keratocytes without signs of immune rejection and their ability to improve corneal transparency by the reorganization of the stromal collagen lamellae and production of new collagen.[45–47]

Alió del Barrio et al. first evaluated the efficacy and safety of intrastromal injection of 3×10^6 ADASCs in 1 mL in five patients with advanced grade IV keratoconus through a femtosecond laser midstromal 9.5-mm pocket with a follow-up of 6 months. There was slight improvement in BSCVA and BCLVA, while manifest refraction and keratometry remained stable. No complications were recorded. Cellular differentiation and production of collagen was demonstrated by confocal biomicroscopy, viewed as dendritic shape cells in the plane of the pocket, and by OCT, with an increase in CCT of 16.5 microns. The authors concluded that intrastromal implantation of ADASCs is a safe procedure but not sufficient to restore the thickness in a very thin ectatic cornea as in advanced keratoconus cases, because the collagen production by the transplanted cells is limited.[41]

Alió del Barrio et al., in a prospective interventional case series, assessed the efficacy and safety of implantation of a decellularized human stromal laminae of 120 microns and 9 mm in diameter into a 9.5-mm midstromal pocket created by femtosecond laser, with 6 months of follow-up.[48] The stromal laminae from human donor corneas with nonviable endothelium were decellularized with sodium dodecyl sulfate solution,[49] so that they could be used as an acellular scaffold. Nine patients were randomized to receive a recellularized stromal lamina with 1×10^6 autologous ADASCs plus 1×10^6 autologous ADASCs at the time of the surgery from elective liposuction, or a previous acellular stromal lamina without recellularization. Five patients received the stromal lamina without recellularization (group 1) (Fig. 34.5), and four patients were implanted with the recellularized lamina (group 2). Five patients received superficial laminae, including BL (four in group 1 and one in group 2) and the other four patients received deeper laminae without BL. After implantation, slight improvement in unaided VA and BCSVA (>1 line) was recorded, with improvement in refractive sphere, anterior keratometry, and corneal aberrometry. Corneal thickness was almost restored, with a mean pachymetry increase of 124 microns. However, no significant differences were observed between groups 1 and 2 in any of the parameters evaluated nor between patients implanted with superficial versus deeper laminae. Confocal microscopy confirmed host recellularization of implanted laminae. No postoperative complications were recorded nor were there rejection episodes.[48]

The results of these two studies were extended to 1 year of follow-up. Five patients underwent implantation of autologous ADASCs 3×10^6 cell/1 mL alone (group 1), five patients received a decellularized donor 120-micron stromal lamina alone (group 2), and four patients received a recellularized donor 120-micron stromal lamina with 1×10^6 autologous ADASCs plus 1×10^6 ADASCs at the time of the surgery (group 3). All patients showed visual improvement, and no patients experienced any loss of lines of VA. The gains in Snellen lines in BSCVA and BCLVA, respectively, at the end of follow-up were 2.3 and 2.6 lines in group 1, 2.6 and 0.4 lines in group 2, and 0.9 and 1.3 lines in group 3. Improvements in refractive sphere, anterior keratometry, pachymetry, and corneal aberrometry were observed in groups 2 and 3, and these remained relatively stable in group 1.[50]

Stromal regeneration through cell therapy is a new and encouraging approach for the treatment of advanced keratoconus and may represent a future option for the restoration of corneal thickness, shape, and transparency in the keratoconus patient. The preliminary studies have demonstrated that implantation of autologous ADASC cells and decellularized corneal stroma is safe but with moderate efficacy.

Crescent Keratectomy Assisted by Laser

A new surgical approach has been proposed by Carriazo and Cosentino to flatten the cornea, improve corneal curvature profile, and shorten the anterior chamber in eyes with keratoconus.[51,52]

This technique is based on performing a crescent keratectomy using excimer or femtosecond laser at the edge of an 8-mm optical zone, at 80% to 90% of planned pachymetry, with suturing of the edges with interrupted 10-0 nylon. Sutures are passed at 90% depth of the crescentic trench, and suture tension is adjusted using slip knots (Fig. 34.6). These sutures are removed between 6 and 12 months after the procedure, based on corneal topography and refraction (Fig. 34.7). The principle of this surgery is the removal of peripheral corneal tissue to effect *corneal stretching*, which increases its tension and shortens the corneal arc, producing corneal flattening.[53] The calculation

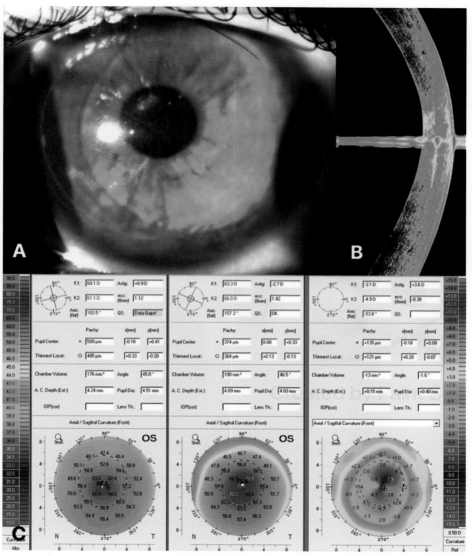

Fig. 34.5 (A) Biomicroscopy of an implant of a decellularized stromal lamina 1 year after surgery; note that total corneal transparency is recovered after procedure although borders of the lamina are still visible. (B) Anterior optical coherence tomography of the same case 6 months after the procedure, in which stromal lenticule is perfectly delimited. (C) Comparative analysis of anterior curvature map 6 months after surgery; note the flattening effect over the anterior curvature and the increase in pachymetry after stromal lamina implantation. (Courtesy Dr. Jorge Alió del Barrio and Prof. Jorge Alió.)

of the length and the width of the resection is performed by specific software and depends on biometry and the degree of keratoconus: the greater the keratoconus, the greater the length and width resection. The resection is wider at the base of the cone, narrowing progressively at the end of the resection. Arc lengths of 180 degrees, 270 degrees, and 360 degrees and resection widths of 300, 400, and 500 microns were planned for keratoconus grades II, III, and IV, respectively.[51,52]

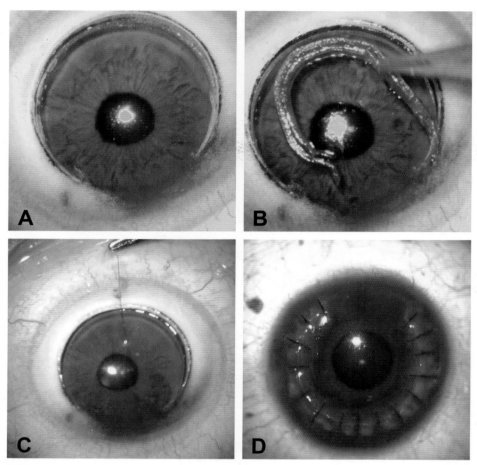

Fig. 34.6 Intraoperative details of crescent keratectomy. (A) Femtosecond laser–assisted parallel side kera-tectomy. (B) Corneal tissue removal. (C) Apposition of the edges with sutures. (D) Interrupted nylon 10-0 sutures in place at the end of surgery. (Courtesy Dr. César Carriazo and Dra. María José Cosentino.)

Moreover, crescentic keratectomy can be combined with laser vision correction procedures to cor-rect residual refractive errors 1 year after removing all sutures and/or CXL.

The first results with this technique were reported in three cases of keratoconus in 2017. The crescent keratectomy was performed then by excimer laser using a conical transparent acrylic mask placed over the cornea. Twelve months after the procedure, all three keratoconus cases showed a decrease in root-mean-square HOAs and coma aberrations, keratometry values, spherical equiva-lent, and anterior chamber depth, with an improvement in BSCVA.[51]

Later, these authors abandoned the use of the excimer laser, developing this technique for the femtosecond laser thereafter, with which it is easier to perform specific resections based on the characteristics of the keratoconus in each patient. They published the results of 69 eyes with keratoconus grades II, III, and IV treated by laser crescentic keratectomy performed with a fem-tosecond laser with a follow-up of 12 to 36 months (Fig. 34.8).

After the procedure, a decrease in root-mean-square HOA and coma aberrations, refractive sphere, and cylinder and anterior chamber depth was observed. For 180-, 270-, and 360-degree arc lengths, 70%, 65%, and 56% of the patients gained two or more lines of BSCVA, respectively.[52]

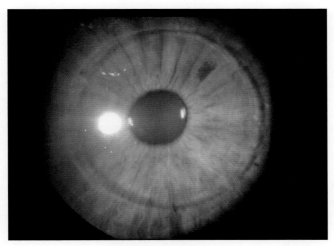

Fig. 34.7 Clinical photograph of a case of keratoconus treated by femtosecond laser–assisted crescent keratectomy after removal of all sutures. (Courtesy Dr. César Carriazo and Dra. María José Cosentino.)

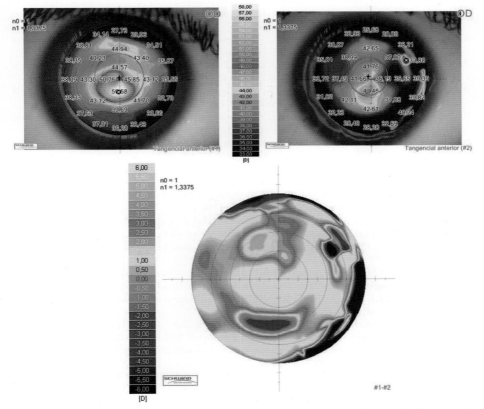

Fig. 34.8 Preoperative tangential anterior topography of a case of keratoconus *(upper left)*. Postoperative tangential anterior topography after surgery *(upper right)*. Difference on tangential anterior curvature before and after surgery *(center bottom)*. (Courtesy Dr. César Carriazo and Dra. María José Cosentino.)

With regard to safety, at 36 months postoperatively, none of the patients lost lines of BSCVA. Adjustment or placing of new sutures in eight cases was needed during follow-up, with no other intraoperative or postoperative complication recorded. However, 14 cases underwent PRK during follow-up.[52]

After analyzing the first 110 cases, the authors found that corneal flattening was achieved in all cases with a decrease in HOA and coma aberrations and with a mean increase in BSCVA of three Snellen lines, with no loss of lines of BSCVA. The anterior chamber depth decreased by 0.4 mm on average. Endothelial cell count decreased less than 5% at 1 year postoperatively.[53]

Crescent laser–assisted keratectomy is a new surgical approach to improve corneal profile and reduce HOAs in keratoconic corneas. Further prospective studies will be required to confirm these initial results and refine the nomograms for this technique in routine practice.

References

1. Rabinowitz YS Keratoconus. *Surv Ophthalmol*. 1998;42(4):297–319.
2. Romero-Jiménez M, Santodomingo-Rubido J, Wolffsohn JS. Keratoconus: a review. *Cont Lens Anterior Eye*. 2010;33(4):157–166 quiz 205.
3. Barnett M, Mannis MJ. Contact lenses in the management of keratoconus. *Cornea*. 2011;30(12):1510–1516.
4. Coskunseven E, Kymionis GD, Tsiklis NS, et al. One-year results of intrastromal corneal ring segment implantation (KeraRing) using femtosecond laser in patients with keratoconus. *Am J Ophthalmol*. 2008;145(5):775–779.
5. Coskunseven E, Kymionis GD, Tsiklis NS, et al. Complications of intrastromal corneal ring segment implantation using a femtosecond laser for channel creation: a survey of 850 eyes with keratoconus. *Acta Ophthalmol*. 2011;89(1):54–57.
6. Wollensak G, Spoerl E, Seiler T. Riboflavin/ultraviolet-a-induced collagen crosslinking for the treatment of keratoconus. *Am J Ophthalmol*. 2003;135(5):620–627.
7. Padmanabhan P, Rachapalle Reddi S, et al. Corneal collagen cross-linking for keratoconus in pediatric patients-long-term results. *Cornea*. 2017;36(2):138–143.
8. Mazzotta C, Traversi C, Baiocchi S, et al. Corneal collagen cross-linking with riboflavin and ultraviolet A light for pediatric keratoconus: ten-year results. *Cornea*. 2018;37(5):560–566.
9. Raiskup F, Spoerl E. Corneal cross-linking with hypo-osmolar riboflavin solution in thin keratoconic corneas. *Am J Ophthalmol*. 2011;152(1):28–32.e1.
10. Chan E, Snibson GR. Current status of corneal collagen cross-linking for keratoconus: a review. *Clin Exp Optom*. 2013;96(2):155–164.
11. Secretariat MA. Intrastromal corneal ring implants for corneal thinning disorders: an evidence-based analysis. *Ont Health Technol Assess Ser*. 2009;9(1):1–90.
12. Wollensak G, Spoerl E, Wilsch M, Seiler T. Endothelial cell damage after riboflavin-ultraviolet-A treatment in the rabbit. *J Cataract Refract Surg*. 2003;29(9):1786–1790.
13. Alió JL, Shabayek MH, Belda JI, Correas P, Feijoo ED. Analysis of results related to good and bad outcomes of Intacs implantation for keratoconus correction. *J Cataract Refract Surg*. 2006;32(5):756–761.
14. Parker JS, van Dijk K, Melles GR. Treatment options for advanced keratoconus: a review. *Surv Ophthalmol*. 2015;60(5):459–480.
15. Olson RJ, Pingree M, Ridges R, Lundergan ML, Alldredge C Jr, Clinch TE. Penetrating keratoplasty for keratoconus: a long-term review of results and complications. *J Cataract Refract Surg*. 2000;26(7):987–991.
16. Arnalich-Montiel F, Alió Del Barrio JL, Alió JL. Corneal surgery in keratoconus: which type, which technique, which outcomes? *Eye Vis (Lond)*. 2016;3:2.
17. Balasubramanian SA, Mohan S, Pye DC, Willcox MD. Proteases, proteolysis and inflammatory molecules in the tears of people with keratoconus. *Acta Ophthalmol*. 2012;90(4):e303–e309.
18. Wilson SE, Hong JW. Bowman's layer structure and function: critical or dispensable to corneal function? A hypothesis. *Cornea*. 2000;19(4):417–420.
19. Mannis MJ, Holland EJ. *Cornea. Fundamentals, Diagnosis and Management*. 4th ed Edinburgh: 2016. Elsevier Health Sciences.
20. Tong CM, van Dijk K, Melles GRJ. Update on Bowmanlayer transplantation. *Curr Opin Ophthalmol*. 2019;30(4):249–255.

21. Dragnea DC, Birbal RS, Ham L, et al. Bowman layer transplantation in the treatment of keratoconus. *Eye Vis (Lond)*. 2018;5:24.
22. Last JA, Thomasy SM, Croasdale CR, Russell P, Murphy CJ. Compliance profile of the human cornea as measured by atomic force microscopy. *Micron*. 2012;43(12):1293–1298.
23. Lie J, Droutsas K, Ham L, et al. Isolated Bowman layer transplantation to manage persistent subepithelial haze after excimer laser surface ablation. *J Cataract Refract Surg*. 2010;36(6):1036–1041.
24. García de Oteyza G, González Dibildox LA, Vázquez-Romo KA, et al. Bowman layer transplantation using a femtosecond laser. *J Cataract Refract Surg*. 2019;45(3):261–266.
25. Ambekar R, Toussaint KC Jr, Wagoner Johnson A. The effect of keratoconus on the structural, mechanical, and optical properties of the cornea. *J Mech Behav Biomed Mater*. 2011;4(3):223–236.
26. Mas Tur V, MacGregor C, Jayaswal R, O'Brart D, Maycock N. A review of keratoconus: diagnosis, pathophysiology, and genetics. *Surv Ophthalmol*. 2017;62(6):770–783.
27. Sherwin T, Brookes NH. Morphological changes in keratoconus: pathology or pathogenesis. *Clin Exp Ophthalmol*. 2004;32(2):211–217.
28. van Dijk K, Parker J, Tong CM, et al. Midstromal isolated Bowman layer graft for reduction of advanced keratoconus: a technique to postpone penetrating or deep anterior lamellar keratoplasty. *JAMA Ophthalmol*. 2014;132(4):495–501.
29. Groeneveld-van Beek EA, Parker J, Lie JT, et al. Donor tissue preparation for Bowman layer transplantation. *Cornea*. 2016;35(12):1499–1502.
30. van Dijk K, Parker JS, Baydoun L, et al. Bowman layer transplantation: 5-year results. *Graefes Arch Clin Exp Ophthalmol*. 2018;256(6):1151–1158.
31. van Dijk K, Liarakos VS, Parker J, et al. Bowman layer transplantation to reduce and stabilize progressive, advanced keratoconus. *Ophthalmology*. 2015;122(5):909–917.
32. Parker JS, Huls F, Cooper E, et al. Technical feasibility of isolated Bowman layer graft preparation by femtosecond laser: a pilot study. *Eur J Ophthalmol*. 2017;27(6):675–677.
33. Melles GR, Lander F, Rietveld FJ, Remeijer L, Beekhuis WH, Binder PS. A new surgical technique for deep stromal, anterior lamellar keratoplasty. *Br J Ophthalmol*. 1999;83(3):327–333.
34. Melles GR, Rietveld FJ, Beekhuis WH. Binder PS. A technique to visualize corneal incision and lamellar dissection depth during surgery. *Cornea*. 1999;18(1):80–86.
35. Tong CM, Parker JS, Dockery PW, Birbal RS, Melles GRJ. Use of intraoperative anterior segment optical coherence tomography for Bowman layer transplantation. *Acta Ophthalmol*. 2019;97(7):e1031–e1032.
36. Zygoura V, Birbal RS, van Dijk K, et al. Validity of Bowman layer transplantation for keratoconus: visual performance at 5-7 years. *Acta Ophthalmol*. 2018;96(7):e901–e902.
37. Luceri S, Parker J, Dapena I, et al. Corneal densitometry and higher order aberrations after Bowman layer transplantation: 1-year results. *Cornea*. 2016;35(7):959–966.
38. Sarezky D, Orlin SE, Pan W, VanderBeek BL. Trends in corneal transplantation in keratoconus. *Cornea*. 2017;36(2):131–137.
39. Ghatak U, Sinha R, Sharma N. Indications and outcome of penetrating keratoplasty. In: Rasik V, ed. *Corneal Transplantation*. United Kingdom: Jaypee-Highlights Medical Publishers, Inc.; 2010.
40. Birbal RS, van Dijk K, Parker JS, et al. Manual mid-stromal dissection as a low risk procedure to stabilize mild to moderate progressive keratoconus. *Eye Vis (Lond)*. 2018;5:26.
41. Alió del Barrio JL, El Zarif M, de Miguel MP, et al. Cellular therapy with human autologous adipose-derived adult stem cells for advanced keratoconus. *Cornea*. 2017;36(8):952–960.
42. Meek KM, Tuft SJ, Huang Y, et al. Changes in collagen orientation and distribution in keratoconus corneas. *Invest Ophthalmol Vis Sci*. 2005;46(6):1948–1956.
43. Ku JY, Niederer RL, Patel DV, Sherwin T, McGhee CN. Laser scanning in vivo confocal analysis of keratocyte density in keratoconus. *Ophthalmology*. 2008;115(5):845–850.
44. Alió del Barrio JL. ¿Se puede regenerar el estroma corneal?. In: Peris Martínez C, Alejandre Alba N, eds. *Actualización en queratocono. Sociedad de superficie ocular y cornea*: Esteve Oftalmología; 2017.
45. Arnalich-Montiel F, Pastor S, Blazquez-Martinez A, et al. Adipose-derived stem cells are a source for cell therapy of the corneal stroma. *Stem Cells*. 2008;26(2):570–579.
46. Du Y, Carlson EC, Funderburgh ML, et al. Stem cell therapy restores transparency to defective murine corneas. *Stem Cells*. 2009;27(7):1635–1642.
47. Liu H, Zhang J, Liu CY, et al. Cell therapy of congenital corneal diseases with umbilical mesenchymal stem cells: lumican null mice. *PLoS One*. 2010;5(5):e10707.

48. Alió Del Barrio JL, El Zarif M, Azaar A, et al. Corneal stroma enhancement with decellularized stromal laminas with or without stem cell recellularization for advanced keratoconus. *Am J Ophthalmol.* 2018;186:47–58.

49. Alio del Barrio JL, Chiesa M, Garagorri N, et al. Acellular human corneal matrix sheets seeded with human adipose-derived mesenchymal stem cells integrate functionally in an experimental animal model. *Exp Eye Res.* 2015;132:91–100.

50. Alió JL, Alió Del Barrio JL, El Zarif M, et al. Regenerative surgery of the corneal stroma for advanced keratoconus: 1-year outcomes. *Am J Ophthalmol.* 2019;203:53–68.

50. Carriazo C, Cosentino MJ. A novel corneal remodeling technique for the management of keratoconus. *J Refract Surg.* 2017;33(12):854–856.

52. Carriazo C, Cosentino MJ. Long-term outcomes of a new surgical technique for corneal remodeling in corneal Ectasia. *J Refract Surg.* 2019;35(4):261–267.

53. Carriazo C, Cosentino MJ. Remodelación corneal: nueva alternativa terapeutica para la ectasia corneal. In: Albertazzi RG, ed. *Queratocono: Pautas para su diagnóstico y tratamiento.* 2nd ed. Ediciones del Cosejo Argentino de Oftalmología 2020:217–232.

CHAPTER 35

Cataract Surgery in the Keratoconus Patient

Enrique O. Graue-Hernández ■ Alejandro Navas ■ Nicolás Kahuam-López

KEY CONCEPTS

- Cataract surgery in the keratoconus patient is challenging. Difficulties in determining accurate measurements for intraocular lens calculations in advanced cases can lead to inaccurate and unpredictable results.

Introduction

Keratoconus (KC) has been classically regarded as a noninflammatory condition characterized by progressive corneal thinning and steepening that results in high irregular astigmatism, myopia, and eventually visual impairment.[1,2] Recent studies have suggested that inflammatory markers are overexpressed in KC patients, even at a subclinical stage.[3-6] The prevalence of KC estimated from population-based studies ranges from 120 to 3300 per 100,000 individuals.[7-14] It may be possible that KC patients are at higher risk of developing cataract sooner when compared with non-KC patients. A plausible explanation, for example might be the frequent use of steroids for allergic conjunctivitis.[15,16] From the standpoint of management of cataract in the KC patient, calculation of the intraocular lens (IOL) power is challenging due to irregular high astigmatism and atypical biometric characteristics (greater axial length, anterior chamber depth, and white-to-white measurements). In this chapter we will review preoperative assessment, IOL power calculation, selection of IOL, considerations during surgery, and special situations encountered in cataract surgery in KC.

Preoperative Assessment

Patients with clinically significant cataract may often complain of glare and loss of contrast. These symptoms are usually present in patients with KC without lens opacification. Therefore, it is crucial to perform a complete and thorough examination to distinguish the precise origin of the visual complaint. The conjunctiva should be carefully examined and both tarsi explored.

Allergic conjunctivitis is commonly present and should be treated and stabilized before surgery is planned. Corneal epithelial irregularities are common in long-standing contact lens users and should be treated with intense lubrication and/or therapeutic contact lens. Corneal subepithelial fibrosis is also common, both as a component of KC and from chronic contact lens touch by apical rigid gas permeable lenses.

Salzmann nodular degeneration may also be present. The decision to treat this condition before surgery is recommended to achieve a proper IOL calculation. Treatment of Salzman´s nodular degeneration before cataract surgery is recommened in order to properly calculate IOL power and alignment. Although outside the scope of this chapter, this can be treated with excimer laser phototherapeutic keratectomy (PTK) ablation, surgical nodulectomy, and anterior lamellar transplantation. The stroma should be examined for anterior scarring or evidence of previous corneal hydrops present as posterior corneal fibrosis. Although KC is largely considered an anterior disease, the endothelium should also be carefully evaluated. Although infrequent, KC may coincide with Fuchs endothelial dystrophy or posterior polymorphous dystrophy. In the first case, slit-lamp examination by specular reflection may show cornea guttata in the central corneal endothelium or edema localized to the posterior stroma. In the latter, biomicroscopy may reveal posterior corneal vesicles and opacities in linear bands and other polymorphous configurations. In patients with abnormal endothelium, specular microscopy should be mandatory.

A complete ophthalmological assessment should be performed with corneal topography/tomography, aberrometry, interferometry, and endothelial cell count. The axial length and the keratometry are the two parameters required by all currently available formulas. The stability, severity, and location of the KC have a great influence on preoperative biometry, resulting in an overestimation of the corneal power and underestimation of the IOL power with consequent postoperative hyperopia.[17]

The irregular corneal shape in eyes with KC makes reliable keratometry difficult to obtain and use because of K values from the apex that differ from the rest of the cornea, displaced visual axis, fixation difficulties during measurements, and variability in K readings between and within devices.[18-21] The Pentacam™ Scheimpflug pachymeter and the Sirius™ system appear to have better repeatability than other devices for K values less than 55 diopter (D).[17,22] Cross-linking or intracorneal ring segments (ICRSs) prior to cataract surgery may improve biometry measurement and final visual outcomes (see Algorithm 35.1, and refer to Combined Procedures section later).

Calculating the corneal power with the standard keratometric index (n = 1.3375) may result in an overestimation of 0.5 to 2.5 D.[23] This index is used to calculate the refractive power of the entire cornea from the anterior corneal curvature, assuming a normal ratio between the anterior and posterior corneal curvature. This assumption is likely disrupted in the corneal ectasias.[24] Camps et al. developed an optimized algorithm that minimizes the error for IOL power calculation in KC.[23]

Intraocular Lens Power Calculation

Formulas for IOL power calculation are the same as those used for patients without KC. The best method for IOL calculation in KC is controversial, Studies have evaluated the predictability of various formulas, including Haigis, Holladay 1, Holladay 2, Hoffer Q, SRK II, SRK/T, Barrett Universal, and Kane formulas, in patients with KC, with variable results.[15,16,25,26] A study by Leccisotti[27] obtained good visual results by calculating IOL power for early-stage KC with the Holladay 2 formula, targeting a residual myopic astigmatism using the steepest meridian over the central 3 mm of the cornea as the K1 and the flattest meridian as the K2. Each meridian power was calculated by averaging the values of its two meridians. Other authors used the Hoffer Q for lower axial lengths and SRK/T for standard axial lengths targeting for emmetropia, resulting in undercorrection of the SRK/T group in contrast with overcorrection of the Hoffer Q.[28] Another study evaluated SRK, SRK II, and SRK/T formulas, and concluded that SRK II was the most accurate formula in mild KC.[16] The predictability of IOL power calculation in eyes with stage 3 and 4 KC is poor. Patients with K values >55 D have more predictable results when using a standard K value (43.25 D) instead of the actual K values.[29,30] Recently, Wang et al. demonstrated Barrett Universal as a predictable formula for different grades of KC.[31] Kane et al. presented good results with the Barrett formula but proposed Kane original and Kane modified (Kane keratoconus) formulas for

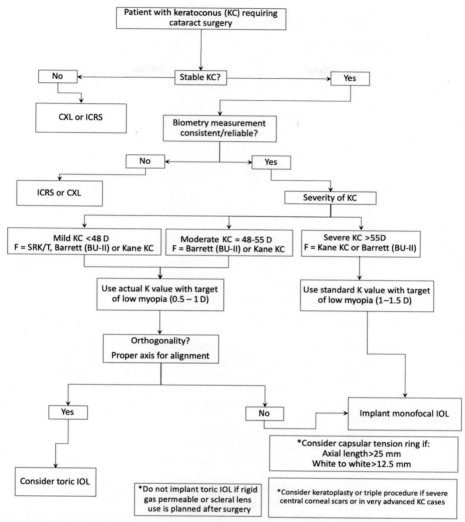

Algorithm 35.1 *BU-II*, Barrett Universal II; *CXL*, corneal collagen cross-linking; *F*, suggested IOL formulas; *ICRS*, intracorneal ring segments; *IOL*, intraocular lens; *K*, keratometries.

all stages of KC,[32] showing less mean absolute prediction error compared with other formulas (Table 35.1).

Some toric calculators use data from predicted lens position and spherical power of the IOL, as well as posterior corneal astigmatism, to derive the suggested lens power.

A review by Gupta and Caty suggested the Barrett calculator, the new Alcon toric calculator (a derivation of the Barrett calculator), and the Holladay toric calculator (integrating the Abulafia-Koch regression formula) as the most accurate methods to calculate toric lens.[33]

Some of the available toric IOLs are Acrysof toric, Rayner toric, Tecnis toric, and Zeiss toric, among others, each with its own online toric IOL calculator (www.acrysoftoriccalculator.com, www.raynertoriccalculator.com, www.tecnisiol.com, www.zcalc.meditec.zeiss.com).

TABLE 35.1 ■ Mean Absolute Prediction Error [a]

Mean Absolute Prediction Error (D)

Formula	Stage 1 $K_m \leq 48$ D	Stage 2 $K_m > 48$ D ≤ 53 D	Stage 3 $K_m > 53$ D
Kane keratoconus	0.49	0.53	1.44
Kane (original)	0.49	1.00	2.64
Barrett	0.54	0.89	2.45
SRK/T	0.56	0.51	2.32
Holladay 1	0.56	1.12	3.07
Hoffer Q	0.57	1.47	3.36
Haigis	0.58	1.34	2.88
Holladay 2 (original)	0.62	1.05	3.01
Holladay 2 (keratoconus adjustment)	0.64	1.41	3.19

[a]Median absolute predicted error of the different formulas divided into keratoconus stage.
Adapted from Kane JX, Connell B, Yip H, et al. Accuracy of intraocular lens power formulas modified for patients with keratoconus. *Ophthalmology*. 2020;127(8):1037–1042.

Intraocular Lens Selection

Deciding between monofocal, spheric, aspheric, toric, multifocal, or trifocal IOLs requires a thorough evaluation. The contour of the KC cornea renders it multifocal, but the visual axis is not at the apex of the cornea, which commonly generates asymmetric astigmatism, a challenge for refractive surgeons. The goal of implanting toric IOLs is to provide less spectacle dependence, better corrected vision, and improved quality of vision. This type of IOL is a suitable option for KC patients with the following characteristics[15,25,28,34–37]:

- Grades 1–2 KC of the Amsler-Krumeich classification.
- Nonprogressive corneal ectasia, at least in the previous 12 months.
- Low possibility of future keratoplasty or postoperative use of rigid gas permeable or scleral lenses.
- Good historical visual acuity (20/40 or better) not dependent on rigid contact lens use.
- Central 4 mm of the cornea without significant irregular astigmatism.
- Orthogonality or a proper axis to align the toric IOL, which is mandatory (Fig. 35.1).

Patients with long axial length (>25 mm) or large white to white (>12.5 mm) have an increased risk of IOL rotation, so these factors should be considered during IOL selection. If a toric IOL is chosen for these patients, a capsular tension ring placement is recommended to avoid IOL rotation (Fig. 35.2).

High astigmatism is a common complication after penetrating keratoplasty (PKP), with amounts greater than 5 D occurring in up to 38% of cases.[38] Despite a clear corneal graft, high astigmatism can lead to poor visual outcomes, and adaptation to contact lens wear may be associated with complications such as epithelial defects or infectious events.[39] A toric IOL can be an effective and safe option for post-PKP stable astigmatism and cataract (Fig. 35.3).[40,41]

Farideh et al. observed good clinical outcomes in five patients with KC grade 1 and 2 (according to the Amsler-Krumeich classification) implanted with trifocal diffractive IOLs.[42] Montano et al. reported successful outcomes in cataract surgery with multifocal toric IOL implantation in forme fruste KC and grade III KC (Fig. 35.4).[43]

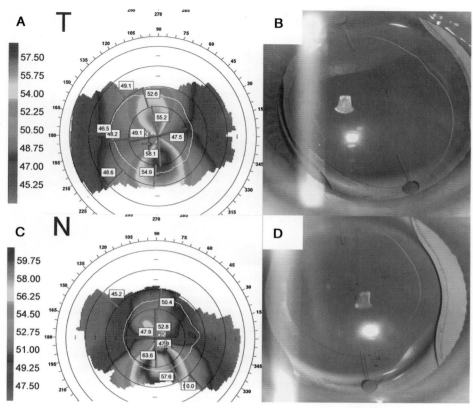

Fig. 35.1 High toric intraocular lens (IOL) implantation in both eyes of a keratoconus patient, despite extreme astigmatism on corneal topography (A, C). There was an identifiable axis to properly align the toric IOLs. Notice the linear IOL marks coinciding with topographic astigmatism (B, D).

The sphericity of the cornea and IOL is another factor to consider during IOL selection. The cornea asphericity can influence the refractive outcomes of patients following IOL implantation. KC eyes have a large negative Q value owing to their steepness and asphericity. Implanting an IOL with a Q value of 0 or with positive Q value may have better refractive and visual outcomes than implanting an IOL with a negative Q value.[44]

The Xtrafocus pinhole intraocular implant (Morcher GmbH) was released in the European market in 2016 as a new treatment option for irregular corneal astigmatism and other aberrations. Trindade et al. evaluated the effect of the pinhole device in a piggyback configuration for patients with KC and observed a marked improvement in visual function.[45] Nevertheless, further studies and longer follow-up are needed to evaluate this device in KC patients.

Surgical Considerations

The irregular astigmatism caused by KC may generate poor visibility for the surgeon during phacoemulsification. Chanbour et al. have proposed the intraoperative use of a rigid gas permeable contact lens to improve visualization during all steps of phacoemulsification in patients with advanced KC.[46]

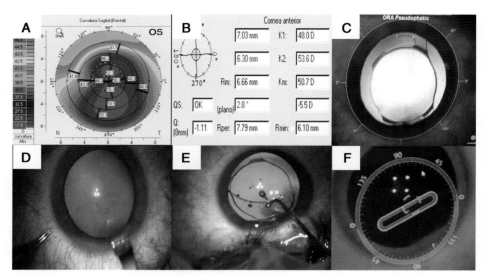

Fig. 35.2 Sagittal curvature topographic map of the left eye of a keratoconus (KC) case (A) and high astigmatism (B). Cataract surgery using intraoperative wavefront aberrometer (C, F), Optiwave Refractive Analysis System (ORA SYSTEM) technology was performed in a patient with stage 4 KC. Intraoperative images showing a single piece −10.00-D lens implanted with a capsular tension ring (D, E) to provide stability due to a 33.52-mm axial length.

Reducing variability in surgically induced astigmatism and keratometry values is strongly recommended to take full advantage of IOL calculation, especially in toric IOLs. Smaller incisions must be constructed in KC patients, because larger incisions can produce a significant amount of surgically induced astigmatism,[47,48] which can result in an unpredictable outcome. Furthermore, patients with KC may have reduced wound healing capacity, which can be managed with sutures in clear corneal incisions.[17]

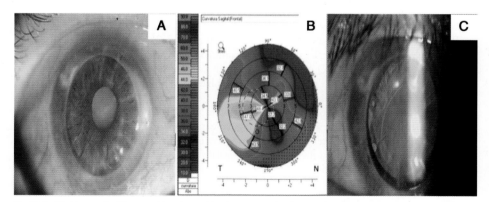

Fig. 35.3 Right eye of a 62-year-old patient with prior penetrating keratoplasty for keratoconus and coexistent mature cataract (A). Scheimpflug axial map of right cornea in the preoperative period showing 14 D of corneal topographical astigmatism (B). Retro-illumination technique shows adequate alignment of toric intraocular lens (according to planned calculation of 23 degrees) into the capsular bag (C).

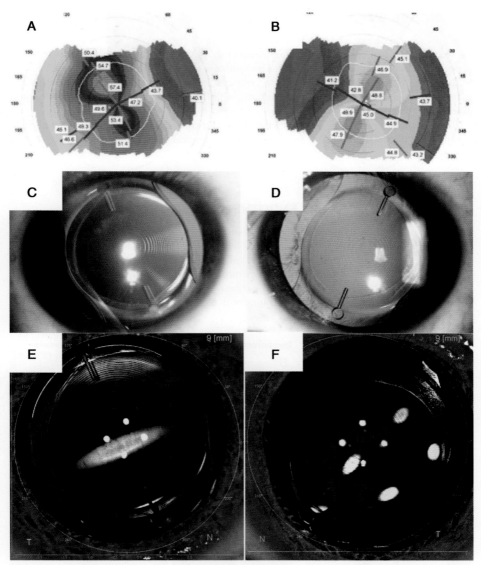

Fig. 35.4 Topographic axial image of forme fruste keratoconus in both eyes and slight enantiomorphism (A, B). Multifocal toric intraocular lens–alignment software calculations with the suggested position according to the astigmatic axis (C, D). No intraocular lens rotation was found during follow-up. Topographic maps overlapped with clinical images, showing proper alignment of the linear marks according to the desired axis (E, F).

Clear corneal incisions should be made as close to the limbus as possible to avoid disruption of the thinner KC cornea, although some surgeons prefer to make modified scleral tunnel incisions with sutures instead of clear corneal incisions.

Combined Procedures

Corneal cross-linking (CXL) or ICRS prior to cataract surgery may improve biometry measurement and final visual outcomes (Fig. 35.5). Sequential CXL with phacoemulsification and IOL placement 6 months later has been studied by Spadea et al. with good outcomes reported.[49]

ICRS to improve corneal shape prior to cataract surgery is a suitable option for clear corneas with high irregular astigmatism and aberrations, with the thinnest point at 6 mm of 400 μm or more.

In contrast, eyes with high irregular astigmatism and corneal scars or with the thinnest point at 6 mm less than 400 μm need to be addressed with a corneal transplant combined with cataract surgery.[50,51]

Special Situations

KC AND FUCHS CORNEAL ENDOTHELIAL DYSTROPHY

Fuchs corneal endothelial dystrophy (FD) is a common corneal dystrophy that is manifest by corneal endothelial dysfunction. FD is dominantly inherited and is characterized by guttate excrescences, representing foci of thickened posterior collagenous layer deposited by dysfunctional corneal endothelial cells between the Descemet membrane and the endothelium.[52] In 1990 Lipman et al. and Orlin et al. were the first to report patients with KC and FD.[53,54] This rare comorbidity was identified in a recent review of the literature with 69 cases of KC with FD[52] treated with PKP,

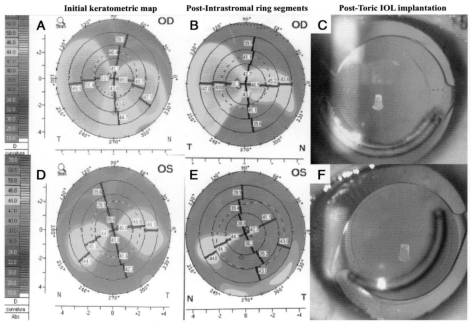

Fig. 35.5 Toric intraocular lenses (*IOLs*) can be considered after intrastromal corneal ring segments. In this image we present a keratoconus case who underwent toric IOL implantation in both eyes after intrastromal ring segments. Initial preoperative keratometric maps of both eyes (A, D). Ideally, waiting at least 6 months after ring segments implantation for stability is advised (B, E). Note the three dots on the toric IOL, aligned with topographic keratometric astigmatism (C, F).

Descemet membrane endothelial keratoplasty, and Descemet stripping automated endothelial keratoplasty. The treatment plan should be individualized considering the aspects previously discussed in this chapter.

Posterior Keratoconus

Posterior KC is a rare corneal disorder characterized by a protrusion (diffuse or localized) of the posterior corneal surface. In most cases, posterior KC has only minimal visual effect and requires no specific treatment, but it may induce a significant error in IOL power calculation and preoperative assessment should be equal to KC.[55]

Patient Expectations

Cataract surgery in an otherwise healthy eye restores visual independence almost immediately with outstanding results. However, as discussed previously in this chapter, cataract surgery in patients with KC may result in an unsatisfied patient if possible outcomes are not thoroughly discussed before surgery. It is important to highlight to the patient that a residual refractive error is more likely the rule than the exception, and if irregular astigmatism is considerable or if the patient was previously a rigid gas permeable contact lens user, a contact lens may still be necessary to fully restore vision after surgery.

Most KC patients are myopic. If the surgeon is faced with the dilemma of choosing IOL power among formulas with very different results, it is wise to err on the myopic side and not overcorrect, as dissatisfaction is likely.

Patient fulfillment depends largely on the truthful information surgeons provide. The adage "underpromise and overdeliver" is particularly true in the context of cataract surgery in KC.

FUTURE DIRECTIONS

Novel IOL designs are developing; intraoperative wavefront aberrometers, supplementary IOLs implanted in the ciliary sulcus, and eye tracking systems are improving. Light adjustable toric, multifocals, or wavefront-customized IOLs could be enhanced in the near future for KC.

Conclusions

Planning, performing, and the postoperative review of cataract surgery in KC patients are challenging. The surgeon must perform an extensive preoperative examination, careful intraoperative planning, and postoperative scrutiny to achieve the best visual outcome for the patients. Residual refractive error or the need to use contact lenses after cataract surgery should be discussed with patients in every case.

Helpful Clinical Tips

- Obtain as much clinical history as possible, including previous refraction, spectacles, and topographies.
- Be familiar with several formulas, calculators, and software, as well as different IOL designs, models, materials. Most of the software is free and confidential.
- Scheimpflug keratometric values are preferred: become familiar with advanced options such as true net power, posterior curvature, and anterior chamber depth that may be helpful in some IOL calculators.
- Use interferometry for axial length, unless not possible because of dense cataract.

- If toric IOL is decided upon, topographies/tomographies or software alignment diagrams should be brought to the operating room.

Potential Pitfalls

- Trypan blue staining is helpful in KC and postkeratoplasty cases. If staining is not used, poor visualization owing to scars, striae, or interfaces could arise in anterior capsule tears.
- Although most cases are older and the possibility of progression is lower, one should try to determine stability in every case, prior to cataract surgery. If stability is not established, progression may require keratoplasty and IOL exchange.
- It is preferable to err toward a myopic residual in IOL power selection. Hyperopic residuals, even mild, will lead to patient dissatisfaction.
- One should discuss the possibility of the need for spectacles or contact lenses after surgery with every KC patient.

References

1. Krachmer JH, Feder RS, Belin MW. Keratoconus and related noninflammatory corneal thinning disorders. *Surv Ophthalmol*. 1984;28(4):293–322.
2. Rabinowitz YS. Keratoconus. *Surv Ophthalmol*. 1998;42(4):297–319.
3. Jun AS, Cope L, Speck C, et al. Subnormal cytokine profile in the tear fluid of keratoconus patients. *PloS One*. 2011;6(1):e16437.
4. Lema I, Sobrino T, Durán JA, Brea D. Díez-Feijoo E. Subclinical keratoconus and inflammatory molecules from tears. *British Journal of Ophthalmology*. 2009;93(6):820.
5. Davidson AE, Hayes S, Hardcastle AJ. Tuft SJ. The pathogenesis of keratoconus. *Eye*. 2013;28(2):189.
6. Behndig A, Karlsson K, Johansson BO, Brännström T, Marklund SL. Superoxide dismutase isoenzymes in the normal and diseased human cornea. *Investigative Ophthalmology & Visual Science*. 2001;42(10):2293.
7. Hashemi H, Beiranvand A, Khabazkhoob M, et al. Prevalence of keratoconus in a population-based study in Shahroud. *Cornea*. 2013;32(11):1441–1445.
8. Hashemi H, Khabazkhoob M, Fotouhi A. Topographic keratoconus is not rare in an Iranian population: the Tehran eye study. *Ophthalmic Epidemiology*. 2013;20(6):385–391.
9. Hashemi H, Khabazkhoob M, Yazdani N, et al. The prevalence of keratoconus in a young population in Mashhad Iran. *Ophthalmic and Physiological Optics*. 2014;34(5):519–527.
10. Hofstetter HW. A keratoscopic survey of 13,395 eyes. *American Journal of Optometry and Archives of American Academy of Optometry*. 1959;36(1):3.
11. Jonas JB, Nangia V, Matin A, Joshi PP, Ughade SN. Prevalence, awareness, control, and associations of arterial hypertension in a rural Central India population: The Central India Eye and Medical Study. *American Journal of Hypertension*. 2010;23(4):347–350.
12. Millodot M, Shneor E, Albou S, Atlani E, Gordon-Shaag A. Prevalence and associated factors of keratoconus in Jerusalem: a cross-sectional study. *Ophthalmic Epidemiology*. 2011;18(2):91–97.
13. Santiago P, Assouline M, Ducoussau F, et al. Epidemiology of keratoconus and corneal topography in normal young male-subjects. *Investigative Ophthalmology & Visual Science*. 1995;36(4):S307.
14. Xu L, Wang YX, Guo Y, You QS, Jonas JB. Prevalence and associations of steep cornea/keratoconus in Greater Beijing. The Beijing Eye Study (prevalence of steep cornea/keratoconus). *PloS One*. 2012;7(7):e39313.
15. Visser N, Gast ST, Bauer NJ, Nuijts RM. Cataract surgery with toric intraocular lens implantation in keratoconus: a case report. *Cornea*. 2011;30(6):720–723.
16. Thebpatiphat MN, Hammersmith JK, Rapuano DC, Ayres JB, Cohen JE. Cataract surgery in keratoconus. *Eye & Contact Lens: Science & Clinical Practice*. 2007;33(5):244–246.
17. Moshirfar DM, Walker CB, Birdsong CO. Cataract surgery in eyes with keratoconus: a review of the current literature. *Current Opinion in Ophthalmology*. 2018;29(1):75–80.
18. McMahon TT, Anderson JR, Joslin EC, Rosas AG. Precision of three topography instruments in keratoconus subjects. *Optometry and Vision Science*. 2001;78(8):599–604.

523

19. Tan B, Baker K, Chen YL, et al. How keratoconus influences optical performance of the eye. *Journal of Vision.* 2008;8(2):1–10.
20. Hashemi H, Yekta A, Khabazkhoob M. Effect of keratoconus grades on repeatability of keratometry readings: comparison of 5 devices. *Journal of Cataract & Refractive Surgery.* 2015;41(5):1065–1072.
21. Yağc ER, Kulak BA, Güler FE, Tenlik FA, Gürağaç FF, Hepşen Fİ. Comparison of anterior segment measurements with a dual Scheimpflug Placido corneal topographer and a new partial coherence interferometer in keratoconic eyes. *Cornea.* 2015;34(9):1012–1018.
22. Lóránt D, Kinga K, Eva J, et al. Evaluation of intereye corneal asymmetry in patients with keratoconus. A Scheimpflug imaging study. *PloS One.* 2014;9(10):e108882.
23. Camps VJ, Piñero DP, Caravaca E, De Fez D. Preliminary validation of an optimized algorithm for intraocular lens power calculation in keratoconus. *Indian Journal of Ophthalmology.* 2017;65(8):690.
24. Aiello F, Nasser QJ, Nucci C, Angunawela RI, Gatzioufas Z, Maurino V. Cataract surgery in patients with keratoconus: pearls and pitfalls. *Open Ophthalmology Journal.* 2017;11(1):194–200.
25. Jaimes M, Xacur-Garcia F, Alvarez-Melloni D, Graue-Hernández EO, Ramirez-Luquín T, Navas A. Refractive lens exchange with toric intraocular lenses in keratoconus. *Journal of Refractive Surgery.* 2011;27(9):658–664.
26. Savini G, Abbate R, Hoffer KJ, et al. Intraocular lens power calculation in eyes with keratoconus. *Journal of Cataract & Refractive Surgery.* 2019;45(5):576–581.
27. Leccisotti A. Refractive lens exchange in keratoconus. *Journal of Cataract and Refractive Surgery.* 2006;32(5):742–746.
28. Alió JL, Peña-García P, Abdulla Guliyeva F, Soria FA, Zein G, Abu-Mustafa SK. MICS with toric intraocular lenses in keratoconus: outcomes and predictability analysis of postoperative refraction. *British Journal of Ophthalmology.* 2014;98(3):365.
29. Bozorg S, Pineda R. Cataract and keratoconus: minimizing complications in intraocular lens calculations. *Seminars in Ophthalmology.* 2014;29(5-6):376–379.
30. Watson MP, Anand S, Bhogal M, et al. Cataract surgery outcome in eyes with keratoconus. *British Journal of Ophthalmology.* 2014;98(3):361.
31. Wang KM, Jun AS, Ladas JG, Siddiqui AA, Woreta F, Srikumaran D. Accuracy of intraocular lens formulas in eyes with keratoconus. *American Journal of Ophthalmology.* 2020;212:26–33.
32. Kane JX, Connell B, Yip H, et al. Accuracy of intraocular lens power formulas modified for patients with keratoconus. *Ophthalmology.* 2020;127(8):1037–1042.
33. Gupta PC, Caty JT. Astigmatism evaluation prior to cataract surgery. *Current Opinion in Ophthalmology.* 2018;29(1):9–13.
34. Nanavaty MA, Lake DB, Daya SM. Outcomes of pseudophakic toric intraocular lens implantation in keratoconic eyes with cataract. *Journal of Refractive Surgery.* 2012;28(12):884.
35. Kwitko S, Marafon SB, Stolz AP. Toric intraocular lens in asymmetric astigmatism. *International Ophthalmology.* 2020;40(5):1291–1298.
36. Allard K, Zetterberg M. Implantation of toric intraocular lenses in patients with cataract and keratoconus: a case series. *International Medical Case Reports Journal.* 2018;11:185.
37. Zvornicanin J, Cabric E, Jusufovic V, Musanovic Z, Zvornicanin E. Use of the toric intraocular lens for keratoconus treatment. *Acta Inform Med.* 2014;22(2):139.
38. Williams KA, Ash JK, Pararajasegaram P, Harris S, Coster DJ. Long-term outcome after corneal transplantation. *Ophthalmology.* 1991;98(5):651–657.
39. Shovlin JP, Argüeso P, Carnt N, et al. 3. Ocular surface health with contact lens wear. *Contact Lens and Anterior Eye.* 2013;36(suppl 1):S14–S21.
40. Allard K, Zetterberg M. Toric IOL implantation in a patient with keratoconus and previous penetrating keratoplasty: a case report and review of literature. *BMC Ophthalmology.* 2018;18(1):215.
41. Lockington D, Wang EF, Patel DV, Moore SP, McGhee CNJ. Effectiveness of cataract phacoemulsification with toric intraocular lenses in addressing astigmatism after keratoplasty. *Journal of Cataract & Refractive Surgery.* 2014;40(12):2044–2049.
42. Farideh D, Azad S, Feizollah N, et al. Clinical outcomes of new toric trifocal diffractive intraocular lens in patients with cataract and stable keratoconus: six months follow-up. *Medicine (Baltimore).* 2017;96(12):e6340.

43. Montano M, López-Dorantes KP, Ramirez-Miranda A, Graue-Hernández EO, Navas A. Multifocal toric intraocular lens implantation for forme fruste and stable keratoconus. *Journal of Refractive Surgery.* 2014;30(4):282–285.
44. Savini G, Hoffer KJ, Barboni P. Influence of corneal asphericity on the refractive outcome of intraocular lens implantation in cataract surgery. *Journal of Cataract & Refractive Surgery.* 2015;41(4):785–789.
45. Trindade CC, Trindade BC, Trindade FC, Werner L, Osher R, Santhiago MR. New pinhole sulcus implant for the correction of irregular corneal astigmatism. *Journal of Cataract & Refractive Surgery.* 2017;43(10):1297–1306.
46. Chanbour W, Harb F, Jarade E. A modified customized rigid gas permeable contact lens to improve visualization during phacoemulsification in ectatic corneas. *Medical Hypothesis, Discovery and Innovation in Ophthalmology.* 2020;9(1):1–6.
47. Oshika T, Nagahara K, Yaguchi S, et al. Three year prospective, randomized evaluation of intraocular lens implantation through 3.2 and 5.5 mm incisions. *Journal of Cataract and Refractive Surgery.* 1998;24(4):509–514.
48. Moon SJ, Lee DJ, Lee KH. Induced astigmatism and high-order aberrations after 1.8-mm, 2.2-mm and 3.0-mm coaxial phacoemulsification incisions. *Journal of the Korean Ophthalmological Society.* 2011;52(4):407.
49. Spadea L, Salvatore S, Verboschi F, Vingolo E. Corneal collagen cross-linking followed by phacoemulsification with IOL implantation for progressive keratoconus associated with high myopia and cataract. *International Ophthalmology.* 2015;35(5):727–731.
50. Wade M, Steinert RF, Garg S, Farid M, Gaster R. Results of toric intraocular lenses for post-penetrating keratoplasty astigmatism. *Ophthalmology.* 2014;121(3):771–777.
51. Lee SJ, Kwon HS, Koh IH. Sequential intrastromal corneal ring implantation and cataract surgery in a severe keratoconus patient with cataract. *Korean Journal of Ophthalmology.* 2012;26(3):226–229.
52. Mylona I, Tsinopoulos I, Ziakas N. Comorbidity of keratoconus and Fuchs' corneal endothelial dystrophy: a review of the literature. *Ophthalmic Research.* 2020;63(4):369–374.
53. Lipman RM, Rubenstein JB, Torczynski E. Keratoconus and Fuchs' corneal endothelial dystrophy in a patient and her family. *Archives of Ophthalmology.* 1990;108(7):993–994.
54. Orlin ES, Raber MI, Eagle CR, Scheie GH. Keratoconus associated with corneal endothelial dystrophy. *Cornea.* 1990;9(4):299–304.
55. Tamaoki A, Kojima T, Hasegawa A, Nakamura H, Tanaka K, Ichikawa K. Intraocular lens power calculation in cases with posterior keratoconus. *Journal of Cataract & Refractive Surgery.* 2015;41(10):2190–2195.

CHAPTER 36

Cellular Therapy of the Corneal Stroma: A New Type of Corneal Surgery for Keratoconus and Corneal Dystrophies—A Translational Research Experience

Jorge L. Alió ■ Mona Zarif ■ Jorge L. Alió del Barrio

KEY CONCEPTS

- Corneal regeneration is a new approach in corneal surgical technique based on advanced therapies using stem cell therapy and bioengineering. In the future, the combination of both will make it possible to renovate the corneal stroma without the need for corneal transplantation.

- Based on experimental animal models and laboratory studies, published work has supported a translational approach to these new therapies.

- Clinical results show that the regeneration of corneal stroma is achievable using stem cells and that the integration of acellular corneal tissue into the human corneal stroma of patients with keratoconus is feasible to improve corneal thickness, biological function, and visual outcomes.

Background: From the Lab to the Patient

The stroma constitutes more than 90% of the corneal thickness. Many features of the cornea, including its strength, morphology, and transparency, are attributable to the anatomy and properties of the corneal stroma.[1] Many diseases such as corneal dystrophies, scars, or ectatic disorders induce a distortion of corneal anatomy or physiology leading to loss of transparency and subsequent loss of vision. In the last decade, enormous efforts have been made to replicate the corneal stroma in the laboratory to find an alternative to classical corneal transplantation. However, this has still not been accomplished because of the extreme difficulty in mimicking the highly complex ultrastructure of the corneal stroma, with substitutes obtained that do not achieve either enough transparency or strength.[2,3]

In the last few years, cell therapy of the corneal stroma using mesenchymal stem cells (MSCs) from either ocular or extraocular sources has gained considerable interest; studies show that MSCs are capable of differentiating into adult keratocytes in vitro and in vivo.[1] Several authors, including from our research group, have demonstrated[4-6] that these stem cells can not only survive and differentiate into adult human keratocytes in xenogeneic scenarios without inducing any inflammatory

TABLE 36.1 ■ Stem Cells Assayed for Corneal Stroma Regeneration: Evidence of Keratocyte or Keratocyte-Like Differentiation and Their Potential Autologous Application

	CSSC	BM-MSC	ADASC	UMSC	ESC	iPSC
Keratocyte differentiation in vitro demonstrated	Yes	Yes	Yes	Yes	Yes	Yes
Keratocyte differentiation in vivo demonstrated	Yes	Yes	Yes	Yes	No	No
Possible autologous use	Yes/No	Yes	Yes	Yes/No	No	Yes

ADASCs, Adipose-derived adult stem cell; BM, bone marrow; CSSCs, corneal stroma stem cells; ESC, embryonic stem cell; iPSC, induced pluripotent stem cell; MSC, mesenchymal stem cell; UMSC, umbilical MSC.

reaction, but also (1) produce new collagen within the host stroma,[4,7] (2) modulate preexisting scars by corneal stroma remodeling,[8,9] and (3) improve corneal transparency in animal models for corneal dystrophies by collagen reorganization, as well as in animal models of metabolopathies by the catabolism of accumulated proteins.[10–13] MSCs have also shown immunomodulatory properties in syngeneic, allogeneic, and even xenogeneic scenarios.[13,14] The first clinical data on the safety and preliminary efficacy of cellular therapy of the corneal stroma from phase 1 human clinical trials are now available,[15,16] and cellular therapy may end up providing a real alternative treatment option for corneal diseases in the near future.

When considering existing scientific evidence, it appears that all types of MSCs behave similarly in vivo (Table 36.1) and are thus able to achieve keratocyte differentiation and modulate the corneal stroma.[17] It has also been recently reported that MSCs secrete paracrine factors such as vascular endothelial growth factor (VEGF), platelet-derived growth factor (PDGF), hepatocyte growth factor (HGF), and transforming growth factor beta 1 (TGFβ1). Although the precise actions of the different growth factors for cornea wound healing are not fully understood, overall they appear to promote cell migration, keratocyte survival by apoptosis inhibition, and upregulation of the expression of extracellular matrix (ECM) component genes in keratocytes, subsequently enhancing corneal reepithelialization and stromal wound healing.[18] MSCs can be obtained from many human tissues, including adipose tissue, bone marrow, umbilical cord, dental pulp, gingiva, hair follicle, cornea, and placenta.[19,20]

Corneal stromal stem cells (CSSCs) are a promising source for cellular therapy as the isolation technique and culture methods have been optimized and refined.[21] Presumably, they should be efficient in differentiating into keratocytes, as they are already committed to the corneal lineage. However, isolating autologous CSSCs is more technically demanding, considering the small amount of tissue from which they are obtained. Furthermore, this technique still requires a contralateral healthy eye, which is not always available (such as in bilateral disease). Therefore these drawbacks may limit its use in clinical practice. Allogeneic CSSC use requires living or cadaveric donor corneal tissue.

Human adult adipose tissue is a good source of autologous extraocular stem cells and fulfils many requirements: easy accessibility to the tissue, high cell retrieval efficiency, and the ability of its adipose-derived adult mesenchymal stem cells (h-ADASCs) to differentiate into multiple cell types (keratocytes, osteoblasts, chondroblasts, myoblasts, hepatocytes, neurons, etc.).[4] This cellular differentiation occurs because of the effect of very specific stimulating factors or environments for each cell type, avoiding the mixure of multiple cell lines within the same niche.

Bone marrow MSCs (BM-MSCs) are the most widely studied MSCs, presenting a similar profile to ADASCs, but their extraction requires a bone marrow puncture, which is a complicated and painful procedure sometimes requiring general anesthesia.

Umbilical MSCs (UMSCs) present an attractive alternative, but their autologous use is currently limited as the umbilical cord is not generally stored after birth.

Embryonic stem cells (ESCs) have great potential, but also present significant ethical issues. However, the use of induced pluripotent stem cell (iPSC) technology[22] could solve such problems, and their capability for generating adult keratocytes has already been proven in vitro.[23]

Finally, it is important to note that the therapeutic effect of MSCs in damaged tissue is not always related to the potential differentiation of the MSCs in the host tissue. Multiple mechanisms might contribute simultaneously to this therapeutic effect: secretion of paracrine trophic and growth factors capable of stimulating resident stem cells, reduction of tissue injury, and activation of immunomodulatory effects. As such, the direct cellular differentiation of the MSCs might not be relevant and could even be nonexistent.[17,24,25]

We will review the different types of stem cells (mesenchymal and others) that have been proposed for the regeneration of the corneal stroma, as well as the current in vitro or in vivo evidence. Finally, we will review the different surgical approaches that have been suggested (in vivo) for the application of stem cell therapy to regenerate the corneal stroma.

Translation to a New Type of Advanced Corneal Therapy

STEM CELL SOURCES USED FOR CORNEAL STROMA REGENERATION

Bone Marrow Mesenchymal Stem Cells

Park et al. reported that human BM-MSCs differentiate in vitro into keratocyte-like cells when they are grown in specific keratocyte differentiation conditions.[26] They demonstrated the strong expression of keratocyte markers such as lumican and aldehyde dehydrogenase (ALDH) along with the loss of expression of MSC markers such as α-smooth muscle actin. However, they could not demonstrate an evident expression of keratocan in these differentiated cells.[26] Trosan et al. showed that mice BM-MSCs cultured in corneal extracts and insulin-like growth factor-I (IGF-I) efficiently differentiate into corneal-like cells with expression of corneal-specific markers such as cytokeratin 12, keratocan, and lumican.[27] The survival and differentiation of human BM-MSCs into keratocytes has also been demonstrated in vivo when these cells are transplanted within the corneal stroma. Keratocan expression was observed without any sign of immune or inflammatory response.[28]

Adipose-Derived Adult Mesenchymal Stem Cells

Human ADASCs (h-ADASCs) cultured in vitro (Fig. 36.1A,B) under keratocyte differentiation conditions express collagens and other corneal-specific matrix components. This expression is quantitatively similar to that achieved by differentiated human CSSCs (h-CSSCs).[29]

The differentiation of h-ADASCs into functional human keratocytes has also been demonstrated in vivo for the first time, in a previous study by our group using the rabbit as a model.[4] These cells, once implanted intrastromally, express not only collagens type I and VI (the main components of corneal ECM), but also keratocyte-specific markers such as keratocan or ALDH, without inducing an immune or inflammatory response. These findings were later reproduced and confirmed by other authors in several research papers.[17]

Umbilical Cord Mesenchymal Stem Cells

Human MSCs isolated from neonatal umbilical cords have exhibited similar differentiation behavior to other types of MSCs when transplanted inside the corneal stroma in vivo, expressing keratocyte-specific markers such as keratocan without inducing immune or rejection responses.[30] Liu et al. reported that the injection of these cells within the corneal stroma of lumican null

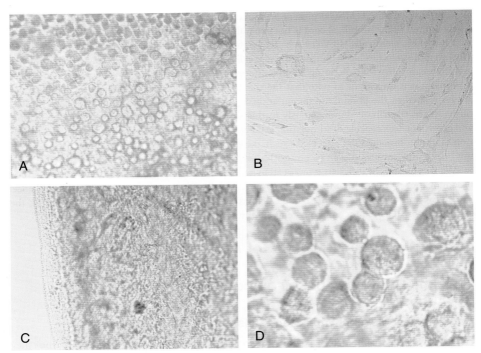

Fig. 36.1 (A) Microscopic appearance (phase-contrast photograph) of human adipose-derived adult mesenchymal stem cells (ADASCs; 10× magnification). (B) Human ADASC in culture. (C) Decellularized human corneal lamina (10× magnification). (D) Recellularized human corneal lamina with ADASCs (0.5 × 10⁶ cells were cultured on each side of the laminas; 10× magnification).

mice improved corneal transparency and increased stromal thickness with reorganized collagen lamellae and also improved host keratocyte function through enhanced expression of keratocan and ALDH in these mice.[11] These data are encouraging, although to date, the autologous use of umbilical cord mesenchymal stem cells (UCMSCs) is not possible as the umbilical cord from new births is not generally stored.

Embryonic Stem Cells

Current experience with these human pluripotent stem cells for corneal stromal regeneration is much more limited. Chan et al. reported that differentiation of these cells into a keratocyte lineage can be induced in vitro, demonstrating upregulation of keratocyte markers including keratocan.[31]

To the best of our knowledge, no in vivo studies with these cells have been performed in the field of regenerative medicine for the corneal stroma. The use of these cells also raises many ethical issues, and together with the lack of in vivo data, discourages their current use in a clinical setting.

Induced Pluripotent Stem Cells

As already discussed, the use of ESCs has been partially abandoned because of ethical concerns, especially since the discovery of iPSCs,[22] which are derived from adult cells. In 2012 Shinya Yamanaka from Japan and John B. Gurdon from the UK received the Nobel Prize in Physiology or Medicine for discovering that mature, specialized cells can be reprogrammed to an immature or stem cell state and then redirected to the required cell lineage using specific factors and environmental stimuli. iPSCs promise to be the future of tissue and cellular engineering.

Regarding their application in the regeneration of the corneal stroma, human iPSCs have demonstrated the capability for differentiating into neural crest cells (the embryonic precursor to keratocytes). By culturing them on cadaveric corneal tissue, their keratocyte differentiation is promoted by the acquisition of a keratocyte-like morphology to express markers similar to corneal keratocytes.[23] iPSC-derived MSCs have also been shown to exert immunomodulatory properties in the cornea similar to those observed with BM-MSCs.[32] To the best of our knowledge, no studies have been published reporting the capability of iPSCs for differentiating into adult keratocytes in vivo in the animal model.

Corneal Stromal Stem Cells

The limbal palisades of Vogt form a niche that contains both limbal epithelial stem cells (LESCs) and CSSCs.[33] CSSCs express genes typical of descendants of the neural ectoderm such as PAX6, adult stem cell markers such as ABCG2, and MSC markers such as CD73 and CD90.[33,34] They exhibit clonal growth, self-renewal properties, and a potential for differentiation into multiple distinct cell types. Unlike keratocytes, h-CSSCs undergo extensive expansion in vitro without losing their ability to adopt a keratocyte phenotype.[33,34] These corneal MSCs have a demonstrated potential for differentiation into corneal epithelium and adult keratocytes in vitro.[33,35] When cultured on a substratum of parallel aligned polymeric nanofibers, h-CSSCs produce layers of highly parallel collagen fibers with packing and fibril diameter indistinguishable from that of the human stromal lamellae.[36] The ability of h-CSSCs to adopt a keratocyte function has been even more striking in vivo. When injected into the mouse corneal stroma, h-CSSCs express keratocyte mRNA and protein, replacing the mouse ECM with human matrix components. These injected cells remain viable for many months, apparently becoming quiescent keratocytes.[10]

These experimental data have raised interest in this novel cell-based therapy for corneal stromal diseases; however, before its application in clinical practice, its efficacy and safety need to be well proven in human clinical trials, and other limitations such as the high laboratory costs and potential therapeutic efficacy differences among different donors have to be given serious consideration.

CORNEAL STROMA REGENERATION TECHNIQUES: EARLY APPLICATION IN CLINICAL PRACTICE

All these types of stem cells have been used in various ways in a variety of research projects to find the optimal procedure for regenerating the human corneal stroma. Corneal MSC implantation has been assayed and studied by direct intrastromal transplantation or after implantation on the ocular surface, intravenously, and into the anterior chamber where cellular migration within the stroma is to be expected. Different cellular carriers have been analyzed to enhance the potential benefits of this therapy.

Ocular Surface Implantation of Stem Cells

Surface implantation of MSCs would be the optimal approach for ocular surface reconstruction and corneal epithelium/limbal stem cell niche regeneration. However, surface implantation of MSCs would play a role in the prevention or modulation of anterior stromal scars after an ocular surface injury (such as a chemical burn). As discussed previously, MSCs secrete paracrine factors that enhance corneal reepithelialization and stromal wound healing.[18] Thus the benefit of MSCs on the ocular surface may be more justified by these paracrine effects rather than by direct differentiation of the MSCs into epithelial cells. In this respect, Di et al. assayed *subconjunctival injections* of BM-MSCs in diabetic mice and reported an increased corneal epithelial cell proliferation as well as an attenuated inflammatory response mediated by tumor necrosis factor-α–stimulated gene 6 (TSG6).[37]

Holan et al. suggested MSC application to the ocular surface using *nanofiber scaffolds*. They reported that BM-MSCs grown on these scaffolds can enhance reepithelialization and suppress neovascularization and local inflammatory reaction when applied to an alkali-injured eye in a rabbit model, and these results were comparable to those obtained with LESCs; both were better than the results obtained with ADASCs.[38] The same group suggested that these results might be improved when these nanofiber scaffolds seeded with rabbit BM-MSCs are covered with cyclosporine-A (CSA)–loaded nanofiber scaffolds, observing an even greater scar suppression and healing results with the combination of both nanofibers (MSC and CSA).[39]

Topical application of a suspension of autologous ADASCs has been reported in an isolated clinical case report in which authors describe the healing of a neurotrophic ulcer unresponsive to conventional treatment.[40] The lack of further scientific evidence for this delivery method since 2012 raises questions about its real efficacy.

Finally, Basu et al. suggested the delivery of MSCs using *fibrin glue*.[21] They resuspended CSSCs in a solution of human fibrinogen, and this was added onto a wounded ocular surface with thrombin on the wound bed. Using this method, they demonstrated the prevention of corneal scarring in the mouse model together with the generation of new collagen organization indistinguishable from that of native tissue. This group is enrolled in a clinical trial to validate these findings, using autologous and heterologous CSSCs from limbal biopsies for cases of chemical burns, neurotrophic ulcers, and established scars. Preliminary reports showed an improvement in visual parameters, corneal epithelialization, corneal neovascularization, and corneal clarity.[41]

Intrastromal Implantation of Stem Cells Alone

Direct in vivo injection of stem cells into the corneal stroma has been assayed in several studies, demonstrating the differentiation of stem cells into adult keratocytes without signs of immune rejection. In our study, we also demonstrated the production of human ECM by immunohistochemistry when h-ADASCs were transplanted inside the rabbit cornea (Figs. 36.1A,B and 36.2A,B).[4] As expected, collagen types I and VI were found expressed in the rabbit corneal stroma, as well as in the transplanted h-ADASCs. Collagen types III and IV, not normally expressed in the corneal stroma, were not detected either in the host corneal stroma or in the transplanted h-ADASCs (see Fig. 36.2C). Du et al.[10] reported restoration of corneal transparency and thickness in lumican null mice (thin corneas, haze, and disruption of normal stromal organization) 3 months after intrastromal transplant of h-CSSCs. They also confirmed that human keratan sulfate was deposited in the mouse stroma, and the host collagen lamellae were reorganized, concluding that delivery of h-CSSCs to the scarred human stroma may alleviate corneal scars without requiring surgery.[10] Very similar findings were reported by Liu et al. who utilized h-UMSCs using the same animal model.[11] Coulson-Thomas et al. found that, in a mouse model for mucopolysaccharidosis, transplanted h-UMSCs participate in extracellular glycosaminoglycans (GAG) turnover and enable host keratocytes to catabolize accumulated GAG products.[12]

Recently, our group has published the first clinical trial in which the preliminary safety and efficacy of the cellular therapy of the human corneal stroma is reported.[15,42] In this pilot clinical trial, we implanted autologous ADASCs (obtained by elective liposuction) in a midstromal femtosecond laser-assisted lamellar pocket in patients with advanced keratoconus (see Fig. 36.1A,B). No signs of inflammation or rejection were observed, confirming all previous evidence reported in the animal model.[15,42]

Intrastromal Implantation of Stem Cells Together With a Biodegradable Scaffold

To enhance the growth and development of the stem cells injected into the corneal stroma, transplantation together with biodegradable synthetic ECM has been performed. Espandar et al. injected h-ADASCs with a semisolid hyaluronic acid hydrogel into the rabbit corneal stroma and

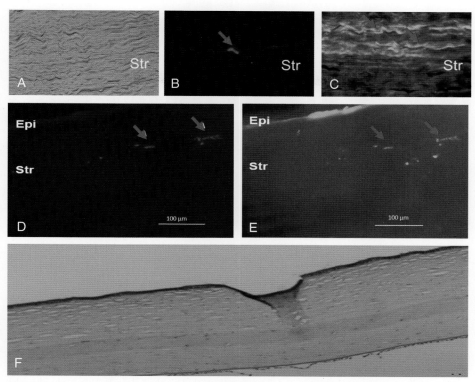

Fig. 36.2 (A–C) Transplantation of human adipose-derived adult mesenchymal stem cells (ADASCs) into the thickness of the rabbit stroma in vivo. (A) Phase-contrast photograph showing a morphologically intact stroma 3 months after transplantation. (B) Same section showing the survival of the implanted cells by detecting the Vybrant CM-Dil dye *(red arrow)*. (C) Same section showing the expression of new human type I collagen inside the rabbit stroma (magnification 400×) *(red arrows)*. (D–F) Corneal stroma enhancement with decellularized human corneal stroma with h-ADASC recellularization in the rabbit animal model. (D) Human cells *(red arrows)*, labeled with CM-Dil, around and inside the implant confirming the presence of living human cells inside the rabbit corneal stroma. (E) Same section showing human keratocan and their eventual differentiation into human keratocytes *(red arrows)* (magnification 400×); (F) Hematoxylin-eosin staining of a rabbit cornea with an implanted graft of decellularized human corneal stroma with h-ADASC colonization; (magnification 200×). *Epi,* Epithelium; *str,* stroma.

reported better survival and keratocyte differentiation of the h-ADASCs when compared with their injection alone (Fig. 36.3A,B).[7] Ma et al. used rabbit ADSCs with a polylactic-co-glycolic (PLGA) biodegradable scaffold in a rabbit model of stromal injury in which they observed newly formed tissue with successful collagen remodeling and less stromal scarring (see Fig. 36.3A–C).[43] At 3 months post implantation, a high extrusion rate of the implant was observed (see Fig. 36.3D,E). Initial data show that these scaffolds may enhance stem cell effects on corneal stroma, although further research is required and warranted.

Intrastromal Implantation of Stem Cells With a Decellularized Corneal Stroma Scaffold

The complex structure of the corneal stroma has still not been replicated and there are well-known drawbacks to the use of synthetic scaffold-based designs: (1) strong inflammatory responses induced with biodegradation and (2) nonspecific inflammatory response induced by all polymer materials.[44]

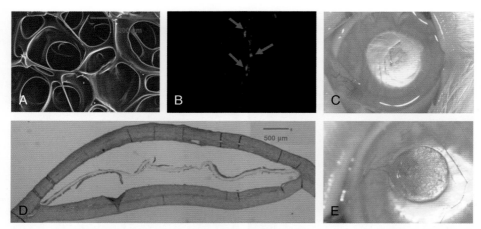

Fig. 36.3 Transplantation of macroporous polyethylacrylate (PEA) membranes together with human adipose-derived adult mesenchymal stem cell (ADASC) into the rabbit stroma in vivo. (A) Electron microscopy image of the PEA. (B) ADASC survivors after 3 months *(red arrows)*. (C) Intrastromal implant in vivo; note its transparency. (D) The absence of a real biointegration leads to the detachment of the sheet of PEA from the surrounding stroma in the histological sections. (E) A high extrusion rate of the implant was observed.

Recently, several corneal decellularization techniques have been described, which provide an acellular corneal ECM (see Fig. 36.1C).[45] These scaffolds have gained attention in the last few years, as they provide a more natural environment for the growth and differentiation of cells when compared with synthetic scaffolds. In addition, components of the ECM are generally conserved among species and are well tolerated by xenogeneic recipients. Moreover, keratocytes are essential for remodeling the corneal stroma and for normal epithelial physiology.[46] This highlights the importance of transplanting a cellular substitute together with the structural support (acellular ECM) to undertake these critical functions in corneal homeostasis. To the best of our knowledge, all attempts to repopulate decellularized corneal scaffolds have used corneal cells.[47–49] However, as already discussed, these cells have significant drawbacks that limit their autologous use in clinical practice (damage to the donor tissue, lack of cells, and more difficulty generating cell subcultures), thus redirecting efforts to find an extraocular source of autologous cells. In a previous study by our group, we showed the perfect biointegration of human decellularized corneal stromal sheets (100-μm thickness) with and without h-ADASC colonization inside the rabbit cornea (see Fig. 36.2D–F) and observed no rejection response despite the graft being xenogeneic.[6] We also demonstrated the differentiation of h-ADASCs into functional keratocytes inside these implants in vivo, which then achieved their proper biofunctionalization (see Fig. 36.2D,E). In our experience, decellularization of the whole (~500 μm) corneal stroma (using sodium dodecyl sulfate anionic detergent) lacks efficacy, as it not possible to completely remove the whole cellular component. However, we demonstrated that this method completely removes the cellular component and preserves the tissue integrity of the corneal stroma when thinner lenticules are treated—a method that has been later confirmed by other authors with the use of electron microscopy.[6,50,51] Others have also assayed the integration of decellularized pig articular cartilage ECM colonized with mice BM-MSCs in the rabbit corneal stroma and reported similar findings, although the transparency of these decellularized scaffolds was not clearly reported.[52]

In our opinion, the implantation of MSCs together with decellularized corneal ECM would be the best technique to restore effectively the thickness of a diseased and severely weakened human cornea, because the implantation of MSCs alone only achieves limited new ECM formation and thickness restoration.[4,15] Moreover, with this technique, and by using autologous MSCs from a given patient, it is theoretically possible to transform allogenic grafts into functional autologous grafts, thus avoiding any risk of rejection. Following this research line, we have recently published the first clinical trial using these decellularized human corneal stroma scaffolds (120-μm thickness and 9.0-mm diameter laminas), with or without autologous ADASC recellularization, in patients with advanced keratoconus (see Fig. 36.1C,D).[16,42]

Decellularized tissues have the drawback of requiring specific laboratory equipment, although eye banks could potentially do this and deliver such grafts to different clinical centers. Keratophakia (intrastromal insertion of an allogeneic lenticule) was originally described by Barraquer in 1964 but was abandoned because of the unpredictability of the refractive outcome and the relatively high frequency of interface haze development.[53] The lack of haze observed in our pilot clinical trial could be due to the absence of donor keratocytes that could potentially activate postoperatively and generate scar tissue. Moreover, rejection episodes have already been described after the implantation of allogeneic lenticules, a risk that is theoretically avoided by the use of decellularized grafts.[51] It is reasonable to consider that as long as human decellularized tissue is used, there will be no risk for zoonotic diseases.

Anterior Chamber Injection of Stem Cells

Demirayak et al. reported that BM-MSCs and ADASCs, suspended in phosphate-buffered solution (PBS) and injected into the anterior chamber after a penetrating corneal injury in a mouse model, are able to colonize the corneal stroma and increase the expression of keratocyte-specific markers such as keratocan, with a demonstrated increase in keratocyte density by confocal microscopy.[9] Conversely, the possible side effects of this MSC injection into the anterior chamber for the lens epithelium and trabecular meshwork are highly questionable, as it may induce scarring and a subsequent glaucoma. Considering this, the potential clinical use of this approach, in our opinion, is limited.

Intravenous Injection of Stem Cells

Systemic use of MSCs by intravenous injection has also been tested. Intravenous injection of BM-MSCs in mice after an allograft corneal transplant led to colonization of the transplanted cornea and conjunctiva but not the contralateral ungrafted cornea, simultaneously decreasing immunity and significantly improving allograft survival rate.[54] Yun et al. recently reported similar findings with the intravenous injection of iPSC-derived MSCs and BM-MSCs after a surface chemical injury, where they observed that the corneal opacity, inflammatory infiltration, and inflammatory markers in the cornea were markedly decreased in the treated mice, without significant differences between both MSC types.[32] In contrast, our group did not observe any benefit in corneal allograft survival and rejection rates after systemic injection of rabbit ADASCs prior to surgery, during surgery, and at various times after surgery in rabbits with vascularized corneas (model more similar to human corneal transplants than those reported in mice). A shorter graft survival compared with the nontreated corneal grafts was noted.[55]

AUTOLOGOUS VERSUS ALLOGENIC MSC

A critical question for future clinical trials to further assess the feasibility of cellular therapy of the corneal stroma is whether the use of autologous MSCs is necessary and whether allogenic MSCs could achieve the same benefit without any risk of inflammation or rejection. If we consider all published evidence in the animal model in which human MSCs were implanted in the corneal stroma, despite being a xenogeneic transplant, no signs of rejection or inflammation have been reported.[4-13] This coincides with the strong evidence on the immunomodulatory and immunosuppressive properties of MSCs, which help them to evade host immune rejection and to survive by inhibiting adhesion and invasion, and which induce cell death of inflammatory cells, partially because of a rich extracellular glycocalyx that contains TSG6.[14,56] TSG6 plays a critical role in the immunosuppressive properties exhibited by MSCs.[13,32,37] Taken together, the use of allogenic MSCs would greatly simplify the clinical application of MSCs, as clinical application centers would not need any specific equipment and potential MSC banks could store and supply stem cells for use in patients. Low-cost systems are already available that are capable of enhancing the preservation of MSCs at hypothermic temperatures while maintaining their normal function, thereby widening the timeframe for distribution between the manufacturing site and the clinic and reducing the waste associated with the limited shelf life of cells stored in their liquid state.[57] Funderburgh et al. recently reported that MSCs from different donors may have different immunosuppressive properties and, consequently, different abilities to regenerate and relieve stromal scars.[58] Considering this important finding, the best donors could be selected by MSC banks to expand and supply only those MSCs with the highest immunosuppressive and regenerative capacity; if so, autologous cells would not be necessary. We should also consider that adult keratocytes obtained from autologous MSCs may carry the same genetic defect that led to the corneal disease, such as in the case of corneal dystrophy. In this scenario, the use of allogenic instead of autologous MSCs would be interesting. A recent study observed gene expression differences between the iPSC-derived keratocytes generated from fibroblasts of both keratoconic and normal human corneal stroma, influencing cellular growth and proliferation, confirming that, at least in keratoconus cases, adult cells obtained from MSCs may still not be functionally normal.[59]

MESENCHYMAL STEM CELL EXOSOMES

Exosomes are nanosized extracellular vesicles that originate from the fusion of intracellular multivesicular bodies with cell membranes and are released into extracellular spaces.[56] They have been implicated in the ability of MSCs to repair damaged tissue. Shojaati et al. recently showed that exosomes isolated from the culture media of h-CSSCs had similar immunosuppressive properties and also significantly reduced stromal scarring in wounded corneas in vivo.[60] This finding suggests that for some diseases, such as prevention or reduction of corneal scars, MSC exosomes may provide a non–cell-based therapy.[58] Zhang et al. suggested that exosomes released by transplanted UCMSCs within the diseased cornea are able to enter into the diseased host corneal keratocytes and enhance their biological functions..[56] The authors experimented in vitro using mucopolysaccharidosis VII mice and discovered that UCMSC-secreted exosomes assisted in the recycling process of accumulated GAGs in the lysosomes of diseased cells.[12] These findings open an exciting new field for research as the use of exosomes may overcome some of the limitations and risks associated with intrastromal cellular injection, given that exosomes can potentially be applied topically.[30]

First Clinical Human Experience in Advanced Keratoconus Cases

Recently, our group performed the implantation of ADASCs and decellularized/recellularized laminas in 14 patients with advanced keratoconus. This clinical experience opened a new and exciting line of therapy for research. As mentioned, the production of new ECM by the implanted MSCs occurs but is not quantitatively enough to be able to restore the thickness of a severely diseased human cornea (as in extreme keratoconic corneas). Meanwhile the implantation of decellularized/recellularized laminae could restore the corneal thickness and the keratometric parameters. However, the direct injection of stem cells may provide a promising treatment modality for corneal dystrophies and corneal stroma progressive opacification in the context of systemic metabolic disorders, and for the modulation of corneal scarring.

STUDY APPROVAL, DESIGN, AND SUBJECTS

This investigation was a prospective series of consecutive cases. The study was conducted in strict adherence to the tenets of the Declaration of Helsinki and was registered in ClinicalTrials.gov (Code: NCT02932852).

Fourteen patients were enrolled in the study, were operated within an interval of 3 months, and were randomly distributed into three study groups: group 1 (G-1) patients were treated with autologous ADASC implantation (n = 5); group 2 (G-2) received decellularized human corneal stroma transplantation (n = 5), and group 3 (G-3) received autologous ADASC recellularized human corneal stroma transplantation (n = 4).

Thirteen patients were included in the clinical follow-up. One patient from G-1 was lost after the first postoperative month because of inability to attend further follow-up for reasons unrelated to the study.

Inclusion and exclusion criteria were defined in previous articles.[15,16,42,61,62] Clinical monitoring of the study of the patients was established for safety purposes at 1 week, and 1, 3, 6, 12, and 36 months for the purpose of the clinical outcomes of the investigation and to observe implant safety for a long time.

METHODOLOGY

Autologous ADASC Isolation, Characterization, and Culture

Patients underwent standard liposuction. Approximately 250 mL of mixed fat was obtained from each patient using local anesthesia. The adipose tissue was processed according to the methods described in the previous articles (see Fig. 36.1A,B).[4,63–65]

Laminas

Human corneal stroma of donor corneas with nonviable endothelium but with negative viral serology was used. The corneas were provided by the eye bank. The quality and safety standards for donation, procurement, testing, processing, conservation, storage, and testing of human cells and tissues were followed. Donor corneas were dissected with IntraLase iFS femtosecond laser (AMO, Santa Ana, CA), two to three consecutive laminas 120-μm thick and 9.0 mm in diameter were obtained. The decellularization protocol was based on previous publications (see Fig. 36.1C).[6,45,66] Twenty-four hours before implantation, the laminas for patients who received recellularized tissue were placed in tissue culture wells for recellularization with autologous ADASC (0.5 × 10^6 cells per 1 mL of PBS were cultured on each side of the laminas). Then the laminas were submerged in PBS at room temperature and transferred to implantation (see Fig. 36.1D).[16,42,62]

Surgical Procedure: Autologous ADASC Implantation

The method for the implantation of the MSCs has been described previously.[15] Topical anesthesia was used. A 60-kHz IntraLase iFS femtosecond laser (AMO Inc, Irvine, CA) was used in single-pass mode for the recipient corneal lamellar dissection. An intrastromal laminar cut of 9.5-mm diameter was created at medium depth of the thinnest preoperative pachymetry point measured by the Visante OCT (Carl Zeiss, Jena, Germany). Three million autologous ADASCs contained in 1 mL PBS were injected into the pocket (Fig. 36.4A,B).

Lenticule Implantation

Topical anesthesia was applied with oral sedation for all surgeries; the 60-kHz IntraLase iFS femtosecond laser was used in single-pass mode. Assisted corneal dissection was done with a 50-degree anterior cut. After opening the corneal intrastromal pocket, the lamina was inserted, centered, and unfolded through gentle tapping and massaging from the epithelial surface of the host. Prior to implantation, a temporary limbal paracentesis was performed to reduce intraocular pressure (see Fig. 36.4C,D). In

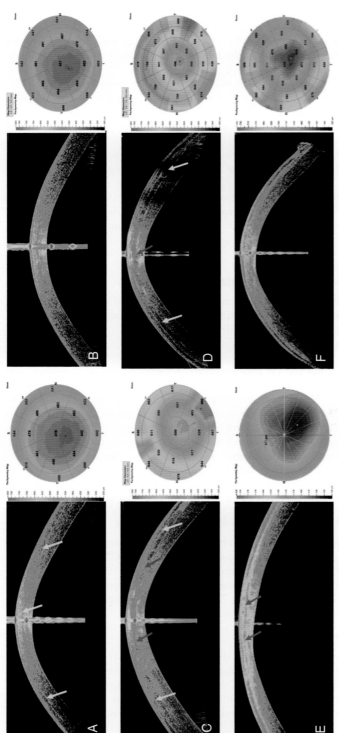

Fig. 36.4 Anterior segment optical coherence tomography (OCT) (Visante OCT). (A) Group 1, case 1 at 1 month postoperative; a formation of some neocollagen in the dissected pocket (*yellow arrows*) can be seen. (B) OCT of group 1, case 1 at 12 months postoperative; note the transparency of the cornea. Note the stability of the pachymetric parameters in group 2, case 7, with modest improvement (C) at 12 months postoperative and (D) at 36 months postoperative. The improvement of the reflective band of neocollagen in the periphery of the implanted lamina (*yellow arrows*) can be seen. *Red arrows* represent the reflectance of the neocollagen band. Note the improvement of the reflectance of this band from 12 months until 3 years postoperative. Group 3, case 11, (E) at 1 month postoperative. The high reflectance of the neocollagen band can be seen (*red arrow*). Capture of the pachymetric map was not possible. (F) Group 3, case 11 at almost 3 years postoperative. The enhancement of the integration of the lamina in the host corneal stroma can be seen. The high reflectance of the band of neocollagen disappeared; an enhancement of the pachymetric map can be seen.

those cases that received a recellularized lamina (G-3) (see Fig. 36.4E,F), to compensate for the cellular damage expected by the implantation process, the pocket was irrigated immediately before and after insertion with a solution containing an additional 1 million autologous ADASCs in 1 mL of PBS, with a 25-G cannula. The incision was then closed with an interrupted 10-0 nylon suture.[16,45]

Postoperative Care and Follow-Up Schedule

Postoperatively, the patients were evaluated monthly to record any evidence of subjective discomfort, ocular inflammation, or sudden unexpected visual loss. For the evaluation of the other clinical parameters, the patients were followed at 1 day, 1 week, and at 1, 3, 6, 12, and 36 months for the following: postoperative unaided distance visual acuity (UDVA), corrected distance visual acuity (CDVA), and rigid contact lens visual acuity (CLVA) (decimal equivalent to the logMAR scale); refractive sphere (Rx Sphr) (D) and refractive cylinder (Rx Cyl) (D); anterior segment OCT-Visante: central corneal thickness (Visante CCT) (µm; Carl Zeiss); Pentacam thinnest point (thinnest point) (µm), cornea volume (CV) (mm^3), and corneal aberrometry with maximum diameter of 6-mm pupils (Pentacam; OCULUS Inc., Wetzlar, Germany): anterior mean keratometry (anterior K_m) (D) and maximum keratometry (K_{max}) (D).

Confocal microscopy was performed up to 12 months postoperatively using HRT3 RCM (Heidelberg) with Rostock Cornea Module and slit-lamp **biomicroscopy**.

Confocal Microscopy Study: Methodology of Count of Cells

An HRT3 confocal microscope with a Rostock Cornea Module RCM (Heidelberg Engineering, Heidelberg, Germany) was used.[67] Brightness and contrast were adjusted to 50%. Cell nuclei were selected with the marker of the device and marked in blue; these nuclei were more illuminated and more refringent (Fig. 36.5A,B).[61,68–70] The selected nuclei had clear well-defined edges.[61,70,71]

The counting of transplanted ADASCs was performed in a way similar to counting normal keratocytes (see Fig. 36.5C). When the decellularized (G-2) or recellularized (G-3) laminas appeared without well-defined cell structures, they were considered totally acellular in the defined chosen area (Fig. 36.6A). All structures that appeared on the anterior surface, posterior surface, and in the midstroma of the lamina, showing similar morphology to a keratocyte nucleus with well-defined edges, were counted as a cell nucleus (Figs. 36.6B and 36.7A–E).[61,70]

Results

AUTOLOGOUS ADASC IMPLANTATIONS: CLINICAL RESULTS

No complications were observed during the 3-year follow-up. No adverse events such as haze and infection were encountered. Full corneal transparency was recovered within the first postoperative day in all patients (Figs. 36.4A,B and 36.8A,B). No patient lost lines of visual acuity. All cases demonstrated an improvement in visual acuity at 6, 12, and 36 months postoperative. All cases improved one to two lines at 36 months postoperative relative to the preoperative values in their UDVA, CDVA, and rigid CLVA. A significant improvement in mean values was recorded at 36 months postop relative to the preoperative mean values; P values and standard deviation are presented in Table 36.2.[62]

Rx Sphr demonstrated a significant improvement at 6, 12, and 36 months postoperative relative to the preoperative mean values. Rx Cyl remained almost stable up to 12 months postoperative followed by a change of 0.5 D at 36 months postoperative relative to the preoperative mean values; *P* values are presented in Table 36.2.[62] Visante CCT (see Fig. 36.4A,B), Pentacam thinnest point, and CV (Fig. 36.9A,B) showed a significant increase in mean values; all results were significantly better when comparing G-2 and G-3 with G-1 at 36 months postop relative to the preoperative mean values (see Table 36.2).[62]

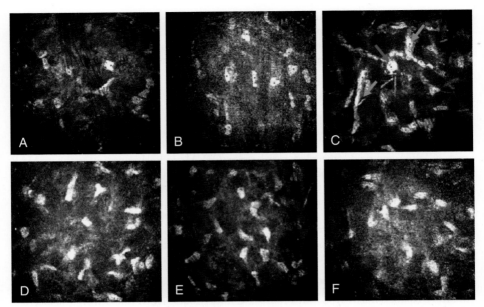

Fig. 36.5 Confocal microscopy findings in group 1 with implantation of adipose-derived adult mesenchymal stem cells (ADASCs). (A, B) shows the small numbers of keratocytes preoperatively in case 1. (A) Anterior stroma; (B) midstroma. (C) Confocal microscopy in the surgical plane at 3 months postoperative in case 4 shows the morphology of implanted ADASCs as rounded in shape *(red arrow)*, and more refringent and voluminous *(blue arrows)*. (D) shows the high number of keratocytes in case 1, at 12 months postoperative in the midcorneal stoma, with morphology similar to normal corneal cells. (E, F) show the high number of keratocytes in the anterior and posterior stroma, respectively, in case 2. Note the different morphology of keratocytes preoperatively compared with 12 months after surgery.

The mean values of third-order aberration root mean square (RMS) (3rd order RMS) (μm) and high-order aberration RMS (HOA RMS) (μm) were statistically significantly better when comparing G-2 and G-3 with G-1; mean values of fourth-order aberration RMS (4th order RMS) (μm) and low-order aberration RMS (LOA RMS) (μm) improved at 36 months postop compared to preoperative values (see Table 36.2).[62]

In adition, anterior Km presented an average improvement of 1D at 12 and 36 months postop. A flattening in mean values of 2 D in K_{max} was found at 12 months postoperative, followed by 1 D at 36 months postoperative in relation to the preoperative mean values; more results were recorded in previous publications.[62]

LAMINA IMPLANTATION: CLINICAL RESULTS

No complications were recorded during the 3-year follow-up, with the exception that the implanted laminas showed a mild early haze during the first postoperative month; this issue was related to a mild lenticular edema. Corneal recovery and full transparency were observed by the third postoperative month in all patients. No adverse events of any type were observed over the 3-year follow-up (see Figs. 36.4C–F and 36.8C–F).[62]

All patients with decellularized or recellularized laminas demonstrated improvement at 6, 12, and 36 months postoperative in mean values relative to the preoperative values. **UDVA** was enhanced by up to 0.13 in decimal value, which was nearly equivalent to one line of the log-MAR scale, with decellularized and recellularized laminas. **CDVA** increased by up to 0.2 with

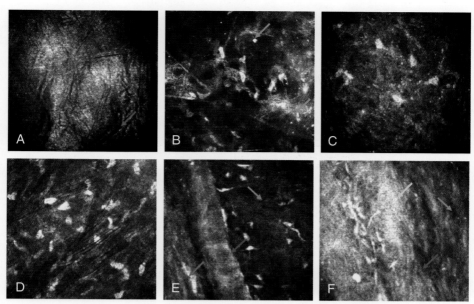

Fig. 36.6 Confocal microscopy findings with implantation of decellularized laminas in group 2. (A) Anterior surface of the decellularized lamina in case 7 at 1 month postoperative. Note the acellular aspect of the laminas. (B) Posterior surface of the decellularized lamina with case 5 at 12 months postoperative with high number of cells type-keratocytes. *Green arrows* show the presence of highly reflective dots. (C) Anterior stoma in case 5 with a very small number of keratocytes preoperative. (D) Anterior stroma in case 5 with a very high number of keratocytes at 12 months postoperative. Note the different morphology of keratocytes between (C) and (D). (E, F) Transition area between the decellularized lamina *(red arrows)* and the host stroma *(blue arrows)* in case 7, at 12 months postoperative. Note the migrating keratocytes *(pink arrows)* from the host stroma toward the decellularized implanted tissue. (E) Shows the absence of fibrotic tissue on the periphery of the lamina. (F) Shows the presence of the fibrotic tissue *(yellow arrow)*.

decellularized and recellularized laminas, equivalent to two lines of the logMAR scale; rigid **CLVA** mean improvement was up to 0.23 with decellularized and recellularized laminas, which was nearly equivalent to two lines of logMAR scale. **CV** demonstrated an improvement in mean values of 2 to 3 mm^3 in both groups at 6, 12, and 36 months postoperative relative to the preoperative values.[62]

Besides the **Rx Sphr, Rx Cyl, Visante CCT** (see Fig. 36.4C–F), Pentacam **thinnest point** (Figs. 36.10 and 36.11), **3rd-order RMS, 4th-order RMS, HOA RMS** (Fig. 36.12), **LOA RMS, anterior K$_m$** (see Figs. 36.10B and 36.11A), posterior mean keratometry (**posterior K$_m$**) (D), **K$_{max}$**, and topographic cylinder (**topo cyl**) (D) with decellularized and recellularized laminas all results close results with implantation of ADASCs.[62]

CONFOCAL MICROSCOPY STUDY

ADASC Results

Morphological Results. The ADASCs appeared rounded in shape and voluminous, and more refringent and luminous than the host keratocytes in G-1 (see Fig. 36.5C). However, the shape of the ADASCs changed from round to fusiform 6 months after surgery (see Fig. 36.5D).

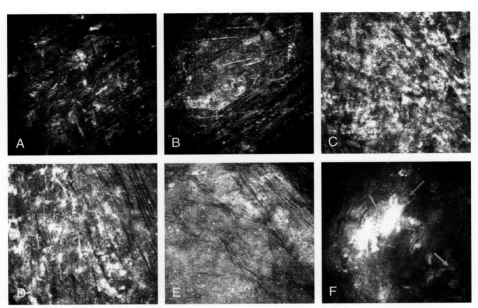

Fig. 36.7   Confocal microscopy findings with implantation of recellularized laminas in group 3. (A–D) Confocal findings of case 13. (A) Anterior surface of the recellularized lamina at 1 month postoperative. note the presence of few adipose-derived adult mesenchymal stem cell (ADASCs, marked in *blue*). (B) Posterior surface of the recellularized lamina 1 month after surgery: note the presence of few ADASCs, more similar in morphology to keratocytes. (C) Anterior surface of the recellularized lamina at 12 months postoperative: note the abundant number of stromal cells. (D) Posterior surface of the recellularized lamina at 12 months after surgery: note the high number of stromal cells. (E) Midstroma of the lamina in case 11 at 12 months postoperative. Note the presence of keratocytes (marked in *blue*). The light gray reflective color of the lamina *(yellow arrows)* indicates the formation of neocollagen. (F) Transition area between the recellularized lamina *(red arrows)* and the host stroma *(blue arrows)* in case 10, at 3 months postoperative. Note the high reflective fibrotic tissue with presence of fibroblasts or myofibroblasts (active state of keratocytes).

A change in morphology of the host keratocytes was observed in the anterior, mid, and posterior stroma; corneal cells acquired a more fusiform shape, very similar to the keratocytes of a normal corneal stroma (see Fig. 36.5D–F).[15,61,70]

Moreover, the confocal microscopy study showed the presence of fibrotic tissue at 3 months postoperative in two of four patients, followed by full recovery of the corneal stroma at 12 months follow-up.[61]

Statistical Results.   A gradual statistically significant increase in cellular density was seen at 12 months after surgery in the anterior, mid, and posterior host stroma compared with the preoperative values (Table 36.3).[61]

Lamina Results

Morphological Results.   Decellularized laminas appeared acellular in the first months (see Fig. 36.6A), unlike the recellularized ones that in some determined areas of interest showed similar structures to corneal keratocytes (see Fig. 36.7A,B). The number of cells increased during the 12-month follow-up. The anterior, mid, and posterior surfaces of the decellularized and recellularized laminas became more colonized by keratocyte-type cells, until they showed similar

TABLE 36.2 ■ *P* Values of the Results of 3 Years of Clinical Outcomes Among G-2/G-1, G-3/G-1, and G-2/G-3, and Standard Deviation (σ) of the Preoperative Time

	(G-2)/(G-1)	(G-3)/(G-1)	(G-2)/(G-3)	σ
UDVA	$P = 0.054$	$P = 0.069$	$P = 0.986$	0.116
CDVA	$P < 0.001$	$P < 0.001$	$P = 0.900$	0.151
CLVA	$P < 0.001$	$P = 0.090$	$P = 0.010$	0.180
Rx Sphr (D)	$P = 0.892$	$P = 0.863$	$P = 0.747$	2.691
Rx Cyl (D)	$P < 0.001$	$P = 0.014$	$P = 0.086$	0.824
Visante CCT (µm)	$P = 0.012$	$P < 0.001$	$P = 0.055$	62.940
Thinnest point (µm)	$P = 0.007$	$P = 0.001$	$P = 0.465$	67.966
CV (mm³)	$P < 0.001$	$P < 0.001$	$P = 0.948$	3.757
K_{max} (D)	$P = 0.949$	$P = 0.387$	$P = 0.391$	8.250
RMS ($n = 3$) (µm)	$P < 0.001$	$P = 0.009$	$P = 0.376$	4.571
RMS ($n = 4$) (µm)	$P = 0.074$	$P = 0.817$	$P = 0.004$	2.515
RMS HOA (µm)	$P < 0.001$	$P = 0.038$	$P = 0.091$	4.530
RMS LOA (µm)	$P = 0.617$	$P = 0.870$	$P = 0.491$	27.299

CDVA, Corrected distance visual acuity; *CLVA*, contact lens visual acuity (decimal equivalent to the logMAR scale); *CV*, cornea volume; *G-1*, group 1; *G-2*, group 2; *G-3*, group 3; *HOA*, high-order aberration; *K*max, maximum keratometry; *LOA*, root mean square low-order aberration; *Rx Cyl*, refractive cylinder; *RMS*, root mean square; *Rx Sphr*, refractive sphere; *thinnest point*, Pentacam thinnest point; *UDVA*, unaided distance visual acuity; *Visante CCT*, anterior segment optical coherence tomography (OCT)-Visante.

morphology to normal corneal keratocytes (see Figs. 36.6B and 36.7C–E).[61,70] We were able to differentiate the morphology of the lamina from the host stroma by the presence of more abundant, dark, and profound striae (see Fig. 36.6A).[70] Some lamina matrix was observed with a light gray color, reflecting more light; this fact could be attributed to the formation of the layer of neo-collagen after the implant of the laminas in the corneal stroma (see Fig. 36.7E).

The morphology and number of cells at the anterior and posterior stroma increased during the 12-month follow-up; then cell density became much closer to that of normal corneal keratocytes (see Fig. 36.6C,D).[61,70]

TABLE 36.3 ■ Results for Cell Density in G-1, G-2, and G-3. *P* Value at 12 Months After Surgery/ Preoperative

	Ante-rior Stroma (Cells/mm²)	Midstroma (Cells/mm²)	Poste-rior Stroma (Cells/mm²)	Anterior Surface of the Lamina (Cells/mm²)	Midstroma of the Lamina (Cells/mm²)	Posterior Surface of the Lamina (Cells/mm²)
Group 1 (G-1)	[$P < 0.001$]	[$P < 0.001$]	[$P < 0.001$]	NA	NA	NA
Group 2 (G-2)	[$P < 0.001$]	NA	[$P < 0.001$]	[$P < 0.001$]	[$P < 0.001$]	[$P < 0.001$]
Group 3 (G-3)	[$P < 0.001$]	NA	[$P < 0.001$]	[$P < 0.001$]	[$P < 0.001$]	[$P < 0.001$]
G-1/G-2/G-3	[$P = 0.025$]	NA	[$P = 0.311$]	NA	NA	NA
G-2/G-3	[$P = 0.025$]	NA	[$P = 0.311$]	[$P = 0.011$]	[$P = 0.011$]	[$P = 0.029$]

Confocal microscopy findings demonstrated the presence of fibrotic tissue in almost all the cases in G-2 and G-3 during the 12-month follow-up (see Figs. 36.6F and 36.7F). All detected fibrotic tissue corresponded with paracentral areas of the decellularized or recellularized implanted laminas. The fibrotic tissue was absent in the central visual axis of the cornea in all the patients from G-2 and G-3 (Figs. 36.6E,F and **36.7F**).[61]

Statistical Results. At 12 months after surgery, in G-2 and G-3, cellular density in the anterior and posterior corneal stroma showed statisticaly significant differences relative to the preoperative values (see Table 36.3).[61] On the anterior surface, posterior surface, and mid decellularized and recellularized laminas, cellular density was statistically significant, close to that found in a normal cornea (see Table 36.3).[61]

However, the statistical results for the fibrotic tissue did not demonstrate a direct and significant association between the recellularization and the presence of such fibrotic tissue on the periphery of the decellularized or recellularized laminas.[61]

Confocal Microscopy Study: Comparison of Results Among G-1, G-2, and G-3

A statistically significant difference in cell density in the anterior stroma was seen among the three groups, with G3 having the highest, followed by G2, and then G1. However, in the posterior stroma, the changes in cell density were not statistically significant among the three groups (see Table 36.3).[61]

In addition, at 12 months postoperative, cell densities in the anterior and posterior surfaces and within the laminas were statistically significantly higher for the recellularized laminas than the decellularized ones (see Table 36.3).[61]

SLIT-LAMP BIOMICROSCOPY

Before surgery only one patient from each group presented with mild paracentral anterior stromal scars (case 2, case 9, and case 11) (see Fig. 36.8A). During the 36-month follow-up, no corneas showed any posterior stromal or pre-Descemet scarring and all presented a fully transparent visual axis (see Figs. 36.4 and 36.8B–F). No case developed any complications such as inflammation or rejection throughout the follow-up period (Figs. 36.4 and 36.8B–F). The transparency of the cornea in G-1 was completely recovered within 24 hours after surgery, and was maintained throughout the 36-month follow-up period (see Figs. 36.4A,B and 36.8A,B) as described in our previous interim report.[15,42,61,62] Case 2 from G-1 presented paracentral anterior stromal scars preoperatively, and we observed progressive improvement of those scars during the 12- and 36-month follow-up after surgery (see Fig. 36.8B).[15,61,62] In G-2 and G-3, the implanted laminas showed a mild early clinical haziness during the first postoperative month that was related to a mild lenticular edema (see Fig. 36.8C). Corneal transparency improved progressively, and complete restoration was observed in all cases toward the third month of follow-up. No patient had visually significant corneal haze or scarring (see Figs. 36.4 and 36.8D–F). In case 11 in G-3, we were able to detect an improvement in the paracentral scar at 36 months postoperative compared with the preoperative examination; more findings have been described in our previous interim publications.[61,62]

Discussion and Conclusions

Alió et al. demonstrated for the first time the feasibility of the implantation of ADASCs into the corneal stromal pocket in cases of advanced keratoconus. They confirmed the appearance of new collagen in the injected areas. This new collagen could be useful for repairing corneal dystrophies

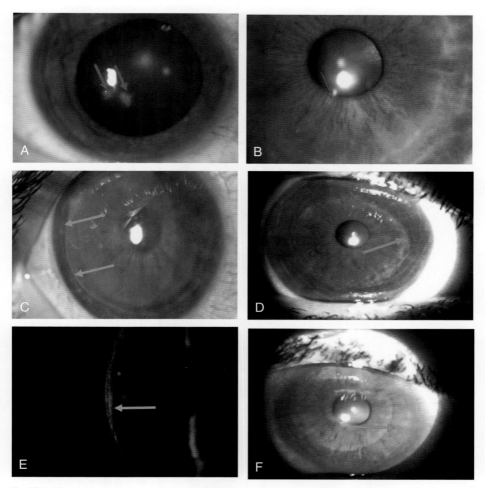

Fig. 36.8 Biomicroscopic changes between the preoperative and up to 36 months postoperative in group 1 (G-1), group 2 (G-2), and group 3 (G-3). (A) Case 2, G-1. Note the presence of paracentral scars *(red arrows)* at the preoperative time. (B) Case 2, G-1 at 36 months postoperative shows the transparency of the cornea and the marked improvement of the paracentral scars *(red arrow)*. (C) Case 5, G-2, 1 day postoperative, shows the reduced transparency of the implanted lamina, *blue arrows* represent the border of the lamina. (D) Case 5, G-2, 36 months postoperative, presents improvement of the transparency of the implanted tissue. *Blue arrows* represent the border of the lamina. (E) G-3, case 12, at 12 months postoperative. The *blue arrow* indicates the implanted recellularized lamina. (F) G-3, case 12, at 36 months postoperative. The *blue arrow* indicates the periphery of the recellularized lamina. Note the improvement of the transparency of the implanted tissue.

and scars, and for slightly increasing corneal thickness, but this enhancement is insufficient for reversing corneal disease in advanced keratoconus.[15]

Decellularized laminas of a human corneal stroma, colonized or not by autologous ADASCs, can be implanted on a clinical basis in the corneal stroma for therapeutic purposes. Also, studies have demonstrated the safety and feasibility of the use of femtosecond laser to dissect the cornea in advanced keratoconus, even when a large 9.5-mm corneal pocket was formed in the middle of the corneal stroma.[16,42,62] After 3 years of follow-up, no patient showed inflammation, rejection,

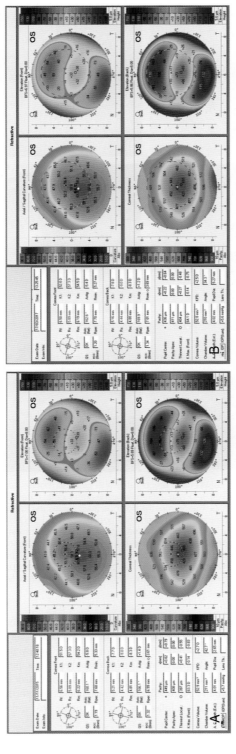

Fig. 36.9 Four-map corneal topography (Pentacam) comparison between preoperative in group 1 (G-1) and 12 months postoperative. (A, B) Four-map corneal topography (Pentacam), G-1, case 4. (A) At the preoperative; (B) 12 months postoperative. A modest improvement in the pachymetric parameters and near stability in the keratometric results can be seen.

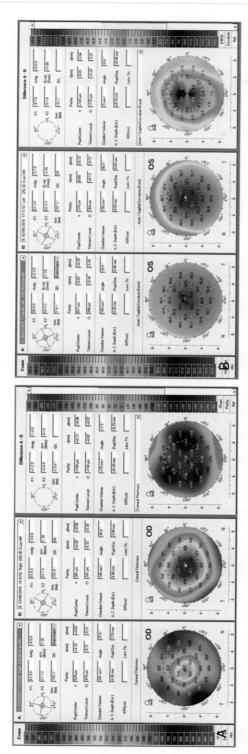

Fig. 36.10 Corneal topography (Pentacam) comparison pachymetric examinations for group 2 (G-2) between preoperative and 12 and 36 months postoperative. (A) Corneal topography (Pentacam) comparison (*right image*) between the preoperative (*middle image*) and almost 12 months postoperative (*left image*) in patient case 9, G-2. Note the enhancement of the pachymetric parameters. (B) Corneal topography (Pentacam) comparison (*right image*) between the preoperative (*middle image*) and almost 3 years postoperative (*left image*), in patient case 7, G-2. Note the enhancement of the keratometric parameters.

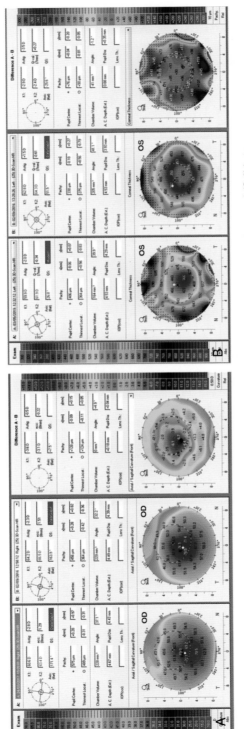

Fig. 36.11 Corneal topography (Pentacam) comparison pachymetric examinations in group 3 (G-3) between preoperative and 12 and 36 months postoperative. (A) Corneal topography (Pentacam) comparison between preoperative and 12 months in G-3, case 12. Note the enhancement of the keratometric parameters. (B) Corneal topography (Pentacam) comparison between preoperative and almost 3 years postoperative, in G-3, patient case 12. Note the enhancement of the pachymetric parameters.

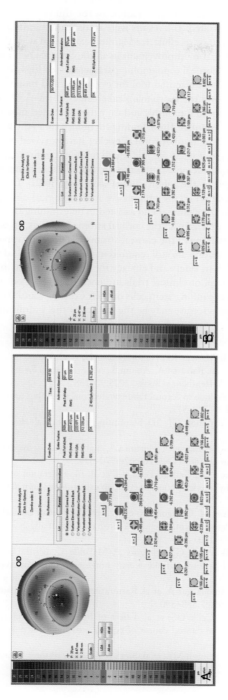

Fig. 36.12 Corneal aberrometries (Pentacam) in group 2, case 5. (A) Preoperatory high-order aberration (HOA) root mean square. (B) Almost three postoperative years HOA. Note the enhancement of 3.888 μm.

or any evidence of scarring or haze (see Figs. 36.4 and 36.8). Furthermore, after 3 years of follow-up all cases showed improvement in all the visual parameters, with one to two lines of logMAR. A significant increase in central corneal thickness in the thinnest portion of the cornea and in corneal volume was demonstrated. The results were statistically significantly better in the groups with implanted decellularized or recellularized laminas compared with the group with implanted ADASCs alone. There was also an improvement in all the corneal aberrations (see Fig. 36.12) and stability or enhancement of corneal topographic parameters (see Figs. 36.9–36.11).[62]

Confocal microscopy was an essential tool for evaluating and monitoring "in vivo" the evolution of the ADASC nuclei and the morphological changes of the ASASCs. These were rounded and highly refringent cells up to 6 months, and they demonstrated more fusiform structures and less nucleus refringent at 12 months. These findings demonstrate in the human clinical model that the ADASCs implanted in the human corneal pocket have survived and have been able to differentiate into keratocytes (see Fig. 36.5C).[61,70] Such findings confirm the previous animal studies in which postmortem analysis demonstrated the survival of these human cells and their capacity to produce human collagen in the rabbit cornea (see Figs. 36.2B–D and 36.3B).[4,44] Confocal microscopy allowed observation of the progressive morphological changes that occurred in the decellularized and recellularized laminas and assisted in determining the change in the cell densities in the grafted tissue as well as in all the corneal stroma (see Figs. 36.6A–D and 36.7A–E).[61,70]

In conclusion, cellular therapy of the corneal stroma is a novel treatment modality for stromal diseases. Although further studies are still required in the form of clinical trials with larger sample sizes to definitively establish its safety and efficacy for different stromal diseases, the initial results obtained from the first few pilot clinical trials are encouraging. In our opinion, the creation of cellular banks storing and expanding stem cells or their exosomes and their shipping and delivery to the various clinical centers for use may be the future for this promising treatment modality.

References

1. De Miguel MP, Casaroli-Marano RP, Nieto-Nicolau N, et al. Frontiers in regenerative medicine for cornea and ocular surface. In: Rahman A., Anjum S., eds. *Frontiers in Stem Cell and Regenerative Medicine Research*. Vol. 1, 1st ed. PA: Bentham e-Books; 2015:92–138
2. Ruberti JW, Zieske JD. Prelude to corneal tissue engineering—gaining control of collagen organization. *Prog Retin Eye Res*. 2008;27:549–577.
3. Isaacson A, Swioklo S, Connon CJ. 3D bioprinting of a corneal stroma equivalent. *Exp Eye Res*. 2018;173:188–193.
4. Arnalich-Montiel F, Pastor S, Blazquez-Martinez A, et al. Adipose-derived stem cells are a source for cell therapy of the corneal stroma. *Stem Cells*. 2008;26:570–579.
5. Alió del Barrio JL, Chiesa M, Gallego Ferrer G, et al. Biointegration of corneal macroporous membranes based on poly(ethyl acrylate) copolymers in an experimental animal model. *J Biomed Mater Res A*. 2015;103:1106–1118.
6. Alió del Barrio JL, Chiesa M, Garagorri N, et al. Acellular human corneal matrix sheets seeded with human adipose-derived mesenchymal stem cells integrate functionally in an experimental animal model. *Exp Eye Res*. 2015;132:91–100.
7. Espandar L, Bunnell B, Wang GY, Gregory P, McBride C, Moshirfar M. Adipose-derived stem cells on hyaluronic acid-derived scaffold: a new horizon in bioengineered cornea. *Arch Ophthalmol*. 2012;130:202–208.
8. Mittal SK, Omoto M, Amouzegar A, et al. Restoration of corneal transparency by mesenchymal stem cells. *Stem Cell Reports*. 2016;7:583–590.
9. Demirayak B, Yüksel N, Çelik OS, et al. Effect of bone marrow and adipose tissue-derived mesenchymal stem cells on the natural course of corneal scarring after penetrating injury. *Exp Eye Res*. 2016;151:227–235.
10. Du Y, Carlson EC, Funderburgh ML, et al. Stem cell therapy restores transparency to defective murine corneas. *Stem Cells*. 2009;27:1635–1642.

11. Liu H, Zhang J, Liu CY, et al. Cell therapy of congenital corneal diseases with umbilical mesenchymal stem cells: lumican null mice. *PLoS One.* 2010;5:e10707.
12. Coulson-Thomas VJ, Caterson B, Kao WW. Transplantation of human umbilical mesenchymal stem cells cures the corneal defects of mucopolysaccharidosis VII mice. *Stem Cells.* 2013;31:2116–2126.
13. Kao WW, Coulson-Thomas VJ. Cell therapy of corneal diseases. *Cornea.* 2016;35(suppl 1):S9–S19.
14. De Miguel MP, Fuentes-Julián S, Blázquez-Martínez A, et al. Immunosuppressive properties of mesenchymal stem cells: advances and applications. *Curr Mol Med.* 2012;12:574–591.
15. Alió del Barrio JL, El Zarif M, de Miguel MP, et al. Cellular therapy with human autologous adipose-derived adult stem cells for advanced keratoconus. *Cornea.* 2017;36(8):952–960.
16. Alió del Barrio JL, El Zarif M, Azaar A, et al. Corneal stroma enhancement with decellularized stromal laminas with or without stem cell recellularization for advanced keratoconus. *Am J Ophthalmol.* 2018;186:47–58.
17. Harkin DG, Foyn L, Bray LJ, Sutherland AJ, Li FJ, Cronin BG. Concise reviews: can mesenchymal stromal cells differentiate into corneal cells? A systematic review of published data. *Stem Cells.* 2015;33(3):785–791.
18. Jiang Z, Liu G, Meng F, et al. Paracrine effects of mesenchymal stem cells on the activation of keratocytes. *Br J Ophthalmol.* 2017;101(11):1583–1590.
19. Hendijani F. Explant culture: an advantageous method for isolation of mesenchymal stem cells from human tissues. *Cell Prolif.* 2017;50(2):e12334.
20. Górski B. Gingiva as a new and the most accessible source of mesenchymal stem cells from the oral cavity to be used in regenerative therapies. *Postepy Hig Med Dosw (Online).* 2016;70(0):858–871.
21. Basu S, Hertsenberg AJ, Funderburgh ML, et al. Human limbal biopsy-derived stromal stem cells prevent corneal scarring. *Sci Transl Med.* 2014;6(266):266ra172.
22. Takahashi K, Yamanaka S. Induction of pluripotent stem cells from mouse embryonic and adult fibroblast cultures by defined factors. *Cell.* 2006;126:663–676.
23. Naylor RW, McGhee CN, Cowan CA, Davidson AJ, Holm TM, Sherwin T. Derivation of corneal keratocyte-like cells from human induced pluripotent stem cells. *PLoS One.* 2016;11(10):e0165464.
24. Yao L, Bai H. Review: mesenchymal stem cells and corneal reconstruction. *Mol Vis.* 2013;19:2237–2243.
25. Caplan AI. Mesenchymal stem cells: time to change the name! *Stem Cells Transl Med.* 2017;6(6):1445–1451.
26. Park SH, Kim KW, Chun YS, Kim JC. Human mesenchymal stem cells differentiate into keratocyte-like cells in keratocyte-conditioned medium. *Exp Eye Research.* 2012;101:16–26.
27. Trosan P, Javorkova E, Zajicova A, et al. The supportive role of insulin-like growth factor-I in the differentiation of murine mesenchymal stem cells into corneal-like cells. *Stem Cells Dev.* 2016;25(11):874–881.
28. Liu H, Zhang J, Liu CY, Hayashi Y, Kao WW. Bone marrow mesenchymal stem cells can differentiate and assume corneal keratocyte phenotype. *J Cell Mol Med.* 2012;16:1114–1124.
29. Du Y, Roh DS, Funderburgh ML, et al. Adipose-derived stem cells differentiate to keratocytes in vitro. *Mol Vis.* 2010;16:2680–2689.
30. Ziaei M, Zhang J, Patel DV, McGhee CNJ. Umbilical cord stem cells in the treatment of corneal disease. *Surv Ophthalmol.* 2017;62(6):803–815.
31. Chan AA, Hertsenberg AJ, Funderburgh ML, et al. Differentiation of human embryonic stem cells into cells with corneal keratocyte phenotype. *PloS One.* 2013;8:e56831.
32. Yun YI, Park SY, Lee HJ, et al. Comparison of the anti-inflammatory effects of induced pluripotent stem cell-derived and bone marrow-derived mesenchymal stromal cells in a murine model of corneal injury. *Cytotherapy.* 2017;19(1):28–35.
33. Pinnamaneni N, Funderburgh JL. Concise review: stem cells in the corneal stroma. *Stem Cells.* 2012;30(6):1059–1063.
34. Du Y, Funderburgh ML, Mann MM, SundarRaj N, Funderburgh JL. Multipotent stem cells in human corneal stroma. *Stem Cells.* 2005;23(9):1266–1275.
35. Katikireddy KR, Dana R, Jurkunas UV. Differentiation potential of limbal fibroblasts and bone marrow mesenchymal stem cells to corneal epithelial cells. *Stem Cells.* 2014;32(3):717–729.
36. Wu J, Du Y, Watkins SC, Funderburgh JL, Wagner WR. The engineering of organized human corneal tissue through the spatial guidance of corneal stromal stem cells. *Biomaterials.* 2012;33(5):1343–1352.
37. Di G, Du X, Qi X, et al. Mesenchymal stem cells promote diabetic corneal epithelial wound healing through TSG-6-dependent stem cell activation and macrophage switch. *Invest Ophthalmol Vis Sci.* 2017;58(10):4344–4354.

38. Holan V, Trosan P, Cejka C, et al. A comparative study of the therapeutic potential of mesenchymal stem cells and limbal epithelial stem cells for ocular surface reconstruction. *Stem Cells Transl Med.* 2015;4(9):1052–1063.

39. Cejka C, Cejkova J, Trosan P, Zajicova A, Sykova E, Holan V. Transfer of mesenchymal stem cells and cyclosporine A on alkali-injured rabbit cornea using nanofiber scaffolds strongly reduces corneal neovascularization and scar formation. *Histol Histopathol.* 2016;31(9):969–980.

40. Agorogiannis GI, Alexaki VI, Castana O, Kymionis GD. Topical application of autologous adipose-derived mesenchymal stem cells (MSCs) for persistent sterile corneal epithelial defect. *Graefes Arch Clin Exp Ophthalmol.* 2012;250(3):455–457.

41. Basu S. Limbal stromal stem cell therapy for acute and chronic superficial corneal pathologies: early clinical outcomes with the Funderburgh technique. Oral presentation at: The Association for Research, Vision and Ophthalmology (ARVO). *Annual Meeting*, Baltimore (USA); 2017.

42. Alió J, Alió Del Barrio J, El Zarif M, et al. Regenerative surgery of the corneal stroma for advanced keratoconus: 1-year outcomes. *Am J Ophthalmol.* 2019;203:53–68.

43. Ma XY, Bao HJ, Cui L, Zou J. The graft of autologous adipose-derived stem cells in the corneal stromal after mechanic damage. *PloS One.* 2013;8:e76103.

44. Alió del Barrio JL, Chiesa M, Gallego Ferrer G, et al. Biointegration of corneal macroporous membranes based on poly(ethyl acrylate) copolymers in an experimental animal model. *J Biomed Mater Res A.* 2015;103:1106–1118.

45. Lynch AP, Ahearne M. Strategies for developing decellularized corneal scaffolds. *Exp Eye Research.* 2013;108:42–47.

46. Wilson SE, Liu JJ, Mohan RR. Stromal-epithelial interactions in the cornea. *Prog Retin Eye Res.* 1999;18:293–309.

47. Choi JS, Williams JK, Greven M, et al. Bioengineering endothelialized neo-corneas using donor-derived corneal endothelial cells and decellularized corneal stroma. *Biomaterials.* 2010;31:6738–6745.

48. Shafiq MA, Gemeinhart RA, Yue BY, Djalilian AR. Decellularized human cornea for reconstructing the corneal epithelium and anterior stroma. *Tissue Eng Part C Methods.* 2012;18:340–348.

49. Gonzalez-Andrades M, de la Cruz Cardona J, Ionescu AM, Campos A, Del Mar Perez M, Alaminos M. Generation of bioengineered corneas with decellularized xenografts and human keratocytes. *Invest Ophthalmol Vis Sci.* 2011;52:215–222.

50. Yam GH, Yusoff NZ, Goh TW, et al. Decellularization of human stromal refractive lenticules for corneal tissue engineering. *Sci Rep.* 2016;6:26339.

51. Liu YC, Teo EPW, Ang HP, et al. Biological corneal inlay for presbyopia derived from small incision lenticule extraction (SMILE). *Sci Rep.* 2018;8(1):1831.

52. Bai H, Wang LL, Huang YF, Huang JX. An experimental study of mesenchymal stem cells in tissue engineering scaffolds implanted in rabbit corneal lamellae to increase keratoprosthesis biointegration. *Zhonghua Yan Ke Za Zhi.* 2016;52(3):192–197.

53. Barraquer JI. Keratophakia. *Trans Ophthalmol Soc UK.* 1972;92:499–516.

54. Omoto M, Katikireddy KR, Rezazadeh A, Dohlman TH, Chauhan SK. Mesenchymal stem cells home to inflamed ocular surface and suppress allosensitization in corneal transplantation. *Invest Ophthalmol Vis Sci.* 2014;55(10):6631–6638.

55. Fuentes-Julián S, Arnalich-Montiel F, Jaumandreu L, et al. Adipose-derived mesenchymal stem cell administration does not improve corneal graft survival outcome. *PLoS One.* 2015;10(3):e0117945.

56. Zhang L, Coulson-Thomas VJ, Ferreira TG, Kao WW. Mesenchymal stem cells for treating ocular surface diseases. *BMC Ophthalmol.* 2015;15(suppl 1):155.

57. Swioklo S, Constantinescu A, Connon CJ. Alginate-encapsulation for the improved hypothermic preservation of human adipose-derived stem cells. *Stem Cells Transl Med.* 2016;5(3):339–349.

58. Funderburgh JL. Assessing the potential of stem cells to regenerate stromal tissue. Oral presentation at: The Association for Research, Vision and Ophthalmology (ARVO) Annual meeting, Baltimore (USA); 2017.

59. Joseph R, Srivastava OP, Pfister RR. Modeling keratoconus using induced pluripotent stem cells. *Invest Ophthalmol Vis Sci.* 2016;57:3685–3697.

60. Shojaati G, Funderburgh ML, Mann M, Khandaker I, Funderburgh JL. Regenerative potential of stem cell-derived exosomes. Oral presentation at: The Association for Research, Vision and Ophthalmology (ARVO) Annual meeting, Baltimore (USA); 2017.

61. El Zarif M, Abdul Jawad K, Alió Del Barrio JL, et al. Corneal stroma cell density evolution in keratoconus corneas following the implantation of adipose mesenchymal stem cells and corneal laminas: an in vivo confocal microscopy study. *Invest Ophthalmol Vis Sci.* 2020;61(4):22.

62. El Zarif M, Alió JL, Alió Del Barrio JL, et al. Corneal stromal regeneration therapy for advanced keratoconus: long term outcomes at 3 years. *Cornea.* 2021;40(6):741–754.

63. Zuk P, Zhu M, Mizuno H, et al. Multilineage cells from human adipose tissue: implications for cell-based therapies. *Tissue Eng.* 2001;7(2):211–228.

64. Zuk P, Zhu M, Ashjian P, et al. Human adipose tissue is a source of multipotent stem cells. *Mol Biol Cell.* 2002;13(12):4279–4295.

65. Bourin P, Bunnell B, Casteilla L, et al. Stromal cells from the adipose tissue-derived stromal vascular fraction and culture expanded adipose tissue-derived stromal/stem cells: a joint statement of the International Federation for Adipose Therapeutics and Science (IFATS) and the International Society for Cellular Therapy (ISCT). *Cytotherapy.* 2013;15(6):641–648.

66. Ponce Márquez S, Martínez VS, McIntosh Ambrose W, et al. Decellularization of bovine corneas for tissue engineering applications. *Acta Biomater.* 2009;5(6):1839–1847.

67. Guthoff R, Klink T, Schlunck G, Grehn F. Die sickerkissenuntersuchung mittels konfokaler in-vivo mikroskopie mit dem rostocker cornea modulerste erfahrungen. *Klin Monatsbl Augenheilkd.* 2005;222:R8.

68. Ali Javadi M, Kanavi M, Mahdavi M, et al. Comparison of keratocyte density between keratoconus, post-laser in situ keratomileusis keratectasia, and uncomplicated post-laser in situ keratomileusis cases. A confocal scan study. *Cornea.* 2009;28(7):774–779.

69. Mastropasqua L, Nubile M. Normal corneal morphology. In: *Confocal Microscopy of the Cornea.* Thorofare, NJ: SLACK; 2002:7–16.

70. El Zarif M, Abdul Jawad K, Alió JL. *Corneal regeneration therapy and surgery.* 1st ed. In: Alió JL, Alió del Barrio JL, Arnalich-Montiel F, eds. Springer; 2019: 363-386.

71. Ku J, Niederer R, Patel D, Sherwin T, McGhee C. Laser scanning in vivo confocal analysis of keratocyte density in keratoconus. *Ophthalmology.* 2008;115(5):845–850.

CHAPTER 37

Medical and Surgical Management of Corneal Hydrops

Andrea L. Blitzer ■ Asim V. Farooq ■ Marian S. Macsai

KEY CONCEPTS

- Acute corneal hydrops (ACH) is characterized by sudden-onset corneal edema, typically in the setting of a corneal ectatic disorder.
- It is a vision-threatening complication of keratoconus that can result in permanent scarring and may be the presenting sign of keratoconus.
- In this chapter an overview of ACH, followed by a discussion of its medical and surgical management, is provided.

Introduction

Acute corneal hydrops (ACH) is characterized by sudden-onset corneal edema, typically in the setting of a corneal ectatic disorder. It is a vision-threatening complication of keratoconus that can result in permanent scarring and may even be the presenting sign of keratoconus.[1] A clinical description of ACH in keratoconus patients can be found as early as 1854 in the treatise by Dr. John Nottingham.[2] The term "acute hydrops," however, was not introduced until 1940 when Drs. Ralph Rychener and Daniel Kirby were able to reproduce acute corneal edema by surgically inducing breaks in the posterior corneas of rabbits.[3]

Epidemiology and Risk Factors

The reported incidence of ACH varies widely, from 0.2% to 2.8% in keratoconus patients.[4,5] Notably, it may occur in up to 11% of patients with keratoglobus and pellucid marginal corneal degeneration.[6,7] Most patients present in the third or fourth decade of life.[8] Some studies have shown that males with keratoconus have nearly double the risk of ACH compared with females.[1,8]

Atopic disease and eye rubbing have been identified as risk factors for ACH.[5] A recent case-control study identified nonocular atopic conditions as risk factors for the development of ACH in keratoconus patients.[8] In addition to its association with atopy, eye rubbing may also be an independent risk factor.[1] Not surprisingly, patients with steeper keratometry prior to hydrops were also found to be at increased risk of ACH.[5,8] There are, however, a number of patients whose first presentation to an ophthalmologist is after an acute episode of hydrops and whose baseline visual acuity and keratometry are unknown.

Patients with prior ACH in one eye have a greater than six-fold increased risk of hydrops in the other eye.[8] ACH is found at increased rates in patients with learning disabilities and is more likely to present bilaterally in patients with Down syndrome.[8,9] A retrospective case series in New Zealand has found that those of Pacific ethnicity had a higher risk of hydrops compared with White Europeans.[1] In a population-based survey in the United Kingdom, South Asian and Black patients had a higher prevalence of both keratoconus and ACH.[4]

Imaging, particularly with anterior segment optical coherence tomography (AS-OCT), has revealed anatomic risk factors for the development of ACH.[10] Corneas with epithelial thickening, stromal thinning at the keratoconus cone, hyperreflective anomalies within Bowman's layer (BL), and an absence of corneal scarring are more likely to experience an episode of ACH.

Natural History

Acute hydrops presents clinically as a marked decrease in visual acuity accompanied by pain and photophobia. Slit-lamp examination will reveal an edematous cornea, which may be Seidel positive (Fig. 37.1).[11,12] In most cases, the edema resolves spontaneously over the course of weeks to months.[13] Deturgescence is thought to occur after endothelial cells migrate to cover the exposed stroma.[14] There is often a flattening of the cornea following an episode of ACH, which may induce a beneficial refractive change and allow for improved contact lens fitting in keratoconic eyes.[15,16]

As the cornea heals, haze and scar formation may occur, which may be vision-impairing. A worse prognosis is seen in cases with large areas of the cornea involved, or in episodes with a prolonged duration of edema.[17] Prognosis is particularly poor for corneas that develop neovascularization. In episodes of ACH with edema lasting longer than 11 weeks, corneal neovascularization may be seen in up to 75% of patients.[17] Additional risk factors for corneal neovascularization include the severity of hydrops, edema located at the limbus, and the presence of intrastromal clefts.[18,19] Vision-limiting scars that cannot be aided by a contact lens may require corneal transplantation.

Pathogenesis

Classically, ACH has been thought to occur after a spontaneous break in Descemet membrane (DM) and the endothelium. Early reports using slit-lamp examination of patients with keratoconus and histopathologic samples taken from patients undergoing penetrating keratoplasty (PKP) after ACH were able to identify breaks in the DM of some patients.[14] Since then, there have been many descriptions of DM scrolls in ACH.

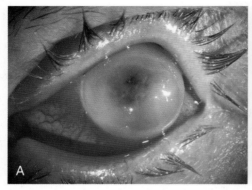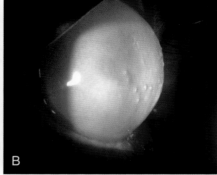

Fig. 37.1 (A) Conjunctival injection and diffuse corneal edema with microbullae during an episode of acute corneal hydrops. (B) Side view of the same patient demonstrates anterior corneal protrusion. (Courtesy James J. Reidy, MD.)

Intraocular pressure (IOP) has been suggested as an etiologic factor in ACH. IOP elevated to approximately twice the baseline level has been shown to significantly increase corneal steepening in keratoconic eyes but does not create any significant change in normal corneas.[20] Eye rubbing, a known risk factor for keratoconus and an independent risk factor in the development of ACH, also transiently increases IOP. A recent in vivo study on nonhuman primates showed that eye rubbing can cause IOP increases that exceed 300 mmHg and average 109 mmHg above baseline.[21] These repeated increases in IOP may increase the risk of ACH development.[9]

There is some evidence that, in addition to DM, disruption of a layer of posterior stroma may be involved in some cases of ACH. Stone et al. published the first case series that examined ACH with electron microscopy, demonstrating a tear in DM that curled anteriorly around a small amount of separated stroma.[15] More recently, a role of posterior stromal rupture has been suggested by Parker et al.[22] Two groups of patients with keratoconus were compared: (1) patients with coexisting Fuchs dystrophy who were undergoing Descemet membrane endothelial keratoplasty (DMEK) and (2) patients undergoing BL transplantation who had inadvertent rupture through the posterior stroma. All eyes with inadvertent rupture through the posterior stroma during BL transplantation developed ACH, but edema was not seen in those patients undergoing DMEK.

In reviewing published histopathology, we have encountered multiple examples where DM rupture appears to be accompanied by adherent posterior stroma.[14,15,23-28] Though the scrolling of DM is thought to be due to its elastic nature,[15] evaluation of the mechanical properties of rabbit corneas showed that DM is relatively stiff compared with the rest of the cornea, whereas the posterior stroma is the least stiff corneal tissue.[29] Taken together, there is evidence that the posterior stroma may be ruptured in some cases of ACH and may participate in its pathogenesis. It is unclear if involvement of the posterior stroma may affect prognosis or preferred management.

Diagnosis

The diagnosis of ACH is made via the history of present illness, focused clinical examination, and corroborating imaging.

HISTORY

Cases of ACH are often described as spontaneous, although they may be unknowingly precipitated by episodes of eye rubbing, coughing, sneezing, and other potential mechanisms of IOP elevation.[9] There is evidence of bilateral involvement in up to 18% of cases,[5] suggestive of a direct causative mechanism.

Patients present with acutely decreased vision, photophobia, and pain. They may have a known history of keratoconus, although in many cases, ACH may be the initial presentation of keratoconus.[1] In a study of New Zealanders with ACH, the acute episode was the first visit to an eyecare provider in 30% of patients.[1] This may be even higher in regions without a national public health service. When obtaining a history, emphasis should be placed on the presence of known risk factors of ACH, including a history of atopy and eye rubbing.

CLINICAL EXAMINATION

In addition to visual acuity, IOP (which may be artificially low in the presence of corneal edema), and pupil responses, particular attention should be paid to anterior segment examination. The degree of edema and extent of corneal involvement should be measured. A tear involving DM may be observed, although corneal edema may preclude detailed evaluation of the posterior cornea. Seidel testing should be performed and, when positive, may indicate transudation of aqueous humor through the cornea, rather than a perforation. An ectatic appearance may be observed in either the involved or contralateral cornea.

IMAGING

AS-OCT can reveal rupture of DM as well as other corneal abnormalities including possible posterior stromal rupture, and can determine the extent of detachment from the rest of the cornea.[30,31] These findings may provide useful prognostic indicators, as eyes with larger DM detachments have been shown to require more time for resolution of hydrops and are subsequently at increased risk for scarring.[26] Likewise, the presence of a tear involving the posterior stroma may decrease the likelihood of spontaneous clearance.[31] AS-OCT of an edematous cornea may produce shadowing that can preclude detailed imaging of the posterior stroma, and repeat AS-OCT images may be necessary to fully visualize the extent of pathology (Fig. 37.2). In addition to aiding diagnosis, AS-OCT may be a useful approach for monitoring resolution after treatment. Serial AS-OCT images may be used to localize the DM (and possible posterior stromal) tear, demonstrate later reattachment of DM, follow resolution of edema, monitor intrastromal clefts, identify areas of absent DM, and visualize scar formation.

In vivo confocal microscopy (IVCM), another noninvasive imaging modality, allows for detailed evaluation of the cornea at the cellular level. Serial examination with IVCM of eyes with hydrops has been used to follow the presence of presumed inflammatory cells in the cornea.[32] Their presence may indicate a poorer prognosis. Although they are found only in a minority of cases of ACH, their prolonged presence beyond 4 weeks is associated with subsequent development of neovascularization. Confocal microscopy requires greater technical skill than other imaging techniques and may be particularly challenging to interpret in an eye with hydrops.

Imaging during ACH by ultrasound biomicroscopy (UBM) may reveal a DM tear, seen as the absence of the normally brightly intense DM spike, even when evaluation of the posterior cornea is precluded by other methods.[33,34] This is also a useful method for evaluation of intrastromal clefts and monitoring of DM reapposition.[33,34]

Corneal tomography provides detailed evaluation of the anterior and posterior corneal surfaces as well as assessment of the distribution of corneal thickness. Corneal tomography has characteristic findings in keratoconus and can be used to monitor progression of the disease. Tomography of the uninvolved eye may be particularly useful for diagnosing ACH in patients who present in the absence of a known history of ectasia.

Management

Many potential treatments have been tried to decrease the duration and visual impact of ACH. In the first half of the 20th century, treatment was aimed primarily at decreasing IOP, and was accomplished by sclerectomy, keratotomy, iridectomy, and frequent paracentesis.[3,35] Despite these

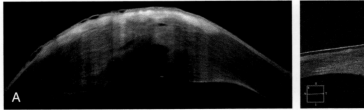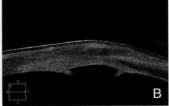

Fig. 37.2 (A) Anterior segment optical coherence tomography (AS-OCT) 10 days after presentation of acute corneal hydrops reveals stromal edema and bullae in the epithelium. Visualization of the posterior cornea is partially precluded by shadowing from the edema. (B) AS-OCT of the same cornea 5 weeks later shows improved corneal edema. There are tissue protrusions posteriorly in the area of the initial break representing scrolled Descemet membrane, possibly with adherent posterior stroma.

various treatments, it was noted that visual improvement seemed to follow the same course in most cases.[3] Although our understanding of ACH has improved, its treatment remains quite varied.

MEDICAL MANAGEMENT

Because many episodes of ACH resolve spontaneously within 2 to 4 months, early treatment is often conservative. There is a lack of case-control studies of topical treatments for ACH, and evidence of the efficacy of topical treatments is largely anecdotal.[6,18] Treatment should be started promptly, on the day of presentation. Initial management depends on the presence of Seidel positivity. In cases of aqueous leak, we recommend consideration of an aqueous suppressant and combination antibiotic–steroid ointment with pressure patching between instillation of medications. Patients should be followed closely, every few days, until the cornea is found to be Seidel negative. After resolution of the aqueous leak, this initial regimen may be discontinued.

Following management of Seidel positivity or in its absence, frequently used topical measures include ocular antihypertensive therapy, hypertonic saline, cycloplegia, and an antibiotic.[6] Topical corticosteroids have been added in some cases to inhibit the development of corneal neovascularization, but previous studies of ACH complicated by neovascularization did not demonstrate an inhibitory benefit from steroids.[18] Our preferred regimen is hypertonic saline 5% drops four times daily and hypertonic saline 5% ointment at bedtime. In patients with photophobia, cycloplegia may be helpful. In cases that do not resolve within the first few weeks, we recommend adding prednisolone acetate 1% four times a day. At this stage, we typically see patients every 1 to 3 weeks. Serial imaging is helpful in monitoring resolution. We recommend consideration of AS-OCT at each visit if possible. AS-OCT may reveal reattachment of DM and improvement in corneal edema in cases that resolve with conservative medical management. Imaging may also guide the need for a procedural intervention. In addition to AS-OCT, corneal tomography should be obtained in the fellow eye, including in cases without a known history of ectasia.

To summarize, because hydrops often improves without procedural interventions, we recommend conservative medical management with close follow-up initially, followed by evaluation every 1 to 3 weeks. Patients are evaluated for improvement based on symptoms, clinical examination, and imaging. If the edema fails to resolve, or if the level of corneal haze stabilizes without further improvement, procedural intervention may be considered.

SURGICAL MANAGEMENT

Although patients with keratoconus tend to have a very favorable prognosis following corneal transplant, the risk of endothelial rejection is increased in eyes that have a history of hydrops.[5,25] The risk of graft rejection is further increased by the presence of neovascularization.[36] The goal of procedural intervention is two-fold: to hasten DM reattachment and corneal deturgescence in cases with persistent edema, and to address scar formation after resolution of ACH.

If AS-OCT reveals that DM is detached and widely separated from the rest of the cornea, a pneumatic descemetopexy may be considered to aid in reattachment. The use of air or gas injection into the anterior chamber has been used to aid in reapposition of DM.[37–40] Early trials of acute hydrops treated with intracameral injection of air found that treatment shortened the period of corneal edema compared with conservative medical treatment.[37] Similar effects have been shown with perfluoropropane (C3F8) and sulfur hexafluoride (SF6) gas injection.[38–40] The benefit of gas injection is its longer duration in the anterior chamber, which may reduce the need for reinjection, but likewise patients require a longer duration of supine positioning and have increased risk for complications. Gases should be used at the isoexpansile concentration of 14% C3F8 or 20% SF6 with a typical volume of 0.2 mL injected into the anterior chamber.

There are two potential mechanisms for hastening resolution after air and gas injection.[37] One possibility is that the air or gas acts as a tamponade, preventing aqueous humor from entering the corneal stroma. The air or gas may also act by unrolling and reapproximating the DM tear to allow for faster migration of endothelial cells over the area of rupture.[37] Though air and gas may speed edema resolution by approximately 1 month, there appears to be no difference in final visual acuity or need for transplantation.[41] Adverse events after the use of air or gas are uncommon but include pupillary block glaucoma, intrastromal migration of gas, cataract, and endothelial cell loss. Patients should be followed closely until the bubble resorbs.[41]

Corneal compression sutures have been described as another method for attempting reapproximation of the rupture, both in isolation[42] and in combination with intracameral gas.[43,44] With either technique, corneal edema was found to resolve significantly faster, often within the first week, and appeared to offer particular benefits in corneas with intrastromal clefts.[42–44] Both full thickness[42,43] and pre-DM[44] sutures have been used with success. Identifying the DM tear may be improved intraoperatively with air injection. When visualized, 10-0 nylon sutures may be placed perpendicular to the tear. The number of sutures used is variable (between 2 and 13), partly depending on the extent of the tear.

New evidence suggests a potential role for intracameral injection of eye platelet-rich plasma (E-PRP) in the management of ACH.[45] E-PRP is an autologous conditioned plasma that contains high levels of growth factors and cytokines and has been used for the treatment of ocular surface disorders.[46] In a single case report using intracameral E-PRP during ACH, resolution of edema occurred within the first week.[45]

Treatment of visually debilitating scar formation after ACH resolution is traditionally accomplished with PKP. Success of PKP is reduced in keratoconus patients following ACH, and further reduced in patients who have developed corneal neovascularization.[5,25] Given the relatively young age of ACH patients and the significant risks of PKP, including long-term graft failure, the use of partial thickness corneal transplantation has gained popularity in recent years. Modifications of deep anterior lamellar keratoplasty (DALK) to replace stroma up to the pre-Descemet layer have been used successfully to restore vision in patients after ACH.[47–52]

Recent evidence suggests that early endothelial keratoplasty (EK) after an episode of acute hydrops may hasten deturgescence, restore vision, and may theoretically decrease the need for later PKP or DALK. Descemet stripping automated EK (DSAEK)[31,53–55] and DMEK[56,57] have been used successfully to resolve edema in ACH cases with large DM detachment or with suspected posterior stromal rupture. By restoring the normal posterior corneal anatomy and endothelial pump function, EK may decrease the duration of edema and reduce the formation of stromal scarring that would otherwise require more extensive transplantation. Following EK, vision may improve over the course of weeks, and visual acuity has been preserved without the need for further intervention. Patients may need a rigid contact lens to achieve best-corrected acuity.

Conclusion

Despite its relative rarity, ACH is a vision-threatening complication seen in the setting of corneal ectasia. It presents acutely, often without any obvious precipitating factor, with marked corneal edema, pain, and photophobia. The etiology of ACH is traditionally described as DM rupture in a susceptible cornea, but careful review of established literature as well as recently reported observations in keratoconus patients have suggested that the posterior stroma may be involved in some cases. Typically, ACH is self-limited with deturgescence occurring in weeks to months, and medical management may include the use of aqueous suppressants, hypertonic saline/ointment, cycloplegia, and topical steroids. Corneal imaging, including AS-OCT, can be helpful in disease assessment, including identifying possible posterior stromal rupture, and in documentation of resolution. Various procedural interventions, including intracameral injection of air or gas, compression sutures, and EK, have been employed to hasten recovery and reduce scar formation. Traditionally, patients have undergone PKP for vision-limiting scars, but recent case series have shown successful visual outcomes with modified DALK. Many of the current medical and surgical therapies used in the treatment of ACH have not been studied systematically, and further research is needed to determine optimal treatment strategies.

References

1. Fan Gaskin JC, Good WR, Jordan CA, Patel DV, McGhee CN. The Auckland keratoconus study: identifying predictors of acute corneal hydrops in keratoconus. *Clin Exp Optom.* 2013;96(2):208–213.
2. Nottingham J. *Practical Observations on Conical Cornea, and on the Short Sight, and Other Defects of Vision Connected With It.* London: John Churchill; 1854.
3. Rychener RO, Kirby DB. Acute hydrops of the cornea complicating keratoconus. *Arch Ophthalmol.* 1940;24(2):326–343.
4. Barsam A, Petrushkin H, Brennan N, et al. Acute corneal hydrops in keratoconus: a national prospective study of incidence and management. *Eye (Lond).* 2015;29(4):469–474.
5. Tuft SJ, Gregory WM, Buckley RJ. Acute corneal hydrops in keratoconus. *Ophthalmology.* 1994;101(10):1738–1744.
6. Grewal S, Laibson PR, Cohen EJ, Rapuano CJ. Acute hydrops in the corneal ectasias: associated factors and outcomes. *Trans Am Ophthalmol Soc.* 1999;97:187–198.
7. Sridhar MS, Mahesh S, Bansal AK, Nutheti R, Rao GN. Pellucid marginal corneal degeneration. *Ophthalmology.* 2004;111(6):1102–1107.
8. Barsam A, Brennan N, Petrushkin H, et al. Case-control study of risk factors for acute corneal hydrops in keratoconus. *Br J Ophthalmol.* 2017;101(4):499–502.
9. McMonnies CW. Mechanisms for acute corneal hydrops and perforation. *Eye Contact Lens.* 2014;40(4):257–264.
10. Fuentes E, Sandali O, El Sanharawi M, et al. Anatomic predictive factors of acute corneal hydrops in keratoconus: an optical coherence tomography study. *Ophthalmology.* 2015;122(8):1653–1659.
11. Nicoli C, Wainsztein RD, Trotta LP. Corneal topography of spontaneous perforation of acute hydrops in keratoconus. *J Cataract Refract Surg.* 1999;25(6):871–872.
12. Farooq AV, Soin K, Williamson S, Joslin CE, Cortina MS, Tu EY. Corneal ectasia and hydrops in ocular hypotony: the corneal crease. *Cornea.* 2015;34(9):1152–1156.
13. Sharma N, Maharana PK, Jhanji V, Vajpayee RB. Management of acute corneal hydrops in ectatic corneal disorders. *Curr Opin Ophthalmol.* 2012;23(4):317–323.
14. Chi HH, Katzin HM, Teng CC. Histopathology of keratoconus. *Am J Ophthalmol.* 1956;42:847–860.
15. Stone DL, Kenyon KR, Stark WJ. Ultrastructure of keratoconus with healed hydrops. *Am J Ophthalmol.* 1976;82(3):450–458.
16. Ueno H, Matuzawa A, Kumagai Y, Takagi H, Ueno S. Imaging of a severe case of acute hydrops in a patient with keratoconus using anterior segment optical coherence tomography. *Case Rep Ophthalmol.* 2012;3(3):304–310.
17. Al Suhaibani AH, Al-Rajhi AA, Al-Motowa S, Wagoner MD. Inverse relationship between age and severity and sequelae of acute corneal hydrops associated with keratoconus. *Br J Ophthalmol.* 2007;91(7):984–985.
18. Rowson NJ, Dart JK, Buckley RJ. Corneal neovascularisation in acute hydrops. *Eye (Lond).* 1992;6 (Pt 4):404–406.
19. Feder RS, Wilhelmus KR, Vold SD, O'Grady RB. Intrastromal clefts in keratoconus patients with hydrops. *Am J Ophthalmol.* 1998;126(1):9–16.
20. McMonnies CW, Boneham GC. Corneal responses to intraocular pressure elevations in keratoconus. *Cornea.* 2010;29(7):764–770.
21. Turner DC, Girkin CA, Downs JC. The magnitude of intraocular pressure elevation associated with eye rubbing. *Ophthalmology.* 2019;126(1):171–172.
22. Parker JS, Birbal RS, Van dijk K, Oellerich S, Dapena I, Melles GRJ. Are Descemet membrane ruptures the root cause of corneal hydrops in keratoconic eyes? *Am J Ophthalmol.* 2019;205:147–152.
23. Wolter JR, Henderson JW, Clahassey EG. Ruptures of Descemet's membrane in keratoconus causing acute hydrops and posterior keratoconus. *Am J Ophthalmol.* 1967;63(6):1689–1692.

24. Bains RA, Stein RM, Tokarewicz AC, Willis NR, Heathcote JG. Posterior stromal changes following acute corneal hydrops in keratoconus. *Can J Ophthalmol.* 1994;29(1):22–24.

25. Basu S, Reddy JC, Vaddavalli PK, Vemuganti GK, Sangwan VS. Long-term outcomes of penetrating keratoplasty for keratoconus with resolved corneal hydrops. *Cornea.* 2012;31(6):615–620.

26. Basu S, Vaddavalli PK, Vemuganti GK, Ali MH, Murthy SI. Anterior segment optical coherence tomography features of acute corneal hydrops. *Cornea.* 2012;31(5):479–485.

27. Rosa RH Jr, Bloomer MM, Gombos DS, et al. Ectatic disorders: keratoconus. In: Rosa Jr, et al. (eds). *Basic and Clinical Science Course (BCSC) Section 4: Ophthalmic Pathology and Intraocular Tumors.* American Academy of Ophthalmology; 2018:95

28. Loh IP, Fan Gaskin JC, Sherwin T, McGhee CNJ. Extreme Descemet's membrane rupture with hydrops in keratoconus: clinical and histological manifestations. *Am J Ophthalmol Case Rep.* 2018;10:271–275.

29. Thomasy SM, Raghunathan VK, Winkler M, et al. Elastic modulus and collagen organization of the rabbit cornea: epithelium to endothelium. *Acta Biomater.* 2014;10(2):785–791.

30. Gokul A, Vellara HR, Patel DV. Advanced anterior segment imaging in keratoconus: a review. *Clin Experiment Ophthalmol.* 2018;46(2):122–132.

31. Blitzer AL, Liles CA, Harocopos GJ, Reidy JJ, Farooq AV. Severe corneal hydrops with suspected posterior stromal rupture managed with ultra-thin Descemet-stripping automated endothelial keratoplasty. *Cornea.* 2021;40(4):513–515.

32. Lockington D, Fan Gaskin JC, McGhee CN, Patel DV. A prospective study of acute corneal hydrops by in vivo confocal microscopy in a New Zealand population with keratoconus. *Br J Ophthalmol.* 2014;98(9):1296–1302.

33. Nakagawa T, Maeda N, Okazaki N, Hori Y, Nishida K, Tano Y. Ultrasound biomicroscopic examination of acute hydrops in patients with keratoconus. *Am J Ophthalmol.* 2006;141(6):1134–1136.

34. Sharma N, Mannan R, Jhanji V, et al. Ultrasound biomicroscopy-guided assessment of acute corneal hydrops. *Ophthalmology.* 2011;118(11):2166–2171.

35. Berner GE. Conical cornea complicated by acute ectasia. *Am J Ophthalmol.* 1934;17:22.

36. Belghmaidi S, Hajji I, Ennassiri W, Benhaddou R, Baha Ali T, Moutaouakil A. [Management of corneal neovascularization prior to corneal transplantation: report of 112 cases]. *J Fr Ophthalmol.* 2016;39(6):515–520.

37. Miyata K, Tsuji H, Tanabe T, Mimura Y, Amano S, Oshika T. Intracameral air injection for acute hydrops in keratoconus. *Am J Ophthalmol.* 2002;133(6):750–752.

38. Shah SG, Sridhar MS, Sangwan VS. Acute corneal hydrops treated by intracameral injection of perfluoropropane (C3F8) gas. *Am J Ophthalmol.* 2005;139(2):368–370.

39. Panda A, Aggarwal A, Madhavi P, et al. Management of acute corneal hydrops secondary to keratoconus with intracameral injection of sulfur hexafluoride (SF6). *Cornea.* 2007;26(9):1067–1069.

40. Basu S, Vaddavalli PK, Ramappa M, Shah S, Murthy SI, Sangwan VS. Intracameral perfluoropropane gas in the treatment of acute corneal hydrops. *Ophthalmology.* 2011;118(5):934–939.

41. Fan Gaskin JC, Patel DV, McGhee CN. Acute corneal hydrops in keratoconus—new perspectives. *Am J Ophthalmol.* 2014;157(5):921–928.

42. García-Albisua AM, Davila-Avila N, Hernandez-Quintela E, et al. Visual and anatomic results after sole full-thickness sutures for acute corneal hydrops. *Cornea.* 2020;39(5):661–665.

43. Rajaraman R, Singh S, Raghavan A, Karkhanis A. Efficacy and safety of intracameral perfluoropropane (C3F8) tamponade and compression sutures for the management of acute corneal hydrops. *Cornea.* 2009;28(3):317–320.

44. Yahia Chérif H, Gueudry J, Afriat M, et al. Efficacy and safety of pre-Descemet's membrane sutures for the management of acute corneal hydrops in keratoconus. *Br J Ophthalmol.* 2015;99(6):773–777.

45. Alio JL, Toprak I, Rodriguez AE. Treatment of severe keratoconus hydrops with intracameral platelet-rich plasma injection. *Cornea.* 2019;38(12):1595–1598.

46. Alio JL, Rodriguez AE, Wróbeldudzińska D. Eye platelet-rich plasma in the treatment of ocular surface disorders. *Curr Opin Ophthalmol.* 2015;26(4):325–332.

47. Ramamurthi S, Ramaesh K. Surgical management of healed hydrops: a novel modification of deep anterior lamellar keratoplasty. *Cornea.* 2011;30(2):180–183.

48. Anwar HM, Anwar M. Pre-Descemetic dissection for healed hydrops—judicious use of air and fluid. *Cornea.* 2011;30(12):1502–1509.

49. Nanavaty MA, Daya SM. Outcomes of deep anterior lamellar keratoplasty in keratoconic eyes with previous hydrops. *Br J Ophthalmol*. 2012;96(10):1304–1309.
50. Fuest M, Mehta JS. Strategies for deep anterior lamellar keratoplasty after hydrops in keratoconus. *Eye Contact Lens*. 2018;44(2):69–76.
51. Zhao Z, Li J, Zheng Q, Lin W, Jhanji V, Chen W. Wet-peeling technique of deep anterior lamellar keratoplasty with hypotonic water and blunt dissection for healed hydrops. *Cornea*. 2017;36(3):386–389.
52. Goweida MB, Sobhy M, Seifelnasr M, Liu C. Peripheral pneumatic dissection and scar peeling to complete deep anterior lamellar keratoplasty in eyes with healed hydrops. *Cornea*. 2019;38(4):504–508.
53. Gorovoy MS, Gorovoy IR, Ullman S, Gorovoy JB. Descemet stripping automated endothelial keratoplasty for spontaneous Descemet membrane detachment in a patient with osteogenesis imperfecta. *Cornea*. 2012;31(7):832–835.
54. Kolomeyer AM, Chu DS. Descemet stripping endothelial keratoplasty in a patient with keratoglobus and chronic hydrops secondary to a spontaneous Descemet membrane tear. *Case Rep Ophthalmol Med*. 2013;2013:697403.
55. Palioura S, Chodosh J, Pineda R. A novel approach to the management of a progressive Descemet membrane tear in a patient with keratoglobus and acute hydrops. *Cornea*. 2013;32(3):355–358.
56. Tu EY. Descemet membrane endothelial keratoplasty patch for persistent corneal hydrops. *Cornea*. 2017;36(12):1559–1561.
57. Bachmann B, Händel A, Siebelmann S, Matthaei M, Cursiefen C. Mini-Descemet membrane endothelial keratoplasty for the early treatment of acute corneal hydrops in keratoconus. *Cornea*. 2019;38(8):1043–1048.

Case Studies

Case Studies

CHAPTER 38

Central Keratoconus: Case Study

Luis Izquierdo Jr. ■ Mauricio Vélez

Case Study

A 27-year-old female presented for follow-up for keratoconus (KC) after collagen cross-linking in both eyes 6 months previously. Her best-corrected visual acuity (BCVA) on the Snellen chart was 20/50 in both eyes with spectacles. Manifest refraction was −9.75 cyl −5.75 × 60 and −1.25 cyl −2.75 × 150, respectively. Central cornea thicknesses were 486 and 502 microns, respectively. A slit-lamp examination revealed the presence of a Fleischer ring in her right eye and a normal examination in her left eye.

Corneal tomography was obtained via the Pentacam Comprehensive Eye Scanner (OCU-LUS Optikgeräte GmbH, Wetzlar, Germany). Her right eye Fig. 38.1 showed a moderate central hyperprolate (nipple-type) KC (level 4 as per Amsler-Krumeich classification) with a K_{max} 55.62 diopters (D) and over 5 D of irregular astigmatism. The thinnest pachymetry reading was abnormal at 486 microns, and the inferior-superior (I-S) index was at 5.26 D. The anterior and posterior corneal elevation maps were abnormal Fig. 38.2. The Belin-Ambrósio Enhanced Ectasia

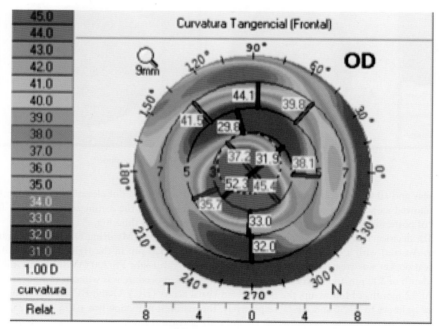

Fig. 38.1 Moderate central keratoconus.

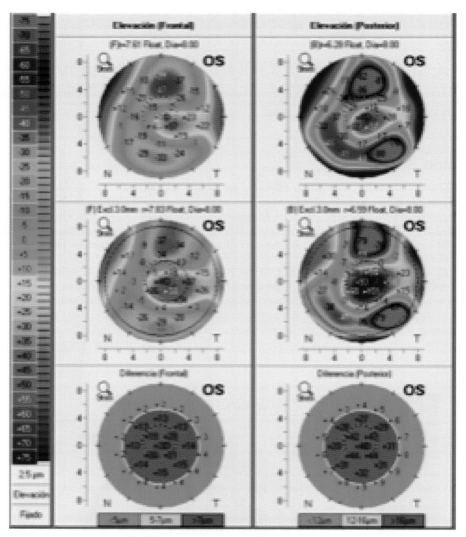

Fig. 38.2 Abnormal elevations maps (anterior and posterior).

Display and all tomographic indices for KC were positive. The anterior elevation map in her left eye showed an abnormal elevation, with a peak of 15 microns in the 3-mm zone Fig. 38.3. This area of posterior elevation coincided with the location of corneal thinning.

The decision was made to implant a circular intrastromal ring (MyoRing DIOPTEX GmbH, Linz, Austria) with a diameter of 5 mm and thickness of 320 μm in the right eye Fig. 38.4. A corneal pocket was created with the femtosecond laser WaveLight FS 200 (WaveLight GmbH) at a depth of 300 μm and with a diameter of 8.5 mm. The procedure was without complications.

At 12 months of follow-up, the uncorrected visual acuity (UCVA) and BCVA had improved in her right eye to 20/50 and 20/25, respectively. The manifest refraction was +0.75 cyl –1.25 × 75. K_{max} by Pentacam was reduced for 7.2 D, and central corneal thickness remained unchanged at 475 microns.

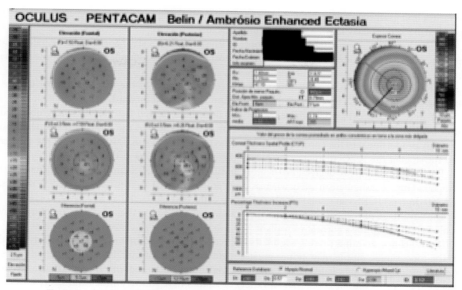

Fig. 38.3 Abnormal D Value and anterior elevation map showed at the BAD Display.

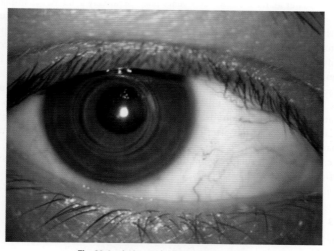

Fig. 38.4 360 circular Intrastromal Ring.

Discussion

KC often leads to high myopia and astigmatism with significant visual impairment.[1,2]

If spectacle or contact lens correction is not feasible in cases of advanced KC, surgical options include deep anterior lamellar keratoplasty, intracorneal ring segments (ICRSs), or penetrating keratoplasty. Although penetrating keratoplasty is associated with a high success rate, there can be significant complications including immune rejection, secondary cataract, glaucoma, microbial keratitis, and graft dehiscence.[3-6] Moreover, visual rehabilitation or recovery of visual acuity after penetrating keratoplasty may be slow and unsatisfactory.

ICRS implantation represents another option. These segments are made of polymethyl methacrylate (PMMA) and are implanted within the corneal stroma to induce a change in the geometry and the refractive power of the corneal tissue.

ICRS implantation induces flattening of the central portion of the anterior corneal surface, and the peripheral area adjacent to the ring insertion is displaced forward.

Theoretical models based on finite element analysis have proven that the flattening observed after ICRS implantation is directly proportional to the thickness of the implanted segment and inversely proportional to the corneal diameter of the implantation site. This means that the thicker and the smaller the ICRS diameter, the higher the corneal flattening effect.[7]

The short arc length (90 degrees, 120 degrees, and 130 degrees) ICRS can correct low-to-moderate compound myopic astigmatism safely, whereas larger arc length (210 degrees, 340 degrees, 355 degrees, and 360 degrees) ICRS can result in higher spherical correction.

The advantage of corneal rings is that they can improve vision in these patients and may delay or obviate the need for a corneal transplant.[8-10]

In oval cones, asymmetric ring segments or even single ring segments placed inferiorly based on the topographic profile may induce greater regularization. However, in cases of central cones, the use of long arc rings is likely to produce a maximum flattening effect. Circular rings were proposed for such cases in 2008,[11] and a variety of studies have shown efficacy and safety of these rings with no loss of BCVA related to implantation.[12,13]

It should be noted, however, that implantation of corneal rings does not stop the progression of KC. Vega-Estrada et al. have shown at 5 years postoperatively after ICRS implantation a significant regression of the positive effect, which negatively affected the vision of young patients.[14]

It is for this reason that corneal cross-linking (CXL) as an adjunct to ICRS implantation may be necessary to halt the disease. The application of CXL significantly increases corneal rigidity immediately after treatment, with an 80% increase of Young's modulus and a 450% increase in the thinner human cornea at 6% strain.[1,2,15,16]

In this case study, we have a patient with advanced and progressive KC (grade 4). Our approach was to perform the cross-linking first, followed in 6 months by ICRS implantation. Once stabilization after cross-linking is achieved, rings can safely be placed.[2] We have not had difficulty implanting corneal rings after cross-linking either with the use of a femtosecond laser or with the manual technique.

In this case, we chose a circular ring because it better corrects central KC and achieves a more significant flattening effect.

References

1. Rabinowitz YS. Keratoconus. *Surv Ophthalmol*. 1998;42(4):297–319.
2. Henriquez MA, Izquierdo L. Jr. Bernilla C, McCarthy M. Corneal collagen cross-linking before Ferrara intrastromal corneal ring implantation for the treatment of progressive keratoconus. *Cornea*. 2012;31(7):740–745.
3. Brierly SC, Izquierdo L. Jr, Mannis MJ. Penetrating keratoplasty for keratoconus. *Cornea*. 2000;19(3):329–332.
4. Shetty R, D'Souza S, Khamar P, Ghosh A, Nuijts RMMA, Sethu S. Biochemical markers and alterations in keratoconus. *Asia Pac J Ophthalmol*. 2020;9(6):533–540.
5. Henriquez MA, Cerrate M, Hadid MG, Cañola-Ramirez LA, Hafezi F, Izquierdo L Jr. Comparison of eye-rubbing effect in keratoconic eyes and healthy eyes using Scheimpflug analysis and a dynamic bidirectional applanation device. *J Cataract Refract Surg*. 2019;45(8):1156–1162.

6. Moon J, Yoon CH, Kim MK, Oh JY. The incidence and outcomes of recurrence of infection after therapeutic penetrating keratoplasty for medically-uncontrolled infectious keratitis. *J Clin Med.* 2020;9(11):3696.

7. Moscovici BK, Rodrigues PF, Rodrigues RAM, et al. Evaluation of keratoconus progression and visual improvement after intrastromal corneal ring segments implantation: a retrospective study. *Eur J Ophthalmol.* 2021;31(6):3483–3489.

8. Izquierdo L. Jr, Mannis MJ, Mejías Smith JA, Henriquez MA. Effectiveness of intrastromal corneal ring implantation in the treatment of adult patients with keratoconus: a systematic review. *J Refract Surg.* 2019;35(3):191–200.

9. Lisa C, Fernández-Vega Cueto L, Poo-López A, Madrid-Costa D, Alfonso JF. Long-term follow-up of intrastromal corneal ring segments (210-degree arc length) in central keratoconus with high corneal asphericity. *Cornea.* 2017;36(11):1325–1330.

10. Yousif MO, Said AMA. Comparative study of 3 intracorneal implant types to manage central keratoconus. *J Cataract Refract Surg.* 2018;44(3):295–305.

11. Daxer A, Mahmoud H, Venkateswaran RS. Intracorneal continuous ring implantation for keratoconus: one-year follow-up. *J Cataract Refract Surg.* 2010;36(8):1296–1302.

12. Mahmood H, Venkateswaran RS, Daxer A. Implantation of a complete corneal ring in an intrastromal pocket for keratoconus. *J Refract Surg.* 2011;27(1):63–68.

13. Izquierdo L. Jr, Rodríguez AM, Sarquis RA, Altamirano D, Henriquez MA. Intracorneal circular ring implant with femtosecond laser: pocket versus tunnel. *Eur J Ophthalmol.* 2022;32(1):176–182.

14. Vega-Estrada A, Alió JL, Plaza-Puche AB. Keratoconus progression after intrastromal corneal ring segment implantation in young patients: five-year follow-up. *J Cataract Refract Surg.* 2015;41(6):1145–1152.

15. Seiler T. Keratoconus and corneal crosslinking. *J Cataract Refract Surg.* 2021;47(3):289–290.

16. Saleh S, Koo EB, Lambert SR, Manche EE. Outcomes after corneal crosslinking for keratoconus in children and young adults. *Cornea.* 2021. doi:10.1097/ICO.0000000000002730.

CHAPTER 39

Very Early Keratoconus: Case Study

Shyam Patel ■ W. Barry Lee

KEY CONCEPTS

- This chapter reviews a case of keratoconus in one eye and early keratoonus in the contralateral eye.
- A review of corneal imaging systems and their abmormal parameters to detect keratoconus is performed.

Case Study

A 40-year-old male presented for follow-up for keratoconus and for evaluation for corneal collagen cross-linking in his right eye. His best-corrected visual acuity on the Snellen chart was 20/20 in both eyes with a rigid gas permeable lens in his right eye and spectacle correction in his left eye. Manifest refraction was −8.50 + 5.00 × 180 and −2.25 + 1.75 × 25 for right and left eye, respectively. Central cornea thicknesses were 487 and 575 microns for right and left eye, respectively. Slit-lamp examination showed apical thinning with a Fleischer ring in his right eye and a normal examination in his left eye.

Corneal topography via the Galilei Dual Scheimpflug topographer (Ziemer Ophthalmic Systems, Port, Switzerland) was obtained. His right eye (Fig. 39.1) showed clinical keratoconus with a K_{max} over 60 diopters (D) and over 6 D of irregular astigmatism with significant inferior thinning and steepening. The thinnest pachymetry reading was abnormal at 466 microns, and the I-S index was elevated at 10.26 D. The elevation maps of both the anterior and posterior cornea were abnormal. The keratoconus probability (KP) and keratoconus prediction index (KPI) were both 100%. Collagen cross-linking was planned for the right eye as topography showed evidence of progression.

Corneal topography of the left eye (Fig. 39.2) showed inferior steepening corresponding to the thinnest corneal thickness with a borderline I-S index at 1.51 D and an elevated KP and KPI. The thinnest corneal thickness was 559 microns. The posterior elevation map showed an abnormal elevation of 15 microns in the 3 mm zone. This area of posterior elevation coincided with the area of corneal thinning. The anterior elevation maps were normal. The percent probability of keratoconus (PPK) was abnormal at 42.9%. Given these findings on topography, he was diagnosed with subclinical keratoconus (SCK) in his left eye. The plan for this eye was continued observation.

Introduction

Early keratoconus (keratoconus suspect) can be classified as either SCK or *forme fruste* keratoconus (FFKC). These terms are frequently interchanged in the literature. However, there is consensus that the specific term FFKC should only be used when the eye in question combines normal topography, normal slit-lamp examination, and keratoconus in the fellow eye. SCK refers to those eyes with normal slit-lamp examination, topographic/tomographic signs of keratoconus

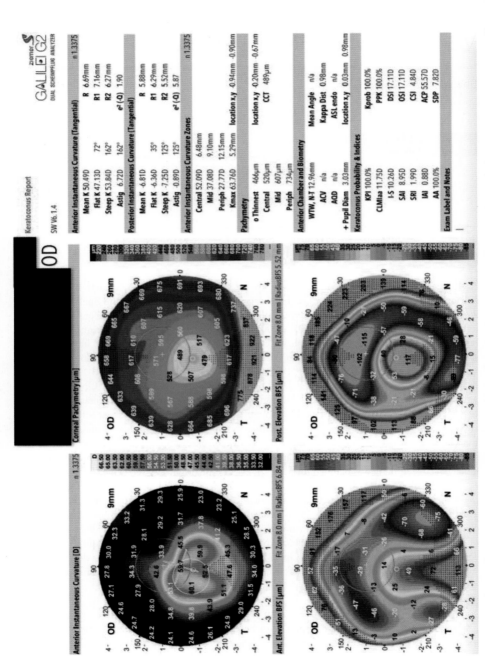

Keratoconus Report

SW V6.1.4

OD

GALILEI G2
ziemer
DUAL SCHEIMPFLUG ANALYZER

Anterior Instantaneous Curvature [D]   n 1.3375

Corneal Pachymetry [µm]

Ant. Elevation BFS [µm]   Fit Zone 8.0 mm | Radius BFS 6.84 mm

Post. Elevation BFS [µm]   Fit Zone 8.0 mm | Radius BFS 5.52 mm

Anterior Instantaneous Curvature (Tangential)   n 1.3375

		R	6.69mm
Mean K	50.49D		
Flat K	47.13D	R1	7.16mm
Steep K	53.84D	R2	6.27mm
Astig	6.72D	e²(-Q)	1.90

Posterior Instantaneous Curvature (Tangential)

		R	5.88mm
Mean K	-6.81D		
Flat K	-6.36D	R1	6.29mm
Steep K	-7.25D	R2	5.52mm
Astig	-0.89D	e²(-Q)	5.87

Anterior Instantaneous Curvature Zones   n 1.3375

Central	52.09D	6.48mm
Mid	37.08D	9.10mm
Periph	27.77D	12.15mm
Kmax 63.76D	5.29mm	

Pachymetry

o Thinnest	466µm	location x,y	-0.94mm	-0.90mm
Central	520µm	CCT	489µm	
Mid	607µm			
Periph	734µm			

Anterior Chamber and Biometry

WTW, N-T 12.96mm	Mean Angle	n/a
ACV n/a	Kappa Dist	0.98mm
AOD n/a	ASL endo	n/a
+ Pupil Diam 3.03mm	location x,y	0.03mm	0.98mm

Keratoconus Probability & Indices

	Kprob 100.0%
KPI 100.0%	PPK 100.0%
CLMIaa 11.75D	DSI 17.10D
I-S 10.26D	ISI 17.11D
SAI 8.95D	CSI 4.84D
SRI 1.99D	ACP 55.57D
IAI 0.88D	SDP 7.82D
AA 100.0%	

Exam Label and Notes

Fig. 39.1 Galilei topographic image of a right eye with clinical keratoconus. The scan shows steepening on the anterior instantaneous curvature map with steepening on both anterior and posterior elevation maps.

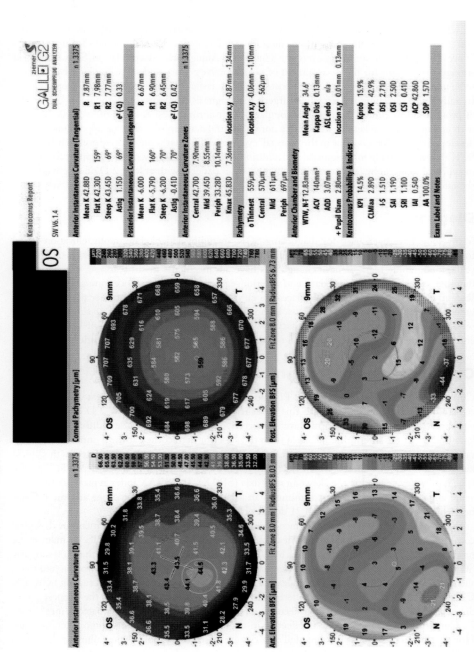

Fig. 39.2 Galilei topographic image of a left eye with subclinical keratoconus. Anterior instantaneous curvature and anterior elevation maps show no abnormalities. Posterior elevation map shows an abnormal elevation of 15 microns within the 3-mm zone.

or suspicious topography (but not enough to define as keratoconus), and keratoconus in the fellow eye. Without symptoms or definite clinical findings, SCK and FFKC can be challenging to detect and to differentiate from normal eyes.

Clinical keratoconus in the fellow eye represents the primary risk factor for SCK and FFKC. The correct diagnosis is obtained when screening for risk factors for SCK, and ranges from 1% to 6% of eyes being screened for myopic refractive surgery.[1-4] Along with a deep ablation, SCK is the next strongest risk factor for the development of postrefractive ectasia, and some studies have found it to be present in up to 88% of eyes with postrefractive ectasia.[5,6] The diagnosis is purely topographic. In addition to screening for refractive surgery, the diagnosis is important, as there is a higher rate of progression to clinical keratoconus compared with normal eyes. A study of over 100 patients with unilateral clinical keratoconus with a normal contralateral eye showed that approximately 50% developed clinical keratoconus in the "normal" eye, suggesting that some of these eyes may have had SCK that was initially misdiagnosed.[7] In addition to refractive surgery, there is support for acquiring corneal topography for diagnosing keratoconus in patients with at least 2 D of astigmatism, as the rates of clinical keratoconus and SCK in this population are 6.3% and 7.8%, respectively.[8]

Diagnosis

Many tools have been used for diagnosing SCK, including videokeratography, elevation-based topography, corneal biomechanics, wavefront aberrations, and various scoring systems. Over the years, topographic markers have changed, as have advancements in slit scanning and Scheimpflug imaging, posterior corneal data, and anterior segment optical coherence tomography (OCT). Recently, more emphasis has been placed on elevation-based topography rather than curvature-based topography and corneal thickness. It should be emphasized that there is no single parameter or technology that has a 100% sensitivity and specificity (area under the curve of 1.00) for SCK, and many experts suggest the approach of using multiple parameters and modalities.

Curvature-Based Topography

Curvature-based topography includes Placido imaging and videokeratography: a variety of indices are used to diagnose SCK with this modality. Central keratometry >47.2 D or >1 D compared with the contralateral normal eye is suggestive of SCK. An I-S index (difference in mean keratometry of the inferior hemicornea from the superior hemicornea at the 3-mm corneal ring) ranging from 1.4 to 1.9 also supports SCK. Anything greater than 1.9 is associated with clinical keratoconus. Another measurement that may have to be manually calculated depending on the topography device used is the skewed radial axis (SRAX). The SRAX index represents the most acute angle between the steepest semimeridian axis in the superior hemicornea and the inferior hemicornea. Any value greater than 21 degrees rules out keratoconus.

KISA% index is a calculation that incorporates many of the values previously mentioned: central corneal power, I-S index, simulated corneal astigmatism, and SRAX index. The KISA% index is the product of these four variables multiplied by 0.3. Any value greater than 60 and less than 100 supports SCK, whereas a value greater than 100 suggests clinical keratoconus. Additional formulas and tools, such as the Cone and Location Map Index (CLMI), may also assist providers in detecting SCK. The CLMI is an index that refers to the difference of the average corneal curvature in the steepest 2-mm diameter circle from the average corneal curvature of the area outside of the designated 2-mm circle.[9]

Curvature-based topography is effective in diagnosing and confirming clinical keratoconus. However, it can miss SCK. The downfall of curvature-based topography is the failure to characterize the posterior cornea and to provide elevation-based maps. It is now evident that the posterior cornea can show elevation in early SCK before showing any abnormalities on curvature-based topography. Therefore the trend has been toward elevation-based topography and the use of multiple modalities in recent years, especially when screening for laser refractive surgery.

Elevation-Based Topography

The main advantages of elevation-based topography are that it includes a broader image of the cornea (9 mm) and provides posterior corneal data with corneal thickness. Posterior corneal changes that would be missed on curvature-based topography have been shown to be associated with SCK.

Two techniques can provide elevation-based topography: slit scanning and Scheimpflug imaging. In the slit-scanning technique two scans of 20 projections are performed on both sides of the eye. The Scheimpflug image is created by a rotating camera that moves around the optical axis. The Orbscan II (Bausch and Lomb, Inc., Rochester, NY), the Pentacam (OCULUS Inc., Arlington, WA), and the Galilei instruments all employ Scheimpflug imaging.

ORBSCAN

The Orbscan II was one of the first slit-scanning topographies on the market. It provides pachymetry, curvature, and elevation values simultaneously. In 2014, Jafarinasab et al. conducted a study using the Orbscan II on patients with clinical keratoconus, SCK, and normal eyes.[10] Many variables, such as anterior and posterior best-fit-spheres, were statistically significantly different between SCK and normal eyes. For example, mean posterior corneal elevation was 106.80 microns, 36.60 microns, and 22.80 microns in clinical keratoconus, SCK, and normal eyes, respectively.[10] However, it was difficult to find a specific cutoff in either anterior or posterior corneal elevation that had a high sensitivity and specificity in detecting SCK (Table 39.1).

In addition, the Screening Corneal Objective Risk of Ectasia (SCORE) analyzer is an algorithm that incorporates data from the Orbscan to calculate a score. A positive score indicates subclinical or clinical keratoconus. Multiple variables are used, including the I-S index, thinnest corneal thickness, and maximum posterior elevation. The SCORE analyzer has been found to have good sensitivity and specificity in differentiating SCK, approaching 92% to 96%.[11]

GALILEI

The Galilei Dual Scheimpflug system provides traditional Placido-based imaging along with pachymetry, net corneal power, anterior chamber depth, and elevation maps. It also provides a specialized keratoconus report (see Figs. 39.1 and 39.2) that is helpful for screening and monitoring keratoconus and provides values such as KP, KPI, CLMI, and PPK.

Feizi et al. conducted a study in 2016 assessing the Galilei's predictive ability for differentiating subclinical and clinical keratoconus from normal eyes.[12] All 24 studied variables were effective (area under curve > 0.80) in differentiating clinical keratoconus from normal eyes using the Galilei. However, only four variables remained effective in distinguishing SCK from normal eyes. These four parameters were the radii of both the anterior and posterior best-fit-sphere, flat keratometry, and mean keratometry (see Table 39.1). The radius of the posterior best-fit-sphere cutoff of 6.27 had a sensitivity and specificity of 87%, and the highest area under the curve. The most sensitive parameter (sensitivity of 91.3%) was the maximum posterior elevation of 12.5 microns in a 5-mm zone.[12] Our case, as seen in Fig. 39.2, had a maximum posterior elevation of 15 microns in the left eye. No single set of indices (elevation, surface, pachymetric, and keratometric indices) could completely detect SCK. Combining three of the sets (elevation, surface, and keratometric data) showed a sensitivity of 97.7% and specificity of 84.6% with an area under the curve of 0.952.[12] This combination was stronger than any of the other combinations studied.

Values such as the KP and KPI are stronger at detecting clinical keratoconus than SCK. Both of these values had higher specificity with poor sensitivity for SCK, which is not ideal for screening (see Table 39.1). A KPI above 5.0 and KP above 11.6 had sensitivities of 56.5% and

TABLE 39.1 ■ **Sensitivities and Specificities of Various Parameters for the Diagnosis of Subclinical Keratoconus**

Parameter	Device(s)	Cutoff Value	Sensitivity	Specificity	AUC
Maximum anterior elevation in 5-mm zone[12]	Galilei	4.5	82.6	36.1	0.615
Maximum posterior elevation in 5-mm zone[12]	Galilei	12.5	91.3	38.3	0.619
Keratoconus probability[12]	Galilei	11.6	39.1	95.5	0.669
Maximum anterior elevation in 3-mm zone[12]	Galilei	3.5	87	43.6	0.678
Keratoconus prediction index[12]	Galilei	5	56.5	83.5	0.71
Maximum posterior elevation in 3-mm zone[12]	Galilei	11.5	60.9	77.4	0.718
Radius of anterior best-fit-sphere (mm)[12]	Galilei	7.645	82.6	69.7	0.828
Mean keratometry[12]	Galilei	45.49	65.2	94.7	0.833
Flat keratometry[12]	Galilei	43.8	82.6	72.9	0.84
Radius of posterior best sphere (mm)[12]	Galilei	6.27	87	87.1	0.892
Three-model structure (elevation + surface indices + pachymetry data)[12]	Galilei	Not available	93.8	80.8	0.936
Three-model structure (elevation + surface indices + keratometry data)[12]	Galilei	Not available	97.7	84.6	0.952
Posterior corneal elevation[10]	Orbscan	≥14	92.86	9.93	0.698
Anterior corneal elevation[10]	Orbscan	≥10	75	31.21	0.698
Posterior corneal elevation[10]	Orbscan	≥27	75	57.45	Not available
Anterior corneal elevation[10]	Orbscan	≥14	64.29	78.01	Not available
Fifth order vertical coma aberration of front cornea[17]	Pentacam	≥0.023	70.6	61.8	0.72
Index surface variance[17]	Pentacam	≥22	74.5	61.8	0.8
Index vertical asymmetry[17]	Pentacam	≥0.14	82.3	73.2	0.86
BAD_D[17]	Pentacam	≥1.54	81.1	73.2	0.86
BAD_D + IVA + ISV + fifth order vertical coma aberration of front cornea[17]	Pentacam	Cutoffs are displayed above	83.6	96.9	0.96
Inferior superior value[22]	Pentacam	0.51	53.3	75	0.599
Index height decentration[22]	Pentacam	0.0075	76.7	51.7	0.604
Index vertical asymmetry[22]	Pentacam	0.115	70	66.7	0.722
Pachymetry apex[22]	Pentacam	531	66.7	75	0.732

TABLE 39.1 ■ **Sensitivities and Specificities of Various Parameters for the Diagnosis of Subclinical Keratoconus**—(Continued)

Parameter	Device(s)	Cutoff Value	Sensitivity	Specificity	AUC
ART_{max}[22]	Pentacam	363.5	56.7	88.3	0.739
BAD_D[22]	Pentacam	1.01	80	66.7	0.754
IVA + pachymetry apex + IHD + ART_{max} + ISV[22]	Pentacam	Cutoffs are displayed above	83	83	0.86
13 Variables[22,a]	Pentacam+ SD OCT	See reference	100	100	1
Epithelium standard deviation[22]	SD OCT	1.35	73.7	58.2	0.671
Epithelium minimum-maximum[22]	SD OCT	−6.5	68.4	65.5	0.676
11 Variables[22,a]	SD OCT	See reference	89	89	0.96

[a]References for each variable are denoted by superscript following the parameter and are listed under the References. Please see referenced paper for more information.
ART_{max}, Ambrósio relational thickness maximum; *AUC*, area under curve; *BAD_D*, Belin Ambrósio Enhanced Ectasia Display Deviation; *IHD*, index of height decentration; *ISV*, index surface variance; *IVA*, index vertical asymmetry; *OCT*, optical coherence tomography; *SD*, standard deviations.

39.1% and specificities of 83.5% and 95.5%, respectively.[12] Both of these cutoff values were met in our patient (see Fig. 39.2). No single variable from the Galilei was found to be very accurate in diagnosing SCK, and a combination of data points had the highest yield.

PENTACAM

The Pentacam is a Scheimflug-based topographer that is widely used and has a different display profile from the Galilei. It employs the Belin Ambrósio Enhanced Ectasia Display (BAD) (Fig. 39.3[13]) that carefully looks at the anterior and posterior elevation maps, corneal thickness, and corneal thickness spatial profiling. It also uses an enhanced best-fit-sphere model that excludes the central ectatic 4 mm, which was found to increase the sensitivity in diagnosing SCK.[14] In Fig. 39.3, this is the middle (second) row; along with the enhanced maps, the middle posterior elevation is accentuated and readily detected compared with the borderline best-fit-sphere maps (top row). The bottom row for both anterior and posterior corneal elevations is the difference between the best-fit-sphere map and the enhanced best-fit-sphere map, which shows how much the enhanced best-fit-sphere map accentuates the central cornea elevation.

The percentage increase in corneal thickness away from the thinnest point of the cornea positively correlates with subclinical and clinical keratoconus, which is displayed in the corneal thickness spatial profiling and percentage thickness increase chart.[14,15] In the BAD, this is shown in the bottom right (see Fig. 39.3). At the bottom right are the D (standard deviations [SDs] from mean) values of five parameters (change in anterior elevation, change in posterior elevation, corneal thickness at the thinnest point, thinnest point displacement, and pachymetric progression). The final D value (most bottom right value, D) shows an overall value incorporating the previously mentioned 5 D parameters. Any value from 1.6 SD to 2.6 SD is borderline, and any value above 2.6 SD is abnormal.[16] In Fig. 39.3, this value is 4.00, which supports the diagnosis of SCK and is therefore highlighted in red in the display. The overall D value is also known as the BAD Deviation (BAD_D).

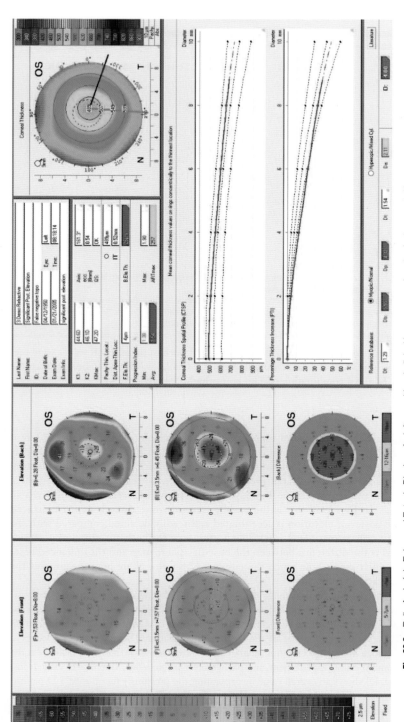

Fig. 39.3 Belin Ambrósio Enhanced Ectasia Display of a left eye with subclinical keratoconus. Anterior *(column on left)* maps are relatively normal. Posterior maps *(second column)* show abnormalities, especially the enhanced best-fit-sphere map showing centrally posterior elevation *(red)*. The percentage thickness increase chart on the bottom right is abnormal as it deviates outside of the three reference marks. (Retrieved and used with permission from www.pentacam.com.)

Hashemi et al. conducted a study in 2016 that found that BAD_D, Index of Vertical Asymmetry, Index of Surface Variance, and fifth order coma aberration of the front surface were the best parameters to diagnosis SCK. When combining all four variables, the sensitivity, specificity, and area under the curve were 83.6%, 96.9%, and 0.96, respectively (see Table 39.1).[17]

Similar to other devices, grading systems have been created for better assessment of keratoconus. The ABCD score (anterior radius of curvature, posterior ["back"] radius of curvature, corneal thickness at thinnest point, and distance best-corrected vision) was created to simplify and characterize the severity of keratoconus based on the score.[18] Even though an ABCD score is displayed on the Pentacam, there has been no evaluation of the score in relation to diagnosing SCK.

No major studies have been performed comparing any of the three previously mentioned devices that evaluate the posterior cornea in terms of diagnosing SCK. Both the Pentacam and the Galilei have been studied in comparison, and there was a significant correlation between these two topographies for all variables studied besides anterior chamber angle and volume and pupil size.[19] These three variables do not have a known effect on the diagnosis of SCK. A study also found that the Orbscan II tends to have higher posterior vault measurements compared with the Pentacam; however, which one is actually more accurate is unknown.[20] No one elevation-based topographer has been found to be superior to the other.

Optical Coherence Tomography

Anterior segment OCT may be used for many purposes, but its role in the diagnosis of keratoconus is not as well established. It is able to measure the corneal thickness and, more specifically, the epithelium and stromal thickness. It has been hypothesized that the corneal epithelium tries to make the corneal surface more regular and, subsequently, the corneal epithelial thickness may be thinner in the location of the apex and thicker surrounding it. Epithelial thickness pattern standard deviation (PSD) has been found to have the best separation between normal and SCK eyes when compared with total corneal thickness PSD and stromal PSD. Epithelial thickness PSD had the highest diagnostic power for SCK with a sensitivity of 96% and a specificity of 100%.[21]

Using OCT along with elevation-based maps has also been evaluated. Hwang et al. studied the use of Pentacam and anterior segment spectral domain OCT in both SCK and normal eyes.[22] Using a set of multiple variables from the Pentacam or OCT alone had sensitivities and specificities all in the range of 80% to 90%. Combining three variables from the Pentacam and 10 variables from the OCT increased both the sensitivity and specificity to 100% (see Table 39.1).[22] However, many realistic obstacles exist, such as the need to use both elevation-based topography and anterior segment OCT, which are very costly. In addition, all combined 13 variables would need to be evaluated from both modalities. A single combined display or calculator of these variables would make it more practical in a clinical setting.

In summary, multiple modalities may be required to diagnose SCK accurately. Table 39.1 supports this by showing that the parameter that contains multiple variables has the highest area under the curve (ranging from 0.86 to 1.00). Elevation-based topography likely gives the most information, as it contains both anterior and posterior corneal readings and thickness maps. Also depending on the elevation-based topographer used, Placido displays are additionally given. There is strong evidence for the use of anterior segment OCT in terms of assessing epithelial corneal thickness in the diagnosis of SCK.

Treatment

The treatment of SCK includes treating the refractive error and monitoring for progression. The refractive error can often be treated with spectacles and soft contact lenses, as these patients are asymptomatic and have not progressed to the point at which they require rigid or scleral contact lens correction. In addition, clarifying circumstances that would increase the risk of further ectasia is important. These include the treatment of allergies or other atopic conditions, cessation of eye rubbing, and the avoidance of laser refractive surgery. Frequency of follow-up for SCK has not been standardized. However, if progression to clinical keratoconus does occur, other treatments such as corneal cross-linking can be employed.

References

1. Wilson SE, Klyce SD. Screening for corneal topographic abnormalities before refractive surgery. *Ophthalmology*. 1994;101:147–152.
2. Ambrósio R Jr, SD Klyce, Wilson SE. Corneal topographic and pachymetric screen of keratorefractive patients. *J Refract Surg*. 2003;19:24–29.
3. Nesburn AB, Bahri S, Salz J, et al. Keratoconus detected by videokeratography in candidates for photorefractive keratectomy. *J Refract Surg*. 1995;11:194–201.
4. Varssano D, Kaiserman I, Hazarbassanov R. Topographic patterns in refractive surgery candidates. *Cornea*. 2004;23:602–607.
5. Randleman JB, Russell B, Ward MA, Thompson KP. Stulting RD. Risk factors and prognosis for corneal ectasia after LASIK. *Ophthalmology*. 2003;110(2):267–275.
6. Tatar MG, Kantarci FA, Yildirim A, et al. Risk factors in post-LASIK corneal ectasia. *J Ophthalmol*. 2014;2014:204191.
7. Li X, Rabinowitz YS, Rasheed K, Yang H. Longitudinal study of the normal eyes in unilateral keratoconus patients. *Ophthalmology*. 2004;111:440–446.
8. Serdarogullari H, Tetikoglu M, Karahan H, Altin F, Elcioglu M. Prevalence of keratoconus and subclinical keratoconus in subjects with astigmatism using Pentacam derive parameters. *J Ophthalmic Vis Res*. 2013;8(3):213–219.
9. Mahmoud AM, Roberts CJ, Lembach RG, et al. CLEK Study Group CLMI: the cone location and magnitude index. *Cornea*. 2008;27(4):480–487.
10. Jafarinasab MR, Shirzadeh E, Feizi S, Karimian F, Akaberi A, Hasanpour H. Sensitivity and specificity of posterior and anterior corneal elevation measure by Orbscan in diagnosis of clinical and subclinical keratoconus. *J Ophthalmic Vis Res*. 2015;10(1):10–15.
11. Saad A, Gatinel D. Validation of a new scoring system for the detection of early forme of keratoconus. *Int J Keratoconus Ectatic Corneal Dis*. 2012;1(2):100–108.
12. Feizi S, Yaseri M, Kheiri B. Predictive ability of Galilei to distinguish subclinical keratoconus and keratoconus from normal corneas. *J Ophthalmic Vis Res*. 2016;11(1):8–16.
13. Oculus Inc. Belin/Ambrósio Enhanced Ectasia Display. Retrieved and obtained permission from www.pentacam.com.
14. Belin MW, Khachikian SS, Ambrósio R Jr, Salomão M. Keratoconus/ectasia detection with the Oculus Pentacam: Belin/Ambrósio Enhanced Ectasia Display. *Highl Ophthalmol*. 2008;35(6):5–12.
15. Ambrósio R, Alonso RS, Luz A. Coca Velarde LF. Corneal-thickness spatial profile and corneal-volume distribution: tomographic indices to detect keratoconus. *J Cataract Refract Surg*. 2006;32(11):1851–1859.
16. Belin MW. The brains behind the. BAD; 2009. https://www.pentacam.com/fileadmin/user_upload/pentacam.de/downloads/publikationen/artikel/2009-Article_Supplement_Pentacam_The_brains_behind_the_BAD-09.2009.pdf.
17. Hashemi H, Beiranvand A, Yekta A, Maleki A, Yazdani N, Khabaskhoob M. Pentacam top indices for diagnosing subclinical and definite keratoconus. *J Curr Ophthalmol*. 2016;28:21–26.
18. Belin MW, Duncan JK. Keratoconus: the ABCD grading system. *Klin Monatsbl Augenheilkd*. 2016;233(6):701–707.
19. Baradaran-Rafii A, Motevasseli T, Yazdizadeh F, Karimian F, Fekri S, Baradran-Rafii A. Comparison between two Scheimpflug anterior segment analyzers. *Ophthalmic Vis Res*. 2017;12(1):23–29.
20. Quisling S, Sjoberg S, Zimmerman B, Goins K, Sutphin J. Comparison of Pentacam and Orbscan II on posterior curvature topography measurements in keratoconus eyes. *Ophthalmology*. 2006;113(9) 1629–1632.
21. Qin B, Chen S, Brass R, et al. Keratoconus diagnosis with an optical coherence tomography-based pachymetric scoring system. *J Cataract Refract Surg*. 2013;39(12):1864–1871.
22. Hwang ES, Perez-Straziota CE, Kim SW, Santhiago MR, Randleman JB. Distinguishing highly asymmetrical keratoconus eyes using combined Scheimpflug and spectral-domain OCT analysis. *Ophthalmology*. 2018;125(12):1862–1871.

CHAPTER 40

Advanced Keratoconus: Case Study

Nicolas Cesário Pereira

CASE STUDY 1

A 14-year-old female patient with a history of ocular allergy controlled with eye drops and progressive advanced keratoconus (KC) in both eyes presented for evaluation, complaining of worsening of the vision in both eyes in the last 6 months. Despite having new rigid contact lenses (RCLs), she was unable to wear them long enough to perform her daily activities. On her examination, best spectacle-corrected visual acuity (BSCVA) was 20/100 in both eyes. The slit-lamp examination demonstrated corneal ectasia with mild Vogt's striae and central corneal thinning with mild paracentral anterior corneal opacity in both eyes. Tomographic evaluation confirmed advanced KC with a simulated steep K of 64.3 diopter (D) in the right eye (Fig. 40.1) and 64.2 D in the left eye (Fig. 40.2), with the thinnest point of 329 μm in the right eye (see Fig. 40.1) and 385 μm in the left eye (see Fig. 40.2).

As the patient had low BSCVA and was unable to adapt to RCLs in both eyes, intrastromal corneal ring segments (ICRS) were indicated. Because the patient was at a higher risk age for progression of ectasia and already had high keratometric values, combined corneal cross-linking (CXL) was recommended to decrease the risk of progression. As the pachymetry without epithelium would be less than 400 μm in both eyes, accelerated CXL using 9 mW/cm^2 for 10 minutes with hypo-osmolar riboflavin was performed. Because the tomographic examinations showed high keratometric values, long-arc ICRS were implanted (Figs. 40.3 and 40.4) in both eyes to achieve the greatest possible applanation effect.

Three months after the procedure her BSCVA improved to 20/40 in the right eye and 20/30 in the left eye, with the tomographic examinations showing 10.7 D of applanation in the simulated steep K of the right eye (Fig. 40.5) and 11.6 D of applanation in the left eye (Fig. 40.6), remaining stable during follow-up.

CASE STUDY 2

A 25-year-old female patient with history of ocular allergy controlled with eye drops and advanced KC with well-adapted RCLs in both eyes presented for evaluation complaining of worsening vision and frequent need to change the RCL of the left eye in the last year. She said that in the follow-up carried out in her city of origin, the examinations had shown stability of the KC in the right eye and progression in the left eye, but that they did not indicate CXL in the left eye, because of a very thin cornea. On her examination, best contact lens–corrected visual acuity (BCLVA) was 20/30 in both eyes. The slit-lamp examination demonstrated corneal ectasia with Vogt's striae and central corneal thinning with mild central anterior corneal opacity in both eyes. The tomographic evaluation confirmed advanced KC with a simulated K of 62.9 D in the left eye, with the thinnest point of 279 μm (Fig. 40.7) and around 220 μm without epithelium, measured by optical coherence tomography (OCT) (Fig. 40.8).

Although the patient had good BCLVA and was well adapted to contact lenses, the left eye was progressing but did not have sufficient corneal thickness to perform CXL; thus Bowman's layer transplantation (BLT) assisted by femtosecond laser (FSL) was indicated in the left eye.

Three months after the procedure her BCLVA was maintained at 20/30 in the left eye, with the well-positioned BLT graft visible on the OCT (Fig. 40.9) and the tomographic examinations showing 2.9 D of applanation in the simulated K (Fig. 40.10), remaining stable during follow-up.

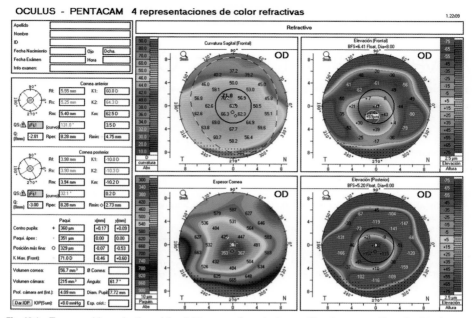

Fig. 40.1 Tomographic evaluation of the right eye confirmed advanced keratoconus, with a simulated steep K of 64.3 D with the thinnest point of 329 μm.

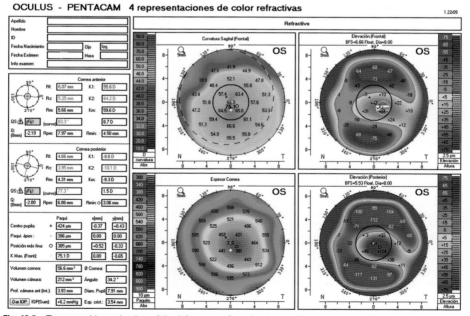

Fig. 40.2 Tomographic evaluation of the left eye confirmed advanced keratoconus, with a simulated steep K of 64.2 D with the thinnest point of 385 μm.

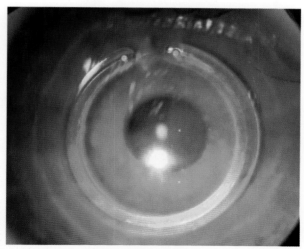

Fig. 40.3 Long-arc intrastromal corneal ring segment implanted in the right eye.

CASE STUDY 3

A 27-year-old male patient with history of ocular allergy controlled with eye drops and advanced KC presented for evaluation, complaining of worsening vision of the left eye that began 1 year ago, after an episode of corneal hydrops. He had stable vision in the right eye, wearing scleral contact lenses with good tolerance. On his examination, BSCVA was 20/400 in the right eye and counting fingers at 1 m in the left eye, with a BCLVA of 20/40 in the right eye and 20/160 in the left eye. The intraocular pressures were within normal limits. The slit-lamp examination demonstrated corneal ectasia with Vogt's striae and central corneal thinning, with central anterior corneal opacity in both eyes and a hydrops corneal scar near the visual axis.

The patient had good BCLVA and was well fit with scleral contact lenses in the right eye, but the left eye had low BCLVA owing to important anterior corneal opacity. Thus, deep anterior lamellar keratoplasty (DALK) was indicated in the left eye, even in the presence of a hydrops scar, as it had adequate endothelial function.

Only 1 month after the procedure his BSCVA was 20/25 in the left eye, with a refractive astigmatism of −1.75 D with all sutures in place (Fig. 40.11).

Introduction

In the management of patients with advanced keratoconus (KC) who did not achieve adequate vision with glasses or contact lenses, penetrating keratoplasty (PK) was the surgical treatment of choice in the last century. However, the surgical treatment of KC has greatly evolved in the last two decades, with new procedures being described that postpone or even prevent corneal transplantation.[1,2] Less invasive procedures have been developed to reshape the cornea and increase its stiffness, improving vision and stabilizing progressive ectasias, enabling better prognosis with lower risks in the surgical management of patients with KC.[1,2]

The management of KC currently consists of visual rehabilitation and stabilization of the ectasia.[1,2] All patients with KC, regardless of their severity, should initially be instructed on the importance of not rubbing the eyes, to decrease the risk of progression.[1,3] As eye rubbing is frequently associated with ocular allergy and dry eye, patients should be treated with topical antiallergic medication and lubricants as needed.[1,3] Visual rehabilitation starts with spectacles and

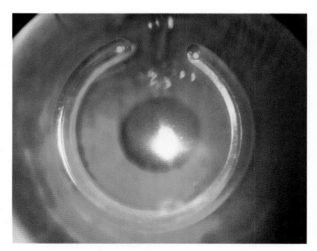

Fig. 40.4   Long-arc intrastromal corneal ring segment implanted in the left eye.

if the vision is not satisfactory, contact lenses should be introduced.[1,2] If achieving adequate vision with contact lenses is not possible, a surgical procedure such as intrastromal corneal ring segment (ICRS) implantation or corneal transplantation is necessary for visual rehabilitation.[1,2] Besides visual rehabilitation, patients must have the evolution of their KC evaluated and if progression is detected should undergo a procedure to stabilize the cornea, such as corneal cross-linking (CXL) and Bowman's layer transplantation (BLT).[1,2]

Intrastromal Corneal Ring Segments

KC patients who have unsatisfactory visual acuity with spectacles and contact lenses can benefit from ICRS implantation to reshape the cornea and improve vision.[4] This procedure can be performed by dissecting intrastromal corneal tunnels manually or with the aid of a femtosecond laser (FSL), which makes the procedure more precise, reproducible, and subject to fewer complications.[5]

Different models of ICRS are available with variation of design, optical zone, arc length, and thickness. A greater flattening effect is achieved in segments of smaller optical zone, with greater arc length and thickness. In advanced KC, long arc-length segments with a small optical zone are generally required for greater flattening effect.[6] Thicker segments may have a greater flattening effect in advanced KC, but a segment thickness limit of 50% to 60% of the thinnest point in the tunnel area must be respected to reduce the risk of complications such as segment extrusion, and patients with corneas thinner than those limits are not good candidates for ICRS.[7,8]

Although the applanation effect of ICRS is described as greater in the higher corneal curvatures of patients with advanced KC, poorer visual results are expected, with more patients requiring contact lens for visual rehabilitation postoperatively.[6,8] Furthermore, complications such as extrusion and progression of ectasia are more expected in advanced KC.[7,8] Therefore, properly informing patients about the prognosis is vital, reinforcing that it is a less invasive and less risky attempt than a corneal transplantation. As the risk of progression after ICRS implantation is higher in more advanced KC cases, some authors recommend performing ICRS combined with CXL,[8] especially in patients under 19 years of age, who are also at higher risk. The combined procedure not only reduces the risk of progression but may also enhance the flattening effect.[8]

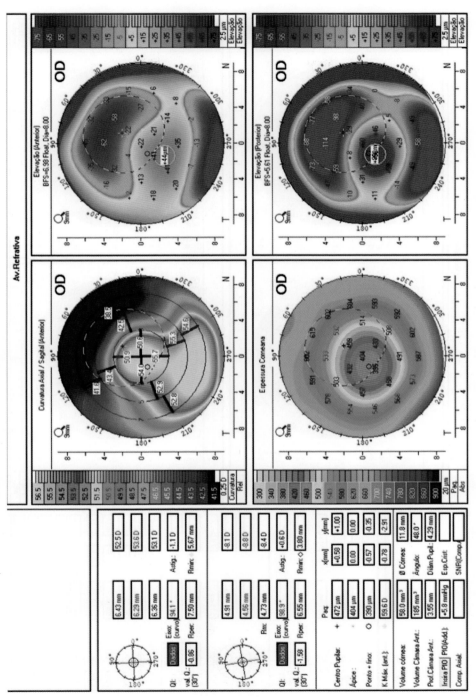

Fig. 40.5 Tomographic examinations showing 10.1 D of applanation in the simulated steep K of the right eye.

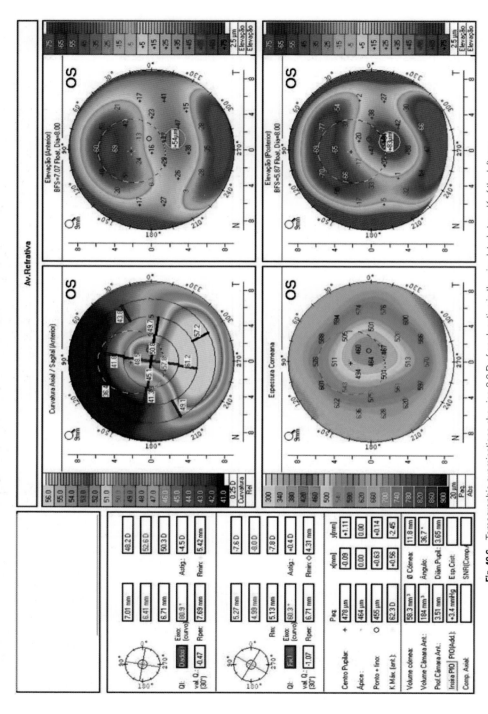

Fig. 40.6 Tomographic examinations showing 8.3 D of applanation in the simulated steep K of the left eye.

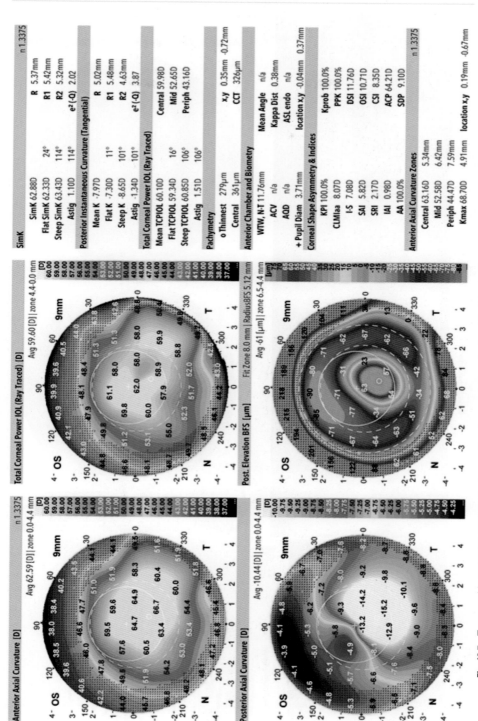

Fig. 40.7 Tomographic evaluation confirmed advanced keratoconus with a simulated K of 62.9 D in the left eye, with the thinnest point of 279 μm.

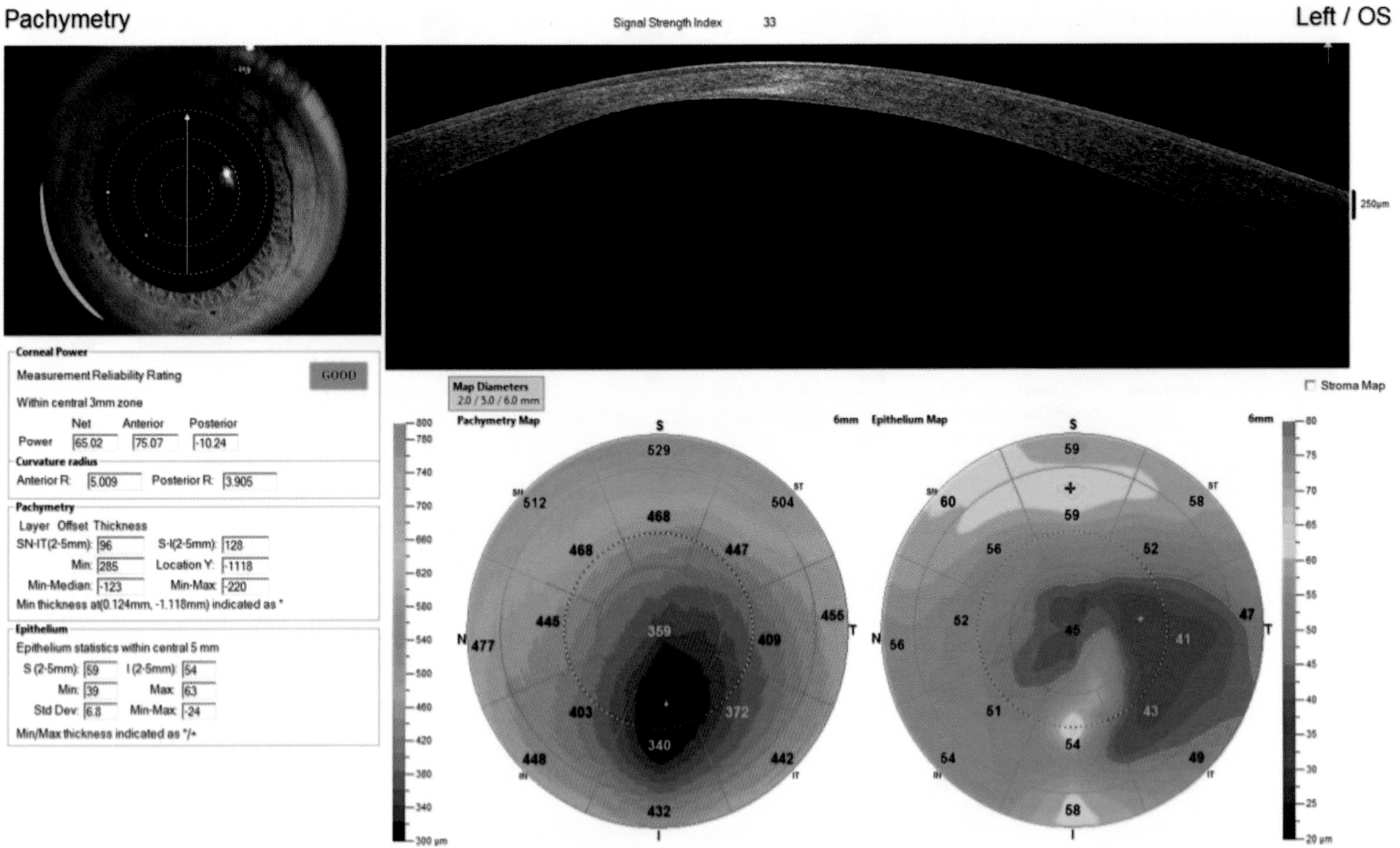

Fig. 40.8 Optical coherence tomography showed a thinnest point around 220 μm without epithelium.

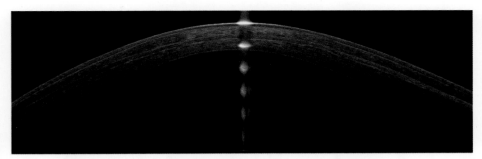

Fig. 40.9 Well-positioned Bowman's layer graft visible with optical coherence tomography.

Bowman's Layer Transplantation

BLT has been described to stabilize progressive advanced KC when CXL cannot be performed because of significant corneal thinning.[9] The procedure is performed by inserting a Bowman's layer graft into a recipient intrastromal corneal pocket.[9] In the original technique, the graft is prepared with a manual dissection of the Bowman's layer, which is challenging and time-consuming and presents a high graft preparation failure rate.[10] The recipient corneal pocket is also dissected manually in the original technique, which is challenging and carries a risk of intraoperative perforation of recipient Descemet membrane preventing the procedure.[9,11]

Despite the technical difficulty of the manual procedure, good stabilization was described in a series with up to 7 years of follow-up.[12] Some patients had corneal flattening and even improved contact lens fitting.[12,13] So with this procedure, it is possible to postpone or avoid corneal transplantation in patients with advanced progressive KC who have adequate vision with contact lenses.[12,13]

Graft preparation using an FSL has been described and shown to be reproducible. However, a thicker graft was achieved compared with the manual technique.[14] These grafts were not used in BLT, so evaluating the clinical results was not possible.[14] A successful recipient pocket dissection with an FSL was described in two cases, but with a manually dissected graft.[15] A BLT study with both graft preparation and recipient corneal pocket performed with an FSL was carried out at Sorocaba Eye Hospital.[16] In addition to the technique being highly reproducible, promising initial results were found with a good stabilization rate in a series with up to 3 years of follow-up.[16]

Deep Anterior Lamellar Keratoplasty and Penetrating Keratoplasty

Corneal transplantation such as PK and deep anterior lamellar keratoplasty (DALK) is only indicated when adequate vision with contact lenses is no longer possible, and ICRS implantation is no longer viable.[1] PK and DALK are more invasive procedures and are the last resource in the management of advanced KC.[1] Both present slow visual rehabilitation and may need contact lenses for adequate vision postoperatively.[1] Their refractive results are unpredictable, with a mean refractive astigmatism of 3 to 5 D, increasing in long-term follow-up.[1,17,18] They can also lead to changes in the ocular surface, in addition to the risk of suture-related complications such as vascularization and infection.[17,18]

DALK is a less invasive procedure than PK, as the recipient endothelium is maintained and the surgery is performed in a closed system. In DALK, fewer topical corticosteroids are used postoperatively compared with PK, decreasing the risk of secondary glaucoma and cataract.[17,18] With DALK, risk of graft rejection is lower, with better graft survival and greater resistance to trauma postoperatively.[1,17,18] DALK presents the same visual results as PK when the interface is properly dissected, thus DALK is indicated whenever possible.[1,17,18]

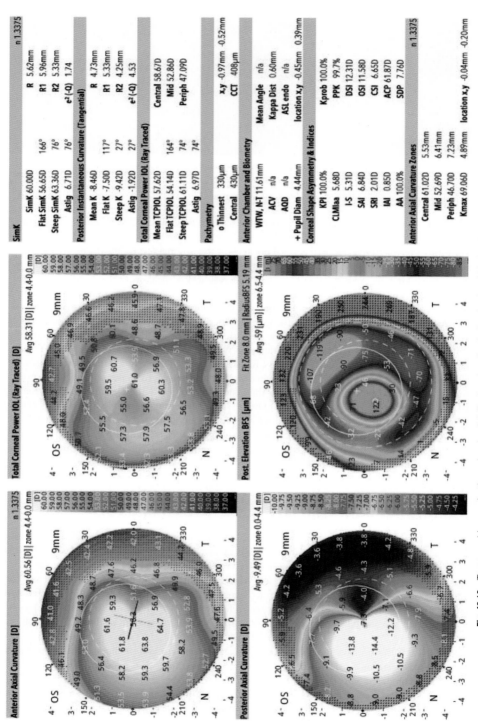

Fig. 40.10 Tomographic examinations showing 2.9 D of applanation in the simulated K after Bowman's layer transplantation.

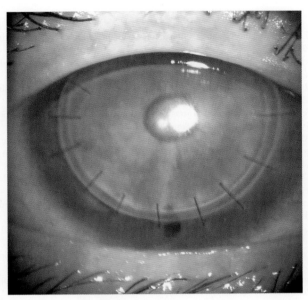

Fig. 40.11 One month after deep anterior lamellar keratoplasty in the left eye of a patient with previous corneal hydrops, with a refractive astigmatism of −1.75 D and a spectacle-corrected visual acuity of 20/25, with all sutures in place.

When the patient with advanced KC needs corneal transplantation, DALK is not always possible.[18] If the recipient cornea does not have adequate endothelial function, PK is required. Patients with hydrops scarring can be managed with DALK by more experienced surgeons, but large scars on the visual axis may require PK for visual rehabilitation.[19] Even in cases in which DALK is possible, inadvertent perforation of the recipient Descemet membrane may occur intraoperatively, which may require conversion to PK.[17]

Conclusions

New advances in the management of advanced KC have completely changed the prognosis of these patients. Besides the advances in corneal imaging improving diagnosis and follow-up of KC patients, minimally invasive procedures have been developed, such as ICRS, in which the cornea can be reshaped and vision improved, and CXL and BLT can be performed to stabilize progressive ectasias. Contact lenses have also evolved, with their use even in more advanced corneal ectasias and irregularities becoming possible.

Despite all these advances, some patients with KC do not adapt to contact lenses with adequate vision and are not eligible for minimally invasive procedures, thus requiring corneal transplantation for visual rehabilitation. For these patients, DALK has evolved considerably, offering the same visual results as PK with fewer risks and better long-term prognosis. Currently, performing DALK in very thin corneas is possible, even with a previous hydrops scar, and the risk of converting to PK intraoperatively has also decreased, especially in the hands of more experienced corneal surgeons.

New procedures such as corneal remodeling, lenticule implantation, corneal allogenic intrastromal ring segment (CAIRS), pinhole intraocular lens, pinhole pupilloplasty, and cell therapy are being evaluated for application in advanced KC and are promising options to assist in the management of these patients. This field is constantly evolving, requiring the knowledge of the corneal specialist to be up to date to enable them to offer each patient the best management.

References

1. Gomes JAP, Tan D, Rapuano CJ, et al. Global consensus on keratoconus and ectatic diseases. *Cornea.* 2015;34:359–369.
2. Parker JS, van Dijk K, Melles GR. Treatment options for advanced keratoconus: a review. *Surv Ophthalmol.* 2015;60:459–480.
3. Najmi H, Mobarki Y, Mania K, et al. The correlation between keratoconus and eye rubbing: a review. *Int J Ophthalmol.* 2019;12:1775–1781.
4. Torquetti L, Ferrara G, Almeida F, et al. Intrastromal corneal ring segments implantation in patients with keratoconus: 10-year follow-up. *J Refract Surg.* 2014;30:22–26.
5. Monteiro T, Alfonso JF, Freitas R, et al. Comparison of complication rates between manual and femtosecond laser-assisted techniques for intrastromal corneal ring segment implantation in keratoconus. *Curr Eye Res.* 2019;1:1–8.
6. Torquetti L, Cunha P, Luz A, et al. Clinical outcomes after implantation of 320°-arc length intrastromal corneal ring segments in keratoconus. *Cornea.* 2018;37:1299–1305.
7. Khan MI, Injarie A, Muhtaseb M. Intrastromal corneal ring segments for advanced keratoconus and cases with high keratometric asymmetry. *J Cataract Refract Surg.* 2012;38:129–136.
8. Izquierdo L Jr, Mannis MJ, Mejias Smith JA, et al. Effectiveness of intrastromal corneal ring implantation in the treatment of adult patients with keratoconus: a systematic review. *J Refract Surg.* 2019;35:191–200.
9. Van Dijk K, Parker J, Tong CM, et al. Midstromal isolated Bowman layer graft for reduction of advanced keratoconus. *JAMA Ophthalmol.* 2014;132:495–501.
10. Groeneveld-van Beek EA, Parker J, Lie JT, et al. Donor tissue preparation for Bowman layer transplantation. *Cornea.* 2016;35:1499–1502.
11. van Dijk K, Liarakos VS, Parker J, et al. Bowman layer transplantation to reduce and stabilize progressive, advanced keratoconus. *Ophthalmology.* 2015;122:909–917.
12. Zygoura V, Birbal RS, van Dijk K, et al. Validity of Bowman layer transplantation for keratoconus: visual performance at 5-7 years. *Acta Ophthalmol.* 2018;96:e901–e902.
13. van Dijk K, Parker JS, Baydoun L, et al. Bowman layer transplantation: 5-year results. *Graefes Arch Clin Exp Ophthalmol.* 2018;256:1151–1158.
14. Parker JS, Huls F, Cooper E, et al. Technical feasibility of isolated Bowman layer graft preparation by femtosecond laser: a pilot study. *Eur J Ophthalmol.* 2017;27:675–677.
15. García de Oteyza G, González Dibildox LA, Vázquez-Romo KA, et al. Bowman layer transplantation using a femtosecond laser. *J Cataract Refract Surg.* 2019;45:261–266.
16. Pereira NC, Gonçalves TB, Forseto AS, et al. Femtosecond laser assisted Bowman layer transplantation for advanced keratoconus. Presented at SINBOS (International Symposium of Sorocaba Eye Bank) 2017 and 2019, CBO (Brazilian Ophthalmology Congress) 2018, 2019 and 2020, *ASCRS 2019 Symposium of Challenging Cases, and accepted as a paper presentation at the World Cornea Congress*; 2020.
17. Gadhvi KA, Romano V, Fernández-Vega Cueto L, et al. Deep anterior lamellar keratoplasty for keratoconus: multisurgeon results. *Am J Ophthalmol.* 2019;201:54–62.
18. Han DC, Mehta JS, Por YM, et al. Comparison of outcomes of lamellar keratoplasty and penetrating keratoplasty in keratoconus. *Am J Ophthalmol.* 2009;148:744–751.
19. Fuest M, Mehta JS. Strategies for deep anterior lamellar keratoplasty after hydrops in keratoconus. *Eye Contact Lens.* 2018;44:69–76.

INDEX

Note: Page numbers followed by '*f*' indicate figures those followed by '*t*' indicate tables and 'b' indicate boxes.